Protocols for High-Risk Pregnancies

An Evidence-Based Approach

Protocols for High-Risk Pregnancies

An Evidence-Based Approach

EDITED BY

John T. Queenan MD

Professor and Chairman, Emeritus
Department of Obstetrics & Gynecology
Georgetown University School Medicine
Washington, DC, USA

John C. Hobbins MD

Professor, Department of Obstetrics & Gynecology
University of Colorado Health Sciences Center
Denver, CO, USA

Catherine Y. Spong MD

Bethesda, MD, USA

FIFTH EDITION

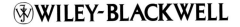

A John Wiley & Sons, Ltd., Publication

This edition first published 2010, © 1982, 1987, 1996, 2005, 2010 by Blackwell Publishing Ltd

Blackwell Publishing was acquired by John Wiley & Sons in February 2007.
Blackwell's publishing program has been merged with Wiley's global Scientific, Technical and Medical business to form Wiley-Blackwell.

Registered office: John Wiley & Sons Ltd, The Atrium, Southern Gate, Chichester, West Sussex, PO19 8SQ, UK

Editorial offices: 9600 Garsington Road, Oxford, OX4 2DQ, UK
111 River Street, Hoboken, NJ 07030-5774, USA
The Atrium, Southern Gate, Chichester, West Sussex, PO19 8SQ, UK

For details of our global editorial offices, for customer services and for information about how to apply for permission to reuse the copyright material in this book please see our website at www.wiley.com/wiley-blackwell

Library of Congress Cataloging-in-Publication Data
Protocols for high-risk pregnancies / edited By John T. Queenan, John C. Hobbins, Catherine Y. Spong.—5th ed.
       p. ; cm.
    Includes bibliographical references and index.
    ISBN 978-1-4051-9650-5 (alk. paper)
    1. Pregnancy—Complications—Handbooks, manuals, etc. I. Queenan, John T.
II. Hobbins, John C., 1936– III. Spong, Catherine Y.
    [DNLM: 1. Pregnancy Complications. 2. Pregnancy, High-Risk.
WQ 240 P967 2010]
    RG571.P73 2010
    618.3—dc22
                                                                        2010011908

ISBN: 9781405196505

A catalogue record for this book is available from the British Library.

Set in 9.5/13pt Meridien by MPS Limited, A Macmillan Company, Chennai, India

Printed and bound in Singapore by Fabulous Printers Pte Ltd

1   2010

Contents

Part 5 Obstetric Problems, 367

Part 6 Labor and Delivery, 489

Contributors

Richard M.K. Adanu MB ChB, FWACS, MPH
Senior Lecturer, Consultant Obstetrician & Gynecologist
University of Ghana Medical School
Accra, Ghana

Ray Bahado-Singh MD
Department of Obstetrics and Gynecology
Wayne State University and Hutzel Women's Center
Detroit, MI, USA

Antonio Barbera MD
Assitant Professor, Obstetrics and Gynecology
Denver Health Medical Center
University of Colorado Denver
School of Medicine
Denver, CO, USA

Vincenzo Berghella MD
Professor of Obstetrics and Gynecology
Director of Maternal-Fetal Medicine
Thomas Jefferson University
Philadelphia, PA, USA

Richard L. Berkowitz MD
Department of Obstetrics and Gynecology
Columbia University Medical Center
New York, NY, USA

Robert L. Brent MD, PhD, DSc (Hon.)
Distinguished Professor of Pediatrics, Radiology, and Pathology
Louis and Bess Stein Professor of Pediatrics
Thomas Jefferson University and
Alfred I. duPont Hospital for Children
Wilmington, DE, USA

Catalin S. Buhimschi MD
Director Perinatal Research
Yale University School of Medicine
New Haven, CT, USA

Brian M. Casey MD
Professor, University of Texas Southwestern Medical Center
Dallas, TX, USA

Patrick M. Catalano MD
Professor and Chair, Reproductive Biology
Case Western Reserve University
Metrohealth Medical Center
Cleveland, OH, USA

Nancy Chescheir MD
Clinical Professor, University of North Carolina
Department of Obstetrics & Gynecology
Chapel Hill, NC, USA

James F. Clapp MD
Emeritus Professor Reproductive Biology
Department of Reproductive Biology and the
Schwartz Center for Metabolism and Nutrition
Case Western Reserve University at
MetroHealth Medical Center
Cleveland, Ohio, USA

Joshua A. Copel MD
Professor of Obstetrics, Gynecology and Reproductive Sciences, and
Professor of Pediatrics
Yale University School of Medicine
New Haven, CT, USA

F. Gary Cunningham MD
Professor, Department of Obstetrics and Gynecology
University of Texas Southwestern Medical Center
Dallas, TX, USA

Mary E. D'Alton MD
Chair, Department of Obstetrics and Gynecology
Columbia University College of Physicians and Surgeons
New York Presbyterian Hospital
New York, NY, USA

Mara J. Dinsmoor MD, MPH
Clinical Professor, Department of Obstetrics and
Gynecology
Pritzker School of Medicine
University of Chicago, Chicago, IL and
North Shore University Health System
Evanston, IL, USA

Patrick Duff MD
Professor and Program Director, Department of
Obstetrics and Gynecology
University of Florida College of Medicine
Gainesville, FL, USA

Gary S. Eglinton MD
Chairman, Department of Obstetrics and
Gynecology, New York Hospital Queens;
Associate Professor of Obstetrics and
Gynecology
Weill Medical College of Cornell University
Flushing, NY, USA

Mark I. Evans MD
Director, Comprehensive Genetics PLLC
Professor of Obstetrics and Gynecology
Mount Sinai School of Medicine
New York, NY, USA

Roger K. Freeman MD
Professor of Gynecology
University of California Irvine
Long Beach, CA, USA

Karin M. Fuchs MD
Department of Obstetrics and Gynecology
Columbia University College of Physicians and
Surgeons
New York Presbyterian Hospital
New York, NY, USA

Steven G. Gabbe MD
Department of Obstetrics and Gynecology
The Ohio State University College of
Medicine
Columbus, OH, USA

Sreedhar Gaddipati MD
Assistant Clinical Professor, Maternal Fetal
Medicine, Department of Obstetrics and
Gynecology
Columbia University Medical Center
New York, NY, USA

Henry L. Galan MD
Professor of Obstetrics & Gynecology
Chief of Maternal-Fetal Medicine
University of Colorado at Denver Health
Sciences Center
Aurora, CO, USA

Stanley A. Gall MD
Professor of Obstetrics and Gynecology
University of Louisville
Louisville, KY, USA

Robert Gherman MD
Head, Division of Maternal Fetal Medicine
Prince George's Hospital Center
Cheverly, MD, USA

Alessandro Ghidini MD
Director, Perinatal Diagnostic Center;
Professor and Executive Director
Department of Obstetrics and Gynecology
INOVA Alexandria Hospital
Alexandria, VA, USA

Martin L. Gimovsky MD
Professor of Obstetrics and Gynecology
Mount Sinai School of Medicine, New York
Vice-Chair and Program Director
Department of Obstetrics and Gynecology
Newark Beth Israel Medical Center
Newark, NJ, USA

Gary D.V. Hankins MD
Jennie Sealy Smith Distinguished Professor
and Chairman, Department of Obstetrics &
Gynecology
University of Texas Medical Branch at
Galveston
Galveston, Texas, USA

Wendy F. Hansen MD
Director, Maternal Fetal Medicine
Associate Professor, Department of Obstetrics
and Gynecology
University of Kentucky
Lexington, KY, USA

James W. Hanson MD
Director, Center for Developmental Biology and
Perinatal Medicine
National Institute of Child Health and Human
Development
Bethesda, MD, USA

Rosemary D. Higgins MD
Program Scientist for the Neonatal Research
Network, Pregnancy and Perinatology Branch
Center for Developmental Biology and Perinatal
Medicine
Eunice Kennedy Shriver National Institute of
Child Health and Human Development
Bethesda, MD, USA

Fred M. Howard MS, MD
Professor and Associate Chair;
Director of Gynecologic Specialties
University of Rochester School of
Medicine and Dentistry
Rochester, NY, USA

Jeffrey R. Johnson MD
Assistant Professor, Dartmouth Hitchcock
Medical Center
Manchester, NH, USA

Charles S. Kleinman MD
Professor of Pediatrics
Columbia University College of Physicians &
Surgeons
New York, NY, USA

Neil K. Kochenour MD
Professor Emeritus, Department of Obstetrics &
Gynecology
University of Utah
Salt Lake City
UT, USA

Mark B. Landon MD
Professor and Interim Chair, Department of
Obstetrics and Gynecology
The Ohio State University College of Medicine
Columbus, OH, USA

Anna Locatelli MD
Assistant Professor, Department of Obstetrics &
Gynecology
University of Milano-Bicocca
Italy

Charles J. Lockwood MD, MHCM
The Anita O'Keeffe Young Professor of
Women's Health and
Chair, Department of Obstetrics, Gynecology
and Reproductive Sciences
Yale University School of Medicine
Chief of Obstetrics & Gynecology
Yale-New Haven Hospital
New Haven, CT, USA

George A. Macones MD, MSCE
Professor and Chairman, Department of
Obstetrics & Gynecology
Washington University School of Medicine
St Louis, MO, USA

Maureen P. Malee PhD, MD
Medical Director, Maternal-Fetal Medicine
Bryan LGH Medical Center
Lincoln, NE, USA

**Fergal D. Malone MD, FACOG, FRCPI,
FRCOG**
Professor and Chairman, Department of
Obstetrics and Gynecology
Royal College of Surgeons in Ireland and
The Rotunda Hospital, Dublin, Ireland

Brian M. Mercer MD, FACOG, FRCSG
Professor Reproductive Biology
Case Western University
Director, Obstetrics and Maternal-Fetal Medicine
MetroHealth Medical Center
Cleveland, OH, USA

Howard Mikoff MD
Chair, Obstetrics and Gynecology, Maimonides
Medical Center
Distinguished Professor
State University of New York (SUNY)
Brooklyn, NY, USA

Kenneth J. Moise, Jr. MD
Professor of Obstetrics and Gynecology
& Professor of Surgery
Baylor College of Medicine
Houston, TX, USA

Thomas R. Moore MD
Department of Reproductive Medicine
University of California at San Diego
CA, USA

John C. Morrison MD
Professor of Obstetrics, Gynecology and
Pediatrics
University of Mississippi Medical Center
Jackson, MS, USA

Michael P. Nageotte MD
Associate Chief Medical Officer, Memorial Care
Center for Women
Miller Children's Hospital, Long Beach, CA
Professor of Obstetrics and Gynecology
University of California
Irvine, CA, USA

Gayle Olson MD
Associate Professor, University of Texas Medical
Branch, Galveston, TX, USA

John Owen MD, MSPH
Bruce A. Harris, Jr. Endowed Professor
Department of Obstetrics and Gynecology
University of Alabama at Birmingham
Birmingham, AL, USA

Yinka Oyelese MD
UMDNJ–Robert Wood Johnson Medical
School
Jersey Shore University Medical Center
Neptune, NJ, USA

Marc R. Parrish MD
Department of Obstetrics, Gynecology and
Pediatrics
University of Mississippi Medical Center
Department of Obstetrics and Gynecology
Jackson, MS, USA

Alan M. Peaceman MD
Professor and Chief, Division of Maternal-Fetal
Medicine
Northwestern University Feinberg School of
Medicine
Chicago, IL, USA

Lawrence D. Platt MD
Professor Obstetrics and Gynecology
David Geffen School of Medicine at UCLA
Director, Center for Fetal Medicine and
Women's Ultrasound
Los Angeles, CA, USA

Manuel Porto MD
Department of Obstetrics and Gynecology
University of California and
Irvine Medical Center
CA, USA

Susan M. Ramin MD
Professor and Chair, Department
of Obstetrics, Gynecology and
Reproductive Sciences
The University of Texas Medical School at
Houston, Houston, TX, USA

Robert Resnik MD
Professor Emeritus of Reproductive Medicine
UCSD School of Medicine
Solana Beach, CA, USA

Jean Rex MD
Instructor, Department of Pediatrics
Washington University School of Medicine
St. Louis, MO, USA

Adam A. Rosenberg MD
Professor of Pediatrics, University of Colorado
Denver School of Medicine
and The Children's Hospital
Aurora, CO, USA

Dwight J. Rouse MD
Attending Physician, Maternal-Fetal Medicine
Division
Women & Infants Hospital of Rhode Island
Professor of Obstetrics and Gynecology
Warren Alpert School of Medicine at Brown
University
Providence, RI, USA

George Saade MD
Professor, Department of Obstetrics and
Gynecology
Chief of Obstetrics and Maternal-Fetal Medicine
Director, Perinatal Research Division
The University of Texas Medical Branch
Galveston, TX, USA

Michael Schatz MD, MS
Chief, Department of Allergy
Kaiser-Permanente Medical Center
San Diego, CA, USA

James R. Scott MD
Professor and Chair Emeritus
Department of Obstetrics and Gynecology
University of Utah Medical Center
Salt Lake City, UT, USA

Jeanne S. Sheffield MD
Director, Maternal-Fetal Medicine Fellowship
University of Texas Southwestern Medical
Center
Dallas, TX, USA

Baha M. Sibai MD
Professor and Director of Clinical Perinatal
Research
University of Cincinnati College of Medicine
Cincinnati, OH, USA

Robert M. Silver MD
Professor of Obstetrics & Gynecology
Chair of Maternal-Fetal Medicine
University of Utah Health Sciences Center
Salt Lake City, UT, USA

Lynn L. Simpson MD
Associate Professor of Obstetrics and
Gynecology
Columbia University Medical Center
New York, NY, USA

Sindhu K. Srinivas MD
Department of Obstetrics & Gynecology
Washington University School of Medicine
St Louis, MO, USA

Jorge E. Tolosa MD MSCE
Associate Professor of Obstetrics and
Gynecology
Oregon Health and Science University
Portland, OR, USA

Carl P. Weiner MD, MBA
K.E. Krantz Professor & Chair, Obstetrics and
Gynecology
Professor, Molecular & Integrative Physiology
University of Kansas School of Medicine
Kansas City, KS, USA

George D. Wendel MD
Professor, Department of Obstetrics &
Gynecology
University of Texas Southwestern Medical
Center
Dallas TX, USA

Katharine D. Wenstrom MD
Professor, Obstetrics & Gynecology
Director, Divison of Maternal-Fetal Medicine
Women & Infants' Hospital of Rhode Island
Brown Alpert Medical School
Providence, RI, USA

Erika Werner MD
Instructor, Yale University School of Medicine
Department of Obstetrics, Gynecology and
Reproductive Sciences
New Haven, CT, USA

Marsha Wheeler MD
Department of Obstetrics & Gynecology
University of Colorado Health Sciences Center
Denver, CO, USA

Deborah A. Wing MD
Professor and Director, Division of Maternal-
Fetal Medicine
Department of Obstetrics and Gynecology
University of California, Irvine, CA, USA

Jerome Yankowitz MD
University of Iowa Hospitals and Clinics
Department of Obstetrics and Gynecology
Division of Maternal-Fetal Medicine and Fetal
Diagnosis and Treatment Unit
Iowa City, IA, USA

Preface

Today's pressures of managed care, rapidly changing technology, and medically sophisticated patients who always expect good outcomes, make it essential to have correct information at hand. The nature and training of physicians instills the constant drive to do the right thing. Therefore, it is necessary to have appropriate, current, and practical information available as protocols to make good decisions. Why use protocols? Having a protocol or guideline organizes essential clinical material in a systematic, logical order and avoids omissions in patient care. It is to that end that we have created *Protocols for High-Risk Pregnancies*

Evaluating all pregnancies for risk factors is an effective way of identifying patients who need additional care. Some patients have factors present from the outset of pregnancy such as diabetes or history of prematurity that place them at increased risk. Others start with a normal pregnancy but subsequently develop risk factors such as pre-eclampsia or premature rupture of the membranes. This may develop quickly and therefore, it is important to have a protocol for management. Of course, care must be taken to be sure that the term "high risk" does not cause alarm or anxiety for your patient.

Since the 4th edition was published, advances in medical knowledge and technology have dictated changes in management. Thus, in this 5th edition all original protocols have been updated. New ones have been added to cover such advances as nuances in Doppler and sonography, as well as changes in the approach to prematurity, diabetes, hypertension, prophylactic immunizations, among others. We have also included protocols in areas of critical importance to the developing world, such as malaria, tuberculosis, and chronic anemia. For each protocol we have invited the physicians whom we believe to be the outstanding authorities on the topics. They start with a brief introduction and pathophysiology and write the protocols as if they were working up their patient and following her through the various stages of management. We require that each protocol is evidence-based to the extent that is possible. In areas where no evidence exists we have asked the experts to make recommendations. There is some intentional overlap in protocols, as medicine is an art as well as a science. All protocols represent the individual thoughts and opinions of these experts.

We realize that the future will bring new medical advances and that new editions of *Protocols* will need to be published in a timely fashion, thus we welcome your comments for future incorporation. We thank Martin Sugden, Lewis O'Sullivan, and the excellent editorial and production staff at Wiley-Blackwell for their professional skills.

This edition, as with the others, was created to be practical, cost effective and clearly presented: a format that is easy to carry with you on rounds and consultations. We have designed this book to help you in your practice. Make it you own!

John T. Queenan
John C. Hobbins
Catherine Y. Spong

PART 1

Hazards to Pregnancy

Developmental Toxicology and Teratology

James W. Hanson

Center for Developmental Biology and Perinatal Medicine, National Institute of Child Health and Human Development, Bethesda, MD, USA

Exposures to potentially hazardous agents during pregnancy are common. Such agents include drugs (both therapeutic agents and abused substances), environmental chemicals, infectious agents, physical agents (radiation, heat and mechanical factors) and maternal health conditions. Many of these exposures are not readily avoidable, as pregnancy is often not planned or recognized for an extended period after conception, or because there is a continuing need for maternal treatment for health conditions (e.g. epilepsy, infection, asthma, chronic cardiovascular disorders). Exposure to various agents in the home or workplace, or as a consequence of maternal lifestyles and self-medication, is almost universal, and pre-conception planning only rarely provides an opportunity to identify exposures of concern. As a consequence, questions about the significance of such an exposure, whether stated or not, are often a source of concern to pregnant women or their care provider.

Not all developmental toxicants need result in permanent adverse outcomes for the fetus or newborn. Some agents may have at least partially reversible or transient effects if recognized early, such as fetal growth restriction from tobacco smoking. It is important to recognize that structural birth defects resulting from exposure to human teratogens are not the only manifestations of exposure to developmental toxicants. Fetal or postnatal growth disorders, functional developmental disorders including cognitive and behavioral deficits, abnormalities of placental function putting the fetus at increased risk, and death (embryonic, fetal, perinatal or postnatal) are all among potential manifestations of exposures. Furthermore, some adverse outcomes may not become apparent until many years later (e.g. reproductive consequences and cancer from exposure to diethylstilbestrol).

Protocols for High-Risk Pregnancies, 5th edition. Edited by J.T. Queenan, J.C. Hobbins and C.Y. Spong. © 2010 Blackwell Publishing Ltd.

Pathogenetic factors in evaluation of risk from exposure to teratogens and other developmental toxicants

When evaluating the likely significance of exposure to potentially hazardous agents, it is essential to consider the following issues in the context of the known or likely pathogenetic mechanisms for adverse fetal outcomes.

Dose and duration of exposure
- In general, the larger the dose, the more likely an effect, and the more likely the effect will be significant.
- Likewise, the longer the duration of exposure, the greater the chance that susceptible periods of organogenesis and development will be encountered.

Timing
- Timing of exposure is critical: certain organ systems may have a limited period of susceptibility for damage.
- Although it is commonly thought that damage can only result during the period of organogenesis, i.e. during the first trimester, this is not correct. Some organ systems (e.g. the brain) undergo developmental processes later in pregnancy and can be damaged throughout the prenatal period.

Pathogenetic mechanism(s)
- Teratogens and developmental toxicants produce their adverse effect by specific mechanisms. As these mechanisms are often important in multiple tissues and organs, it is not surprising that several specific types of damage may result.
- Those agents that affect basic morphogenetic processes commonly are related to first trimester exposures. However, those agents which act through mechanical pressures are likely to have the greatest impact during the third trimester, and those agents that produce necrosis through inflammation and/or hemorrhage can potentially destroy normally developing structures throughout pregnancy.

Host susceptibility
- Variability in the genetic factors related to metabolism of drugs and chemicals may result in differential susceptibility of the host. These pharmacogenetic factors must be expressed at a relevant time in the tissue or organ system affected.
- There are two potentially relevant 'hosts' to be considered. Mother and embro/fetus only share 50% of the genome. Thus, depending on the pathogenesis of the adverse outcome, maternal or fetal (or perhaps both) genotype may be more important.

Exposures to human teratogens and developmental toxicants commonly are manifest across a wide spectrum of effects. At the severe end, a clinically recognizable pattern of effects (a 'syndrome') may be identified. However, variability of manifestations within the scope of specific adverse outcomes comprising a syndrome is the rule. Among the population of exposed and affected infants, less severe and less pervasive manifestations are often more frequent. Thus infants exposed to alcohol prenatally may have outcomes ranging from mild effects on cognition and behavior from smaller amounts consumed on a few occasions, to the full-blown fetal alcohol syndrome.

Table 1.1 presents a list of agents, including therapeutic agents, for which substantial human data is available establishing a risk for humans.

Table 1.1 Important human teratogens

Agent	Dose	Susceptible period
Medications		
Acitretin	Usual therapeutic	1st trimester
Aminopterin	Usual therapeutic	1st trimester
Amodarone	Usual therapeutic	12 weeks–term
Androgens (including danazol)	Usual therapeutic	Unknown
Angiotensin II receptor inhibitors (candesartan, eprosartan, irbesartan, losartan, olmesartan, tasosartan, telmisartan, valsartan)	Usual therapeutic	2nd and 3rd trimesters
Angiotensin-converting enzyme inhibitors (benazepril, captopril, cilazapril, enalapril, enalaprilat, fosinopril, lisinopril, moexipril, perindopril, quinapril, ramipril, trandolapril)	Usual therapeutic	2nd and 3rd trimesters
Carbamazepine	Usual therapeutic	1st trimester
Clonazepam	Usual therapeutic	1st trimester
Coumarin anticoagulants	Usual therapeutic	1st trimester
Cyclophosphamide	Usual therapeutic	1st trimester
Diethylstilbestrol	1.5–150 mg/d	1st and 2nd trimesters
Ethosuximide	Usual therapeutic	1st trimester
Etretinate	Usual therapeutic	1st trimester
Fluconazole	Chronic, parenteral, 400–800 mg/d	1st trimester
Indomethacin	Usual therapeutic	2nd and 3rd trimesters
Isotretinoin	Usual therapeutic (oral)	1st trimester
Lithium	Usual therapeutic	1st trimester
Methimazole	Usual therapeutic	1st trimester (malformations) 12 weeks–term (hypothyroidism, goitre)
Methotrexate	≥12.5 mg/wk	1st trimester

(Continued)

Table 1.1 (Continued)

Agent	Dose	Susceptible period
Methylene blue	Intra-amniotic injection	2nd trimester
Misoprostol	Usual therapeutic	1st and 2nd trimesters
Penicillamine	Usual therapeutic	Unknown
Phenobarbital	Usual therapeutic	1st trimester
Phenytoin	Usual therapeutic	1st trimester
Primidone	Usual therapeutic	1st trimester
Quinine	$\geq$2g/d	Entire pregnancy
Tetracyclines (chlortetracycline, demeclocycline, doxycycline, methacycline, minocycline, oxytetracycline, tetracycline)	Usual therapeutic	1st trimester
Thalidomide	Usual therapeutic	41–54 days
Trimethadione, paramethadione	Usual therapeutic	1st trimester
Trimethoprim	Usual therapeutic	1st trimester
Valproic acid	Usual therapeutic	1st trimester
Agents of abuse		
Alcohol	Abuse	Unknown
Cigarette smoking	Risks greater with heavy smoking	Entire pregnancy
Cocaine	Abuse	Entire pregnancy
Toluene	Abuse (inhalation)	Unknown
Environmental exposures		
Methyl mercury	Associated with maternal methylmercury concentration $\geq$0.1 μg/mL	Unknown
PCBs	Toxic exposure	Unknown
Infections		
Varicella	Primary infection (much smaller risk with recurrent infection)	Entire pregnancy (but higher in 2nd trimester)
Parvovirus B19	Primary infection	Entire pregnancy (but higher in 2nd trimester)
Cytomegalovirus	Primary infection (much smaller risk with recurrent infection)	Entire pregnancy (but much higher in first half)
Syphilis	–	2nd and 3rd trimester
HIV	–	3rd trimester, especially during labor
LMCV	–	Unknown
Toxoplasmosis	Primary infection	Entire pregnancy

(Continued)

Table 1.1 (Continued)

Agent	Dose	Susceptible period
Rubella	Primary infection (rarely secondary infection)	1st and 2nd trimester (but much higher in 1st trimester)
Maternal illnesses and conditions		
Maternal diabetes mellitus	–	1st trimester
Maternal autoantibodies (Rh, SLE, platelet)	–	2nd and 3rd trimester
Maternal endocrinopathies	–	Unknown
Maternal phenylketonuria	Untreated	Unknown
Maternal obesity	Risk greater with severe obesity than with mild obesity	1st trimester
Physical agents		
Chorionic villus sampling	–	<10 weeks
Early amniocentesis	–	<14 weeks
Ionizing radiation	>10–20 cGy	Entire pregnancy (but highest in 1st trimester)
Radioactive iodine	Therapeutic	12 weeks–term

Table 1.2 Information resources: computerized databases

Database	Contact
REPROTOX	(202) 687-5137
TERIS	(206) 543-2465

The list continues to grow as new research reveals more details about the magnitude and nature of risks associated with many of these and other newly recognized agents. Thus it is important to check the current literature before counseling an exposed family. A variety of information resources, ranging from Internet-based computerized databases and commercially available information resources, to standard reference resources for further reading are listed in Table 1.2.

For the clinician whose practice only rarely encounters these questions, or for those who encounter a question for which current data is limited or difficult to access, consultation with a specialist may be an appropriate option. Many states or academic centers have established Teratogen Information Services to help meet this need. Table 1.3 presents a current listing of these resources.

Table 1.3 Teratogen information services in North America

Service	Telephone number
Alabama Birth Defects Surveillance	(800) 423-8324 or (334) 460-7691
Arizona Teratogen Information Program	(888) 285-3410 or (520) 626-3410 (in Tucson)
Arkansas Teratogen Information Service	(800) 358-7229 or (501) 296-1700
CTIS Pregnancy Risk Information	(800) 532-3749 (CA only)
IMAGE: Info-Medicaments en Allaitement et Grossesse, Province of Quebec, Canada	(514) 345-2333
Motherisk Program, Ontario, Canada	(416) 813-6780
Connecticut Pregnancy Exposure Information Service	(800) 325-5391 (CT only) or (860) 679-8850
Reproductive Toxicology Center, District of Columbia, MD	(301) 620-8690 or (301) 657-5984
Illinois Teratogen Information Service	(800) 252-4847 (IL only) or (312) 981-4354
Indiana Teratogen Information Service	(317) 274-1071
Massachusetts Teratogen Information Service (MaTIS)	(800) 322-5014 (MA only) or (781) 466-8474
Genetics & Teratology Unit, Pediatric Service, Massachusetts General Hospital	(617) 726-1742
Missouri Teratogen Information Service (MOTIS)	(800) 645-6164 or (573) 884-1345
Nebraska Teratogen Project	(402) 559-5071
Pregnancy Healthline, Southern New Jersey Perinatal Cooperative	(888) 722-2903 (NJ) or (856) 665-6000
Pregnancy Risk Network	(800) 724-2454 (then press 1) (NY only) or (716) 882-6791 (then press 1)
PEDECS, Rochester, NY	(716) 275-3638
NCTIS Pregnancy Exposure Riskline	1-800-532-6302 (NC)
North Dakota Teratogen Information Service	(701) 777-4277
Texas Teratogen Information Service	(800) 733-4727 or (940) 565-3892
Pregnancy RiskLine, Salt Lake City, UT	(801) 328-2229 or (800) 822-2229
Pregnancy Risk Information Service	800-531-9800 (VT only) and 800-932-4609
CARE Northwest, Seattle, WA	(888) 616-8484
West Virginia University Hospitals	(304) 293-1572
Wisconsin Teratogen Information Service	(800) 442-6692
Workplace Hazards to Reproductive Health, Madison, WI	(608) 266-2074

For information regarding the Teratology Information Service in your area, contact the Organization of Teratology Information Services (OTIS) at: (866) 626-6847 or http://www.otispregnancy.org.

Suggested readings

Bennett PN. *Drugs and Human Lactation*. Amsterdam: Elsevier, 1988.

Briggs GG, Freeman RK, Yaffe SJ. *Drugs in Pregnancy and Lactation*, 6th edn. Baltimore: Williams & Wilkins, 2001.

Friedman JM, Hanson JW. Protocol 39. Clinical teratology. In: Rimoin DL, Connnor JM, Pyeritz R, Korf, B (eds) *Emory & Rimoin's Principles and Practice of Medical Genetics*, 4th edn. London: Churchill Livingstone, 2002.

Paul M: *Occupational and Environmental Reproductive Hazards*. Baltimore: Williams & Wilkins, 1993.

Schardein JL. *Chemically Induced Birth Defects*. 3rd edn. New York: Marcel Dekker, 2001.

Scialli AR. *A Clinical Guide to Reproductive and Developmental Toxicology*. Boca Raton: CRC Press, 1992.

Shepard TH. *Catalog of Teratogenic Agents*, 10th edn. Baltimore: Johns Hopkins, 2001.

Tobacco, Alcohol and the Environment

Jorge E. Tolosa[1] and George Saade[2]

Department of Obstetrics and Gynecology, Division of Maternal-Fetal Medicine, Oregon Health & Science University, Portland, OR, USA[1] and University of Texas Medical Branch, Galveston, TX, USA[2]

Tobacco

Clinical significance

About 250 million women worldwide are daily smokers. The prevalence of tobacco smoking among women in developed countries is 22% while it is 9% in developing countries. In 2003, 10.7% reported smoking during pregnancy, a decrease from 11.2% when compared to 2002. Women 18–19 years old (17.1%) show the highest prevalence; 26% smoked half a pack or more of cigarettes a day. Women are more likely to smoke if they have a higher parity, less than 12 years of education, a lower socio-economic status, poor coping skills, or are exposed to domestic violence. Tobacco exposure in pregnancy is associated with an increased rate of adverse outcomes including low birthweight resulting from preterm birth and/or fetal growth restriction. In 2003 in the United States, non-smokers had a rate of 7.7% of low-birthweight babies compared with 12.4% born to smokers. Tobacco dependence is a chronic addictive condition that requires repeated intervention for cessation. Although a light smoker is defined as a cigarette smoker of fewer than 10 per day, smoking is unsafe at all levels. Tobacco cessation in pregnancy results in reduction in preterm birth, fetal growth restriction, low birthweight and perinatal death, as well as in improved neonatal outcomes. It is the most important preventable cause of low birthweight.

Pathophysiology

Tobacco smoke contains thousands of compounds that may have adverse effects. The major compounds suspected of causing harm to the developing fetus are nicotine and carbon monoxide. Nicotine crosses the placenta and can be detected in the fetal circulation at levels that exceed maternal concentrations by 15%, while amniotic fluid concentrations of nicotine are 88% higher than maternal plasma. The actions of nicotine include vasoconstriction and decreased uterine artery blood flow. Carbon monoxide also crosses the placenta rapidly and is detectable in the fetal circulation at levels that are 15% higher than maternal. It has a higher affinity for hemoglobin than oxygen to form the compound carboxyhemoglobin that shifts the oxygen dissociation curve to the left. Consequently, the availability of oxygen to fetal tissues is decreased. Levels of cyanide in the circulation are higher in smokers, a substance which is toxic to rapidly dividing cells. In addition, smokers frequently have other clinical characteristics that may account for some adverse pregnancy outcomes, e.g. poor nutrition, alcohol or drug abuse.

Screening for tobacco exposure and increasing tobacco cessation

Smoking cessation interventions for pregnant women result in fewer low-birthweight newborns and perinatal deaths; fewer physical, behavioral and cognitive problems during infancy and childhood, and important health benefits for the mothers. Women who discontinue smoking even as late as 30 weeks of gestation have infants with higher birthweight than those who continue smoking. In contrast, 'cutting down' seems to improve fetal growth only slightly.

Smoking cessation interventions should be included as part of prenatal care. Women are more likely to quit smoking during pregnancy than at any other time in their lives. An office-based cessation counseling session of 5–15 minutes, when delivered by a trained provider with the provision of pregnancy-specific educational materials, increases rates of cessation among pregnant smokers by 20%. Trials have shown that a five-step intervention program (the 5 As) is effective.

1 **Ask** pregnant women about smoking status using a multiple-choice question method to improve disclosure.
2 **Advise** women who smoke to quit smoking, with unequivocal, personalized and positive messages about the benefits for her, the baby and family. Review the risks associated with continued smoking. Congratulate women who have quit and reinforce the decision by reviewing the benefits resulting from not smoking.
3 **Assess** the woman's willingness to make an attempt to quit smoking within the next 30 days. If the woman wants to try to quit, the provider should move to the next step, Assist. For women who are unwilling to attempt cessation, the advice, assessment and assistance should be offered at each future visit.

4 Assist
- Provide self-help smoking cessation materials that contain messages to build motivation and confidence in support of a cessation attempt.
- Suggest and encourage the use of problem-solving methods and skills for cessation for issues that the woman believes might adversely influence her attempt to quit. Avoid 'trigger situations'.
- Arrange social support in the smoker's environment by helping her identify and solicit help from family, friends, co-workers and others who are most likely to be supportive of her quitting smoking.
- Provide social support as part of the treatment. This means that the counselor is encouraging, communicates care and concern, and encourages the patient to talk about the process of quitting.

5 Arrange follow-up. Smoking status should be monitored throughout pregnancy, providing opportunities to congratulate and support success, reinforce steps taken towards quitting, and advise those still considering a cessation attempt.

Pharmaceutical cessation aids such as nicotine replacement therapy (NRT), varenicline, or bupropion SR have efficacy as first-line agents in the general non-pregnant population. *The use of these medications is not yet routinely recommended in pregnancy*, as there is inconclusive data of their effectiveness and safety. *Nicotine replacement therapy* is available in transdermal patch, nasal spray, chewing gum or lozenge. If used, it should be with extreme caution and women should be warned of uncertain side effects in pregnancy. *Bupropion SR* is an atypical antidepressant which has been approved by the FDA for use in smoking cessation. It is contraindicated in patients with bulimia, anorexia nervosa, use of MAO inhibitors within the previous 14 days, or a known or history of seizures. It carries a black box warning due to an association of antidepressant medications with suicidality in children, adolescents and young adults under the age of 24. *Varenicline* is approved for smoking cessation in the general population. Serious neuropsychiatric symptoms have been associated with its use including agitation, depression and suicidality. The FDA issued a public health advisory in 2008 cautioning its use in populations with a history of psychiatric illness.

Complications

Pregnancies among women who smoke have been associated with increased risks for miscarriage, ectopic pregnancy, fetal growowth restriction, placenta previa, abruptio placentae, preterm birth, premature rupture of the membranes and low birthweight. Overall, the perinatal mortality rate among smokers is 150% greater than is seen in non-smokers.

The progeny of smoking mothers face additional risks during childhood. There is a strong association between maternal smoking and sudden infant death syndrome, and a clear dose–response relationship has been demonstrated. Prenatal and postnatal tobacco smoke exposure also has been associated with increased risk of persisting reduced lung function, respiratory infections and childhood asthma. Recent studies suggest that infants born to women who smoke during pregnancy may be at increased risk for childhood obesity. In addition, there is evidence suggesting a neurotoxic effect of prenatal tobacco exposure on newborn behavior, i.e. being more excitable and hypertonic. The behavioral and cognitive deficits associated with in utero exposure to tobacco seem to continue into late childhood and adolescence with increased risk for attention deficit hyperactivity disorder and conduct disorder.

Follow-up and prevention

It is essential to identify the pregnant woman who is a smoker, ideally pre-conception, when the risks associated with smoking in pregnancy should be discussed and the benefits of smoking cessation emphasized. Cotinine, a metabolite of nicotine, is an accurate assay for nicotine exposure and can be part of a cost-effective cessation program. Studies indicate higher success rates when participants are aware that complicance is measured with biochemical tests. Postnatal relapse rates are high, averaging 50–80% in the first year after delivery. Counseling should be continued at each postpartum visit including unequivocal, personalized and positive messages about the benefits to the patient, her baby and family resulting from smoking cessation. If indicated, pharmacotherapy could be recommended to the lactating woman, after giving consideration to the risk for the nursing infant of passage of small amounts of the medications through breast milk, compared to the increased risks associated with smoking for children such as sudden infant death syndrome, respiratory infections, asthma and middle ear disease.

Alcohol

Clinical significance

In the mother, chronic alcohol abuse is associated with pneumonia, hypertension, hepatitis and cirrhosis, among other serious medical complications. For the fetus, it is a known teratogen. *Alcohol exposure in pregnancy is the leading known cause of mental retardation and the leading preventable cause of birth defects in western societies.* As many as 1 in 100 births are affected in the United States. Fetal alcohol syndrome is characterized by fetal growth restriction, central nervous system abnormalities and facial dysmorphology, with an average IQ of 70. Functionally, the spectrum of disease even when fetal alcohol syndrome is not fully expressed includes hyperactivity, inattention, memory deficits, inability to solve problems, and mood disorders.

It has been estimated that the risk of fetal alcohol syndrome is 20% if the pregnant woman consumes four drinks per day, increasing to 50% with eight drinks per day. No safe level of exposure to alcohol has been identified, thus alcohol consumption during pregnancy should be avoided.

Public health warnings about the importance of avoiding alcohol in pregnancy were initiated 30 years ago. Despite this, the 2007 National Survey on Drug Use and Health found that among pregnant women between 15 and 44 years, 11.6% used alcohol in the previous 30 days and 0.7% were classified as heavy drinkers (five or more drinks on one occasion, on 5 or more days in the last 30 days) and 6.6% reported binge drinking in the first trimester.

Screening for alcohol abuse in pregnancy

Identifying women who drink during pregnancy is difficult. While a recent report reveals that 97% of women are asked about alcohol use as part of their prenatal care, only 25% of practitioners use standard screening tools.

There is no validated biological marker for alcohol available for use in the clinical setting. Healthcare providers have to rely on self-reported use, resulting in significant underreporting. Of available screening tools, the T-ACE is validated for pregnant women.

Tolerance (T): The first question is 'How may drinks can you hold?' A positive answer, scored as a 2, is at least a 6-pack of beer, a bottle of wine or 6 mixed drinks. This suggests a tolerance of alcohol and very likely a history of at least moderate to heavy alcohol consumption.

Annoyed (A): 'Have people annoyed you by criticizing your drinking?'

Cut down (C): 'Have you felt you ought to cut down on your drinking?'

Eye opener (E): 'Have you ever had a drink first thing in the morning to steady your nerves or get rid of a hangover?'

These last three questions, if answered positively, are worth 1 point each. A score on the entire scale of 2 or higher is considered positive for excessive or risk drinking. Follow-up of a positive screen should include questions about volume and frequency. A report of more than seven standard drinks per week, less if any single drinking episode involves more than three standard drinks, should be considered at risk. A standard drink is defined as 12 ounces of beer, 5 ounces of wine or 1.5 ounces of liquor in a mixed drink. The T-ACE has been reported to identify 90% or more of women engaging in risk drinking during pregnancy.

Treatment of risk drinking in pregnancy

Advice by the healthcare provider is valid, effective and feasible in the clinical office setting. Brief behavioral counseling interventions with follow-up in the clinical setting have been demonstrated to produce significant reductions in alcohol consumption lasting at least12 months. Practitioners need to be aware of the possibility of concurrent psychiatric and or social problems. Consultation with mental health professionals and social workers is indicated and can be powerful adjuvants to assist women to discontinue use of alcohol.

Brief interventions for pregnancy risk drinking generally involve systematic counseling sessions, approximately 5 minutes in length, which are tailored to the severity of the identified alcohol problem. In the first intervention, the provider should state her/his concern, give advice, and help to set a goal. Educational written materials should be provided. Routine follow-up is essential and should involve encouragement, information and re-evaluation of goals at each prenatal visit. Women who are actually alcohol-dependent may require additional assistance to reduce or eliminate consumption during pregnancy. For these women, referral for more intensive intervention and alcohol treatment needs to be recommended. No randomized clinical trials for pregnant women enrolled in alcohol treatment in pregnancy have been conducted to test the use of pharmacological or psychosocial interventions as reported by the Cochrane collaboration.

Environmental hazards

In 1970, the Occupational Safety and Health Act was implemented with a surge of interest in the reproductive effects of working and the workplace. While an adult worker with an occupational exposure is best served by referral to an occupational medicine specialist, workplace exposures of pregnant women tend to be avoided by occupational physicians and the responsibility for these issues thus falls to the obstetrician. In their *Guidelines for Perinatal Care*, the American Academy of Pediatrics and the American College of Obstetricians and Gynecologists include environmental and occupational exposures among the components of the preconceptional and antepartum maternal assessment and counseling. Help is available in the form of Teratogen Information Services, accessed through local health departments, and via the databases, such as REPROTOX (http://reprotox.org/) and TERIS (http://depts.washington.edu/~terisweb/teris/), which were set up to provide information to physicians and the Teratogen Information Services on potential teratogens from any source, including the workplace.

Physical agents
Heat
The metabolic rate increases during pregnancy, and the fetus's temperature is approximately 1°C above the mother's. Because pregnant women have

to eliminate the physiological excess heat, they may be less tolerant of high environmental temperatures. Exposure to heat and hot environments can occur in many occupations and industries. Few studies specifically address the hazards of occupational heat stress in pregnancy. Data from animal studies and fever during pregnancy indicate that core temperature elevations to 38.9°C or more may increase the rate of spontaneous abortion or birth defects, most notably neural tube defects. Women with early pregnancy hyperthermic episodes should be counseled about possible effects and offered alpha-fetoprotein screening and directed sonogram studies.

Ionizing radiation

The effects of prenatal irradiation depend on the exposure dose and the timing of exposure during pregnancy as well as the repair capabilities of the developing organism. Information on the reproductive and developmental effects of ionizing radiation derives from studies in animals, atomic bomb survivors, and those who have been medically irradiated. Preimplantation exposures are thought to result in an 'all or none' phenomenon. Either the insult is great enough to destroy the embryo or, if sublethal, allows the totipotential cells to effectively repair the conceptus. Sensitivity to radiation is greatest during the late first and early second trimester.

Virtually all ionizing radiation exposures in the workplace are well below those expected to result in fetal loss or deficit. Occupational exposure most often occurs in the medical field, in mining, and in power plants. It is thought that while doses less than 5 rad (0.05 Gy) might cause a genetic effect, this would be indistinguishable from the background burden of adverse developmental outcomes. According to the American College of Radiology, no single diagnostic x-ray procedure results in radiation exposure to a degree that would threaten the well-being of a developing pre-embryo, embryo, or fetus.

Occupational exposure to radiation is regulated by a number of federal agencies. The current limit for whole-body radiation is 5 rem (0.05 Sv). The Nuclear Regulatory Commission limits the total dose to the fetus at 500 mrem (5 mSv) once pregnancy is established, not to exceed 50 mrem (0.5 mSv) in any gestational month. The radiation dose can be limited by time, distance and proper shielding. A pregnant worker must work with the physician to estimate the dose, frequency and timing of exposure in gestation. All radiation worksites should have radiation safety personnel and availability of experts to provide quantitative estimates of the dose to the fetus. With exposures to the conceptus of less than 5 rad (0.05 Gy), no intervention is recommended. If higher doses are documented the patient must be counseled, utilizing the datasets outlined above, and offered sonogram screening for microcephaly. The normalcy of these tests cannot guarantee the neurological status of the infant.

Chemical exposures
Hairstylists

Hair colorants and dyes contain aromatic amines that may be absorbed through the skin. These agents are mutagenic but are not teratogenic in rats and cause embryotoxicity in mice only at high doses that are also maternally toxic. Permanent wave solutions may cause maternal dermatitis but are not known to be teratogenic in animals.

There is no direct evidence that hair dyes and permanent wave solutions are teratogenic in human pregnancy, but very limited data are available. One study found a higher rate of spontaneous abortion among cosmetologists. Exposure to these agents should be minimized by the use of gloves and, if possible, reduction of chronic exposures in the first trimester.

Painters and artists

Organic and inorganic pigments may be used in paints. The raw materials for organic pigments may contain aromatic hydrocarbons, such as benzene, toluene, napthalene, anthracene and xylene. Inorganic pigments may contain lead, chromium, cadmium, cobalt, nickel, mercury and manganese. Workers in battery plants and those involved in the removal of old paint are also exposed to lead salts.

Reproductive concerns about inorganic pigments is focused primarily on lead, which is readily transferred across the placenta. Inorganic lead salts have been associated with increased spontaneous abortion, infant cognitive impairment, and stillbirth rates in humans, and central nervous system abnormalities and clefting in rodents. Women at risk of lead exposure should be monitored for blood lead levels before becoming pregnant. If blood lead concentration is greater than 10 μg/mL, the patient should be removed from exposure and chelation considered before pregnancy. Chronically exposed workers will have significant bone lead stores and should remain in a lead-free environment until safe lead levels are reached before attempting pregnancy. There is no consensus on how to manage elevated blood lead levels during pregnancy as chelation will at least temporarily elevate blood lead levels by releasing bone stores. Further, the chelating agent, calcium edetate, may be developmentally toxic, probably by decreasing zinc stores.

Solvent workers

Some organic hydrocarbons may cause a fetal dysmorphogenesis syndrome comparable to fetal alcohol syndrome if ingested in large amounts. This has best been evaluated for gasoline, in a group of individuals who habitually 'sniffed' the fuel for its euphoric effects. An excess of mental retardation, hypotonia and microcephaly was found in the offspring.

The effects of lower levels of gasoline are not known. Similar effects were reported with toluene sniffing.

Ethylene glycol is another solvent used in a large number of industrial processes (paint, ink, plastics manufacture). No human studies exist, but in rodents many studies report abnormal development and skeletal and central nervous system abnormalities. If a woman has a considerable exposure level as determined by blood and urine levels or abnormal liver function tests, increased monitoring of fetal development is recommended.

Pesticide workers

Pesticides are often encountered in agricultural workers and landscape artists. Two common agents are carbaryl and pentachlorophenol. A suspected workplace exposure may be quantitated by urine levels. Human studies for these agents are not available but animal studies suggest that high doses, particularly those that produce maternal toxicity, may impair reproductive success and be responsible for skeletal and body wall defects. These outcomes may be related to maternal toxicity and may not be a specific developmental effect.

Exposure to inhalational anesthetics

The studies that have suggested an association between occupational exposure to inhalational anesthetics and adverse reproductive outcomes have been heavily criticized. The available scientific evidence, while weak, does lead to concern over occupational exposure to inhalational anesthetics in the trace concentrations encountered in adequately scavenged operating rooms. Recommending limitation of exposure may be reasonable in environments where scavenging equipment is not available, such as some dentists' offices.

Other occupational hazards
Air travel

The environment in passenger cabins of commercial airlines is maintained at the equivalent of 5000–8000 feet. While living at high altitude has significant effects on maternal and fetal physiology, air travel has not been associated with harmful fetal effects because of the short duration of most flights. Adequate hydration is essential as the humidity is also reduced to less than 25% in most cabins. Intermittent ambulation and changing posture is recommended in order to prevent deep vein thrombosis. Reports indicate that flight attendants experience twice the incidence of first trimester spontaneous abortions as other women, but not other employed women. Most airlines restrict the working air travel of flight attendants after 20 weeks of gestation, and restrict commercial airline pilots from flying once pregnancy is diagnosed. Counseling for women with medical or obstetrical complications should be individualized. It should be noted that air travel can contribute to background radiation. The magnitude of in-flight exposure to radiation depends on altitude and the solar cycle. A round trip between New York and Seattle can result in exposure to 6 mrem (0.06 mSv), well below the safe upper limit accepted by most experts. Because the effect may be cumulative, frequent flyers need to keep track of their exposure. Patients and physician can consult the FAA's radiation estimation software (http://jag.cami.jccbi.gov./cariprofile.asp) to calculate the exposure and the National Oceanic and Atmospheric Administration (http://www.sec.noaa.gov) to check for solar flares.

Suggested reading

Tobacco

American College of Obstetricians and Gynecologists. Smoking Cessation During Pregnancy. *ACOG Committee Opinion No. 316*. Washington (DC): ACOG; 2005.

Fiore MC, Jaén CR, Baker TB, *et al. Treating Tobacco Use and Dependence: 2008 Update.* Clinical Practice Guideline. Rockville, MD: US Department of Health and Human Services, Public Health Service, May 2008.

Martin JA, Hamilton BE, Sutton PD, Ventura SJ, Manacker F, Munson ML. Births: Final Data for 2003: *National Vital Statistics Reports*; 54(2). Hyattsville, MD: National Center for Health Statistics; 2005. DHHS Publication (PHS) 2005–1120. http://www.cdc.gov/nchs/data/nvsr/nvsr54/nvsr54_02.pdf. Accessibility verified April 16, 2009.

Department of Health and Human Services. Women and Smoking: A report of the Surgeon General. Rockville: US Department of Health and Human Services, Public Health Service, Office of the Surgeon General, 2001.

Department of Health and Human Services. The Health Benefits of Smoking Cessation: US Department of Health and Human Services, Public Health Service, Centers for Disease Control, Center for Chronic Disease Prevention and Health Promotion, Office on Smoking and Health, 1990.

Lumley J, Oliver S, Chamberlain C, Oakley L. Interventions for promoting smoking cessation during pregnancy. *Cochrane Database Syst Rev* 2004 (4).

Alcohol

Sokol RJ, Martier S, Ager J. The T-ACE questions: practical prenatal detection of risk-drinking. *Am J Obstet Gynecol* 1989;160:863–70.

Lui S, Terplan M, Smith EJ. Psychosocial interventions for women enrolled in alcohol treatment during pregnancy. *Cochrane Database Syst Rev* 2008 (3).

Chang G. Screening and brief intervention in prenatal care settings. *Alcohol Research & Health* 28(2): 80–84, 2004. (24 refs.)

Substance Abuse and Mental Health Services Administration. *Results from the 2007 National Survey on Drug Use and Health.* (www.oas.samhsa.gov/nsduh/reports.htm).

At-Risk Drinking and Illicit Drug Use: Ethical Issues in Obstetric and Gynecologic Practice. *ACOG Committee Opinion # 422*, Dec. 2008.

Environmental agents

Barish RJ. In-flight radiation exposure during pregnancy. *Obstet Gynecol* 2004;103:1326–30.

Chamberlain G. Women at work in pregnancy. In: Chamberlain G (ed.) *Pregnant Women at Work*. New York: Macmillan, 1984.

Frazier LM, Hage ML (eds) *Reproductive Hazards of the Workplace*. New York; Chichester: John Wiley & Sons, 1998.

Mittlemark RA, Dorey FJ, Kirschbaum TH. Effect of maternal exercise on pregnancy outcome. In: Mittlemark RA, Drinkwater BL (eds) *Exercise in Pregnancy*, 2nd edn. Baltimore: Williams & Wilkins, 1991.

Paul M (ed.) *Occupational and Environmental Reproductive Hazards: A Guide for Clinicians*. Baltimore: Williams & Wilkins, 1993.

Scialli AR. The workplace. In: Scialli AR (ed.) *A Clinical Guide to Reproductive and Developmental Toxicology*. Boca Raton: CRC Press, 1992.

PROTOCOL 3

Ionizing Radiation

Robert L. Brent

Thomas Jefferson University, Alfred I. duPont Hospital for Children, Wilmington, DE, USA

What are the reproductive and developmental risks of in utero exposure to ionizing radiation?

1 Birth defects, mental retardation and other neurobehavioral effects, growth retardation and embryonic death are deterministic effects (threshold effects). This indicates that these effects have a NOAEL (no adverse effect level). Almost all diagnostic radiological procedures provide exposures that are below the NOAEL for these developmental effects. Diagnostic radiological studies rarely exceed 10 rad (0.1 Gy), while the threshold for congenital malformations or miscarriage is >20 rad (0.2 Gy) (Table 3.1).

2 In order for the embryo to be deleteriously affected by ionizing radiation when the mother is exposed to a diagnostic study, the embryo has to be exposed above the NOAEL to increase the risk of deterministic effects. This rarely happens when pregnant women undergo x-ray studies of the head, neck, chest or extremities.

3 During the pre-implantation and pre-organogenesis stages of embryonic development the embryo is least likely to be malformed by the effects of ionizing radiation because the cells of the very young embryo are omnipotential and can replace adjacent cells that have been deleteriously affected. This early period of development has been designated as the 'all or none' period.

4 Protraction and fractionation of exposures of ionizing radiation to the embryo decrease the magnitude of the deleterious effects of deterministic effects.

5 The increased risk of cancer following high exposures to ionizing radiation exposure to adult populations has been demonstrated in the atomic bomb survivor population. Radiation-induced carcinogenesis is assumed to be a stochastic effect (non-threshold effect) so that there is theoretically a risk at low exposures. While there is no question that

Protocols for High-Risk Pregnancies, 5th edition. Edited by J.T. Queenan, J.C. Hobbins and C.Y. Spong. © 2010 Blackwell Publishing Ltd.

Table 3.1 Radiation exposure and risk at different gestational phases. There is no evidence that radiation exposure in the diagnostic ranges (<0.10 Gy, <10 rad) is associated with measurably increased incidence of congenital malformation, stillbirth, miscarriage, growth and mental retardation

Stage, gestation weeks	Effect
1st and 2nd weeks after 1st day of the last menstrual period (LMP) (prior to conception)	First 2 weeks after 1st day of the last menstrual period. This is a preconception radiation exposure. Mother has not yet ovulated
3rd and 4th week of gestation (first 2 weeks post conception)	Minimum human acute lethal dose (from animal studies) approx 0.15–0.20 Gy. Most sensitive period for the induction of embryonic death
4th to 8th week of gestation (2nd to 6th week post conception)	Minimum lethal dose (from animal studies) – at 18 days post conception = 0.25 Gy (25 rad); after 50 days post conception = >0.50 Gy (50 rad).
	Embryo is predisposed to the induction of major malformations and growth retardation. Minimum dose for growth retardation: at 18–36 days = 0.20–0.50 Gy (20–50 rad) and at 36–110 days = 0.25–0.5 Gy (25–50 rad). But the induced growth retardation during this period is not as severe as during mid-gestation from similar exposures
8th to 15th week of gestation	Most vulnerable period for irreversible whole body growth retardation, microcephaly and severe mental retardation. Threshold for severe metal retardation is 0.35–0.50 Gy (35–50 rad).[1] Miller[2] indicated that the threshold was >50 rad (1999). Decrease in IQ may occur at lower exposures but is difficult to document. There is probably no increased risk for mental retardation with exposures <0.10 Gy
16th week of gestation to term	Higher exposures can produce growth retardation and decreased brain size and intellect, although the effects are not as severe as what occurs from similar exposures during mid-gestation. There is no risk for major anatomical malformations. The threshold dose for lethality (from animal studies) from 15 weeks to term is >1.5 Gy (150 rad).
	Minimum dose for severe mental retardation: at 15 weeks to term = >1.50 Gy, but decrease in IQ can occur at lower exposures

high exposures of ionizing radiation can increase the risk of cancer, the magnitude of the risk of cancer from embryonic exposures following diagnostic radiological procedures is very controversial. Recent publications and analyses indicate that the risk is lower for the irradiated embryo than for the irradiated child, which surprised many scientists interested in this subject.

Evaluating the risks

The responsibility for evaluating risks of environmental toxicants to the pregnant patient and her embryo frequently lies with the obstetrician. When evaluating the risks of ionizing radiation, the physician is faced with several different clinical situations, as outlined below.

1 The pregnant patient presents with clinical symptoms that need to be evaluated. What is the appropriate utilization of diagnostic radiological procedures that may expose the embryo or fetus to ionizing radiation?

A pregnant or possibly pregnant woman complaining of gastrointestinal bleeding, abdominal or back pain, or an abdominal or pelvic mass that cannot be attributed to pregnancy deserves the appropriate studies to diagnose and treat her clinical problems, including radiological studies. Furthermore, these studies should not be relegated to one portion of the menstrual cycle if she has not yet missed her period. The studies should be performed at the time they are clinically indicated whether or not the woman is in the first or second half of the menstrual cycle.

2 The patient has completed a diagnostic procedure that has exposed her uterus to ionizing radiation. Her pregnancy test was negative. She now believes she was pregnant at the time of the procedure. What is your response to this situation?

Explain that you would have proceeded with the necessary x-ray diagnostic test whether she was pregnant or not, since diagnostic studies that are indicated in the mother have to take priority over the possible risk to her embryo, because almost 100% of diagnostic studies do not increase the risks to the embryo (Table 3.1). Second, she must have been very early in her pregnancy, since her pregnancy test was negative. At this time, obtain the calculated dose to the embryo and determine her stage of pregnancy. If the dose is below 10 rad (0.1 Gy, 0.1 Sv), you can inform the mother that her risks for birth defects and miscarriage have not been increased. In fact the threshold for these effects is 20 rad (0.2 Gy) at the most sensitive stage of embryonic development (Tables 3.1 and 3.2). Of course, you are obligated to tell her that every healthy woman is at risk for the background incidence of birth defects and miscarriage, which is 3% for birth defects and 15% for miscarriage. Every woman faces these risks.

Table 3.2 Risk of 5 rad (5 rem, 50 mSv, 5000 mrem) to embryo

Risk	0 rad exposure	Additional risk of 5 rad exposure
Risk of very early pregnancy loss, before the first missed period	350,000/10^6 pregnancies	0
Risk of spontaneous abortion in known pregnant women	150,000/10^6 pregnancies	0
Risk of major congenital malformations	30,000/10^6	0
Risk of severe mental retardation	5000/10^6	0
Risk of childhood leukemia/year	40/10^6/year	<2/10^6/year
Risk of early- or late-onset genetic disease	100,000/10^6	Very low risk is in next generation and is not measurable increased with small populations
Prematurity	(5.6% to 12.4%) 60,000/10^6	0
Growth retardation	30,000/10^6 pregnancies	0
Stillbirth	20–2000/10^6 pregnancies	0
Infertility	7% of couples	0

3 A woman delivers a baby with serious birth defects. On her first postpartum visit, she recalls that she had a diagnostic x-ray study early in her pregnancy. What is your response when she asks you whether the baby's malformation could be caused by the radiation exposure?

In most instances, the nature of the clinical malformations will rule out radiation teratogenesis. At this time, a clinical teratologist or radiation embryologist could be of assistance. On the other hand, if the exposure is below 10 rad (0.1 Gy), it would not be scientifically supportable to indicate that the radiation exposure was the cause of the malformation. As mentioned before, the threshold for malformations is 20 rad (0.20 Gy). Dose, timing, and the nature of the malformation would enter into this analysis.

In order to appropriately and more completely respond to these questions, the obstetrician should rely on the extensive amount of information that has accumulated on the effects of radiation on the embryo. In fact, there is no environmental hazard that has been more extensively studied or on which more information is available.[1–9] (See Tables 3.1 and 3.2.)

Radiation risks to the embryo

There is no question that an acute exposure to ionizing radiation above 50 rad represents a significant risk to the embryo, regardless of the stage of gestation.[6–11] The threshold dose for low LET (low energy transfer) ionizing radiation that results in an increase in malformations is approximately 20 rad (0.2 Gy) (Table 3.1). Although congenital malformations are unlikely to be produced by radiation during the first 14 days of human development, there would be a substantial risk of embryonic loss if the dose is high. From approximately the 18th day to the 40th day post-conception, the embryo would be at risk for an increased frequency of anatomical malformations if the embryonic exposure is greater than 20–25 rad (0.2–0.25 Gy). Up until about the 15th week, the embryo maintains an increased susceptibility to central nervous system (CNS) effects, major CNS malformations early in gestation, and mental retardation in mid-gestation. Of course, with very high doses, in the 100s of rads, mental retardation can be produced in the latter part of gestation. While it is true that the embryo is sensitive to the deleterious effects of these mid-range exposures of ionizing radiation, the measurable effects fall off rapidly as the exposure approaches the usual exposures that the embryo receives from diagnostic radiological procedures (<10 rad; 0.1 Gy). The threshold of 20 rad at the most sensitive stage of development (20–25 days post-conception) is raised by protraction of the radiation exposure, for example, following several clinical diagnostic radiological procedures occurring over a period of days.[6,10,11]

That is why the recommendation of most official organizations, including the National Council on Radiation Protection and Measurements (NCRP),[6,8,9] indicates that exposures in the diagnostic range will not increase the risk of birth defects or miscarriage. The risks of radiation exposure to the human embryo when the exposure exceeds the no-effect dose (20 rad) are:

- embryonic loss
- growth retardation
- congenital malformations
- carcinogenesis (the magnitude of the risk is controversial)[6]
- microcephaly and mental retardation
- sterility.

Because all of the above effects are threshold phenomena, except for carcinogenesis, radiation exposure below 10 rad (0.1 Gy) literally presents no measurable risk to the embryo. Even if one accepts the controversial concept that the embryo is more sensitive to the carcinogenic effects of radiation than the child, the risk at these low exposures is much smaller that the spontaneous risks.[3] Furthermore, other studies indicate that Stewart's[12] estimate of the risk involved is exaggerated.[13–15]

Table 3.2 compares the spontaneous risks facing an embryo at conception and the risks from a low exposure of ionizing radiation (5 rad, 50 mGy, 5000 mrad).

Therefore, the hazards of exposures in the range of diagnostic roent-genology (2000–10,000 mrad; 0.02–0.1 Gy) (0.2 mGy–0.1 Gy) present an extremely low risk to the embryo, when compared with the spontane-ous mishaps that can befall human embryos (Table 3.2). Approximately 30–40% of human embryos abort spontaneously (many abort before the first missed menstrual period). Human infants have a 2.75% major mal-formation rate at term, which rises to approximately 6–10% once all mal-formations become manifest. In spite of the fact that doses of 1–3 rad can produce cellular effects and the fact that diagnostic exposure during preg-nancy has been associated with malignancy in childhood, the maximum theoretical risk to human embryos exposed to doses of 10 rad or less is extremely small. When the data and risks are explained to the patient, the family with a wanted pregnancy invariably continues with the pregnancy.

The difficulty that frequently arises is that the risks from diagnostic radiation are evaluated outside the context of the significant normal risks of pregnancy. Furthermore, many physicians approach the evaluation of diagnostic radiation exposure with either of two extremes: a cavalier attitude or panic. The usual procedures in clinical medicine are ignored, and an opinion based on meager information is given to the patient. Frequently, it reflects the physician's bias about radiation effects or his or her ignorance of the field of radiation biology. We have records in our files of scores of patients who were not properly evaluated but were advised to have an abortion following radiation exposure. The following case history is a typical example.

Case report

A 27-year-old woman (gravida 3, pars 2, abortus 0) called on a Friday afternoon because she was 8 weeks pregnant and was scheduled for a therapeutic abortion on Monday morning. Her obstetrician and a pediatric genetic counselor had advised her to have a therapeutic abortion because at the time of conception she had had several x-ray examinations of the abdomen, and they were concerned that the embryo would be malformed. Dosimetry had not been performed, and an evaluation had not been ini-tiated. It took about 10 minutes on the telephone to determine that she became pregnant after the diagnostic radiation studies had been completed and that her two previous boys had developmental problems (hemangi-oma and pyloric stenosis). She canceled the abortion, and she delivered a normal full-term girl. She was adequately warned that we could not guarantee the outcome of the pregnancy – that there are 27.5 serious mal-formations per 1000 births as a minimum. She had another determining factor in that she had a serious problem with varicose veins and planned a tubal ligation after either the abortion or the delivery. This case history illustrates the inadequate amount of data that was collected by the physicians before counseling the patient. There was an added feature in this case. The paternal family was religiously devout and the consideration of an abortion was causing much dissension within the family.

Evaluating the patient

Case histories similar to this are transmitted to our laboratory frequently. In most instances, the dose to the embryo is <10 rad (0.1 Gy) and frequently is <1 rad (0.01 Gy). Our experience has taught us that there are many variables involved in radiation exposure to a pregnant or potentially pregnant woman. Therefore, there is no routine or predetermined advice that can be given in this situation. However, if the physician takes a systematic approach to the evaluation of the possible effects of radiation exposure, he/she can help the patient make an informed decision about continuing the pregnancy. This systematic evaluation can begin only when the following information has been obtained:

- stage of pregnancy at the time of exposure
- menstrual history
- previous pregnancy history
- family history of congenital malformations
- other potentially harmful environmental factors during the pregnancy
- ages of the mother and father
- type of radiation study, dates and number of studies performed
- calculation of the embryonic exposure by a medical physicist or competent radiologist
- status of the pregnancy: wanted or unwanted.

An evaluation should be made of the information, with both patient and counselor arriving at a decision. The physician should place a summary of the following information in the medical record. It should state that the patient has been informed that every pregnancy has a significant risk of problems and that the decision to continue the pregnancy does not mean that the counselor is guaranteeing the outcome of the pregnancy. The use of amniocentesis and ultrasound to evaluate the fetus is an individual decision that would have to be made in each pregnancy.

The carcinogenic effects of radiation

The carcinogenic risk of in utero radiation is an important topic that cannot be addressed adequately in this publication. Alice Stewart[12] published the results of her case–control study indicating the diagnostic radiation from pelvimetry increased the risk of childhood leukemia by 50% (Table 3.2).

Table 3.3 Follow-up of adults with solid cancers in Hiroshima and Nagasaki who were in utero at the time of detonation of the A-bombs in 1945 (Preston *et al.* 2008)

Dose in Sv (rads)	No. of patients	No. of cancers	Person-years	% with solid cancers
<0.005 (<0.5)	1 547	54	49,326	3.5
0.005–<0.1 (0.5–10)	435	16	14,005	3.7
0.1–<0.2 (10–<20)	168	6	5 041	3.6
0.2–<0.5 (20–<50)	172	8	5 496	4.6
0.5–<1.0 (50–<100)	92	7	2 771	7.6
>1.0	48	3	1 404	6.2
Total	2 452	94	94	3.5

Table 3.4 Follow-up of adults with solid cancers in Hiroshima and Nagasaki who were in children at the time of detonation of the A-bombs in 1945 (Preston *et al.* 2008)

Dose in Sv (rads)	No. of patients	No. of cancers	Person-years	% of cancers
<0.005 (<0.5)	8 549	318	247,744	3.7
0.005–<0.1 (0.5–<10)	4 528	173	134,621	3.8
0.1–<0.2 (10–<20)	853	38	25,802	4.4
0.2–<0.5 (20–<50)	859	51	25,722	5.9
0.5–<1.0 (50–<100)	325	21	9 522	6.5
>1.0	274	48	7 620	17.5
Total	15,388	649	451,031	4.2

That would change the annual risk of childhood leukemia from 4 cases per 100,000 children to 6 cases per 100,000 children in the population of exposed fetuses. This has been a very controversial subject.[10–15] A recent publication by Preston *et al.*[16] presented data from the in utero population of the A-bomb survivors which indicated that the embryo was less vulnerable to the oncogenic effects of ionizing radiation than the child. It appears that the embryo is much less vulnerable to the oncogenic effects of radiation than previous investigators have believed. Patients can be told that the fetal risks are extremely small, so small that we cannot measure the risks because such a large exposed population would be necessary (Tables 3.3 and 3.4).

Diagnostic or therapeutic abdominal radiation in women of reproductive age

In women of reproductive age, it is important for the patient and physician to be aware of the pregnancy status of the patient before performing any type of x-ray procedure in which the ovaries or uterus will be exposed. If the embryonic exposure will be 10 rad or less, the radiation risks to the embryo are very small when compared with the spontaneous risks (Table 3.2). Even if the exposure is 10 rad, this exposure is far from the threshold or no-effect dose of 20 rad. The patient will accept this information if it is offered as part of the *preparation* for the x-ray studies at a time when both the physician and patient are aware that a pregnancy exists or may exist. The pregnancy status of the patient should be determined and noted.

Because the risks of 10 rad fetal irradiation are so small, the immediate medical care of the mother should take priority over the risks of diagnostic radiation exposure to the embryo. X-ray studies that are essential for optimal medical care of the mother and evaluation of medical problems that need to be diagnosed or treated should not be postponed. Elective procedures such as employment examinations or follow-up examinations, once a diagnosis has been made, need not be performed on a pregnant woman even though the risk to the embryo is very small. If other procedures (e.g., MRI or ultrasound) can provide adequate information without exposing the embryo to ionizing radiation, then of course they should be used. Naturally, there is a period when the patient is pregnant but the pregnancy test is negative and the menstrual history is of little use. However, the risks of 10 rad or less are extremely small during this period of gestation (all-or-none period,[6] first 2 weeks). The patient will benefit from knowing that the diagnostic study was indicated and should be performed in spite of the fact that she may be pregnant.

Scheduling the examination

In those instances in which elective x-ray studies need to be scheduled, it is difficult to know whether to schedule them during the first half of the menstrual cycle just before ovulation or during the second half of the menstrual cycle, when most women will not be pregnant. The genetic risk of diagnostic exposures to the oocyte or the embryopathic effects on the preimplanted embryo is extremely small, and there are no data available to compare the relative risk of 10 rad to the oocyte or the preimplanted embryo. If the diagnostic study is performed in the first 14 days of the menstrual cycle, should the patient be advised to defer conception for several months, based on the assumption that the deleterious effect of radiation to the ovaries decreases with increasing time between radiation exposure and a subsequent ovulation? The physician is in a quandary because he may be warning the patient about a very-low-risk phenomenon. On the other hand, avoiding conception for several months is not an insurmountable hardship. This potential genetic hazard is quite speculative for man, as indicated by the report by the NCRP and BEIR committee report dealing with preconception radiation:[3,8]

> It is not known whether the interval between irradiation of the gonads and conception has a marked effect on the frequency of genetic changes in human offspring, as has been demonstrated in the female mouse. Nevertheless, it may be advised for patients receiving high doses to the gonads (>25 rad, 0.25Gy) to wait for several months after such exposures before conceiving additional offspring.[3]

Because the patients exposed during diagnostic radiological procedures absorb considerably less than 25 rad, the recommendations made here may be unnecessary, but it involves no hardship to the patient or physician. Because both the NCRP and ICRP have previously recommended that elective radiological examinations of the abdomen and pelvis be performed during the first part of the menstrual cycle (10-day rule, 14-day cycle) to protect the zygote from possible but largely conjectural hazards, the recommendation to avoid fertilization of recently irradiated ova perhaps merits equal attention.

Importance of determining pregnancy status of patient

If exposures <10 rad do not measurably affect the exposed embryos, and it is recommended that diagnostic procedures should be performed at any time during the menstrual cycle, if necessary, for the medical care of the patient, why expend energy to determine the pregnancy status of the patient?

There are several reasons why the physician and patient should share the burden of determining the pregnancy status before performing an x-ray or nuclear medicine procedure that exposes the uterus:

1 If the physician is forced to include the possibility of pregnancy in the differential diagnosis, a small percentage of diagnostic studies may no longer be considered necessary. Early symptoms of pregnancy may mimic certain types of gastrointestinal or genitourinary disease.

2 If the physician and patient are both aware that pregnancy is a possibility and the procedure is still performed, it is much less likely that the patient will be upset if she subsequently proves to be pregnant.

3 The careful evaluation of the reproductive status of women undergoing diagnostic procedures will prevent many unnecessary lawsuits. Many lawsuits are stimulated by the factor of surprise. In some instances, the jury is not concerned with cause and effect but with the fact that something was not done properly by the physicians.[17,18] In this day and age, failure to communicate adequately can be interpreted as less-than-adequate medical care. Both these factors are eliminated if the patient's pregnancy status has been evaluated properly and the situation discussed adequately with the patient. Physicians are going to have to learn that practicing good technical medicine may not be good

enough in a litigation-prone society. Even more important, the patient will have more confidence if the decision to continue the pregnancy is made before the medical x-ray procedure is performed, because the necessity of performing the procedure would have been determined with the knowledge that the patient was pregnant.

In every consultation dealing with the exposure of the embryo to diagnostic studies involving ionizing radiation (x-ray, CT scans, use of radionuclides) in which her reproductive risks or developmental risks for her fetus have not been increased by the radiation exposure, the patient should be informed that every healthy woman with a negative personal and genetic family reproductive history has background reproductive risks which are 3% for birth defects and 15% for miscarriage. We cannot change these background risks, which every woman faces.

References

1 Otake M, Schull WJ. In utero exposure to A-bomb radiation and mental retardation: a reassessment. *Br J Radiol* 1984;57:409–14.
2 Miller RW. Discussion: Severe mental retardation and cancer among atomic bomb survivors exposed in utero. National Council on Radiation Protection and Measurements, Bethesda, MD. *Teratology* 1999;59:234–5.
3 Committee on the Biological Effects of Ionizing Radiation. *BEIR VII Report: The Effects on Populations of Exposure to Low Levels of Ionizing Radiation*. Washington, DC: National Academy of Science Press, 2005; pp. 1–524.
4 National Council on Radiation Protection and Measurements. *Basic Radiation Criteria, Report No. 39*. Washington, DC: NCRP, 1971.
5 Brent RL. Radiations and other physical agents. In: Wilson JG, Fraser FC (eds) *Handbook of Teratology, Vol 1*. New York: Plenum Press, 1977; pp. 153–223.
6 Brent RL. Utilization of developmental basic science principles in the evaluation of reproductive risks from pre- and postconception environmental radiation exposures. Paper presented at the Thirty-third Annual Meeting of the National Council on Radiation Protection and Measurements. The Effects of Pre- and Postconception Exposure to Radiation, April 2–3, 1997, Arlington, Virginia. *Teratology* 1999;59: 182–204.
7 Brent RL. The effects of embryonic and fetal exposure to x-rays and isotopes. In: Barron WM, Lindheimer MD (eds) *Medical Disorders During Pregnancy*, 3rd edn. St. Louis, MO: Mosby-Yearbook, 2000; pp. 586–610.
8 National Council on Radiation Protection and Measurements. *Medical Radiation Exposure of Pregnant and Potentially Pregnant Women*, Report No. 54, Washington, DC: NCRP, 1977; pp. 1–32.
9 Mettler FA Jr, Brent RL, Streffer C, Wagner L. Pregnancy and medical radiation. In: Valentin J (ed.) *Annals of the International Commission on Radiological Protection (ICRP)*, Publication 84, Tarrytown, NY: Elsevier Science, Vol. 30(1), 2000.
10 Brent RL. Lauriston S. Taylor Lecture: Fifty years of scientific research: the importance of scholarship and the influence of politics and controversy. *Health Physics* 2007;93(5):348–79.

11 Brent RL. Saving lives and changing family histories: appropriate counseling of pregnant women and men and women of reproductive age, concerning the risk of radiation exposures during and before pregnancy. *Am J Obstet Gynecol* 2009; 200(1):4–24.

12 Stewart A, Webb D, Giles D, *et al.* Malignant disease in childhood and diagnostic irradiation in utero. *Lancet* 1956;2:447.

13 McMahon B, Hutchinson GB. Prenatal X-ray and childhood: a review. *Acta Union Int Contra Cancrum* 1964;20:1172.

14 Boice JD Jr, Miller RW. Childhood and adult cancer after intrauterine exposure to ionizing radiation. *Teratology* 1999;59(4):227–33.

15 Wakeford R, Little MP. Risk coefficients for childhood cancer after intrauterine irradiation: a review. *Int J Radiat Biol* 2003;79:203–9.

16 Preston DL, Cullings H, Suyama A, *et al.* Solid cancer incidence in atomic bomb survivors exposed in utero or as young children. *J Natl Cancer Inst* 2008;100:428–36.

17 Brent RL. The effect of embryonic and fetal exposure to X-ray, microwaves, and ultrasound: counseling the pregnant and non-pregnant patient about these risks. *Semin Oncol* 1989;16:347–69.

18 Brent RL. Litigation-produced pain, disease and suffering: an experience with congenital malformation lawsuits. *Teratology* 1977;16:1–14.

PROTOCOL 4

Exercise during Pregnancy: Risks and Benefits

James F. Clapp

Department of Reproductive Biology and the Schwartz Center for Metabolism and Nutrition, Case Western Reserve University at MetroHealth Medical Center, Cleveland, Ohio, USA

Overview

Over the last 50 years the medical complications associated with a sedentary lifestyle have been well documented, as have the health benefits of regular exercise. This first became common knowledge in the 1960s and immediately the general public's awareness about the value of maintaining an active lifestyle increased. Unfortunately, beginning in the 1970s, there was little or no information available to support that decision and there were many theoretical concerns that strenuous exercise might harm the fetus and/or the mother-to-be. By 1985, the American College of Obstetricians and Gynecologists decided that the benefits of regular exercise outweighed the risks for healthy women with normal pregnancies and published guidelines for exercise during pregnancy based on theory and therefore necessarily conservative. Unfortunately, their multiple limitations and exclusions were not well accepted by many active women, which created conflict with their healthcare providers and occasional guilt. With additional evidence, ACOG's recommendations were revised in 1994 and again in 2002.[1]

Regular exercise during pregnancy appears to benefit both mother and fetus. Beginning or continuing a structured exercise regimen is strongly recommended by both the American and Canadian Colleges of Sports Medicine and their respective Obstetrical Societies.[2] However, the type of exercise performed, its duration, its intensity and its frequency remain controversial.

Physiological responses to exercise during pregnancy

Maternal responses
The maternal physiological responses to exercise are modified by the adaptations to pregnancy. In addition, exercise training augments many of the

---

Protocols for High-Risk Pregnancies, 5th edition. Edited by J.T. Queenan, J.C. Hobbins and C.Y. Spong. © 2010 Blackwell Publishing Ltd.

positive physiological adaptations to pregnancy and negates many of the negative ones. As a result, regular exercise during pregnancy appears to be physiologically protective to both mother and fetus.[3,4]

Thermal

Pregnancy drastically blunts the exercise-induced increase in body temperature, primarily by increasing the capacity for heat loss. It increases both skin blood flow and skin temperature which increases heat loss through convection and radiation. Indeed, where a pregnant woman dressed in usual exercise apparel rests quietly in a thermoneutral environment, her core body temperature actually decreases because her rate of heat loss exceeds her heat production and, when she starts exercise, there is another abrupt decrease when the cooler peripheral blood returns to her core. Pregnancy also lowers the threshold for sweating, which improves evaporative heat loss. All these responses are further augmented in the trained recreational or competitive athlete. As a result, only prolonged, strenuous endurance exercise (interval training, Versa climbers, and pleometrics are three examples) elevates maternal core temperature above 100.5°C.

Blood volume expansion, cardiac output and vascular reactivity

Vascular reactivity decreases dramatically in early pregnancy that, in turn, increases peripheral venous pooling and decreases both venous return and functional blood volume. Thus, hypotension and tachycardia are common responses to hemodynamic stress during early pregnancy. These changes also trigger a rapid increase in blood volume that progressively blunts these responses with advancing gestation. Exercise training also increases blood volume and alters vascular reactivity so women who exercise prior to pregnancy have a hemodynamic advantage and the differential between them and those who are sedentary is maintained throughout pregnancy if they continue to exercise.

In both sedentary and active women, however, heart rates during and immediately after exercise in early pregnancy are usually 20–40 beats higher and postural hypotension is common at rest in the upright position immediately after exercise. The magnitude of both responses is less in regularly exercising women and both decrease with advancing gestation. However, exercise which involves arm movement above shoulder level continues to accentuate the maternal heart rate response. Thus, one should avoid sudden cessation of exercise followed by quiet standing or sitting, and exercise heart rates are a poor index of exercise intensity during pregnancy. Indeed, heart rate monitoring is not recommended as a method for assessing exercise intensity during pregnancy.

During pregnancy cardiac output increases and splanchnic, renal, uterine and skin blood flows rise while blood pressure and total peripheral resistance fall. During exercise, the magnitude of blood flow redistribution away from the splanchnic and uterine beds to those in exercising muscle is undoubtedly buffered by these changes and is definitely reduced during late pregnancy in well-trained women. Again, this is due to the additive effects of exercise training and pregnancy on blood volume, blood pressure, cardiac output and flow redistribution requirements. An additive benefit is that many of these changes persist postpartum in exercising women, resulting in improved exercise capacity. Thus, pregnancy has a training effect in active women that may explain the improved performance of elite women athletes after their index pregnancy. Regular exercise also accentuates the vascular remodeling within the uterine circulation which increases placental size and also magnifies the pregnancy-associated increases in uterine blood flow.

Metabolic

Pregnancy is a growth process that increases oxygen consumption and glucose utilization and decreases gluconeogenesis and insulin sensitivity. The latter shifts the balance of maternal substrate utilization towards lipid oxidation, which increases the availability of carbohydrate for fulfilling feto-placental energy needs. The magnitude of these changes increase with advancing gestation. Exercise also increases oxygen consumption and glucose utilization while suppressing insulin secretion but increases sympathetic output and gluconeogenesis. The combined effects of exercise and pregnancy alter the glucose response to exercise from a hyperglycemic to a hypoglycemic one. The magnitude of the hypoglycemia increases with advancing gestation and is also augmented when exercise is performed in the 2-hour postprandial period. Thus, the timing of exercise sessions relative to nutrient intake is an important consideration for the active pregnant woman, as is the type and amount of nutrient intake during and immediately after an exercise session.

Concomitant progesterone-induced changes in the sensitivity of the respiratory center produce a respiratory alkalosis which augments oxygen transfer across the lung and into tissue both at rest and during exercise.

The effects of exercise training on the magnitude of these metabolic adaptations is unknown but the usual physiological adaptations to exercise training in the non-pregnant state (greater reliance on lipid for energy, improved insulin sensitivity, and enhanced oxygen transfer) suggest that continuing exercise training during pregnancy should have similar beneficial effects. Indeed, regular exercise during pregnancy decreases TNF_α levels, suggesting that it increases insulin sensitivity. However, short-term exercise training in late pregnancy does not appear to change insulin sensitivity but does appear to reduce insulin requirements in gestational diabetics.

Muscle, ligament and bone

The combination of maternal weight gain, protuberant abdomen, changing center of gravity and ligamentous laxity alter posture, decrease mobility and balance and increase musculoskeletal stress. Bone turnover is increased but bone density is unchanged and the effect of pregnancy on muscle mass is unknown. In sedentary women these changes make physical activity more difficult, often uncomfortable and are associated with a high incidence of low back pain. Women who exercise regularly, however, gain less weight, experience very little change in posture, maintain their abdominal muscle tone and feel better.

Feto-placental responses

Response to decreased uterine blood flow

Direct measurement of uterine blood flow during or immediately after exercise is not yet available but indirect indices indicate that uterine blood flow falls significantly during exercise and, if the exercise is moderately intense for more than 10 minutes, fetal heart rate invariably increases. This is a manifestation of an acute fetal stress or sympathetic response to a small decrease in fetal Po_2 and the magnitude of the heart rate increase is directly related to the intensity and duration of the exercise and the muscle mass utilized. Other components are an increase in fetal cardiac output and a change in the distribution of cardiac output which maintains adequate oxygenation of critical tissues (brain, heart, adrenal and placenta). Transfer of oxygen into and carbon dioxide out of fetal tissues is improved by the concomitant shift in the oxyhemoglobin dissociation curve. The chronic pregnancy-associated increase in alveolar ventilation increases maternal arterial Po_2 and decreases Pco_2 which further enhances placental transfer of both gases.

Regular exercise increases maternal and fetal placental blood volumes and surface areas which is estimated to improve placental transfer function by 20% or more. Regular exercise training during pregnancy augments the usual pregnancy-associated increase in maternal blood volume and cardiac output. This reduces the magnitude of the decrease in uterine blood flow by reducing the need for flow redistribution to supply the needs of exercising muscle.

How effective is this combined response to recurrent sustained exercise-induced decreases in uterine blood flow? In normal singleton pregnancy, these flow perturbations do not produce short- or long-term evidence of fetal distress or tissue hypoxia. The fetal biophysical profile does not decrease and the amount of time the fetus spends breathing and moving is either unchanged or increased. The incidence of meconium-stained amniotic fluid is actually decreased in fetuses born of women who exercised right up until the day of delivery and, at delivery, fetal cord blood and amniotic fluid erythropoietin levels are not increased. Both findings indicate that fetal tissue oxygenation was well maintained during exercise in late pregnancy. Finally, the offspring of regularly exercising women experienced normal to superior neurodevelopment in various domains throughout the first 5 years of life.

However, it appears that, under specific circumstances, the combined response may not be entirely adequate. Several investigators report that episodes of bradycardia occurred in some of the fetuses of untrained women immediately after an acute bout of strenuous cycle ergometer exercise. This suggests that either severe fetal hypertension or hypoxic myocardial depression occurred. It is unclear, however, if this response was related to the exercise *per se* or to the effects of exercise plus the effects of superimposed maternal postural hypotension immediately after stopping exercise.

Response to decreased nutrient delivery
The fetus and placenta normally respond to a recurrent or chronic decrease in nutrient availability by decreasing their growth rate which matches fetal demands to the supply available. As regular exercise sessions intermittently decrease both blood flow and glucose levels one might expect that regular exercise would initiate a similar response. Detailed studies summarized elsewhere[5] indicate that the effects of regular exercise on feto-placental growth vary depending on the type, frequency, duration and intensity of the exercise, the total exercise volume performed at different times during pregnancy and concomitant maternal carbohydrate intake. Thus, different exercise regimens and food intakes can increase, decrease or not alter fetal growth, size at birth and neonatal body composition.

Briefly, current evidence indicates that non-weight-bearing forms of exercise (biking, swimming) have no effect on size at birth. Continuing common weight-bearing types of exercise (running, aerobics classes, cross-country skiing) during pregnancy stimulate placental growth while their effect on fetal growth varies with the effects of exercise on 24-hour substrate availability. The latter is a function of maternal exercise volume and diet. Several examples follow. Women who start exercise in early pregnancy and eat to appetite have significantly larger babies than those who remain sedentary. Women who train hard or increase their exercise volume throughout pregnancy are delivered of offspring with normal lean body masses who have experienced normal axial and head circumferential growth in utero. However, growth of their fat organ is restricted which, if it persists, may be of value later in life. Women who train hard in early pregnancy and then cut back have large infants with significantly increased fat mass, suggesting overgrowth. Finally, women who exercise and eat a high glycemic index diet deliver large infants (over 4 kg) while those who eat a low glycemic index diet are delivered of fetuses who weigh about 3.2 kg.[6]

Risks

Initial concern was that the effects of maternal exercise on body temperature, uterine blood flow, substrate utilization, catecholamine release and shear stress placed the embryo, fetus and/or placenta at risk for multiple complications. During pregnancy these included spontaneous abortion, congenital abnormality, hypoxia, growth restriction, cord entanglement, preterm labor, placental insufficiency, premature membrane rupture and placental abruption. There also was concern that the offspring might experience abnormalities in postnatal growth and neurodevelopment. The main risks for the pregnant woman appeared to be difficulty with conception, energy drain and either acute or chronic injuries (arthritis, dislocation, hernia, diastisis, etc.). To date, it appears that neither these nor other unanticipated negative outcomes have occurred but there are many forms of exercise yet to be studied and risk may vary in women who lead different lifestyles or who experience a variety of complications during pregnancy.

Benefits

The major benefit of regular exercise during pregnancy is that it enhances the normal physiological adaptations to pregnancy while negating many of their musculoskeletal side effects. Additional maternal benefits of most forms of exercise studied to date include an improved body image and sense of well-being, improved productivity, a decrease in the incidence and magnitude of common pregnancy discomforts, a decrease in the incidence of situational depression both during and after pregnancy, and improved fitness. Specific feto-placental benefits of most forms of maternal exercise have not been studied in detail. Thus, at present they are limited to the feto-protective effects of the enhanced maternal adaptations to pregnancy and perhaps improved placental growth and function.

However, other specific maternal and feto-placental benefits have been identified in women who continue moderate to high volume weight-bearing recreational exercise regimens throughout pregnancy.[3] For the mother these include: limited weight gain and fat retention; shorter, less complicated labors; shorter recovery times after the birth; and improved maximal aerobic capacity. For the fetus, infant and young child these include: a decreased incidence of clinically diagnosed fetal distress before or during labor; a decrease in the growth rate of the fat organ which persists for the first 5 years of life; improved neonatal behavioral profile and normal to superior cognitive development.

Potential preventive value of exercise

The enhanced physiological adaptations to pregnancy suggest that regular exercise might be of value in women with a history of poor outcome (preterm labor, growth restriction, implantation abnormalities) and, when combined with diet, its effects on feto-placental growth could be of value. Initial studies indicate that it is of value in the prevention and treatment of gestational diabetes mellitus and in the prevention of pregnancy-induced hypertension and preterm labor.

Recommendations

It should be emphasized that currently these recommendations apply only to otherwise healthy women with clinically normal pregnancies.

1 A regular exercise regimen should be recommended as part of prenatal care and should be started in the first trimester.
2 The frequency of the exercise sessions should be 3 or more times a week with each session lasting at least 20–30 minutes.
3 The exercise should be continuous and conducted at a moderate to hard level of perceived exertion.
4 The overall weekly volume of exercise should be individualized based on a woman's exercise volume prior to pregnancy and her exercise tolerance. A beginner should start a moderate intensity regimen 3 times a week, increasing frequency and duration but not intensity over time. An athlete should avoid serious competition, limit interval training and not exceed a weekly exercise volume equal to 120% of that performed prior to pregnancy. Chronic fatigue and/or other signs of over-training suggest that overall exercise volume should be reduced.
5 Exercise sessions should occur 2 or more hours after a meal and include a planned post-exercise snack.
6 Quiet standing or sitting immediately after exercise should be avoided and each individual regimen should include time for warm-up and cool-down.
7 Exercising in a hot, humid environment should be avoided, hydration encouraged and interval training periods should be short.
8 Sanctioned guidelines view stationary biking and swimming as the best forms of exercise during pregnancy but, to date, experience with many

other forms of weight-bearing exercise indicate that they are well tolerated and not associated with injury.

9 The exercise regimen should be re-evaluated and changed if clinical,
pregnancy-related problems develop or local pain and tenderness occur.

References

1 American College of Obstetricians and Gynecologists. Committee Opinion No. 267:
   Exercise during pregnancy and the postpartum period. *Obstet Gynecol* 2002;99:171–3.
2 Davies GA, Wolfe LA, Mottola MF, MacKinnon C. Joint SOGC/CSEP clinical practice guideline: exercise in pregnancy and the postpartum period. *Can J Appl Physiol*
   2003;28:330–41.
3 Clapp JF. *Exercising Through Your Pregnancy*. Omaha, NB: Addicus Books, 2002.
4 Wolfe LA, Weissgerber TL. Clinical physiology of exercise in pregnancy: a literature
   review. *J Obstet Gynaecol Can* 2003;25:473–83.
5 Clapp JF. The effects of maternal exercise on fetal oxygenation and feto-placental
   growth. *Eur J Obstet Gynaecol Reprod Biol* 2003;110:S80–5.
6 Clapp JF. Maternal carbohydrate intake and pregnancy outcome. *Proc Nutr Soc*
   2002;61:45–50.

PART 2
Antenatal Testing

PROTOCOL 5

Routine and Prenatal Screening

Lawrence D. Platt

Department of Obstetrics and Gynecology, David Geffen School of Medicine at UCLA and Center for Fetal Medicine and Women's Ultrasound, Los Angeles, CA, USA

Introduction

Pregnancy provides a unique opportunity to assess a woman's general health. The objective of routine antenatal laboratory tests is to recognize an unknown condition. Pregnancy can initiate dramatic changes in various systems, and routine antenatal laboratory tests help detect alterations from what is considered normal for pregnancy. Ideally, routine laboratory and screening tests in the preconceptional period would help identify the pregnancy at risk and provide an opportunity to institute preventive measures. The goal is to maintain the health of the mother in order to assure the optimal outcome for a pregnancy.

For practical purposes, various routine laboratory screening endeavors will be broken up according to trimesters.

First trimester

Tests during the first visit
This represents the provider's first contact with the patient, ideally in the first trimester.

Blood type and Rh factor
Every pregnant woman must have her blood type and Rh factor determined. Records of previous determinations have a 0.4–3.0% error rate (either mislabelling, laboratory error or a transcription error). If the patient's blood type is O or Rh-negative, or both, her husband's blood type and Rh should be determined. If the patient is Rh-negative and her husband is Rh-positive, there may be Rh incompatibility. If the patient's

Protocols for High-Risk Pregnancies, 5th edition. Edited by J.T. Queenan, J.C. Hobbins and C.Y. Spong. © 2010 Blackwell Publishing Ltd.

blood is type O and her husband's is A, B, or AB, there may be ABO incompatibility.

Antibody screen for sensitisation

Every pregnant woman must have her serum screened for antibodies formed from exposure to major or minor blood group antigens. Exposure may have occurred naturally or from a transplacental hemorrhage, abortion, or blood transfusion. If the screen is positive, the antibody must be identified and titered. See Protocol 52 for management. In Rh-negative patients, if the screen is negative, repeat the antibody screen at 28 weeks preparatory to Rh-immune prophylaxis administration.

Hemoglobin and hematocrit

During pregnancy, the blood volume increases by 30–50%. Since plasma volume increases more than red cell volume, hemoglobin (Hb) and hematocrit (Hct) will fall. Mild anemia is defined as Hb <11 gm/dL (Hct 27–33%); severe anemia is Hb <9 gm/dL (Hct <27%).

Anemia during pregnancy is usually due to iron-deficiency type (see Protocol 18). A folic acid-deficient state may coexist with iron deficiency. Hemoglobin and hematocrit testing should be repeated at 28 weeks.

Leukocyte count

This test is used primarily as a screen to rule out leukemia and infection. Normal values may reach 16,000 in pregnancy.

Platelet count

The platelet count may detect unrecognized thrombocytopenia. Although gestational thrombocytopenia occurs, levels of 80,000–100,000 may be pathologic, but most likely is a finding of minimal clinical significance (see Protocol 20).

Serology

This test is carried out to diagnose maternal syphilis. The common VDRL (Venereal Disease Research Laboratory) is a screening test. If it is positive, the more specific fluorescent treponemal antibody (FTA) test is performed (see Protocol 35).

Rubella titer

The purpose of the rubella titer is to determine whether the mother is susceptible to rubella or is immune. If performed during the preconceptional period, it does not need to be repeated. If the patient is not immune before pregnancy, vaccination should be advised and pregnancy avoided for 3 months (see Protocol 35).

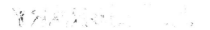

Hepatitis B surface antigen and hepatitis C
All pregnant women should be screened for hepatitis B. The infants of hepatitis B surface antigen (HBs Ag)-positive mothers need immunoprophylaxis at delivery. If possible, women at risk (drug abusers, homosexuals, health care workers) should be tested during the preconceptual period, and vaccination is advised. Women with high risk factors should be tested for hepatitis C.

Special considerations
Human immunodeficiency virus
Testing for human immunodeficiency virus (HIV) should be offered to all patients. Screening should be repeated at 36 weeks in the at-risk patient (see Protocol 38).

Illicit drug screening
Screening for illicit drugs should be offered to all patients.

Other screening tests
The following screening tests should be considered preconceptionally or in high-risk patients:
- Toxoplasmosis (see Protocol 35)
- Cytomegalovirus (see Protocol 35)
- Tuberculosis skin test (some providers skin test all patients with a negative history of tuberculosis) (see Protocol 36)
- Hemoglobin electrophoresis for patients at risk of sickle cell trait, thalassemia, or other hemoglobinopathies
- Tay-Sachs screening for individuals of Jewish ancestry; if only one of the couple is Jewish, it is recommended that the Jewish partner be screened, and if he or she is a carrier, the other partner should also be screened
- Cystic fibrosis screening
- Thyroid screening in women with history of hypothyroid or prior prescription for hyperthyroidism.

Routine urine tests
Urinalysis should be performed on clean-catch specimens:
- *Microscopy* Microscopic examination of a centrifuged specimen can identify bacteria, leukocytes, and erythrocytes, which may indicate infection. Casts or red cells, or both, may indicate chronic pyelonephritis. A complete urinalysis should be repeated at 28–30 weeks' gestation.
- *Glucose* Glycosuria may occur in pregnancy because of increased glomerular filtration rate. However, it may also indicate carbohydrate intolerance. The test should be repeated; if positive (>1+), further testing should be performed. Repeat this test at each visit.

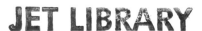

- *Protein* A value over 1+ is abnormal. The cause should be identified (urinary tract infection, pregnancy-induced hypertension, renal disease). This test should be repeated at each visit.
- *Leukocyturia* The leukocyte esterase reagent test strip is helpful in identifying patients with significant leukocyturia which suggests infection.

Urine culture
- A urine culture can be obtained on the first visit. However, some consider the leukocyte esterase test as the first step and, if it is negative, then routine culture should be avoided (see Protocol 41).

Cervical vaginal–rectal examination evaluation
- *Papanicolaou smear* to identify cancer of the cervix, as well as cervical herpes and papillomavirus. A positive result requires further evaluation.
- *Culture for gonorrhea* is recommended at the initial visit. At 36 weeks' gestation, a repeat culture may be indicated in an at-risk patient. A positive culture requires treatment with appropriate antibiotics and a follow-up culture 2 weeks after therapy to assure a cure.
- *Culture for herpes* should be done only when a woman has active herpes to confirm the diagnosis (see Protocol 35).
- *Culture for Group B Streptococci*. Vaginal and rectal GBS screening cultures at 35–37 weeks' gestation for all pregnant women (unless patient had GBS bacteriuria during the current pregnancy or a previous infant with invasive GBS disease). Indications for prophylaxis are covered in Protocol 40.

Special consideration
- *Assessment for the risk of bacterial vaginosis* Bacterial vaginosis (BV) is a common alteration of vaginal flora, occurring in 10–25% of women, with over half asymptomatic. Although some trials have found an association between BV and preterm birth, treatment has not been universally effective. There is insufficient evidence to suggest screening and treating women either low or high risk will reduce the rate of preterm birth.

Ultrasound
1 Early sonography provides optimal dating and assessment of fetal number.
2 Sonography between 8 and 12 weeks, involving the measurement of crown rump length (CRL), will provide the best documentation of fetal age, and, since at least 10% of patients will have dates erroneously

based on menstrual history alone, this is enough to justify this practice as "routine".

3 A nuchal translucency (NT) assessment, if available, can be used to screen for aneuploidy (see Protocol 7).

First trimester biochemistry

Human chorionic gonadotropin (hCG) is a product of the placenta which is generally found in high levels in fetuses with Down syndrome (average 1.83 MOM (Multiple of Median)). Pregnancy associated plasma protein A (PAPP-A), another product of the placenta, is generally found in lower levels in Down syndrome (average 0.39 MOM). These two analytes can be used in combination with NT ("combined" first trimester screening), or alone (first trimester serum screening). The sensitivity of the combined test is about 85–90 for Down syndrome at a screen positive rate of 5%. First trimester biochemical screening alone has reported a 65% sensitivity at a screen positive rate of 5% (see Protocol 7).

Second trimester

Serum screening (16–20 weeks)

1 Maternal serum alpha feto protein (MSAFP). The observation that levels of this analyte are elevated in about 85% of pregnancies complicated by fetal open neural tube defects (NTD) has led to universal screening. MSAFP elevation is also seen with ventral wall defects, skin disorders such as epidermolysis ballosa, or in Finnish congenital nephrosis. Ultrasound examination of the fetal cranium (especially the posterior fossa) and spine in those with elevated MSAFP should result in virtually a 100% identification rate for open NTDs.

2 Biochemical combination testing for aneuploidy (see Protocol 7)

Levels of MSAFP were noted by Merkatz to be depressed in Down syndrome. Later, hCG (which tends to be elevated) and estriol (which is decreased) were added to the screening regimen to form the commonly used "triple screen". By adding inhibin-A, which is elevated in Down syndrome, to the mix the "quad screen" was created. If used alone, these four analyte serum tests will screen in approximately 85% of Down syndrome fetuses at a 5% screen positive rate.

Although triple screens are still used in some areas of the country, most providers are now using the quad screen as a routine screening tool. It is controversial as to whether the full quad screen adds enough to a screening regimen for Down syndrome to warrant doing it if a comprehensive first trimester algorithm has already been used to predict the risk for Down syndrome.

Table 5.1 Quad markers and adverse pregnancy outcomes

Outcome	Markers	Odds ratio
Spontaneous loss <24 weeks	AFP	7.8
Fetal death ≥24 weeks	Inhibin-A	3.7
Preterm birth ≤32 weeks	Inhibin-A	5.0
Preterm PROM	AFP	1.9
Preeclampsia	Inhibin-A	3.8
Gestational hypertension	Inhibin-A	2.7
Abruption	AFP	1.9
Previa at delivery	AFP	3.1
IUGR	Inhibin-A	3.0
Birthweight ≤5th percentile	Inhibin-A	2.3
Delivery ≤37 weeks	Inhibin-A	8.0
Delivery ≤32 weeks	Inhibin-A	18.6

This is covered in more detail in Protocol 7, but the above biochemistry can be used in combination with first trimester biochemistry ("combined serum screening"), or with first trimester NT and biochemistry ("modified sequential screen"); the latter have over a 90% sensitivity at a screen positive rate of 5%.

All of the algorithms consider the patient's age, and the time of gestation, in order to give patients an individual risk for Down syndrome which allows each patient to weigh her risk of fetal Down syndrome against the risk of amniocentesis or chorionic villus sampling (CVS), if the first trimester results are not reassuring.

3 Biochemical screening for adverse pregnancy outcome

There are tendencies among first and second trimester biochemical analytes to be somewhat predictive of adverse pregnancy outcome. Although this would not be considered a standard strategy, the above first and second trimester serum analytes can be used singly, or in combination, to predict adverse pregnancy outcomes such as intrauterine demise, fetal growth restriction, preeclampsia, or early delivery. Table 5.1 demonstrates which analytes are most predictive of the various types of adverse pregnancy outcome (Table 5.1).

Second trimester ultrasound examination (16–24 weeks)

Most providers will obtain a standard ultrasound examination between 16 and 24 weeks. The specifics of this exam will be discussed in Protocol 6, but the intent is to establish the position of the placenta; determine the adequacy of amniotic fluid; document gestational age; and attempt to rule out major congenital abnormalities.

Patients at higher risk for fetal anomalies, such as a history of previous anomalies, diabetes, suspicious medications, multiple gestations, pregnancy through assisted reproductive technology (ART), etc., might benefit from a "targeted exam" to focus on a particular anomaly in question. Also, patients of advanced maternal age (>34 years of age) often will add a "genetic sonogram", which consists of a search for markers for Down syndrome, to the usual requirements of the standard ultrasound examination.

Cervical length (CL) exam by transvaginal ultrasound may be measured at 18 to 24 weeks in women with a history of PTB. If the CL is >3.0 cm, the likelihood of PTB is extremely low. (See protocol 46)

Early third trimester testing (24–30 weeks)

1 *Glucose screening* A 1 hour glucose screen should be performed at 26–28 weeks since about 5% of pregnant patients will be glucose intolerant (see Protocol 28).

The current screening regimen consists of an oral glucose load of 50 g and the 1 hour plasma glucose threshold most commonly used today is 130 mg%. This will identify 90% of diabetics at a 15% positive rate. If 140 mg% is used, then 100% would be picked up, unfortunately, at a 25% false positive rate. If the threshold is exceeded, the next step would be to have a full 3 hour glucose tolerance test with 100 g oral glucose load, with the cut offs for fasting, 1 hour, 2 hour, and 3 hour serum levels of 95 mg%, 180 mg%, 155 mg%, and 140 mg%, respectively (Coustan and Carpenter). If two or more of these values are exceeded, then the patient would be considered a diabetic. Patients with a strong family history of diabetes, or a history of delivering a macrosomic infant, or one with neonatal hypoglycemia, might benefit from earlier glucose screening. Also, patients who are noted to have a 1 hour screen that is abnormal and a 3-hour glucose tolerance test is "negative", will often become "positive" later in pregnancy, especially if their fetuses are large for gestational age.

2 *Antibody screening* Women who are Rh negative, should have an antibody screen repeated at about 28 weeks' gestation (see Protocol 52), preparatory to administering Rh-immune prophylaxis.

Summary

Screening tests are staged according to when the information is most important and/or when in pregnancy the test is most efficient in accomplishing

Table 5.2 Routine laboratory tests to be obtained at the first visit

Routine blood test
Blood type and Rh factor
Antibody screen for sensitization
Hemoglobin and hematocrit
Leukocyte count
Platelet count
Red cell count and indices
Differential smear
Serology
Rubella titer
Hepatitis B surface antigen and hepatitis C
Glucose screening test
First trimester screening
Maternal serum markers in the first and second trimester

Special considerations
Human immunodeficiency virus
Illicit drug screening

Other screening tests
Toxoplasmosis
Cytomegalovirus
Tuberculosis skin test
Hemoglobin electrophoresis for patients at risk for sickle cell trait, thalassemia, or other
hemoglobinopathies
Jewish panel, including Tay-Sachs, Familial Dysautonomia, and other commonly associated
diseases
Ethnic specific conditions
Cystic fibrosis
Thrombophilia screening
Thyroid screening in women with history of hypothyroid or prior prescription for hyperthyroid
See special considerations (in section on cervical-vaginal-rectal examination evaluation) for the
assessment of risk for vaginal infections secondary to bacterial vaginosis

Ultrasound screening
As described above

Routine urine tests
Urinalysis (microscopy, glucose, protein, leukocyturia)
Urine culture

Cervical-vaginal-rectal examination
Papanicolaou smear
Culture for gonorrhea
Culture for herpes
Culture for group B streptococci
Intrapartum prophylaxis as indicated by GBS screening culture history
Special consideration: assessment for risk of bacterial vaginosis

the screening goal. The majority of requisite blood and urine tests are performed at the first visit.

Concisely, the following represents a synopsis of screening events:

8–12 weeks
- Requisite blood and urine tests (Table 5.2).
- First trimester ultrasound examination (CRL, prenatal screening if desired)

16–22 weeks
- Biochemistry for aneuploidy if desired
- Standard ultrasound examination
- Cervical length in those at risk for PTB

26–28 weeks
- Screen for diabetes
- Repeat antibody screen in Rh negative patients

28–30 weeks
- Repeat complete urinanalysis

30–36 weeks
- Repeat glucose screen in those with strong predisposition, but initially negative test

Suggested reading

Andrews JI, Diekema DJ, Yankowitz J. Prenatal testing for infectious disease. *Clin Lab Med* 2003;23:295–315.

Assessment of Risk Factors for Preterm Birth. ACOG Practice Bulletin #31, October 2001.

Gjerdingen D, Fontaine P, Bixby M *et al*. The impact of regular vaginal pH screening on the diagnosis of bacterial vaginosis in pregnancy. *J Fam Pract* 2000;49:39–43.

Wapner R, Thom E, Simpson JL *et al*. First-trimester screening for trisomies 21 and 18. *N Engl J Med* 2003;349:1405–13.

Chen Min, Lee CP, Lam YH *et al*. Comparison of Nuchal and Detailed Morphology Ultrasound Examinations in Early Pregnancy for Fetal Structural Abnormality Screening: A Randomized Controlled Trial. Ultrasound Obstet Gynecol 2008;31: 136–46.

Levi S. Ultrasound in prenatal diagnosis: polemics around routine ultrasound screening for second trimester fetal malformations. Prenatal Diag 2002;22:285–95.

Malone FD, Canick JA, Ball RH *et al*. First-Trimester or Second-Trimester Screening, or Both, for Down's Syndrome. *N Engl J Med* 2005;353:2001–11.

Bromley B, Lieberman E, Shipp TD *et al*. The Genetic Sonogram: A Method of Risk Assessment for Down Syndrome in the Second Trimester. J Ultrasound Med 2002; 21:1087–1096.

Dugoff, Lorraine MD; Hobbins *et al*. for the FASTER Trial Research Consortium. Quad Screen as a Predictor of Adverse Pregnancy Outcome. Obstet Gynecol 2005;106: 260–267.

American College of Obstetricians and Gynecologists. 2009 Compendium of Selected Publications. ACOG, Washington, DC.

Canick JA, Lambert-Messerlian GM, Palomaki GE *et al.* First and Second Trimester Evaluation of Risk (FASTER) Trial Research Consortium. Obstet Gynecol 2006;108: 1192–9.

PROTOCOL 6

Sonographic Screening for Fetal Anomalies

John Hobbins

Department of Obstetrics and Gynecology, University of Colorado Health Sciences Center, Denver, CO, USA

Overview

In most of the world, the prevalence of major fetal anomalies is about 20–30/1000 births. Being aware of the presence of an anomaly can be beneficial to those continuing their pregnancies by adjusting their management to optimize outcome, and by preparing parents for the birth of a child with an anomaly. However, it also can put pressure on the provider not to miss a fetal anomaly during an ultrasound examination, and, as pointed out below, the public must become more accepting of the fact that screening for anomalies is still less than perfect.

Although there are many ways in which ultrasound can be used in pregnancy, the type of examination undertaken will be dictated by the diagnostic question that needs to be answered. The most basic examination is the 'limited' scan, which is generally a one-task venture, such as determining placental position in a patient with vaginal bleeding, determining fetal presentation in early labor, or assessing amniotic fluid volume. The most comprehensive examination is the 'targeted' scan which is used when there is a high suspicion of a fetal anomaly. The examination which is undertaken in almost every pregnancy is the 'standard' ultrasound scan which involves:

1 obtaining fetal biometry for gestational age and size
2 amniotic fluid
3 fetal position and number
4 evaluating the maternal adnexa.

In addition to the above components, the most important function of the standard examination is to screen for fetal anomalies. In 1990, in a collaborative effort, the American Institute of Ultrasound in Medicine (AIUM), the American College of Radiology (ACR) and the American

Protocols for High-Risk Pregnancies, 5th edition. Edited by J.T. Queenan, J.C. Hobbins and C.Y. Spong. © 2010 Blackwell Publishing Ltd.

College of Obstetricians and Gynecologists (ACOG) drafted guidelines for the performance of the standard examination, including the fetal anatomy survey. These guidelines have been later amended, resulting in the current product summarized below.

Components of the fetal survey

Head
Biparietal diameter (BPD)
An axial plane through the head at the level of the thalami will allow measurement of the BPD and visualization of the cavum septi pellucidi and a portion of the frontal horns.

Lateral ventricles
The downside ventricle can be imaged in a plane that is just above the BPD. The distance between the medial and lateral walls of the ventricle should not exceed 1 cm. A measurement between 1.0 and 1.25 cm indicates 'mild', between 1.25 and 1.50 cm 'moderate', and greater than 1.5 cm 'severe' ventriculomegaly (or hydrocephaly).

Posterior fossa
With an angled axial view through the posterior fossa, one can view the cisterna magna, the cerebellar hemispheres, as well as the cerebral peduncles, thalami and the third ventricle. Imaging these three planes will allow the vast majority of anomalies of the central nervous system (CNS) to be detected.

Face
During the standard examination one can isolate coronally the triad of nose, upper lip and mouth to exclude a cleft lip. The palate is more difficult to examine and involves a cross-section of the face at the level of the alveolar ridge and hard palate.

Heart
The original guidelines only included the standard four-chamber view. The current recommendations are that an attempt be made to image both outflow tracts.

Spine
The standard procedure involves imaging as much of the spine as possible in one longitudinal slice. Some practitioners will document the integrity

of the spine with three cross-sections along it. Any effort to rule out an open spinal defect should be combined with evaluation of the posterior fossa, since virtually all open defects will have disruption of this area.

Abdomen

Both kidneys can be identified with a transverse slice through the abdomen. Occasionally the downside kidney will be shadowed by the spine, but its presence can be documented by imaging both renal arteries with color Doppler. Also, the umbilical cord insertion can be seen on cross-section, ruling out a ventral wall defect. The presence of two umbilical arteries can be documented with color Doppler as they split to enclose the bladder.

Extremities

The current guidelines require an attempt to image both lower extremities to rule out clubbing. However, the hands can be difficult to image precisely in a moving fetus.

The efficacy of screening for fetal anomalies with ultrasound

Screening for all anomalies

It is clear that over the past 20 years there has been an improvement in identifying or, at least, screening in major fetal abnormalities, but it has been difficult to quantify the actual sensitivity of this process because of the heterogeneity of the many studies in the literature. For example, studies that scrupulously exclude high-risk patients (the RADIUS study) rather than evaluating an unselected group (the Eurofetus study) will have different results because of differences in prevalence. Also, studies in which patients are scanned by highly skilled practitioners are going to have better results than patients who are scanned by those with less training and who may only see two or three anomalies per year. In the RADIUS trial, 35% of major fetal anomalies were found in teaching centers, compared with 13% by practitioners. Also, retrospective studies based on birth data, such as the Euroscan study, do not take into account diagnoses that were correctly made in fetuses that were either spontaneously lost or aborted. However, the Eurofetus study, which involved over 200,000 patients being screened in 60 centers throughout Europe over a 3-year period, can act as a realistic model regarding what can easily be accomplished today. In this study, where the majority of the scans were performed by those in non-tertiary care settings, the overall detection rate of major anomalies was 61%.

Improvement in identification rates over time

There is no doubt that the detection rate has improved over the last three decades, perhaps because of more experience, better equipment, and the addition of a more expanded examination (outflow tracts, extremities, and a more comprehensive evaluation of the brain and face). For example, in a review in 2002, Levi noted that the average sensitivity of all studies in the literature rose from 33% prior to 1992 to 40% in studies over the next 7 years.

Comparison of screening performance according to organ systems

The best sensitivities for ultrasound screening are obtained for anomalies of the fetal central nervous system and gastrointestinal tract. The poorest performance has been for cardiac anomalies.

Central nervous system

The central nervous system lends itself to screening because most abnormalities of the head and spine are accompanied by ventriculomegaly. For example, in the Eurofetus study 88% of central nervous system anomalies were identified.

Face

Facial abnormalities are on the lower end of the performance scale. One large study in the United States showed a screening detection rate of 33% for cleft lip and palate, 20% for cleft lip alone, and 0.3% for cleft palate alone.

Heart

Norwegian investigators have found that in their large study population the overall sensitivity for the detection of cardiac anomalies has been 67% for those with associated defects and 48% for isolated abnormalities. Unfortunately, others have found that less than one-third of cardiac anomalies are identified before birth. However, this can be misleading since the poorest identification rates have come from older studies, and there has been a significant improvement over time, as evidenced by the last 10 years of the Norwegian study. Also, they and others have found that the more severe cardiac defects are less apt to escape detection, and more than half of the ductal-dependent anomalies are identified before birth. By adding the outflow tracts to screening protocols, a detection rate has recently been reported to be as high as 65% in a study involving 15 obstetric units in Italy in low-risk patients.

Genitourinary tract

Most abnormalities involve the finding of pyelectasis. A cut-off of 4 mm in the anteroposterior dimension in the second trimester will screen for obstructive abnormalities and reflux. However, the most sensitive indicator of the need for surgery in childhood is a dilation of the renal pelvis that exceeds 10 mm after 30 weeks. Interestingly, 89% of genitourinary abnormalities were identified in the Eurofetus study.

Skeletal dysplasias

Screening-in skeletal dysplasias depends predominantly on recognition of short limbs. However, the ultimate diagnosis of specific dysplasias can be very difficult, and is dependent upon a collaborative approach and the use of many diagnostic modalities. The most commonly diagnosed conditions are thanatophoric dysplasia and osteogenesis imperfecta.

Deterrents to screening performance
Obesity

The rate of obesity has skyrocketed in the United States. In one very recent study involving 10,000 Texas women, only 38% were in the 'normal' range for BMI (<25). Thirty-four percent were 'overweight' (BMI 25–30), and 26% were 'obese' (BMI >30).

   This study demonstrated the difficulty obesity plays in the performance of a standard fetal survey. Using a 10-task requirement for a complete fetal survey, the authors found that this could be accomplished in 72% of those of normal weight, but only in 57% of those with BMI between 30 and 35, and in a dismal 30% when BMIs were over 40. Unfortunately, the quality of an ultrasound image is inversely proportional to the distance between the transducer and the target. The heart is a particularly difficult organ to examine when a patient is obese and, in some cases, the best chance to image the fetal heart may be between 13–15 weeks, using transvaginal sonography.

Late developing anomalies

Some anomalies do not become manifest until later in pregnancy. One classic example is duodenal atresia. With this anomaly, the stomach may not increase in size and the duodenum may not dilate until well after 20 weeks. Another example is infantile polycystic kidney disease, where the kidneys may not become enlarged or 'echogenic' in appearance until after the 20th week. Also, structures like the corpus callosum or cerebellar vermis will not be fully formed until 22 weeks.

Screening for anomalies prior to 16 weeks with transvaginal sonography

Many patients would like to know as early as possible about the status of their fetuses. On the other hand, many organs, by their size alone, are generally easier to visualize as pregnancy progresses. Transvaginal sonography has revolutionized the ability to image the fetus earlier in pregnancy.

Accompanying the advent of nuchal translucency (NT) sonography, screening for aneuploidy has become an increased interest in the earlier diagnosis of structural anomalies. Several authors have explored the possibility of conducting a thorough fetal survey between 11 and 14 weeks with or without a standard second trimester anatomic evaluation. Some authors have reported an excellent ability to image various fetal anatomic structures and anomaly detection rates ranging from 18% to 85%. However, since most of the patients in these studies were in higher-risk categories, the results may have been skewed by a more focused approach to the study design.

Perhaps the best insight comes from a very recent randomized clinical trial by Chen *et al.* These authors found that by adding a first trimester anatomic survey to their NT protocol, the first trimester anomaly detection rate rose from 32% to 47%. However, after a second trimester anatomy scan was added to both groups, the detection rates were similar (64% vs 67%).

The fetal heart has lent itself to thorough scrutiny in more recent studies, with successful visualization of the four-chamber view being accomplished in 69–97% at 12 weeks and outflow tracts being visualized between 56% and 98% of fetuses at that time.

These studies show that an anatomic survey *can* be accomplished in the first trimester and, especially if an anomaly is suspected by history, NT size, or by a suspicious finding during the NT scan, a fetal problem can be identified in many cases.

Three-dimensional sonography

At the moment, the role of three-dimensional in diagnostic protocols is controversial, especially regarding in which circumstances this technology would be considered essential, helpful, or superfluous. There is little doubt that with a three-dimensional planar reconstruction, one can now visualize midline cranial structures, as well as the palate, which were previously inaccessible with two-dimensional technology. Also, one can pinpoint the exact level of an open spinal defect with this modality. For those using it, it is clear that 3-D is invaluable as an adjunctive tool in the diagnosis of *many* anomalies, but, as of now, its usefulness has been downplayed as a screening tool and emphasized more as providing a valuable adjunctive role in the targeted approach to anomaly detection. However, it could have great potential as a way to provide high-volume screening 'off-line', utilizing the few 3-D sweeps obtained by sonographers in remote sites.

Summary

Over the past 20 years, the fetal anomaly identification rate has improved with increased experience and an expanded scope of the fetal survey. With a standard fetal survey, it is possible to identify at least two-thirds of major fetal anomalies in the second trimester. Once an anomaly is suspected, a targeted scan and adjunctive tests, including 3-D and MRI, should pinpoint the problem with excellent accuracy.

Suggested reading

1 Levi S. Ultrasound in prenatal diagnosis: polemics around routine ultrasound screening for second trimester malformations. *Prenat Diag* 2002;22:285–95.

2 Crane JP, Lefevre MI, Winborn RC, *et al*. A randomized trial of prenatal ultrasonographic screening: impact on the detection, management, and the outcome of anomalous fetuses: The RADIUS Study Group. *Am J Obstet Gynecol* 1994;171:392–9.

3 Grandjean H, Larroque, Levi S. The performance of routine ultrasonographic screening of pregnancies in the Eurofetus study. *Am J Obstet Gynecol* 1999;181:446–54.

4 Johnson CY, Honein MA, Hobbs CA, Rasmussen SA. Prenatal diagnosis of orofacial clefts, National Birth Defects Prevention Study 1998–2004. *Prenat Diag* 2009; DOI: 10.1002/pd.2293.

5 Tegnander E, Williams W, Johansen OJ, Blaas HG, Eik-Nes SH. Prenatal detection of heart defects in a non-selected population of 30,149 fetuses: detection rates and outcome. *Ultrasound Obstet Gynecol* 2006; 7:252–65.

6 Fadda GM, Capobianco G, Balata A, *et al*. Routine second trimester ultrasound screening for prenatal detection of fetal malformations in Sassari University Hospital, Italy: 23 years of experience in 42,256 pregnancies. *Eur J Obstet Gynecol Rep Biol* 2009;144:110–14.

7 Dashe JS, McIntire DD, Twickler DM. Maternal obesity limits the ultrasound evaluation of fetal anatomy. *J Ultrasound Med* 2009;28:1025–30.

8 Timor-Tritsch I.E., Bashiri A, Monteagudo A, Arslan AA. Qualified and training sonographers in the US can perform early fetal anatomy scans between 11 and 14 weeks. *Am J Obstet Gynecol* 2004;191(4):1247–52.

9 Chen M, Lee CP, Lam YH, *et al*. Comparison of nuchal and detailed morphology ultrasound examinations in early pregnancy for fetal structural abnormality screening: a randomized controlled trial. *Ultrasound Obstet Gynecol* 2008;31(2):136–46.

10 Goncalves LF, Lee W, Espinosa J, Romero R. Three- and 4-dimensional ultrasound in obstetric practice: does it help? *J Ultrasound Med* 2005;24:1599–624.

Sonographic Detection of Aneuploidy

Fergal D. Malone

Department of Obstetrics and Gynecology, Royal College of Surgeons in Ireland and The Rotunda Hospital, Dublin, Ireland

Overview

Fetal aneuploidy refers to an abnormal number of chromosomes, other than the usual diploid complement of 46 chromosomes. Presence of a single additional chromosome, known as trisomy, is an important cause of congenital malformations. The most common autosomal trisomies are Down syndrome (trisomy 21), Edwards syndrome (trisomy 18) and Patau syndrome (trisomy 13). Trisomy 21 is the most common of these chromosomal syndromes, and is one of the most important causes of congenital mental retardation, affecting approximately one in 800 to one in 900 live births. Trisomy 18 and trisomy 13 are considered lethal malformations, with 95% of trisomy 18 infants dying by 1 year of age, and almost all trisomy 13 infants dying by 3 months of age. The incidence of trisomies 18 and 13 is approximately one in 3000 live births and one in 5000 live births, respectively. Antenatal sonographic-based screening can be used to detect over 90% of cases of trisomies 21, 18 and 13.

Pathophysiology

The phenotype of trisomy 21 occurs when there is a triplication of genes at a particular part of chromosome number 21, known as band 21q22. Nondisjunction of the pair of chromosomes number 21 during egg or sperm meiosis accounts for 95% of cases of trisomy 21. In the vast majority of cases the extra chromosome is maternal in origin, and there is a strong correlation between maternal age and the chances of fetal trisomy 21. In less than 5% of cases, the additional chromosome 21

Protocols for High-Risk Pregnancies, 5th edition. Edited by J.T. Queenan, J.C. Hobbins and C.Y. Spong. © 2010 Blackwell Publishing Ltd.

material is a result of an unbalanced translocation, usually affecting chromosomes 14 and 21, but occasionally also involving chromosomes 15 or 22. About 50% of such cases occur as *de novo* translocations and 50% are inherited from one parent who is a carrier of a balanced translocation. Rarer cases of trisomy 21 are mosaic, in which some cell lines carry three copies of chromosome number 21 while others are normal. Trisomies 18 and 13 are also due to meiotic nondisjunction in approximately 85% of cases, while 10% of cases are mosaic and 5% are due to a translocation.

Diagnosis/screening protocol

Sonographic screening and diagnosis of autosomal trisomies is commonly performed during antenatal care. Three options for screening for aneuploidy are now available: first trimester serum and sonographic screening, second trimester serum and sonographic screening, and combining different screens across both first and second trimesters.

First trimester screening

The ability to provide an accurate, patient-specific, risk assessment for fetal trisomy 21 during the first trimester is an established part of routine clinical practice. This allows patients the option of chorionic villus sampling (CVS) to confirm or exclude fetal aneuploidy, and the possibility of pregnancy termination, earlier in gestation. Techniques used to evaluate risk for trisomy 21 during the first trimester include nuchal translucency (NT) sonography, nasal bone sonography, Doppler sonography of the ductus venosus, sonographic evaluation for tricuspid regurgitation, as well as assay of the maternal serum markers pregnancy-associated plasma protein A (PAPP-A) and either the free beta-subunit or the intact molecule of human chorionic gonadotropin (hCG). Additionally, first trimester cystic hygroma can also be used for trisomy 21 risk assessment, as it is the most powerful of all markers for fetal aneuploidy.

Nuchal translucency sonography

Nuchal translucency (NT) refers to the normal space that is visible between the spine and overlying skin at the back of the fetal neck during first trimester sonography (Figs. 7.1 and 7.2). The larger this space, the higher the risk for trisomy 21, while the smaller the space the lower the risk for trisomy 21. Measurement of this NT space has been shown to be a powerful sonographic marker for trisomy 21, when obtained between 10 weeks 3 days and 13 weeks 6 days of gestation. Table 7.1 describes the components of a standardized NT sonographic protocol.

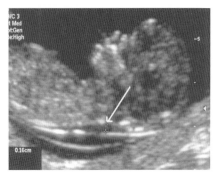

Figure 7.1 Nuchal translucency (NT) ultrasound measurement at 13 weeks in a chromosomally normal fetus, measuring 1.6 mm. Various features of good NT ultrasound technique are evident in this image: adequate image magnification, mid-sagittal plane, neutral neck position, inner to inner caliper placement perpendicular to the fetal body axis (as indicated by white arrow), and separate visualization of the overlying fetal skin and amnion. Reproduced from Malone *et al.*, Obstet Gynecol 2003;102:1066 with permission from Lippincott Williams & Wilkins.

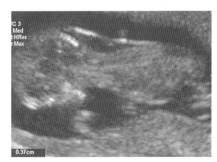

Figure 7.2 Increased nuchal translucency measurement of 3.7 mm at 12 weeks in a fetus with Down syndrome. Reproduced from Malone *et al.*, Obstet Gynecol 2003;102:1066 with permission from Lippincott Williams & Wilkins.

NT sonography can be technically challenging to master initially, and requires considerable effort to maintain quality over time. Sonographers should be comfortable using both transabdominal and transvaginal approaches to NT sonography, as the latter may be required in up to 5% of cases. Additionally, in up to 7% of cases, adequate images of the NT space may not be obtainable, regardless of the sonographic approach. In such cases it may be reasonable to have the patient return in 1 week for re-measurement provided she is still under 14 weeks' gestation, or alternatively, a risk assessment may be calculated based on serum assay results alone.

In order to use an NT measurement to calculate a patient's risk for trisomy 21, a special software program is required to convert the raw millimeter measurement into a multiple of the median (MoM) value. Use of MoM values takes into account the normal gestational age variation in NT size, and allows integration of maternal age and serum results into the final risk assessment.

Table 7.1 Sonographic technique to optimize nuchal translucency (NT) sonography

1 Nuchal translucency ultrasound should only be performed by sonographers or sonologists trained and experienced in the technique

2 Transabdominal or transvaginal approach should be left to the sonographer's discretion, based on maternal body habitus, gestational age and fetal position

3 Gestation should be limited between 10 weeks 3 days and 13 weeks 6 days, which are equivalent to approximate fetal crown : rump lengths of 36–79 mm (some centers use 45–84 mm for eligibility for NT imaging)

4 Fetus should be examined in a mid-sagittal plane

5 Fetal neck should be in a neutral position

6 Fetal image should occupy at least 75% of the viewable screen

7 Fetal movement should be awaited to distinguish between amnion and overlying fetal skin

8 Calipers should be placed on the inner borders of the nuchal fold

9 Calipers should be placed perpendicular to the long axis of the fetal body

10 At least three nuchal translucency measurements should be obtained, with either the maximum or the mean value (depending on the requirements of each laboratory's risk assessment protocol) of those used in risk assessment and patient counseling

11 At least 20 minutes may need to be dedicated to the nuchal translucency measurement before abandoning the effort as failed

12 Nuchal translucency measurements for each sonographer should be monitored as part of an ongoing quality assurance program to ensure optimal screening performance (such as is available with the NTQR Program from the Society for Maternal Fetal Medicine in the US, or the Fetal Medicine Foundation in Europe)

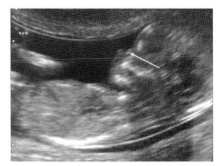

Figure 7.3 Nasal bone image of a euploid fetus at 13 weeks' gestation. Various features of good nasal bone technique are evident in this image: a good mid-sagittal plane, clear fetal profile, downward-facing spine, slight neck flexion, and two echogenic lines, representing the overlying fetal skin and the nasal bone. The white arrow represents the fetal nose bone, which loses its echogenicity distally. Reproduced from Malone *et al.*, Obstet Gynecol 2003;102:1066 with permission from Lippincott Williams & Wilkins.

Nasal bone sonography

If a perfect mid-sagittal image can be obtained of the fetus at 10 to 13 weeks' gestation, with the fetal profile facing upwards, it may be possible to distinguish an echogenic line representing the fetal nasal bones (Fig. 7.3). It has been suggested that failure to visualize this echogenic line, suggesting absence of the fetal nasal bones, may be an independent marker for fetal trisomy 21. However, it should be noted that studies suggesting a role for this marker in the first trimester are derived from select high-risk populations, and more recent research has suggested that nasal bone evaluation may not be a useful tool for general population screening. At this time, first trimester evaluation of the fetal nasal bones for general population screening is not recommended. Instead, many tertiary referral centers use nasal bone sonography as a second-line screening tool to evaluate a patient who has a high-risk first trimester screening result but who is uncertain about whether to proceed with invasive testing. If the nasal bones appear absent then this might be used as an additional indicator to proceed with CVS.

Ductus venosus Doppler sonography

Blood flow patterns in the fetal ductus venosus may be evaluated during the first trimester using Doppler ultrasound. Normally, this vessel shows a triphasic flow pattern, with forward flow reaching peaks during ventricular systole and early ventricular diastole. There should normally be forward flow even during the nadir coinciding with the atrial contraction (Fig. 7.4). Reversal of blood flow during the atrial contraction phase is considered abnormal, and has been suggested as an additional marker for trisomy 21 during the first trimester. However, to date there have been insufficient studies confirming the utility of first trimester ductus

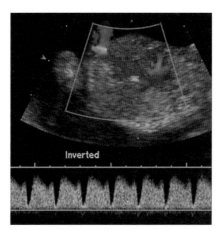

Figure 7.4 Ductus venosus flow velocity waveform in a normal 13-week fetus. The Doppler gate is placed in the ductus venosus between the umbilical venous sinus and the inferior vena cava. Note that there is triphasic pulsatile flow with constant forward flow. The troughs of flow during the atrial contraction also demonstrate forward flow. Reproduced from Malone *et al.*, Obstet Gynecol 2003;102:1066 with permission from Lippincott Williams & Wilkins.

venosus flow assessment for population screening for trisomy 21. Instead, as with nasal bone sonography, many tertiary referral centers use ductus venosus sonography as a second-line screening tool to evaluate a patient who has a high risk first trimester screening result but who is uncertain about whether to proceed with invasive testing. If there is reversed flow in the ductus venosus then this might be used as an additional indicator to proceed with CVS.

Tricuspid regurgitation

Fetuses with trisomy 21 are also more likely to have abnormal blood flow waveforms across the tricuspid valve, with tricuspid regurgitation being described in the first trimester in such pregnancies. Significant tricuspid regurgitation is seen in about 50% of aneuploid fetuses at 11 to 13 weeks, and in about 1% of normal fetuses. It may therefore be a useful second-line screening tool to evaluate a patient who has a high-risk first trimester screening result but who is uncertain about whether to proceed with invasive testing. Presence of tricuspid regurgitation of greater than 60 cm per second may be used as an additional indicator to proceed with CVS.

PAPP-A and fßhCG

Maternal serum levels of PAPP-A are approximately 50% lower in trisomy 21 pregnancies compared with normal pregnancies at 10 to 13 weeks' gestation. By contrast, maternal serum levels of fßhCG are approximately twice as high in trisomy 21 pregnancies compared with normal pregnancies at this gestational age. Depending on which laboratory is used, either total hCG or fßhCG can be used for such first trimester screening. When combined with maternal age, these two serum markers can be used to detect approximately 65% of cases of trisomy 21, for a 5% false-positive rate.

Combined sonographic and serum screening

Because measurement of fetal NT is largely independent of maternal age and the serum markers PAPP-A and fßhCG, the most efficient method of first trimester screening for trisomy 21 involves a combination of these approaches. NT sonography, together with maternal age, PAPP-A and fßhCG will detect 85% of cases of trisomy 21, for a 5% false-positive rate, between 10 and 13 weeks' gestation. It is best to perform such combination screening earlier in the first trimester, as it has been shown to have trisomy 21 detection rates of 87% at 11 weeks, compared with 82% at 13 weeks' gestation, for a 5% false-positive rate.

Cystic hygroma

In about 1 of every 300 first trimester pregnancies, during sonographic evaluation of the fetal nuchal translucency, the NT space will be found to be markedly enlarged, often extending along the entire length of the fetus, with septations clearly visible within the space. This condition is referred to as first trimester septated cystic hygroma and is the most powerful predictor of fetal aneuploidy yet described. In early gestation, this finding is associated with a 50% risk for fetal aneuploidy, with most being trisomy 21, and others including Turner syndrome, trisomy 18, trisomy 13 and triploidy. Of the 50% of such pregnancies that are proven to have a normal fetal karyotype, almost half will be complicated by major structural fetal malformations, such as cardiac defects and skeletal anomalies. Less than 25% of all cases of first trimester septated cystic hygroma will result in a normal liveborn infant. Therefore, this finding should prompt immediate referral for CVS, and pregnancies found to be euploid should be evaluated carefully for other malformations. This should include detailed fetal anomaly scan and fetal echocardiography at 18 to 22 weeks' gestation.

Second trimester screening

The mainstay of risk assessment for fetal trisomy 21 for years has been second trimester serum and sonographic screening. Despite the growing popularity of first trimester methods of risk assessment, second trimester screening will remain necessary because many patients may not present for care sufficiently early to avail of first trimester approaches, and also because many patients may be either wary of the safety of CVS or may not have access to a provider skilled in the performance of CVS. Techniques used to evaluate risk for trisomy 21 during the second trimester include sonographic detection of major structural fetal malformations, sonographic detection of minor markers, and maternal serum assay of alphafetoprotein (AFP), hCG, unconjugated estriol (uE3) and inhibin-A.

Sonographic detection of major malformations

The genetic sonogram is a term used to describe second trimester sonographic assessment of the fetus for signs of aneuploidy. The detection of certain major structural malformations that are known to be associated with aneuploidy should prompt an immediate consideration of genetic amniocentesis. Table 7.2 summarizes the major structural malformations that are associated with the most common trisomies. While the genetic sonogram can be performed at any time during the second and third trimesters, the optimal time is likely to be at about 18 weeks' gestation,

Table 7.2 Sonographic findings associated with trisomies 21, 18 and 13

Trisomy 21	Trisomy 18	Trisomy 13
Major structural malformations		
Cardiac defects:	Cardiac defects:	Holoprosencephaly
• AV canal defect	• double outlet right ventricle	Orofacial clefting
• ventricular septal defect	• Ventricular septal defect	Cyclopia
• tetralogy of Fallot	• AV canal defect	Proboscis
Duodenal atresia	Meningomyelocele	Omphalocele
Cystic hygroma	Agenesis corpus callosum	Cardiac defects:
Hydrops	Omphalocele	• ventricular septal defect
	Diaphragmatic hernia	• hypoplastic left heart
	Esophageal atresia	Polydactyly
	Clubbed or rocker	Clubbed or rocker bottom feet
	bottom feet	Echogenic kidneys
	Renal abnormalities	Cystic hygroma
	Orofacial clefting	Hydrops
	Cystic hygroma	
	Hydrops	
Minor sonographic markers		
Nuchal thickening	Nuchal thickening	Nuchal thickening
Mild ventriculomegaly	Mild ventriculomegaly	Mild ventriculomegaly
Short humerus or femur	Short humerus or femur	Echogenic bowel
Echogenic bowel	Echogenic bowel	Enlarged cisterna magna
Renal pyelectasis	Enlarged cisterna magna	Echogenic intracardiac focus
Echogenic intracardiac focus	Choroid plexus cysts	Single umbilical artery
Hypoplastic nasal bones	Micrognathia	Overlapping fingers
Brachycephaly	Strawberry-shaped head	Growth restriction
Clinodactyly	Clenched or overlapping fingers	
Sandal gap toe	Single umbilical artery	
Widened iliac angle	Growth restriction	
Growth restriction		

which is late enough to maximize fetal anatomical evaluation, yet early enough to allow for amniocentesis results to be obtained. When a major structural malformation is found, such as an atrioventricular canal defect or a double-bubble suggestive of duodenal atresia, the risk of trisomy 21 in that pregnancy can be increased by approximately 20- to 30-fold. For almost all patients, such an increase in their background risk for aneuploidy will be sufficiently high to justify immediate genetic amniocentesis.

Sonographic detection of minor markers
Second trimester sonography can also detect a range of minor markers for aneuploidy. The latter are not considered structural abnormalities of

the fetus *per se* but, when noted, may be associated with an increased probability that the fetus is aneuploid. Table 7.2 also summarizes the minor sonographic markers that, when visualized, may increase the probability of an aneuploid fetus. It should be noted that almost all data supporting the role of second trimester sonography for minor markers for aneuploidy are derived from high-risk populations, such as patients of advanced maternal age or with abnormal maternal serum screening results. The detection of such minor markers in lower-risk patients from the general population will likely have minimal impact on an already low back-ground risk of aneuploidy.

To objectively counsel patients following the prenatal diagnosis of a minor sonographic marker, likelihood ratios can be used to create a more precise risk assessment for the patient that their fetus might be affected with trisomy 21. Table 7.3 summarizes the likelihood ratios that can be used to modify a patient's risk for trisomy 21, depending on which minor marker is detected. If no markers are present, the patient's *a priori* risk can be multiplied by 0.4, effectively reducing their chances of carrying a fetus with trisomy 21 by 60%. The likelihood ratio values listed for each marker assume that the marker is an isolated finding. By contrast, when more than one minor marker is noted in the same fetus different likeli-hood ratios must be used, with the risk for trisomy 21 being increased by a factor of 10 when two minor markers are detected and by a factor of 115 when three or more minor markers are found. It should also be noted that the 95% confidence interval values for each marker's likeli-hood ratios are rather wide. These values should therefore be used only as a general guide for counseling patients, and care should be exercised to avoid implying too much precision in the final risk estimates. Accuracy of risk estimates, however, can be maximized by using the best available

Table 7.3 Likelihood ratios for trisomy 21 when an isolated minor sonographic marker is detected. The patient's *a priori* risk is multiplied by the appropriate positive likelihood ratio to yield an individualized post-test risk for fetal trisomy 21. (Derived from Nyberg et al., *J Ultrasound Med* 2001;20:1053)

Minor marker	Likelihood ratio	95% confidence intervals
Nuchal fold >5 mm	11	6–22
Echogenic bowel	6.7	3–17
Short humerus	5.1	217
Short femur	1.5	0.8–3
Echogenic intracardiac focus	1.8	1–3
Pyelectasis	1.5	0.6–4
Any two minor markers	10	6.6–14
Any three or more minor markers	115	58–229
No markers	0.4	0.3–0.5

a priori risk value for a particular patient, such as the results of maternal serum marker screening, rather than maternal age, when available.

Nuchal fold

Sonographic measurement of the nuchal fold is performed by imaging the fetal head in an axial plane passing through the posterior fossa. Calipers should be placed on the outer aspect of the occipital bone and the outer aspect of the skin. When measured between 15 and 21 weeks' gestation, a cut-off of 5 mm is commonly used to define an abnormally thickened nuchal fold. The finding of an isolated nuchal fold greater than 5 mm is associated with an 11-fold increase in background risk for trisomy 21. Some centers now use second trimester nuchal fold as a continuous variable, with different likelihood ratios for each millimeter measurement.

Echogenic bowel

Sonographic visualization of bright bowel in the fetal abdomen is considered abnormal if the echogenicity is similar to that of fetal bone. A common pitfall with this minor marker is to over-diagnose the finding because of inappropriately high sonographic gain settings. When present, it is associated with a 6.7-fold increase in background risk for trisomy 21.

Humerus and femur length

The expected humerus and femur lengths can be estimated after a measurement of the fetal biparietal diameter (BPD) is obtained, and can be calculated using the formula $- 7.9404 + 0.8492 \times BPD$ for the humerus, or $- 9.645 + 0.9338 \times BPD$ for the femur. A ratio of observed to expected humerus or femur lengths less than 0.90 is considered abnormal. It is likely that separate norms will be needed to interpret long bone length in certain populations, as such biometry tends to be shorter amongst Asian fetuses. The isolated finding of a short humerus or a short femur is associated with a 5-fold and a 1.5-fold increase in background risk for trisomy 21, respectively.

Echogenic intracardiac focus

Calcification of the papillary muscle in the intracardiac ventricles can be demonstrated by sonography as a discrete echogenic dot within the left or right ventricle. The majority of cases are present in the left ventricle, and care should be exercised in imaging the fetal heart from multiple angles to avoid over-diagnosis due to specular reflection. Additionally, echogenic intracardiac focus may be considered a normal variant in certain populations, being present in up to 30% of normal Asian fetuses. When an echogenic intracardiac focus is detected, the background risk for trisomy 21 can be increased by a factor of 1.8.

Pyelectasis

Sonographic measurement of the anteroposterior diameter of the renal pelves from 15 to 20 weeks' gestation should normally reveal a diameter of 3 mm or less. Bilateral pyelectasis, in which both renal pelves measure 4 mm or greater, is associated with a 1.5-fold increase in background risk for trisomy 21.

Nasal bones

Failure to visualize the nasal bone, on a perfect sagittal fetal profile during the second trimester, or visualization of hypoplastic nasal bones, may also be a useful minor marker for trisomy 21. It is likely that this second trimester approach may not be as subjective as first trimester nasal bone evaluation. It has been suggested that the absence or hypoplasia of nasal bones may increase the background risk for trisomy 21 by up to a factor of 8.

Choroid plexus cyst

Sonographic evaluation of the choroid plexus, using an axial view through the upper portion of the fetal head, can frequently reveal the presence of one or more discrete cysts. While debated extensively in the past, it does not appear that isolated choroid plexus cysts represent markers for trisomy 21, although they have been described as being associated with trisomy 18. It is possible that the detection of an isolated choroid plexus cyst might increase the background risk for trisomy 18 by a factor of 7. However, since the background risk for trisomy 18 is generally very low, it is unlikely that the finding of an isolated cyst in a low-risk patient is of any clinical significance. Additionally, it does not appear that the number, size or evolution of choroid plexus cysts has any impact on trisomy 18 risk assessment.

AFP, hCG, uE3 and inhibin-A

Maternal serum levels of AFP and uE3 are both approximately 25% lower in pregnancies complicated by trisomy 21, compared with euploid pregnancies. By contrast, levels of hCG and inhibin-A are approximately twice as high in pregnancies complicated by trisomy 21. Maternal serum levels of AFP, uE3 and hCG all tend to be decreased in pregnancies complicated by trisomy 18. The combination of AFP, uE3 and hCG, commonly known as the triple screen, can detect 70% of cases of trisomy 21, for a 5% false-positive rate. When inhibin-A is added to this test, commonly known as the quad screen, the trisomy 21 detection rate increases to 81%, for a 5% false-positive rate. Performance of serum screening tests can be maximized by accurate ascertainment of gestational age, and, wherever possible, sonographic dating should be used instead of menstrual dating. It is optimal to provide serum screening between 15 and 16 weeks' gestation, thereby allowing the results to be available at the time of second trimester sonographic evaluation.

Combined first and second trimester screening

First trimester combination screening for trisomy 21, using NT, PAPP-A and fßhCG, has very similar performance characteristics to second trimester serum screening using AFP, hCG, uE3 and inhibin-A. In an effort to maximize the performance of both of these forms of risk assessment, it is possible to combine first and second trimester serum and sonographic screening techniques. There are three approaches to combining different screening modalities across different gestational ages, namely: integrated screening, step-wise screening and contingent screening.

Integrated screening

This form of risk assessment refers to a two-step screening protocol, with results not being released until all screening steps are completed. Sonographic measurement of NT, together with serum assay for PAPP-A, are obtained between 10 and 13 weeks' gestation, followed by a second serum assay for AFP, hCG, uE3 and inhibin-A obtained between 15 and 16 weeks' gestation. A single risk assessment is then calculated at 16 weeks' gestation. This 'fully integrated' test has a trisomy 21 detection rate of 95%, for a 5% false-positive rate. A variant of this approach, referred to as the 'serum integrated' test, involves blood tests only, including PAPP-A in the first trimester, followed by AFP, hCG, uE3 and inhibin-A in the second trimester. This latter test, which does not require an NT ultrasound assessment, has a trisomy 21 detection rate of 86%, for a 5% false-positive rate.

For some patients who are anxious to receive rapid screening results, or for those who might wish to avail of a first trimester CVS, it is possible that such integrated screening tests might not be acceptable, as a delay inevitably exists between the time of first trimester screening measurements and release of results in the second trimester. However, for patients who may not be interested in, or have access to, first trimester CVS, the efficiency of being provided with a single trisomy 21 risk assessment result, which maximizes detection and minimizes false positives, may make such integrated screening tests appear attractive.

Step-wise screening

In contrast to integrated screening, step-wise screening refers to multiple different trisomy 21 screening tests being performed, with risk estimates being provided to patients upon completion of each step. A key concept in performing step-wise screening is to ensure that each subsequent screening test that is performed should use the trisomy 21 risk from the preceding test as the new *a priori* risk for later screening. For example, if a patient with an age-related risk for trisomy 21 of 1 in 300 has a first tri-mester screening test resulting in a new trisomy 21 risk of 1 in 1000, it is essential that any subsequent second trimester screening test uses the 1 in 1000 risk in its *a priori* risk calculation, rather than the original age-related risk of 1 in 300. If sequential screening tests are performed independently for trisomy 21, without any modification being made for earlier screening results, the positive predictive value of the later tests will inevitably dete-riorate, and it is likely that the overall false-positive rate will increase.

A potential advantage of step-wise screening over integrated screening is that it allows patients in the first trimester to avail of an immediate CVS, should their risk estimate justify this test, without having to wait until 16 weeks when the integrated screening results are provided. Patients could possibly get the benefit of early diagnosis associated with first tri-mester screening, as well as the higher detection rate for trisomy 21 asso-ciated with integration of both first and second trimester screening tests.

Contingent screening

Contingent screening is a modification of step-wise screening in which patients are counseled in different clinical directions depending on first trimester screening results. With this form of screening, patients have a standard combined first trimester screening test using NT, PAPP-A and fßhCG. Those with high-risk screening results of 1 in 30 or higher have immediate invasive diagnostic testing with CVS, while those with very low-risk results of 1 in 1500 or lower are reassured and have no further screening or diagnostic testing. The remaining patients who have interme-diate first trimester screening results (between 1 in 30 and 1 in 1500 risk) return at 15–16 weeks for quad serum markers. These markers are then combined with the first trimester markers in an integrated test, with those having a final risk of 1 in 270 or higher then undergoing amniocentesis.

The advantage of such contingent screening is that 75% of patients complete aneuploidy screening in the first trimester, with either a diag-nostic test or such low-risk results that there is little value in further screening. Only 25% of patients need to return in the second trimester for further evaluation. Detection rates of at least 90% for a 5% false-positive rate should be achievable with this form of screening.

Conclusion

A wide range of screening tests for fetal aneuploidy, in particular trisomy 21, is now available in both the first and second trimesters. The increasing integration of serum and sonographic screening tests across gestational ages will allow patients and providers access to a panel of risk assessment tools that can be tailored to suit individual patients' needs. Because of the huge array of available tests, and because of the potential for inefficient combinations of screening approaches, it would be ideal if all pregnant patients could be provided with formal pre-test counseling to select the most appropriate risk assessment algorithm for their particular circumstances.

Suggested reading

Bianchi DW, Crombleholme TM, D'Alton ME, Malone FD. *Fetology: Diagnosis and Management of the Fetal Patient*. New York, London: McGraw Hill, 2nd edn. 2010.

Breathnach FM, Malone FD, Lambert-Messerlian G, *et al*. First and second trimester screening: detection of aneuploidies other than Down syndrome. *Obstet Gynecol* 2007:110:651–7.

Bromley B, Lieberman E, Shipp TD, Benacerraf BR. The genetic sonogram: a method of risk assessment for Down syndrome in the midtrimester. *J Ultrasound Med* 2002;21:1087–96.

Cuckle HS, Malone FD, Wright D, *et al*. Contingent screening for Down syndrome. *Prenatal Diag* 2008;28:89–94.

Malone FD, Canick JA, Ball RH, *et al*. A comparison of first trimester screening, second trimester screening, and the combination of both for evaluation of risk for Down syndrome. *N Engl J Med* 2005;353:2001–11.

Malone FD, Ball RH, Nyberg DA, *et al*. First trimester septated cystic hygroma: prevalence, natural history, and pediatric outcome. *Obstet Gynecol* 2005;106;288–94.

Nyberg DA, Souter VL, El-Bastawissi A, Young S, Luthhardt F, Luthy D. Isolated sonographic markers for detection of fetal Down syndrome in the second trimester of pregnancy. *J Ultrasound Med* 2001;20:1053–63.

Nyberg DA, Souter VL. Chromosomal abnormalities. In: Nyberg DA, McGahan JP, Pretorius DH, Pilu G (eds) *Diagnostic Imaging of Fetal Anomalies*. Philadelphia; London: Lippincott Williams & Wilkins, 2003; pp. 861–906.

Smith-Bindman R, Howmer W, Feldstein VA, Deeks J, Goldberg J. Second trimester ultrasound to detect fetuses with Down syndrome: a meta-analysis. *JAMA* 2001;285:1044–55.

Snijders RJ, Noble P, Sebire N, Souka A, Nicolaides KH. UK multicenter project on assessment of risk of trisomy 21 by maternal age and fetal nuchal-translucency thickness at 10–14 weeks of gestation. *Lancet* 1998;351:343–6.

Wald NJ, Watt HC, Hackshaw AK. Integrated screening for Down's syndrome based on tests performed during the first and second trimesters. *N Engl J Med* 1999;341:461–7.

Wald NJ, Rodeck C, Hackshaw AK, Walters J, Chitty L, Mackinson AM. First and second trimester antenatal screening for Down's syndrome: the results of the serum, urine and ultrasound screening study (SURUSS). *J Med Screening* 2003;10:56–104.

Fetal Echocardiography

Joshua A. Copel[1] and Charles S. Kleinman[2]

[1] Department of Obstetrics, Gynecology and Reproductive Sciences, and Pediatrics, Yale University School of Medicine, New Haven, CT, USA

[2] Department of Pediatrics, Columbia University College of Physicians and Surgeons, New York, NY, USA

Overview

Congenital heart disease occurs in approximately 8 of 1000 live births. Of these, approximately half are relatively minor ventricular septal defects or valve stenoses that are of little hemodynamic significance. Some of these can be identified prenatally with sensitive color Doppler flow mapping with little clinical impact,[1] while many others are undetectable prenatally. The remainder are significant lesions that may benefit from prenatal detection, parental counseling and obstetric-pediatric planning for delivery and neonatal care.

Pathophysiology

Most types of congenital heart disease are thought to be inherited in multifactorial fashion, with both genetic and environmental contributions. The indications used for fetal echocardiography, a prenatal ultrasound technique that can detect most significant congenital heart disease, reflect that. Most patients referred for fetal echocardiography have had prior affected children, and the recurrence risk for these families is about 2 to 3%.

The pathophysiology of congenital cardiac anomalies varies with the type of anatomic abnormality that is present. The underlying mechanisms include failures of cell migration, leading to failure of a structure to form, or diminished flow, inhibiting the normal growth of a downstream structure (e.g., poor flow across the foramen ovale and mitral valve predisposing to a coarctation of the aorta).

Protocols for High-Risk Pregnancies, 5th edition. Edited by J.T. Queenan, J.C. Hobbins and C.Y. Spong. © 2010 Blackwell Publishing Ltd.

Structural heart disease

Diagnosis and workup
In patients without risk factors for congenital heart disease, full fetal echocardiography, which is generally more time-consuming and expensive than general obstetric sonography, is not indicated unless cardiac anomalies are suspected. Many risk factors for congenital heart disease have been described (Table 8.1).

The four-chamber view of the heart has been suggested as an easy way of screening for congenital heart disease, although its sensitivity to significant cardiac anomalies has varied in the literature. Approximately one-third

Table 8.1 Indications for fetal echocardiography

Familial risk factors
    History of congenital heart disease
        Previous sibling
        Paternal
    Mendelian syndromes that include congenital heart disease
        Noonan
    Tuberous sclerosis

Maternal risk factors
    Congenital heart disease
    Cardiac teratogen exposure
        Lithium carbonate
        Alcohol
        Phenytoin
        Valproic acid
        Trimethadione
        Carbamazepine
        Isotretinoin
        Paroxetine
    Maternal metabolic disorders
        Diabetes mellitus
        Phenylketonuria
    In vitro fertilization (controversial)

Fetal risk factors
    Extracardiac anomalies
        Chromosomal
        Anatomic
    Fetal cardiac arrhythmia
        Irregular rhythm
        Tachycardia (>200 bpm) in absence of chorioamnionitis
        Fixed bradycardia
    Nonimmune hydrops fetalis
    Lack of reassuring four-chamber view during basic obstetric scan
    Monochorionic twins

Table 8.2 Standard fetal echocardiographic views and what to see

---

Four chamber
   Situs: check fetal position and stomach
   Axis of heart to the left
   Intact interventricular septum
   Atria approximately equal sizes
   Ventricles approximately equal sizes
   Free movement of mitral and tricuspid valves
   Foramen ovale flap (atrial septum primum) visible in left atrium

Long-axis left ventricle
   Intact interventricular septum
     Continuity of the ascending aorta with mitral valve posteriorly
     Interventricular septum anteriorly

Short axis of great vessels
   Vessel exiting the anterior (right) ventricle bifurcates, confirming it is the pulmonary artery

Aortic arch
   Vessel exiting the posterior (left) ventricle arches and has 3 head vessels, confirming it is
   the aorta

Pulmonary artery-ductus arteriosus
   Continuity of the ductus arteriosus with the descending aorta

---

of cases of major heart disease are detected according to a review of the world's literature on screening prenatal ultrasound.[2] Our own experience suggests that it has a very high positive predictive value, with at least half of patients referred for abnormal four-chamber views actually having cardiac anomalies.

Full fetal echocardiography includes obtaining all of the views in the fetus routinely obtained in postnatal echocardiography (Table 8.2) using both real-time grayscale and color Doppler imaging. Additionally, spectral Doppler, cardiac biometry and M-mode data can be obtained as indicated. Fetal echocardiographers use these latter techniques variably. The two-dimensional examination should be sufficient to exclude significant heart disease in the vast majority of affected individuals. The more sophisticated studies are especially useful in cases of suspected structural or functional abnormalities.

Management

When a cardiac anomaly is found, a full detailed fetal scan to detect any other anomalies is mandatory. Many fetal syndromes include cardiac anomalies, and accurate counseling requires complete enumeration of associated anomalies. Fetal karyotype testing should be offered to the parents, as chromosome anomalies are seen in a large segment of fetuses with congenital heart disease. In our experience at Yale, 28% of fetuses with congenital heart disease and an extracardiac anomaly were aneuploid, and 15% of those with congenital heart disease and no identifiable extracardiac anomaly were also chromosomally abnormal. Additional testing for a microdeletion of chromosome 22q11 by FISH can be helpful in fetuses with conotruncal malformations (e.g., tetralogy of Fallot, truncus arteriosus).

Overall survival once a cardiac lesion is found depends on the nature of the cardiac problem, the presence of extracardiac anomalies, the karyotype and the presence of fetal hydrops. Fetal hydrops in association with structural heart disease is virtually universally fatal. Aneuploid fetuses may have dismal prognoses even in the absence of heart disease, and a finding such as trisomy 18 may make repairing even a straightforward ventricular septal defect inadvisable.

Lesions that can be repaired into a biventricular heart carry a better long-term prognosis than those that result in a univentricular heart. Several groups have now reported that infants who are known to have congenital heart disease prenatally do better than those whose cardiac defects are only found after birth.[3–5]

Fetal arrhythmias

Diagnosis and management

The largest group of fetal arrhythmias are intermittent and due to atrial, junctional or ventricular extrasystoles. They carry a small risk of coexistent structural abnormality. A greater risk exists of an unrecognized tachyarrhythmia, or the development of a tachyarrhythmia later in gestation. Atrial extrasystoles predispose the fetus to development of re-entrant atrial tachycardia, which can lead to fetal hydrops. Weekly auscultation of the fetal heart along with avoidance of caffeine or other sympathomimetics is suggested until resolution of the arrhythmia.

Fetal tachycardias represent a management challenge, because determination of the precise electrophysiological cause of the arrhythmia is essential to any rational management strategy, but fetal electrocardiography is not yet clinically practical in the presence of intact membranes. The differential diagnoses of fetal tachycardias include re-entrant atrial tachycardia, atrial flutter and ventricular tachycardia. The treatment of these disorders differs significantly, and appropriate medications for one may be contraindicated for another. The correct diagnosis, which should be based on combinations of M-mode, Doppler and color Doppler–M-mode imaging, is essential to appropriate therapy.

If there is a fetal bradycardia the first step is to determine if there is a regular or an irregular atrial rate. If the atrial rate is regular and slow, that is below 100 beats per minute, there may be sinus bradycardia, which should prompt a complete evaluation of fetal well-being. The most common clinically important fetal bradycardia results from complete heart block, which will demonstrate a normal atrial rate with a slower ventricular rate whose beats do not occur in conjunction with atrial beats. This is usually caused by maternal antibodies associated with lupus erythematosus and Sjogren syndrome, termed SSA/Ro and SSB/La. A smaller group of patients, without maternal antibodies, may present with congenital complete heart block in a setting of complex congenital heart disease involving the central fibrous body of the heart (e.g., left atrial isomerism, corrected transposition of the great arteries). In these patients the prognosis is directly related to the complexity of the heart disease and the association with congestive heart failure. A more benign cause of fetal bradycardia, which may be mistaken for 2:1 heart block, is blocked atrial bigeminy. In such cases the atrial rate is not regular, but rather demonstrates paired beating in which a premature atrial beat follows closely after a normal atrial beat with no ventricular response to the premature beat. This arrhythmia has no significance beyond that of isolated atrial extrasystoles.

Follow-up

The fetus with congenital heart disease should be carefully followed by ultrasound up to delivery. Structural lesions may evolve prenatally even as they do postnatally.[6] It is particularly important to evaluate areas of potential obstruction, and the relationships of the great arteries to the ventricles. Fetuses with significant arrhythmias (including re-entrant tachycardias, atrial flutter and complete heart block) should also be followed at a center with experience in the prenatal medical management of fetal arrhythmias, by a team that includes perinatologists, pediatric cardiologists and adult electrophysiologists. Delivery need not be by cesarean section except in the presence of selected fetal arrhythmias that do not permit adequate fetal heart rate monitoring. For fetuses with lesions that are expected to render the neonate dependent on ductus arteriosus patency for systemic or pulmonary perfusion, prostaglandin E_1 should be available in the nursery at the time of delivery to keep the ductus open.

References

1 Bahtiyar MO, Dulay AT, Weeks BP, Friedman AH, Copel JA. Prenatal course of isolated muscular ventricular septal defects diagnosed only by color Doppler sonography: single-institution experience. *J Ultrasound Med* 2008;27:715–20.

2 Todros T, Faggiano F, Chiappa E, Gaglioti P, Mitola B, Sciarrone A. Accuracy of routine ultrasonography in screening heart disease prenatally. Gruppo Piemontese for Prenatal Screening of Congenital Heart Disease. [Journal Article. Multicenter Study] *Prenatal Diag* 1997;17(10):901–6.

3 Copel JA, Tan AS, Kleinman CS. Does a prenatal diagnosis of congenital heart disease alter short-term outcome? *Ultrasound Obstet Gynecol* 1997;10:237–41.

4 Bonnet D, Coltri A, Butera G, Fermont L, Le Bidois J, Kachaner J, Sidi D. Detection of transposition of the great arteries in fetuses reduces neonatal morbidity and mortality. *Circulation* 1999;99:916–18.

5 Tworetzky W, McElhinney DB, Reddy VM, Brook MM, Hanley FL, Silverman NH. Improved surgical outcome after fetal diagnosis of hypoplastic left heart syndrome. *Circulation* 2001;103:1269–73.

6 Rice MJ, McDonald RW, Sahn DJ. The evolution of congenital heart disease. In: Copel JA, Reed KR (eds) *Doppler Ultrasound in Obstetrics and Gynecology*. New York: Raven, 1995; pp. 219–30.

Suggested readings

Copel JA, Liang RI, Demasio K, Ozeren S, Kleinman CS. The clinical significance of the irregular fetal heart rhythm. *Am J Obstet Gynecol* 2000;182:813–17.

Copel JA, Cullen M, Green J, *et al*. The frequency of aneuploidy with prenatally diagnosed congenital heart disease: an indication for fetal karyotyping. *Am J Obstet Gynecol* 1988;158:409–13.

Copel JA, Pilu G, Green J, *et al*. Fetal echocardiographic screening for congenital heart disease: the importance of the four chamber view. *Am J Obstet Gynecol* 1987;157:648–55.

Copel JA, Pilu G, Kleinman CS. Congenital heart disease and extracardiac anomalies: associations and indications for fetal echocardiography. *Am J Obstet Gynecol* 1985;154:1121–32.

Kleinman CS, Copel JA. Electrophysiological principles and fetal antiarrhythmic therapy. *Ultrasound Obstet Gynecol* 1991;4:286–97.

Kleinman CS, Donnerstein RL, DeVore GR, *et al*. Fetal echocardiography for evaluation of in utero congestive heart failure: a technique for the study of non-immune hydrops fetalis. *N Engl J Med* 1982;306:568–75.

Nora JJ, Nora AH. The genetic contribution to congenital heart diseases. In: Nora JJ, Takao A (eds) *Congenital Heart Diseases: Causes and Processes*. Mount Kisco, NY: Futura, 1984; pp. 3–14.

Silverman NH, Kleinman CS, Rudolph AM, *et al*. Fetal atrioventricular valve insufficiency associated with nonimmune hydrops: a two-dimensional echocardiographic and pulsed Doppler study. *Circulation* 1985;72:825–32.

Smythe J, Copel JA, Kleinman CS. Outcome of prenatally detected cardiac malformations. *Am J Cardiol* 1992;69:1471–4.

Zierler S. Maternal drugs and congenital heart disease. *Obstet Gynecol* 1985;65:155–65.

Clinical Use of Doppler

Henry L. Galan

Department of Obstetrics and Gynecology, University of Colorado at Denver Health
Sciences Center, Aurora CO, USA

Overview

Doppler depends upon the ability of an ultrasound beam to be changed
in frequency when encountering a moving object such as red blood
cells (RBC). The change in frequency (Doppler shift) between the emit-
ted beam and the reflected beam is proportional to the velocity of the
RBC and dependent on the angle between the ultrasound beam and the
vessel. Pulsed-wave Doppler velocimetry provides a flow velocity waveform from which information can be obtained to determine three basic
characteristics of blood flow that are useful in obstetrics: velocity, resistance indices and volume blood flow. Doppler velocimetry is primarily
useful for diagnostic fetal echocardiography and antenatal surveillance of
three high-risk obstetrical conditions: (1) intrauterine growth restriction
(IUGR); (2) rhesus alloimmunization (isoimmunization); and (3) preterm
labor (tocolysis with indomethacin). A more recent application of pulsed-
wave Doppler is its use in evaluation of the ductus venosus flow velocity
waveform (FVW) in first trimester risk assessment for Down's Syndrome,
but is not discussed in this protocol.

Pathophysiology

Normal fetal circulation

The umbilical vein brings oxygen and nutrient-rich blood to the fetus.
The umbilical vein enters the umbilicus and travels anteriorly along the
abdominal wall, diving into the liver and becoming the hepatic portion
of the umbilical vein. The umbilical vein eventually becomes the portal
vein, but first gives off the left inferior and superior portal vein, the ductus venosus (DV), and finally the right portal vein. Approximately 50%
of umbilical vein blood is directed towards the DV and then to an area

Protocols for High-Risk Pregnancies, 5th edition. Edited by J.T. Queenan, J.C. Hobbins and
C.Y. Spong. © 2010 Blackwell Publishing Ltd.

under the diaphragm that is referred to as the subdiaphragmatic vestibulum. The subdiaphragmatic vestibulum also receives blood from the
inferior vena cava and blood exiting the liver via the right, middle and
left hepatic veins. The process of preferential streaming begins in the subdiaphragmatic vestibulum with blood from the ductus venosus and the
left and middle hepatic veins preferentially shunted across the foramen
ovale into the left atrium and left ventricle so that the heart and the head
receive the most oxygenated and nutrient-rich blood. In contrast, blood
coming from the inferior vena cava and the right hepatic vein are preferentially streamed into the right atrium and right ventricle and then
out the pulmonary artery and then shunted across the ductus arteriosus
which then delivers this blood to the descending aorta. Blood leaving the
fetus does so via two umbilical arteries arising from the hypogastric arteries which course around the lateral aspects of the bladder anteriorly and
cephalad, exiting the umbilicus, returning back to the placenta.

There are three primary shunts in the fetus that require closure after
delivery in order for normal postnatal circulation and subsequent adult
circulation to take place. As mentioned above, the ductus venosus
shunts from the umbilical vein towards the heart. The ductus arteriosus
shunts approximately 90% of the blood in main pulmonary artery to the
descending aorta leaving only 10% of pulmonary artery blood to reach
the fetal lungs. The third shunt is the foramen ovale which is maintained
in a patent state in utero to allow the process of preferential streaming to
occur from the right atrium to the left atrium. Failure of any one of these
shunts to close properly may result in adverse cardiopulmonary transition
in the newborn.

Intrauterine growth restriction

Fetuses that fail to reach genetically determined growth potential due to
uteroplacental dysfunction may develop abnormal resistance to blood
flow in the placenta. This abnormal resistance is due to numerous placental vascular abnormalities (poor villous capillarization, reduced number
and branching of stem arteries, luminal reduction and wall hypertrophy),
which can be detected with Doppler velocimetry in the umbilical artery
located upstream from the placenta. Progression of placental disease with
concomitant worsening of blood flow resistance may lead to additional
Doppler velocimetry changes in the precordial venous system or in the
heart. Once the fetus decompensates to that level, acidemia is nearly
always present.

Rh alloimmunization

In Rh disease, a fetal RBC antigen enters the maternal bloodstream and
stimulates antibody production against that RBC antigen. An amnestic

response may occur in a subsequent pregnancy if the same RBC antigen is presented to the mother's immune system and this may lead to a series of events that include fetal anemia, extramedullary hematopoiesis, hydrops fetalis and fetal death. Historically, the degree of fetal anemia and need for fetal RBC transfusion involved an amniocentesis to determine the amniotic fluid ΔOD450 to assess the degree of RBC-derived hemoglobin breakdown products and to estimate of anemia. If moderate to severe anemia is suspected, the fetus should undergo a fetal blood sampling and transfusion.

Preterm labor

Although the pathophysiology of preterm labor is still largely unknown, tocolytic use is widespread. Use of agents that inhibit prostaglandin synthesis can result in premature closure of the ductus arteriosus and oligohydramnios. Doppler velocimetry is useful in assessment of ductus arteriosus closure.

Cardiac abnormalities

Fetuses with known cardiac abnormalities including congenital or structural heart disease, arrhythmias and congestive failure may have intracardiac and outflow tract flow velocity abnormalities that can be detected with Doppler velocimetry. Depending on the nature of the abnormality, this can affect other flow velocity waveforms including the ductus venosus, hepatic veins, inferior vena cava and the umbilical vein.

Diagnosis

Doppler techniques and measurements

As mentioned in the overview, pulse-wave Doppler velocimetry can be used to obtain the following information from a flow velocity waveform:

1 Velocity of the blood – requires an angle of insonation of zero degrees between the transducer and the vessel of interest (Fig. 9.1).
2 Resistance indices (S/D ratio, resistance index, pulsatility index) – these are angle independent measurement such that the value obtained for any one of these indices is not dependent upon the angle between the transducer and the vessel being interrogated (Fig. 9.2).
3 Volume blood flow (milliliters per minute) – this is determined by obtaining the velocity of the blood and multiplying it by the cross-sectional area of the vessel (obtained by two-dimensional ultrasound) times 60 seconds:

$$\textit{Volume flow (mL/min)} = \textit{velocity (cm/sec)} \times \textit{cross-sectional area (cm}^2)$$
$$\times \textit{60 seconds}$$

Velocity

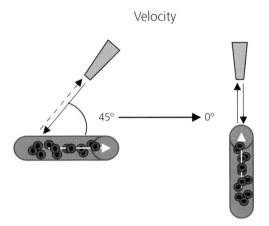

45° ⟶ 0°

Figure 9.1 Schematic representing zero angle of insonation between the Doppler transducer and the vessel of interest.

Doppler indices of resistance

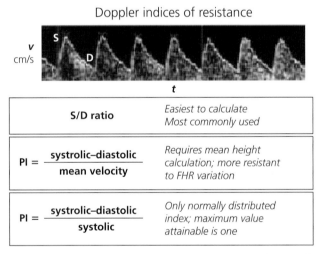

S/D ratio	Easiest to calculate Most commonly used
$PI = \dfrac{\text{systrolic–diastolic}}{\text{mean velocity}}$	Requires mean height calculation; more resistant to FHR variation
$PI = \dfrac{\text{systrolic–diastolic}}{\text{systolic}}$	Only normally distributed index; maximum value attainable is one

Figure 9.2 Flow velocity waveform of the umbilical artery and definitions for the different Doppler indices of resistance.

Cardiac flow velocities

Normal values and blood flow velocity patterns have been previously reported for cardiac Doppler velocities. More specifically, blood flow velocity values and patterns have been described for the pulmonary and aortic outflow tracts, ductus arteriosus, ductus venosus, tricuspid and mitral valve, and the inferior vena cava. Any fetal structural cardiac abnormality or precordial or postcordial vascular abnormality can affect the blood flow velocity and waveform of the aforementioned vessels and valves. Further discussion of detailed fetal echocardiography is beyond the scope of this protocol.

Prediction of adverse pregnancy events

There has been a great deal of excitement during the last decade with the application of maternal Doppler studies of the uterine arteries in the prediction of pre-eclampsia, intrauterine growth restriction, fetal demise and preterm birth. The most distal branches of the uterine artery (spiral arteries) undergo a remarkable transition during the first half of pregnancy from highly muscularized vessels with high resistance to remodeled vessels with low resistance. This is in response to differentiation of cytotrophoblast to non-invasive and invasive cytotrophoblast with the latter literally invading and altering spiral artery muscular architecture. It is this change that leads to the enormous blood flow eventually seen in pregnancy (600–800 mL/min). There are many publications on the use of uterine artery Doppler for predicting adverse pregnancy outcomes in both low- and high-risk populations. In the low-risk population, there does not seem to be a benefit of wide application of this Doppler test as a screening tool for adverse pregnancy events. There may be a role in uterine artery Doppler testing in high-risk pregnancy as it may pick out a subgroup of patients at a particular higher risk for adverse events which may lead to useful additional monitoring during pregnancy or preventative strategies. In addition, the high negative predictive value for adverse pregnancy events can provide reassurance. However, until further studies elucidate not just a clear predictive capability, but also a prevention therapy or strategy, uterine artery Doppler screening will not likely be applied to the general obstetrical population.

Intrauterine growth restriction

The blood flow velocity waveform obtained by pulsed Doppler velocimetry changes in any given vessel throughout gestation. There is a progressive increase in diastolic flow velocity across gestation in the umbilical artery which reflects a decrease in the resistance within the placenta. Depending on the definition, intrauterine growth restriction of placental etiology can affect up to 10% of all pregnancies. A characteristic of intrauterine growth restriction is an increase in blood flow resistance within the placenta. This increase in blood flow resistance can be detected upstream in the umbilical arteries. If the placental disease progresses, the increase within the placenta can be sensed across the cardiac structures and into the "prechordial" venous circulation such that the flow velocity waveform within the inferior vena cava, the ductus venosus and the hepatic veins become abnormal.

Umbilical artery Doppler velocimetry was first introduced into clinical use in the late 1980s and subsequently approved by the American College of Obstetricians and Gynecologists as an adjunct to antenatal testing for the management of intrauterine growth restriction. The use of umbilical artery Doppler velocimetry reduces mortality by approximately one-third

Normal

Abnormal
high resistance

Abnormal
Absent EDF

Abnormal
Reverse EDF

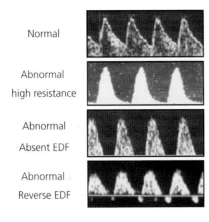

Figure 9.3 Normal and abnormal flow velocity waveforms in the umbilical artery.

when used in surveillance of the growth-restricted fetus. Figure 9.3 shows a normal flow velocity waveform in the umbilical artery and then several abnormal flow velocity waveforms. Reverse end-diastolic flow in the umbilical artery is associated with obliteration of greater than 70% of the placental arteries. Absent or reverse end-diastolic flow is also associated with a high rate (>60–70%) of fetal acidemia. As mentioned before, if the disease process worsens in intrauterine growth restriction, flow velocity waveform in the precordial aspects of the fetus can become abnormal. More specifically, the flow velocity waveform in the inferior vena cava, ductus venosus and hepatic veins can become abnormal. Again, if the disease process worsens further, abnormalities can be detected in the umbilical vein flow velocity waveform. Studies published in 2001 and 2002 showed that the decompensating fetus will proceed to have flow velocity waveform abnormalities in a sequential fashion across different fetal vessels in approximately 50–70% of cases. When flow velocity waveforms are assessed in the decompensating fetus, the first vessels to show abnormalities are the umbilical artery and the middle cerebral artery. The umbilical artery abnormality first noted is an increase in resistance such as an increase in the S/D ratio. Abnormalities in the middle cerebral artery show a decrease in resistance which represents an effort on the part of the fetus to spare its brain by increasing the delivery of blood. Abnormalities then typically proceed in the following sequence: absent end-diastolic in the umbilical vein, an increase in resistance in the ductus venosus, reverse flow in the umbilical artery and abnormalities in the outflow tracts of the heart. Figure 9.4 shows normal and abnormal flow velocity waveforms in the ductus venosus.

Rh sensitization

As previously mentioned, fetal anemia resulting from Rh sensitization was historically detected by amniocentesis and assessment of the ΔOD450 and then confirmed by fetal blood sampling. Assessment of the middle

Ductus venosus flow velocity waveform

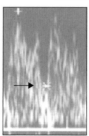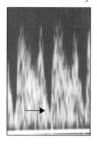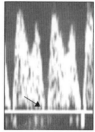

Figure 9.4 Ductus venosus flow velocity waveform deterioration from normal to abnormal as indicated by a decrease in flow at the atrial kick (arrow).

cerebral artery (MCA) peak systolic velocity (PSV) has essentially replaced the ΔOD450 as the gold standard test for fetal anemia. The MCA PSV has greater sensitivity for moderate to severe anemia than does the ΔOD450. Moreover, the ΔOD450 is not useful in Kell sensitization because fetal anemia in this condition is caused by bone marrow suppression rather than hemolysis and thus does not lead to RBC breakdown products in the amniotic fluid normally detected by the ΔOD450.

One of the resultant pathophysiological features present in Rh disease is a reduction in the viscosity of the fetal blood which is secondary to a lower hematocrit. This results in an increase in the velocity of blood flow which can be detected by pulse-wave Doppler velocimetry. One of the vessels branching off the circle of Willis is the middle cerebral artery (MCA). The middle cerebral artery is first identified with the use of color flow Doppler. With an angle of insonation of 0°, pulse-wave Doppler velocimetry is used to obtain the flow velocity waveform. From the flow velocity waveform, one can determine the PSV across serial peaks of the systolic component of the flow velocity waveform profile and obtain a mean systolic peak velocity of the middle cerebral artery flow waveform. Nomograms are available for peak systolic velocity in the middle cerebral artery across gestation. Web-based MCA PSV multiples of the median (MoM) calculators for a given gestational age are also available at Perinatology.com. When the MCA peak systolic velocity surpasses the threshold of 1.55 MoM, there is a high risk of moderate-to-severe anemia in the fetus. The cut-off 1.55 MoM has a sensitivity of 100% and a negative predictive value of 100% for moderate to severe anemia. Once this value is surpassed, the fetus can undergo a blood sampling to determine the actual fetal hematocrit and, from that, one can determine if a transfusion is necessary. Using Doppler to assess peak systolic velocity of the MCA and identifying anemia in the fetus in this fashion avoids the standard invasive procedural risks of amniocentesis (needed for the ΔOD450) including exacerbation of the Rh sensitization.

Table 9.1 Indications for fetal echocardiography

Family history of congenital heart disease
Maternal diabetes
Drug exposure
Teratogenic exposure
Other fetal abnormalities
Chromosomal abnormalities
Rhythm abnormalities
Non-immune hydrops
Maternal phenylketonuria

Management

Congenital heart disease and arrhythmia

A number of clinical scenarios may warrant fetal echocardiography. Please refer to Table 9.1 for a list of indications for fetal echocardiography.

The ideal time to obtain a fetal echocardiogram is between 18 and 22 weeks of gestation; however, there are several specialized perinatal centers performing this in the first trimester. Counseling and management of the patient with a congenital heart defect involves a variety of steps including a karyotypic analysis of the fetus, defining the type and severity of cardiac legion, consideration of the patient's moral and religious disposition, and the presence of extracardiac abnormalities. Management of a patient with congenital heart disease should be a collaborative effort with a team consisting of a perinatologist, genetic counselor, pediatric cardiologist, neonatologist, pediatric cardiothoracic surgeon and the primary obstetrical provider.

Fetal arrhythmias are typically first detected by routine Doppler auscultation during a prenatal clinic visit or by external electronic fetal monitoring. Further identification of the specific type of arrhythmia requires the use of M-mode cardiography and full assessment of the cardiac structure and flow velocities.

Intrauterine growth restriction

Once the fetus has been diagnosed by ultrasound to be growth restricted, a full assessment of the fetus should be performed to exclude fetal anomalies, possible karyotypic abnormalities and congenital infection. Particular attention should be paid to the symmetrically growth-restricted fetus to exclude karyotype abnormalities and congenital infection. Treatment options are limited in intrauterine growth restriction and include modified bed rest, increase fluid intake, and elimination of adverse social habits such as tobacco, alcohol or recreational drug use. In pregnant patients with a history of

- ≥ **36 weeks**
  - o   deliver
- **32-36 weeks**
  - o   **perform NST and Doppler studies**
  - o   **if both tests are reassuring:**
    - repeat in 1 week OR
    - test for fetal lung maturity
      - if immature, repeat in 1 week
      - if mature, deliver
  - o   if either test is non-reassuring
    - deliver*
- **26-32 weeks**
  - o   **perform NST and Doppler studies**
  - o   **efforts should be made to gain time as safely as possible in utero.**
  - o   **if NST is reactive:**
    - perform umbilical artery Doppler studies
    - if reassuring, repeat in 1 week
    - if non-reassuring, perform venous Doppler studies
      - if reassuring, repeat in 1 week
      - if non-reassuring, consider delivery*
  - o   **if NST is non-reactive:**
    - **perform biophysical profile**
      - if ≥ 8, perform umbilical artery Dopplers
      - if 6, repeat 6 – 24 hours and perform umbilical artery Dopplers
      - if ≤ 4, based on gestational age, consider delivery*
    - **perform umbilical artery Doppler studies**
      - if umbilical artery Doppler studies are non-reassuring:
        - o   perform venous Doppler studies
          - if reassuring, repeat in 1 week
          - if non-reassuring, deliver
      - if umbilical artery Doppler studies are reassuring:
        - o   repeat in 1 week

Figure 9.5 Algorithm for the management of intrauterine growth restriction.
*For deliveries less than 34 weeks, maternal steroid administration should be given for fetal benefit.

intrauterine growth restriction in a previous pregnancy, a baby aspirin has been shown to have some benefit in reducing the risk of recurrence.

Surveillance of the growth-restricted fetus includes the use of fetal activity count, serial assessment of fetal growth with ultrasound (every 2 to 3 weeks), non-stress test and/or biophysical profile and Doppler velocimetry. Figure 9.5 demonstrates an algorithm or guideline for the management of the IUGR fetus based on the gestational age. The presence of oligohydramnios warrants additional workup, particularly since this may be a potential sign of significant compromise. Oligohydramnios may represent underperfusion of the kidneys with subsequent decrease in urine output and thus cardiovascular compromise of the fetus. Management of oligohydramnios should include a brief hospitalization to rule out other etiologies for oligohydramnios such a preterm premature rupture of the membranes, maternal dehydration, and pre-eclampsia. The patient with oligohydramnios should be hydrated and undergo fetal surveillance in the hospital. In the case of IUGR with oligohydramnios, delivery should be considered if the fetus is beyond 32–34 weeks and after administration of corticosteroids for fetal benefit. Delivery should be performed in concert with the neonatal team. Recent data suggest that in severe and early intrauterine growth restriction, efforts should be made to gain time in utero as gestational age is the most significant determinant of overall survival and intact survival. Beyond 29 weeks and a birthweight of 600 grams, the ductus venosus Doppler and umbilical artery pH predict neonatal mortality. A growth-restricted fetus with normal Dopplers and amniotic fluid may be constitutionally (normal) small and delaying delivery may be appropriate.

Rh sensitization

The management of Rh sensitization begins with identification of an isoimmunised patient from routine blood type and Rh and antibody screening tests. When the antibody screen shows the presence of an antibody that places the fetus(es) at risk for fetal anemia, the patient needs to undergo serial screening with antibody titers. Once a critical threshold has been reached by a specific titer of that antibody, the patient must undergo evaluation for fetal anemia. Most hospital laboratories use either a 1:16 or 1:32 threshold cut-off and it is essential that each practitioner know the threshold for any given hospital or laboratory. Once the critical threshold has been reached, the patient needs to undergo either (1) an amniocentesis for assessment of ΔOD450 in the amniotic fluid or (2) middle cerebral artery peak systolic velocity assessment using pulse-wave Doppler velocimetry. If the latter is available, it should receive priority over the amniocentesis simply because it avoids the risk associated with the amniocentesis. If an amniocentesis is performed and the ΔOD450 is in the high zone 2 or zone 3 of the Liley or Queenan curve, then that fetus must undergo fetal blood sampling for documentation of the anemia and transfusion (see Protocol 52). Alternatively, if the middle cerebral artery peak systolic velocity is used to assess fetal anemia, a 1.55 multiple of the median (MoM) value should be used as a threshold beyond which fetal blood sampling and transfusion is needed. After one blood transfusion, the MCA PSV threshold for subsequent transfusion should be changed to 1.32 MoM. The MCA PSV becomes less reliable for timing of subsequent transfusions and empiric intervals between transfusions are usually used: 7–10 days after first transfusion, 2 weeks until fetal marrow suppression achieved by Kliehauer-Betke stain and 3 weeks thereafter. Administration of phenobarbitol (30 mg PO TID) to enhance hepatic maturation should be considered at 34 weeks gestation or one week prior to delivery. Delivery of the anemic fetus receiving blood transfusion can generally be accomplished at between 36 and 37 weeks with documentation of fetal lung maturity. If fetal blood sampling will be performed at a very preterm gestation, administration of betamethasone or dexamethasone should be considered.

Preterm labor

Use of anti-prostaglandin medications such as indocin for tocolysis results in inhibition of prostaglandin synthase activity and reduction in prostaglandin synthesis, which may constrict the ductus arteriosus. The effect on the ductus arteriosus is gestational age dependent and generally, indomethacin is not used beyond 32 weeks gestation. A ductus arteriosus effect is not typically seen within the first 48 hours of treatment. Assessment of the velocity within the ductus arteriosus should be performed beyond that time if the patient continues on a prostaglandin synthase inhibitor. Constriction is typically reversible with discontinuation of anti-prostaglandin drugs.

Summary

Color and pulse-wave Doppler velocimetry is a useful component of ultrasound evaluation of fetuses with Rh disease, growth restriction, congenital heart disease and fetal arrhythmias. While Doppler ultrasound has been used in other fetal conditions, no study has demonstrated any clear clinical benefit for its use outside those stated above. Widespread use of the ductus venosus FVW in the diagnosis of Down's Syndrome in the first trimester has not yet occurred. The use of umbilical artery Doppler velocimetry as adjunct to antepartum testing reduces mortality. The use of Doppler velocimetry to interrogate blood flow in the precordial vein of the fetus may assist the practitioner in delivering the very preterm IUGR fetus prior to end-organ injury, and studies evaluating this are in progress. While uterine artery Doppler evaluation of the high-risk pregnancy might identify a subgroup of women who are at higher risk for adverse pregnancy outcome, the use of Doppler should not be considered a standard medical practice in the general population until further studies demonstrate benefit.

Suggested reading

Hecher K, Snijders R, Campbell S, Nicolaides K. Fetal venous, intracardiac, and arterial blood flow measurements in intrauterine growth retardation: Relationship with fetal blood gases. *Am J Obstet Gynecol* 1995;173:10–15.

Rizzo G, Arduini D. Fetal cardiac function in intrauterine growth retardation. *Am J Obstet Gynecol* 1991;165:876–82.

Reed KL, Anderson CF, Shenker L. Changes in intracardiac Doppler blood flow velocities in fetuses with absent umbilical artery diastolic flow. *Am J Obsetet Gyencol* 1987;157:774.

Mari G, Deter RL, Carpenter RL, *et al.* Collaborative Group for Doppler Assessment of the Blood Velocity in Anemic Fetuses. Noninvasive diagnosis by Doppler ultrasonography of fetal anemia due to maternal red-cell alloimmunization. *N Eng J Med* 2000;342:9–14.

Galan HL, Jozwik M, Rigano S, Regnault TRH, Hobbins JC, Battaglia FC, Ferrazzi E. Umbilical vein blood flow in the ovine fetus: comparison of Doppler and steady-state techniques. *Am J Obstet Gynecol* 1999;181:1149–53.

Ferrazzi E, Bellotti M, Bozzo M, Rigano S, Pardi G, Battaglia F, Galan HL. The temporal sequence of changes in fetal velocimetry indices for growth restricted fetuses. *Ultrasound Obstet Gynecol* 2002;19:140–6.

Hecher K, Bilardo CM, Stigter RH, *et al.* Monitoring of fetuses with intrauterine growth restriction: a longitudinal study. *Ultrasound Obstet Gyencol* 2001;18:564–70.

Baschat AA, Genbruch U, Harman CR. The sequence of changes in Doppler and biophysical parameters as severe fetal growth restriction worsens. *Ultrasound Obstet Gynecol* 2001;18:571–7.

Moise KJ, Huhta JC, Sharif DS, *et al.* Indomethacin in the treatment of premature labor: effects on the fetal ductus arteriosus. *N Engl J Med* 1998;319:327.

Ciscione AC, Hayes EJ. Uterine artery Doppler flow studies in obstetric practice. *Am J Obstet Gynecol* 2009;201(2)121–6.

Baschat AA, Cosmi E, Bilardo CM, *et al.* Predictors of neonatal outcome in early-onset placental dysfunction. *Obstet Gynecol* 2007;109:253–61.

Scheier M, Hernandez-Andrade E, Fonseca EB, Nicolaides KH. Prediction of severe fetal anemia in red blood cell alloimmunization after previous intrauterine transfusion. *Am J Obstet Gynecol* 2006;195:1550–6.

Mari G. Opinion. Middle cerebral artery peak systolic velocity for diagnosis of fetal anemia: the untold story. *Ultasound Obstet Gynecol* 2005;25:323–30.

Moise KJ. The usefulness of middle cerebral artery Doppler assessment in the treatment of the fetus at risk for anemia. *Am J Obstet Gynecol* 2008;198:161.e1–e4.

PROTOCOL 10

Antepartum Testing

Michael P. Nageotte

Associate Chief Medical Officer, Miller Children's Hospital, Long Beach, Professor, Department of Obstetrics and Gynecology, University of California, Irvine

Antepartum fetal testing is utilized to assess fetal well-being, especially in the complicated pregnancy. Several tests are utilized including the contraction stress test, the nonstress test, the modified biophysical profile and the biophysical profile.

Contraction stress test

The contraction stress test (CST) was historically the first method of fetal assessment using the non-invasive technique of fetal heart rate monitoring during the antepartum period. The test is based upon the fact that normal uterine contractions will restrict fetal oxygen delivery in a transient manner resulting from stasis of blood flow secondary to compression of maternal blood vessels in the uterine wall. Alterations in respiratory exchange in the maternal-fetal interface at the level of the placenta will result in differing responses of the fetus to interruption of maternal blood flow secondary to uterine contractions. If such contractions result in episodic fetal hypoxia, this will be demonstrated by the appearance of late decelerations of the fetal heart rate.

The CST is performed over a period of 30 to 40 minutes with the patient in the lateral recumbent position while both the fetal heart rate and uterine contractions are simultaneously recorded utilizing an external fetal monitor. A frequency of at least three 40 second or longer contractions in a 10-minute period of monitoring is required and these contractions can be either spontaneous or induced with nipple stimulation or resulting from the intravenous infusion of oxytocin.

The results of the CST are either negative (no late or significant variable decelerations), positive (late decelerations following 50% or more of contractions), equivocal (intermittent late or significant variable decelerations or late decelerations following prolonged contractions of 90 seconds or more or with a contraction frequency of more than every 2 minutes), or unsatisfactory. A major problem associated with the CST is the relatively high frequency of equivocal test results.

Protocols for High-Risk Pregnancies, 5th edition. Edited by J.T. Queenan, J.C. Hobbins and C.Y. Spong. © 2010 Blackwell Publishing Ltd.

The relative contraindications to the CST are those conditions associated with a significant increased risk of preterm labor, preterm rupture of membranes, placenta previa with bleeding or history of classical cesarean delivery or extensive uterine surgery.

The CST has a remarkably low false-negative rate of 0.04% (antepartum stillbirth within 1 week of a negative test) but up to 30% of positive tests when followed by induction of labor do not require intrapartum interventions for continued abnormalities of the fetal heart rate or adverse neonatal outcome.[1,2] Because of the fact that the CST is more labor intensive, takes more time and has a high rate of equivocal test results, this test has generally been abandoned as the primary means of antepartum fetal surveillance. In some centers, the CST remains the primary test for women with type I diabetes. However, the CST remains a very reliable means of either primary or backup fetal surveillance for any number of high-risk pregnancy conditions.

Non-stress test

Although historically not the first form of antepartum assessment of the fetal heart rate, the non-tress test (NST) is currently the most common means of evaluation of fetal oxygenation status during the antepartum period. Less intensive than the CST in many regards, the NST evolved as an excellent means of fetal assessment following observations that the occurrence of two or more accelerations of the fetal heart during a CST most often predicted a negative CST while the absence of these accelerations of baseline fetal heart rate was associated with a positive test and poor perinatal outcome.[3] The basic premise of the NST is that the fetal heart will accelerate its rate with fetal movement if the fetus is not acidotic or depressed neurologically.

The NST utilizes an electronic fetal heart monitor which is applied externally for a period of between 10 and 40 minutes with the patient in the lateral tilt position. Usually, the patient is asked to note when fetal movement is perceived during the period of monitoring. A reactive NST is defined by the presence of two or more accelerations of the fetal heart rate of at least 15 beats per minute lasting for at least 15 seconds within 20 minutes. Other definitions of reactivity have been proposed with a requirement of two or more accelerations in as little as 10 minutes before the test is considered reactive. If such accelerations are not elicited either spontaneously or with repeated vibroacoustic stimulation within 40 minutes of monitoring, the NST is interpreted as non-reactive. Options for further management include admission to the hospital for delivery or extended monitoring or more commonly some form of backup test (e.g. a CST or BPP) is performed immediately. The presence of variable decelerations may occur in up to 50% of NSTs. If the variable decelerations are repetitive or prolonged (lasting greater than 1 minute), the test is read as equivocal and a backup test is indicated at that time. The NST has a false-negative rate of approximately 0.3% but this is influenced by indication for test and testing interval.[4] Of note, most non-reactive NSTs have a normal backup test which allows continuation of the pregnancy in most instances. The current recommendation is that the NST should be performed at least twice weekly.[5]

Biophysical profile

The fetal biophysical profile (BPP) is a frequently utilized method of antepartum fetal surveillance. The BPP score is a composite of four acute or short-term variables (fetal tone, movement, breathing and non-stress test) and one chronic or long-term variable (amniotic fluid index). All four short-term variables of the BPP are regulated by the fetal central nervous system (CNS). The fetal CNS is highly sensitive to decreases in the level of oxygenation and these biophysical variables are directly influenced by changes in the state of oxygenation of the fetus.[6]

The four short-term variables respond to fetal hypoxemia in a predictable fashion. The biophysical parameter that appears earliest in the fetal life, fetal tone, is the last to disappear as a result of fetal hypoxia. In the early intrauterine development, the fetal tone center appears in the cortex, and begins to function at 7–8 weeks followed by fetal movements at 9 weeks of gestation. Fetal breathing becomes regular at 20–21 weeks, whereas fetal heart rate reactivity is controlled by the hypothalamus and medulla, and appears in the late second trimester. As an immediate response to hypoxemia, the fetus decreases its activity to conserve energy and minimize oxygen consumption. This leads to a decrease in fetal movements, which directly correlates with fetal heart rate accelerations. In the presence of progressive hypoxemia, clinical studies have confirmed that reactivity is the first biophysical variable to disappear. This is followed by the loss of fetal breathing and subsequently the loss of fetal movement. Fetal tone is the last variable to be lost in the presence of ongoing in utero hypoxemia.[7,8]

Fetal urine production is the predominant source of amniotic fluid volume and is directly dependent upon renal perfusion. In response to sustained fetal hypoxemia, there is a long-term adaptive response mediated by chemoreceptors located in the aortic arch and carotid arteries. This results in chemoreceptor-mediated centralization of fetal blood flow by differential channeling of blood to vital organs in the fetus (brain, heart, adrenals), at the expense of non-essential organs (lung, kidney) by means of peripheral vasoconstriction. In cases of prolonged or repetitive episodes of fetal hypoxemia, there is a persistent decrease in blood flow to the lungs and kidneys resulting in a reduction in the amniotic fluid production leading to oligohydramnios. Amniotic fluid volume, therefore, is a reflection of chronic fetal condition. On an average, it takes approximately 13 days for a fetus to progress from a normal to an abnormal amniotic fluid volume.[9]

The NST is first performed followed by the sonographic evaluation of fetal biophysical activities including fetal tone, movement and breathing. Amniotic fluid volume is measured by holding the transducer perpendicular to the floor. The largest vertical pocket is selected in each quadrant. The composite of all four quadrants' deepest vertical pockets is the amniotic fluid index (AFI). A total of 30 minutes are assigned for obtaining ultrasound variables. A normal variable is assigned a score of two and an abnormal variable a score of zero (see Table 10.1).[10]

A composite score of 8 or 10 is considered normal and correlates with the absence of fetal acidemia. A score of 6 is equivocal, and the test should be repeated in 24 hours, except in cases of oligohydramnios with intact membranes. In this particular instance, either delivery or close fetal surveillance is indicated depending on the gestational age. BPP scores of 4, 2 or 0 indicate fetal compromise and delivery should be strongly considered. The BPP score correlates linearly with fetal pH. A direct relationship has been shown between the BPP score and fetal blood pH obtained either with antepartum cordocentesis[5] or cord gases at elective cesarean delivery in non-laboring patients.[11] A normal BPP score virtually rules out the possibility of fetal acidemia being present at the time of testing. A normal BPP result is highly reassuring with a stillbirth (false negative) rate of

Table 10.1 Fetal biophysical profile

Biophysical variable	Normal (score = 2)	Abnormal (score = 0)
Non-stress test	Reactive: >2 acclerations of >15 bpm for >15 s in 20 min	Non-reactive: <2 accelerations of >15 bpm for >15 s in 20 min
Fetal breathing movements	>1 episode of >30 s in 30 min	Absence or <30 s in 30 min
Gross body movements	>3 discrete body/limb movements in 30 min	<2 discrete body/limb movements in 30 min
Fetal tone	>1 active extension/flexion of limb, trunk, or hand	Slow or absent fetal extension/flexion
Amniotic fluid volume	>1 pocket of fluid >2 cm in 2 perpendicular planes	No pocket >1 cm in 2 perpendicular planes

Modified from ref 10: Manning FA, Platt LW, Sipos L. Antepartum fetal evaluation: development of a biophysical profile. *Am J Obstet Gynecol* 1980:136;787.

0.8 per 1,000 within one week of the test.[12] The positive predictive value of an abnormal BPP for evidence of fetal compromise (non-reassuring fetal heart rate tracing in labor, acidemia, etc.) is approximately 50%, and a negative predictive value of 99.9% with a normal BPP. A BPP score of 6 has a positive predictive value of 25% while a score of 0 correlates with a compromised fetus in close to 100% of cases.[13] Vibroacoustic stimulation (VAS) can be used as an adjunct in the assessment of BPP score without changing the predictive value of the test. Further, this may reduce unnecessary obstetric interventions.[14] The BPP can either be used as a primary test for fetal well-being in high-risk conditions or, more commonly, a back-up test for a non-reactive NST. In the presence of a reactive NST or negative CST, BPP parameters do not add to the assessment of fetal status. Therefore, the BPP should be used as a back-up test only for patients with non-reactive or equivocal non-stress or contraction stress tests.

Modified biophysical profile

Modified BPP is a commonly employed primary mode of fetal surveillance in many institutions. It takes into consideration the two most important predictors of fetal well-being – fetal heart rate reactivity and the amniotic fluid volume. The NST is an excellent predictor of acute fetal status when reactive. The amniotic fluid assessment is a means to evaluate the chronic uteroplacental function. The NST is performed in the usual manner and interpreted as previously defined. An amniotic fluid index is obtained as in the BPP and a value of greater than 5 is considered to represent a normal amount of amniotic fluid. The combination of the NST and ultrasonographic evaluation of amniotic fluid volume appears to be as reliable as BPP in acutely assessing fetal well-being with a very low incidence of false negativity.[15] Indeed, the rate of stillbirth within 1 week of a normal modified BPP is the same as a normal BPP (0.8 per 1000). Consequently, the modified BPP is reliable, easy to perform and can be utilized as a primary means of surveillance. The testing frequency should be at least once per week.[16] In a setting of an AFI of less than 8 but greater than 5, a repeat evaluation of the amniotic fluid is recommended within 3 to 4 days.

Indications for antepartum fetal surveillance

The American College of Obstetricians and Gynecologists recommends testing in the following situations:[17]
- Women with high-risk factors for fetal asphyxia and stillbirth should undergo antepartum fetal surveillance

- Maternal conditions: antiphospholipid syndrome, hyperthyroidism, hemo-globinopathies, cyanotic heart disease, systemic lupus erythematosus, chronic renal disease, type I diabetes mellitus and hypertensive disorders.
- Pregnancy-related conditions: pre-eclampsia, gestational hypertension, chronic hypertension, decreased fetal movements, oligohydramnios, poly-hydramnios, intrauterine growth restriction, post-term pregnancy, isoim-munization, previous fetal demise, multiple gestation (with significant growth discrepancy), preterm premature rupture of membranes and uter-ine bleeding.
- Testing may be initiated at 32–34 weeks for most patients. However, it may begin as early as 26 weeks of gestation in pregnancies with mul-tiple risk factors, when fetal compromise is suspected. However, the fetal reactivity may be diminished due to early gestational age and not necessarily reflect fetal compromise.
- A reassuring test should be repeated on a weekly or a twice-weekly basis.
- Test should be repeated in the event of significant deterioration in the clinical status regardless of the time elapsed since the last test.

Newer indications for antenatal testing

Clinicians should consider utilizing fetal testing in pregnancies at increased risk of fetal demise. Beyond the traditional indications listed above, several recent publications have correlated an increased risk of stillbirth with various addi-tional and common maternal conditions. These include maternal age greater than 35 years, nulliparity, grand multiparity, obesity, abnormalities of first tri-mester and second trimester genetic risk assessments, pregnancy following assisted reproductive techniques, multifetal gestations even in the absence of fetal growth concerns and various antenatally identified maternal hereditary and acquired thrombophilias.[5] Utilizing such an expanded list of indications would markedly increase the frequency of fetal testing in any population with its attendant costs and consequences. Further, it has not been demonstrated that the use of any form of antenatal fetal surveillance has been associated with a reduction in the incidence of stillbirth in women with such conditions. Consequently, beyond those indications currently listed by the American College of Obstetricians and Gynecologists, utilization of some form of antena-tal testing for other conditions should be determined by the clinician.

References

1 Freeman RK, Anderson G, Dorchester W. A prospective multi-institutional study of antepartum fetal heart rate monitoring. II. Contraction stress test versus non-stress test for primary surveillance. *Am J Obstet Gynecol* 1982;143:778.

2 ACOG practice bulletin. Antepartum fetal surveillance. Number 9, October 1999 (replaces Technical Bulletin number 1988, January 1994). Clinical management guidelines for obstetrician-gynecologists. *Int J Gynecol Obstet* 2000;68:175.

3 Evertson LR, Gauthier RJ, Schifrin BS, Paul RH. Antepartum fetal heart rate testing. I. Evolution of the nonstress test. *Am J Obstet Gynecol* 1979;133:29.

4 Freeman RK, Anderson G, Dorchester W. A prospective multi-institutional study of antepartum fetal heart rate monitoring. I. Risk of perinatal mortality and morbidity according to antepartum fetal heart rate test results. *Am J Obstet Gynecol* 1982;143:771.

5 Signore C, Freeman RK, Spong CY. Antenatal testing-a reevaluation. Executive summary of the Eunice Kennedy Shriver National Institute of Child Health and Human Development Workshop. *Obstet Gynecol* 2009;113:687.

6 Manning FA, Platt LW, Sipos L. Antepartum fetal evaluation: development of a biophysical profile. *Am J Obstet Gynecol* 1980;136:787.

7 Baschat AA, Gembruch U, Harman CR. The sequence of changes in Doppler and biophysical parameters as severe growth retriction worsens. *Ultrasound Obstet Gynecol* 2001;18:571.

8 Manning FA, Morrison I, Harman CR, *et al*. The abnormal fetal biophysical profile score. V. Predictive accuracy according to score composition. *Am J Obstet Gynecol* 1990;162:918.

9 Nicolaides, KH, Peters MT, Vyas S, *et al*. Relation of rate of urine production to oxygen tension in small-for-gestational-age fetuses. *Am J Obstet Gynecol* 1990;162:387.

10 Manning FA, Snijders R, Harman CR, *et al*. Fetal biophysical profile scoring. VI. Correlations with antepartum umbilical venous pH. *Am J Obstet Gynecol* 1993;169:755.

11 Vintzileos A, Campbell W, Nochimson D, *et al*. The use and misuse of biophysical profile. *Am J Obstet Gynecol* 1987;156:527.

12 Dayal AK, Manning FA, Berck DJ, *et al*. Fetal death after normal biophysical profile score: an eighteen year experience. *Am J Obstet Gynecol* 1999;181:1231.

13 Manning FA, Morrison I, Harman CR, *et al*. Fetal assessment based on fetal biophysical profile scoring. IV. Positive predictive accuracy of the abnormal test. *Am J Obstet Gynecol* 1990;162:703.

14 Inglis SR, Druzin ML, Wagner WE, Kogut E. The use of vibroacoustic stimulation during the abnormal or equivocal biophysical profile. *Obstet Gynecol* 1993;82:371.

15 Nageotte MP, Towers CV, Asrat T, Freeman RK. Perinatal outcomes with the modified biophysical profile. *Am J Obstet Gynecol* 1994;170:1672.

16 Miller DA, Rabello YA, Paul RH. The modified biophysical profile: antepartum testing in the 1990s. *Am J Obstet Gynecol* 1996;174:812.

17 American College of Obstetricians and Gynecologists. Antepartum fetal surveillance. ACOG practice bulletin #9. Washington, DC: ACOG, 1999.

PROTOCOL 11

Indices of Maturity

Anna Locatelli

Department of Obstetrics and Gynecology, University of Milano-Bicocca, Italy

Overview

Surfactant is a complex substance containing phospholipids and apoproteins produced by the type II alveolar cells. It reduces surface tension throughout the lung, contributing to its compliance, leading to alveolar stability, and reducing the likelihood of alveolar collapse.

Neonatal respiratory distress syndrome (RDS) occurs when the lungs fail to produce adequate amount of surfactant. RDS affects approximately 1% of live births and complications of its treatment are associated with an increased risk of serious acute and long-term pulmonary and non-pulmonary morbidities. Although the frequency and severity of RDS are worse for delivery remote from term, the pulmonary system is the last organ system to mature, and RDS can occur even near term.

Indications for assessment of fetal pulmonary maturity include:
- preterm labor (as tocolysis is generally contraindicated in the presence of mature fetal lungs)
- iatrogenic preterm delivery
- need to plan delivery at term in the presence of unsure dates or obstetric complications affecting lung maturity.

Several invasive and non-invasive tests are available to establish fetal lung maturity (Table 11.1).

Invasive tests

Given the outward flow of pulmonary secretions from the lungs into the amniotic fluid, several tests can directly determine fetal pulmonary maturity from amniotic fluid samples measuring the concentration of particular components of pulmonary surfactant or the surface-active effects of these phospholipids.

Protocols for High-Risk Pregnancies, 5th edition. Edited by J.T. Queenan, J.C. Hobbins and C.Y. Spong. © 2010 Blackwell Publishing Ltd.

Table 11.1 Accuracy and characteristics of available fetal lung maturity tests in non-diabetic women

Test	Technique	Threshold	Predictive value mature test (%)	Predictive value immature test (%)	Difficulty/cost
L/S ratio	Thin-layer chromatography	2/1	95–100	33–50	High/high
PG	Thin-layer chromatography	Present	95–100	23–53	High/high
PG	Slide agglutination	Positive (>2%)	–	–	Low/low
Surfactant/ albumin ratio	Fluorescence polarization	≥55 mg/g	96–100	47–61	Low/ moderate
LB count	Cell counter	30,000– 40,000/µL	97–98	29–35	Low/low
Amniotic fluid density at 650 nm	Spectrophotometric reading	OD ≥15	98	13	Low/low
FSI	Ethanol dilution	≥47	95	51	Moderate/ moderate

Lecithin/sphingomyelin ratio

The lecithin/sphingomyelin (L/S) ratio for assessment of fetal pulmonary maturity was first introduced by Gluck and colleagues in 1971.[1] The concentrations of these two substances are approximately equal until mid-third trimester of gestation, when the concentration of pulmonary lecithin increases significantly while the non-pulmonary sphingomyelin concentration remains unchanged. The measurement of sphingomyelin serves as a constant comparison for control of the relative increases in lecithin because the volume of amniotic fluid cannot be measured reliably. Determination of the L/S ratio involves thin-layer chromatography after centrifugation to remove the cellular component and organic solvent extraction. The test requires time and expertise to perform and interpret. An L/S ratio of 2.0 or greater predicts absence of RDS in 98% of neonates. With a ratio of 1.5 to 1.9, approximately 50% of infants will develop RDS. Below 1.5, the risk of subsequent RDS increases to 73%. Thus, the L/S ratio, like most indices of fetal pulmonary maturation, rarely errs when predicting fetal pulmonary maturity, but many neonates with an immature L/S ratio will not develop RDS.

A threshold value for prediction of lung maturity should be calculated in individual institutions by correlation with clinical outcome, as the variation within and between laboratories can be considerable. The sample should be kept on ice or refrigerated if transport to a laboratory is required. Improper storage conditions can change the L/S ratio since amniotic fluid contains enzymes that can be affected by temperature. Maternal serum has a L/S ratio ranging from 1.3 to 1.9; thus blood-tinged samples could falsely lower a mature result but should not increase an immature result to a mature value. The presence of meconium can interfere with test interpretation, increasing the L/S ratio by 0.1–0.5, thus leading to an increase in falsely mature results.

Phosphatidylglycerol

Phosphatidylglycerol (PG) is a minor constituent of surfactant that becomes evident in amniotic fluid several weeks after the rise in lecithin.[2] Its presence indicates a more advanced state of fetal lung development and function, as PG enhances the spread of phospholipids on the alveoli. The original PG testing was performed by thin-layer chromatography and required time and expertise. More recently enzymatic assay or slide agglutinations have been used successfully to determine the presence of PG. The results are typically reported qualitatively as positive or negative, where positive represents an exceedingly low risk of RDS. When reported in a quantitative fashion, a value of 0.3 is associated with negligible risk of respiratory distress. The test is usually immature when performed before 36 weeks. PG determination is not generally affected by blood, meconium, or vaginal secretion.

Surfactant/albumin ratio

The fluorescence polarization assay uses polarized light to evaluate the competitive binding of a probe to both albumin and surfactant in amniotic fluid.[3] It provides a quantitative and automated measurement of the amniotic fluid surfactant/albumin ratio by the TDx-FLM analyzer and its subsequent modification, TDx-FLM II. The test is simple, rapid, objective, reproducible, and can be performed with equipment commonly available in clinical laboratories. It is independent of the amniotic fluid volume. An elevated ratio is correlated with the presence of fetal lung maturity. A TDx-FLM value above 50 or 70 has similar predictive ability of pulmonic maturity as positive PG test or L/S of 2 or greater. More recently, a surfactant-to-albumin ratio of 55 has been proposed as a better threshold to indicate maturity.[4] A disadvantage of the TDx-FLM method is the large quantification scale. Values greater than 55 are regarded as mature, however, values of 35 to 55 are considered 'borderline'. There is controversy as to whether gestational age should be used in interpreting the TDx for determining the likelihood of RDS. In general, higher threshold values are needed at earlier gestational ages to determine lung maturity and lower thresholds are required at later gestational ages. Blood and meconium contamination can interfere with test interpretation. As for L/S ratio, red blood cell phospholipids may falsely lower the TDx-FLM result, but a mature test can reliably predict pulmonary maturity.

Lamellar body counts

Lamellar bodies are produced by type II pneumocytes and are a direct measurement of surfactant production because they represent its storage form. In 1989 Dubin[5] described a method for quantifying lamellar bodies with a commercial blood cell analyzer which takes advantage of the similar size between lamellar bodies and platelets. The results can be obtained quickly, with a small fluid volume, and the test is less expensive than traditional phospholipids analysis. Moreover, the platelet counter is accessible in most hospitals with 24-hour availability without need of special training for technologists. The sample should be processed without spinning as centrifugation reduces the number of lamellar bodies. Freezing and instrumentation can affect the enumeration of lamellar bodies.[6] Values of 30,000 to 40,000/μL generally indicate pulmonary maturity. The test compares favorably with L/S and PG with a negative predictive value of a mature cutoff of 97.7% vs 96.8% and 94.7%, respectively.[7] A meta-analysis calculated receiver-operating characteristic curves based upon data from six studies and showed the lamellar body count performed slightly better than the L/S ratio in predicting RDS.[8] Meconium has a marginal impact on lamellar body counts, increasing the count by 5000/μL. Bloody fluid can initially slightly increase the count because the platelets are counted as lamellar bodies. Subsequently the procoagulant activity of amniotic fluid produces an entrapment of both platelets and lamellar bodies, causing a decrease of lamellar body counts.

Amniotic fluid density

An indirect measurement of pulmonary maturity can be performed by measuring optical density of amniotic fluid at a wavelength of 650 nm. It is based upon the concept that increasing opalescence is due to increasing numbers of fetal squamous cells and lamellar bodies, that are dependent on the total amniotic fluid phospholipid concentration rather than directly reflect it. An optical density of 0.15 or greater correlates well with a mature L/S ratio and the absence of RDS.[5] Different authors report that a visual assessment of amniotic fluid turbidity correctly classifies 87% of samples collected for assessment of fetal lung maturity by optical density, L/S and PG, and has a 92% positive and a 87% negative predictive value for a mature TDx-FLM result.

Foam stability index

The foam stability index (FSI) is a simple and rapid predictor of fetal lung maturity based upon the ability of surfactant to generate stable foam in the presence of ethanol. After centrifugation ethanol is added to a sample of amniotic fluid to eliminate the contributions of protein, bile salts and salts of free fatty acids. The mixture is shaken for 30 second and will demonstrate generation of a stable ring of foam if surfactant is present in the amniotic fluid. The FSI is calculated by utilizing serial dilutions of ethanol to quantitate the amount of surfactant present. RDS is very unlikely with an FSI value of 47 or higher.

A positive result virtually excludes the risk of RDS; however, a negative test often occurs in the presence of mature lung. Amniotic fluid samples should not be collected in silicone tubes as the silicone will produce 'false foam'. Contamination of the amniotic fluid specimen by blood or meconium interferes with the FSI results.

Special conditions

Several maternal/fetal clinical or non-clinical circumstances can affect the risk of RDS and modifies the predictive value of pulmonary maturity tests, including:

- Antenatal glucocorticoids to induce maturation can alter the results of tests for predicting fetal lung maturity.
- In African-American race lung maturity is achieved at lower gestational ages and at lower L/S ratios (1.2 or greater) than in Caucasians.
- Female gender is associated with acceleration of lung maturation.
- SGA fetuses with placental insufficiency are characterized by higher L/S rate but the effect of growth restriction or preeclampsia on risk for RDS remains controversial.[9]
- Maternal diabetes and, in particular, poor glycemic control is associated with a delay in fetal lung maturation. Amniocentesis is indicated in patients with poor glucose control if delivery is contemplated at less than 39 weeks of gestation and in patients with good control before 38 weeks. Some authors have recommended the use of higher thresholds of L/S ratio (e.g., a cut-off ratio of 3), presence of a lamellar body count $\geq$50,000/μL, and usual cutoff of TDx-FLM to indicate mature fetal lungs in diabetic women.[10] Presence of PG, which production is delayed, is commonly considered as gold standard for documentation of fetal lung maturity.
- In twin gestations discordant fetal lung maturity values occur more frequently at earlier gestational age.[11] Therefore amniocentesis of both twins should be performed between 30 weeks 0 days and 32 weeks 7 days of gestation while of one twin appears to be sufficient after 32 weeks 7 days.[12] Is commonly recommended that the sac of the male and/or larger twin be sampled at amniocentesis.

Non-invasive tests

Amniocentesis performed under ultrasonographic guidance in experienced hands is associated with low rates of failure or of bloody fluid collection, and a <1% risk of complications, such as emergent delivery.[13] The assessment of fetal pulmonary maturity can be obtained from vaginal pool specimens in presence of premature rupture of membranes. Blood, meconium and mucus can alter the results. In the absence of these contaminants vaginally free-flowing collected fluid can be evaluate for determination of L/S ratio, PG and LBC yielding results similar to those observed with samples obtained with amniocentesis.

None of the described ultrasonographic indicators of fetal maturity (free-floating particles, grade III placenta, imaging of the fetal lung) is specifically predictive of pulmonic maturity. The proposed parameters are in general predictive of gestational age. Lecithin has a characteristic magnetic resonance spectroscopic peak that may be detected in amniotic fluid and lung but this test is actually too expensive and technically challenging.

Indications for assessing pulmonary maturity and role of gestational age

The relative risk of composite neonatal respiratory morbidity for cesarean delivery before labor at 37 weeks 0 days to 37 weeks 6 days compared with 38 weeks 0 days to 38 weeks 6 days is 1.74 (95% confidence interval 1.1–2.8) and at 38 weeks 0 days to 38 weeks 6 days compared with 39 weeks 0 days to 39 weeks 6 days is 2.4 (95% confidence interval, 1.2–4.8).[14] The American College of Obstetricians and Gynecologists has recommended that fetal pulmonary maturity should be confirmed before elective delivery at less than 39 weeks of gestation unless fetal maturity can be deduced from any of the following criteria:[11]

- fetal heart tones have been documented for 20 weeks by non-electronic fetoscope or for 30 weeks by Doppler;
- 36 weeks have elapsed since a serum or urine human chorionic gonadotropin based pregnancy test was reported to be positive;
- ultrasound measurement of the crown–rump length at 6 to 11 weeks of gestation or other ultrasound measurements (e.g., biparietal diameter, femur length) at 12 to 20 weeks of gestation support a clinically determined gestational age equal to or greater than 39 weeks.

Fetal lung maturity assessment in non-elective delivery is more controversial. Pretest probability of RDS is highly dependent on gestational age. After 37 weeks of gestation the risk of respiratory distress syndrome is very low, thus testing is not indicated if prolonging pregnancy will place the mother or fetus at significant risk. Prior to 32 to 34 weeks, the prevalence of neonatal morbidity is sufficiently high that knowledge of fetal lung maturity does not substantially modify obstetric management. Between 32 and 36 weeks of gestation, fetal pulmonary maturity assessment is most useful in managing pregnancies with indications for delivery.[15] Because the probability of RDS is related principally to gestational age and test results, risk tables have been recently proposed and prospectively validated that report the risk of respiratory distress at different GA-stratified TDx-FLM II ratios. These tables can assist physicians to individualize the risk–benefit decisions regarding the execution and delivery of tests.[16]

Multiple tests or cascade?

Faced with different assays for fetal lung maturity, some laboratories perform multiple tests simultaneously, leaving the clinician with the possibility of results both indicative and not of pulmonary maturity from the same amniotic fluid specimen. In general, any 'mature' test result is indicative of fetal pulmonic maturity given the high predictive value of any single test (5% or less of false mature rates). Conversely the use of a 'cascade' approach has been proposed to minimize the risk of delivery of an infant with immature lungs, while avoiding unnecessary delay in delivery and costs. According to this approach, a rapid, easy-to-perform and inexpensive test is done first (e.g., lamellar body count or FSI), with follow-up tests (e.g., L/S ratio or PG) performed only in the face of immaturity of the initial test. However, a recent study showed that L/S ratio does not add any significant information to that already provided by lamellar body count and PG.[6]

Summary

Several methods can be used to establish fetal lung maturity by testing for components of fetal lung secretions in amniotic fluid. Fetal pulmonary maturity should be viewed as a probability that is a function of gestational age, amniotic fluid analysis and clinical maternal/fetal conditions. Most methods have similar diagnostic indices, and the predictive value of a mature test ranges from 95% to 100%. On the contrary the risk of RDS for an immature test varies from 5% to 100%, depending on gestational age and result of the test.[17] The choice and the sequence of tests should be based upon availability, presence or absence of contaminants, and physician and laboratory personnel preference.

References

1 Gluck L, Kulovich MV, Boerer RC Jr, *et al*. Diagnosis of the respiratory distress syndrome by amniocentesis. *Am J Obstet Gynecol* 1971;109:440.
2 Hallman M, Kulovich M, Kirkpatrick E, *et al*. Phosphatidylinositol and phosphatidylglycerol in amniotic fluid: indices of lung maturity. *Am J Obstet Gynecol* 1976; 125:613.

3 Russell JC, Cooper CM, Ketchum CH, *et al.* Multicenter evaluation of TDx test for assessing fetal lung maturity. *Clin Chem* 1989;35:1005.

4 *Standards of Laboratory Practice: Guidelines for the Evaluation and Management of the Newborn.* National Academy of Clinical Biochemistry, 1998.

5 Dubin, SB. The laboratory assessment of fetal lung maturity. *Am J Clin Pathol* 1992; 97:836.

6 Grenache DG, Gronowsky AM. Fetal lung maturity. *Clin Biochem* 2006;39:1–10.

7 Neerhof MG, Haney EI, Silver RK, Ashwood ER, Lee I, Piazze JJ. Lamellar body counts compared with traditional phospholipid analysis as an assay for evaluating fetal lung maturity. *Obstet Gynecol* 2001;97:305–9.

8 Wijnberger LD, Huisjes AJ, Voorbij HA, Franx A, Bruinse HW, Moll BV. The accuracy of lamellar body count and lecithin/sphingomyelin ratio in the prediction of neonatal respiratory distress syndrome: a meta-analysis. *Br J Obstet Gynaecol* 2001;108:585–8.

9 Torrance HL, Voorbijb HAM, Wijnberger LD, vanBel F, Visser GHA. Lung maturation in small for gestational age fetuses from pregnancies complicated by placental insufficiency or maternal hypertension. *Early Human Development* 2008; 84, 465–469.

10 Ghidini A, Spong CY, Goodwin K, Pezzullo JC. Optimal thresholds of lecithin/ sphingomyelin ratio and lamellar body count for the prediction of the presence of phosphatidylglycerol in diabetic women. *J Maternal Fetal Neonatal Med* 2002;12:95–8.

11 American College of Obstetricians and Gynecologists. Fetal lung maturity. ACOG Practice Bulletin #97. *Obstet Gynecol* 2008;112:717–26.

12 Mackenzie MW. Predicting concordance of biochemical lung maturity in the preterm twin gestation. *J Matern Fetal Neonatal Med* 2002;12:50–8.

13 Stark CM, Smith RS, Lagrandeur RM, Batton DG, Lorenz RP. Need for urgent delivery after third-trimester amniocentesis. *Obstet Gynecol* 2000;95:48–50.

14 Hansen AK, Wisborg K, Uldbjerg N, Henriksen TB. Risk of respiratory morbidity in term infants delivered by elective caesarean section: cohort study. *Br Med J* 2008;336:85–87.

15 Myers, ER, Alvarez, JG, Richardson, DK, Ludmir J. Cost-effectiveness of fetal lung maturity testing in preterm labor. *Obstet Gynecol* 1997; 90:824.

16 Melanson SEF, Berg A, Jarolim P, Tanasijevic MJ, McElrath TF. Validation of a formula that calculates the estimated risk of respiratory distress syndrome. *Obstet Gynecol* 2006;108:1471–6.

17 Mercer BM. Assessment and induction of fetal pulmonary maturity. In: Creasy RK, Resnik R, Iams JD, Lockwood CJ, Moore TR (eds) *Maternal-Fetal Medicine: Principles and Practice.* Philadelphia: WB Saunders, 2007:23:419–20.

PART 3

Special Procedures

PROTOCOL 12

Invasive Fetal Testing: Chorionic Villus Sampling and Amniocentesis

Katharine D. Wenstrom

Division of Maternal-Fetal Medicine, Womens & Infants' Hospital of Rhode Island and Brown Alpert Medical School, Providence, RI, USA

Overview

Because genetic disorders can result in considerable morbidity and mortality for reproductive-age women and their families, prenatal genetic screening and diagnosis is an important part of obstetrical practice. The current standard of care is to offer all pregnant women a prenatal screening test to determine their risk of having a fetus with Down syndrome (trisomy 21); many laboratories also provide the risk of trisomies 13 and 18, and Smith Lemli Opitz syndrome. Currently available Down syndrome screening tests can be performed in either the first or second trimester. Based on the results, women may need immediate access to a definitive diagnostic test, thus clinicians who offer screening should be able to provide or refer for either a first trimester diagnostic procedure (chorionic villous sampling) or a second trimester procedure (amniocentesis).

Pre-procedure counseling

Prenatal genetic screening and testing is voluntary. Counseling by a clinician with special expertise in prenatal diagnosis can assist patients in making an informed decision. Among the factors that the patient may consider are the likelihood of fetal aneuploidy as determined by the screening test result or the family history, the severity of the disease in question, treatment options, personal and family values regarding reproductive choices, and the risks of the diagnostic test.

Protocols for High-Risk Pregnancies, 5th edition. Edited by J.T. Queenan, J.C. Hobbins and C.Y. Spong. © 2010 Blackwell Publishing Ltd.

Complications and risks of chorionic villus sampling and amniocentesis

Spotting or a small amount of vaginal bleeding occurs after approximately 7–10% of transcervical CVS procedures and 1% or fewer of those performed transabdominally. It is usually limited in nature and not associated with an increased risk of pregnancy loss. More serious but rare complications include acute rupture of the membranes, leakage of fluid, and the development of chorioamnionitis, each of which occur in fewer than 1 per 1000 procedures. Spotting or leaking of fluid also occurs after 2–3% of amniocenteses; usually fluid leaking is self limited. Rarely, true rupture of the membranes occurs, increasing the risk of chorioamnionitis, complete anhydramnios and pregnancy loss.

CVS and amniocentesis entail a similar low risk of pregnancy loss. Although the rate of miscarriage from the time of CVS until 28 weeks' gestation is generally quoted as approximately 2.5%, the majority of these are early losses that would have occurred whether or not CVS had been performed. The rate of pregnancy loss after second trimester amniocentesis is 1 in 400 to 1 in 1600 based on recent data.

Several international studies in which women were randomly assigned in early pregnancy to either CVS or second trimester amniocentesis and all losses, both spontaneous and procedure-related, were followed, found similar loss rates after either procedure. Studies comparing transcervical to transabdominal CVS have shown that they are equally safe when performed by an experienced operator.

The safety of both amniocentesis and CVS is directly related to the gestational age at which they are performed (discussed below) and the experience and skill of the operator. Many studies have shown that their safety increases along with the number of procedures performed by the operator, and that ongoing performance of a minimum number of procedures each month is necessary to maintain operator skill. In most experienced centers, patients are counseled that the procedure-induced miscarriage rates for CVS and second trimester amniocentesis are equivalent and in the range of 1 in 200 to 1 in 400.

Chorionic villus sampling

Timing

CVS is usually performed between 10 weeks 0 days and 13 weeks 6 days of gestation. CVS performed prior to 63 days post-LMP is associated with an increased incidence of fetal limb reduction defects and oromandibular limb hypogenesis, believed to result from fetal vascular hypoperfusion/reperfusion injury. To assure fetal safety, CVS should be delayed until 70 or more days post LMP. Successful and safe transabdominal procedures can be performed throughout the second and third trimester if a rapid karyotype is needed or severe oligohydramnios is present.

Technique

Chorionic villus sampling can be done using either a transcervical or transabdominal approach. The approach is based primarily on the position of the placenta and the ease with which it can be reached; other considerations include operator preference and the fact that the transabdominal approach may cause greater – although brief – discomfort. Over 95% of patients can be sampled using either approach, but one approach is clearly preferable to the other in about 5% of cases.

Transcervical CVS

A negative cervical culture for *Gonococcus* is suggested prior to the procedure but testing for other organisms such as *Chlamydia* and Group B *Streptococcus* is unnecessary. The patient's blood type and a recent antibody screen should be available so that Rhogam can be administered after the procedure, if appropriate. Existing blood group sensitization is a contraindication to CVS since post-procedure elevations in antibody titers have been described.

The bladder must be partially filled to allow adequate visualization of the cervix and uterus and to displace the uterus favorably. A sonogram is performed to confirm fetal viability and gestational age, to evaluate the size of the bladder, and to determine the position of the uterus and placenta relative to the cervix. The goal is to have the uterus aligned such that the CVS catheter does not have to negotiate a sharp bend to come through the inner cervical os and into the chorion. Alterations in the degree of bladder filling may be needed to achieve this. Once it has been determined that the bladder volume is optimal, the patient is placed in the lithotomy position, a speculum is inserted, and the vagina and cervix are prepared with a povidine-iodine solution. A specially designed polyethylene catheter placed over a malleable stainless steel stylet with a blunt rounded tip is used for sampling. The most frequently used catheter has a 5.7 Fr diameter and is 27 cm long. Prior to insertion, the distal 3 to 4 cm of the catheter is gently curved to facilitate passage through the cervix, taking into account the position of the placenta and the path the catheter will have to take.

The sonographer visualizes the cervix and chorion frondosum simultaneously. The operator then inserts the catheter tip into the cervix until it reaches the internal os. While still under ultrasound guidance, the catheter is advanced into the chorion frondosum parallel to the chorionic membrane. Care must be taken that the catheter does not perforate the membrane or penetrate into the underlying decidua basalis; entering the decidua will cause bleeding and must be avoided. Confirmation that the catheter is in the correct plane comes not only from ultrasound imaging but also tactile sensation. Little to no resistance is encountered when the tip is passed in the appropriate plane, while the underlying decidua has a gritty sensation. The catheter is inserted through a sufficient portion of the chorion frondosum to allow an adequate sample size. Once appropriately placed, the stylet is removed, a 20 mL syringe containing 5 mL of tissue culture medium is attached and suction applied as the catheter is slowly withdrawn.

The collection of adequate tissue can usually be confirmed through direct visualization of the villi within the sampling syringe. The villi appear as white, fluffy, branching tissue with a frond-like appearance which can easily be differentiated from the amorphous-appearing decidua. Alternatively, some operators ask an assistant to be available to inspect the tissue immediately after sampling, using a dissecting microscope. A sufficient volume of villi is usually 10 mg or more. If insufficient tissue is obtained on the initial pass, a second insertion can be performed without additional risk. More than two insertions are associated with an increased risk of miscarriage but may, in rare cases, be necessary.

Transabdominal CVS

For transabdominal CVS, the patient is placed in supine position, and her abdomen is prepared with a povidone-iodine solution and draped appropriately for an abdominal procedure. Using ultrasound guidance, a 20-gauge spinal needle is inserted into the chorion frondosum. Once in place, a 20 mL syringe containing 5 mL of medium is attached and the tip is passed through the body of the frondosum remaining parallel to the chorionic membrane. Three to five 'to and through' aspirations through as much of the frondosum as possible will usually retrieve sufficient tissue before the catheter is removed from the uterus.

Some operators prefer a two-needle technique in which a thin-walled 18-gauge spinal needle is inserted through the maternal abdominal wall into the myometrium. Once in place, the stylet is removed and replaced with a 20-gauge needle, which is then advanced into the frondosum for villus aspiration. This approach has the advantage of allowing repetitive insertions of the aspiration needle without the need for multiple maternal sticks. However, with experience, the single-needle approach can aspirate sufficient tissue in over 90% of cases.

Post-procedure care

Since CVS routinely results in a small fetal to maternal bleed, Rhesus-negative women should receive post-procedure Rhogam. No specific post-procedure care is required, although many operators advise their patients to avoid intercourse and not to lift more than 20 pounds for the remainder of the day. Patients should be made aware of the risk of post-procedure bleeding and spotting, and instructed to report any leakage of amniotic fluid, fever, chills, or malaise occurring within 2 weeks of the procedure.

Tissue analysis

Chorionic villi are composed of multiple tissue components: the cytotrophoblast cells surround a mesenchymal core, within which are fetal blood vessels containing fetal blood cells. Because there are spontaneous mitoses occurring in the cytotrophoblast, villi can be used to create a chromosome spread as quickly as 2 hours, although most laboratories now do a 24-to 48-hour preparation. However, results from this 'rapid prep' should be considered preliminary, because the chromosomes obtained this way are more difficult to analyze, and discrepancies between the 'rapid prep' and the final culture have been reported. Mesenchymal core cell cultures usually produce readable chromosome spreads within 5 to 10 days. The results obtained from cell culture are considered more reliable, although rarely a follow-up amniocentesis may be required for final resolution.

If CVS is being down for the purpose of biochemical or molecular diagnostic tests, the laboratory that will be performing the analysis should be contacted prior to sampling to discuss any specific instructions regarding tissue handling. In general, there is sufficient DNA in the average CVS sample for most routine DNA analyses. The laboratory will do a better job of evaluating the sample if they have been informed of the reason for referral, pertinent family or patient history, and any specialized tests required.

Reliability of results

CVS results reflect those of the fetus in approximately 98% of cases. Rarely, discrepancies occur as the result of contamination of the sample with maternal decidual cells. More commonly, discrepancies are due to 'confined placental mosaicism' (CPM), in which the placenta contains an abnormal cell line as well as a euploid cell line, while the fetus has only one line of cells, usually with a normal karyotype. CPM is associated with poor obstetric outcomes such as perinatal loss, preterm birth, intrauterine growth restriction, or miscarriage, in 10 to 20% of cases. The impact of the aneuploid cell line is determined by the specific chromosome involved, the tissue source (cytotrophoblast or mesenchymal core), and the percent of abnormal cells.

CPM can only be confirmed by ruling out true fetal mosaicism. Although 1% of CVS samples are mosaic, the abnormal cell line is confirmed in the fetus only 10–40% of the time. In cases of placental mosaicism, amniocentesis is required to determine whether the fetus is also mosaic or carries only the abnormal cell line. A normal amniocentesis result significantly reduces the likelihood of fetal chromosomal mosaicism. However, since the fetal cells obtained by amniocentesis come from the skin, gastrointestinal tract, bladder and lungs, and thus do not represent all fetal cell types, false-negative results have occurred.

Genetic amniocentesis

Timing
The ideal time for genetic amniocentesis the time is 14–20 weeks of gestation. At 14 weeks, the amniotic fluid volume is high enough to make the procedure easy to perform, and it continues to increase with each successive week of gestation. Doing the procedure before 18–20 weeks usually leaves enough time to complete cell cultures and evaluate laboratory tests before it is too late to consider pregnancy termination should an abnormality be detected. Technically, the procedure can be performed before 14 weeks. However, early amniocentesis, performed between 11 weeks and 13 weeks 6 days, has been associated with a higher pregnancy loss rate than the traditional procedure, as well as an increased incidence of positional foot deformities. Some reports have also suggested an increased incidence of neonatal respiratory distress after early amniocentesis.

Technique
A full bladder is not necessary for genetic amniocentesis. A scan is performed to confirm fetal viability and gestational age, and to determine the placental location and amniotic fluid volume. The ideal location for needle insertion is then identified; if there is no such site, an area where fluid can be obtained by traversing the thinnest portion of placenta possible should be located.

The area of the abdomen just above the chosen site should then be prepared with a povidone-iodine solution, after which the abdomen can be sterilely draped, if desired. Some operators infiltrate the skin over the site with a local anesthetic. However, many operators skip this step because the site for needle insertion frequently has to be altered due to fetal movement, necessitating infiltration of additional sites, and because the anesthetic numbs only the skin and the uterus is the source of procedure-related pain.

A sterile sleeve (or a sterile glove) is placed over the ultrasound transducer so that it can be used to guide needle insertion. Sterile ultrasound gel is applied and the site for needle insertion is confirmed by inserting a finger under the transducer and pushing down on the uterus while watching the screen to establish where the needle will enter the uterus. Alternatively, many machines have a biopsy guide function that, when activated, indicates on the ultrasound screen the path the needle will take. The operator can also get some idea of how far the needle will need to be inserted by measuring the distance from the skin to the amniotic fluid in the chosen site. Although putting the needle through the placenta should be avoided whenever possible, because the placenta may cover as much as two-thirds of the uterine wall in early pregnancy, it may be necessary to traverse placental tissue to obtain fluid. A 22 gauge needle is ideal for all amniocentesis procedures, but especially when the placenta must be traversed, because it reduces placental trauma.

After alerting the patient that there will be a needle stick, the needle is inserted briskly under ultrasound guidance to the estimated depth, 'popping' through the chorion and amnion. The stylet is removed, a syringe is attached to the needle, and gentle suction applied to draw amniotic fluid into the syringe. If no fluid appears, the needle should be rotated 90° (to clear any membrane from the beveled edge) and suction applied again. Occasionally, the needle pushes the membranes ahead of it (tenting of the membranes), which should be visible by sonography – in this setting, the stylet should be reinserted and the needle briskly advanced a short distance to achieve membrane puncture. The first 3 to 4 mL of fluid should be aspirated into a 5 mL syringe. Because this fluid could be contaminated with maternal cells, it should not be used for genetic studies; it can be used for measurement of amniotic fluid AFP or discarded. A larger (10 or 20 mL) syringe is then attached to the needle, and approximately 20 mL of amniotic fluid is aspirated. If the patient is having anything other than a standard fetal karyotype, contact the laboratory ahead of time to determine how much fluid will be needed.

If the procedure is being done on a multiple gestation and it is not obvious which sac has been sampled, 2 mL of indigo carmine diluted in 8 mL of sterile saline can be injected into the sac *after* the fluid specimen has been collected but *before* the needle has been removed, as a marker. If needle insertion into the next sac yields clear fluid, the original sac has not been entered again.

When sufficient fluid has been collected, disengage the syringe from the needle. After the needle has returned to a neutral position, withdraw it rapidly; it is not necessary to reinsert the stylet. Ultrasound is then used to show the patient the fetal heart rate and post-procedure amniotic fluid volume. If the patient is Rh-negative and unsensitized, 300 μg of Rh-immune globulin is administered. The amniotic fluid can be kept at room temperature and transported to the laboratory as soon as possible (within 24 hours).

Suggested reading

American College of Obstetricians and Gynecologists. Practice Bulletin #77, Screening for fetal chromosomal abnormalities. *Obstet Gynecol* 2007;109(1):217–27.

Alfirevic Z, Sundberg K, Brigham S. Amniocentesis and chorionic villus sampling for prenatal diagnosis. [Review] *Cochrane Database Syst Rev* 2003;(3):CD003252.

Brambati B, Tului L, Camurri L, Guercilena S. Early second trimester (13 to 20 weeks) transabdominal chorionic villus sampling (TA-CVS): a safe and alternative method for both high and low risk populations. *Prenat Diagn* 2002;22(10):907–13.

Canadian Early and Mid-Trimester Amniocentesis Trial (CEMAT) Group. Randomized trial to assess safety and fetal outcome of early and midtrimester amniocentesis. *Lancet* 1998;351:242.

Eddleman KA, Malone FD, Sullivan L, Dukes K, Berkowitz RL, *et al.* Pregnancy loss rates after midtrimester amniocentesis. *Obstet Gynecol* 2006;108:1067.

Jackson LG, Zachary JM, *et al.* Randomized comparison of transcervical and transabdominal chorionic villus sampling. *N Engl J Med* 1992;327:594–8.

Johnson A, Wapner RJ, Davis GH, *et al.* Mosaicism in chorionic villus sampling: An association with poor perinatal outcome. *Obstet Gynecol* 1990;75:573.

Phillips OP, Tharapel AT, Lerner JL, *et al.* Risk of fetal mosaicism when placental mosaicism is diagnosed by chorionic villus sampling. *Am J Obstet Gynecol* 1996;174(3):850.

Romero R, Jeanty P, Reece EA, Grannum P, Bracken M, Berkowitz R, Hobbins J. Sonographically monitored amniocentesis to decrease intraoperative complications. *Obstet Gynecol* 1985;65:426.

Wolstenholme J, Rooney DE, Davison EV. Confined placental mosaicism, IUGR, and adverse pregnancy outcome: a controlled retrospective UK collaborative survey. *Prenat Diagn* 1994;14:345.

Third Trimester Amniocentesis

Nancy Chescheir
University of North Carolina, Department of Obstetrics & Gynecology, Chapel Hill, NC, USA

The techniques for aspiration of amniotic fluid via abdominal needle placement in the third trimester of pregnancy do not differ substantially from the techniques used in the second trimester. The indications and risk–benefit profiles for third trimester amniocentesis are different than those for second trimester procedures.

Indications

While the majority of second trimester amniocenteses are done to obtain fetal cells for chromosomal or DNA analysis, this indication makes up a lesser proportion of indications for third trimester amniocentesis. The primary reasons in the third trimester are:

1 Pulmonary maturity testing prior to planned delivery.
2 Evaluation for infection and pulmonary maturity in patients with preterm labor, premature rupture of the membranes or growth restriction.
3 Bilirubin testing in amniotic fluid of isoimmunized pregnancies.
4 Karyotype analysis or DNA testing after third trimester identification of fetal structural abnormalities, amniotic fluid volume abnormalities, and growth restriction.

Notably, there are limited data upon which to determine a risk of poor outcomes attributable to the procedure itself. Except for those procedures carried out to confirm pulmonary maturity prior to planned delivery in an otherwise uncomplicated pregnancy, one can assume a greater risk of complications among pregnancies with all of the other indications, irrespective of whether an amniocentesis is performed or not.

As with all clinical testing, third trimester amniocentesis should be performed only when the results would provide clinically useful information to the patient and her care provider that might alter treatment strategies.

Protocols for High-Risk Pregnancies, 5th edition. Edited by J.T. Queenan, J.C. Hobbins and C.Y. Spong. © 2010 Blackwell Publishing Ltd.

Risks

Discussions with the patient should include an evaluation of the following risks.

Failure to obtain a sample

Among the studies reporting this complication, 20/1640 total procedures were unsuccessful in obtaining a sample (1.2%).

- In a study of 562 consecutive women undergoing third trimester amniocentesis by operators of different levels, 5 (0.8%) were unsuccessful.[1]
- Stark et al.[2] reported a 98.4% success rate in obtaining a sample among 913 women with complete data following amniocentesis carried out to determine pulmonary maturity.
- Relative to earlier gestations, amniocentesis in the third trimester is more frequently performed in the setting of relatively low amniotic fluid.
- Uterine contractions, such as Braxton-Hicks contractions and premature labor contractions, are common in this setting and can disturb initial needle placement, increasing the risks of failure to maintain intra-amniotic needle placement.

Rupture of the membranes

Among the studies reporting this complication, there were two cases of rupture of the membranes following 1005 procedures (0.2%).

- In the study of 562 consecutive amniocentesis procedures, there was one case of premature rupture of the membranes.[1]
- In a case–control study, Hodor[3] reported that there were no cases of premature rupture of membranes among 167 third trimester amniocenteses.
- Zalud[4] reported a series of 111 third trimester amniocenteses, with one case of rupture of the membranes following the procedure.
- There were no cases of rupture of the membranes reported by O'Donoghue (0/165).[5]

Need for urgent delivery

Among the studies reporting this complication, there were six urgent deliveries of 1802 cases (0.3%).

- Gordon et al.[1] found no incidences of emergency cesarean delivery for non-reassuring heart tones within 48 hours of third trimester amniocentesis among 562 women.
- Stark et al.[2] reported the results of 962 lung maturity amniocenteses. In this series, six (0.7%) required emergency delivery. Three were related to non-reassuring fetal heart tones, one due to placental bleeding, one due to placental abruption and one due to uterine rupture.
- Among 167 amniocenteses, Hodor[3] reported that no patients required urgent delivery following amniocentesis.

Direct fetal or cord injury

Hodor's series[3] of 167 amniocentesis procedures resulted in no direct fetal or cord injuries.

Infection

While infection is the likely etiology of many of the pregnancy losses following second trimester amniocentesis, there is little data to make that assertion in third trimester procedures. Likewise there is little data to argue that intra-amniotic infection occurs less commonly. The majority of pregnancy losses following second trimester amniocentesis occur during the second and third week post-procedure, presumably due to the time necessary for an intra-amniotic infection to become clinically significant. Many patients who undergo third trimester amniocentesis are delivered within 3 weeks of the amniocentesis, thus preempting the development of clinical infection.

Amniocentesis in the setting of maternal HIV is in general contraindicated and should be avoided unless the unquantifiable risk of vertical HIV infection is less than the information to be gained.

Patients with other blood-borne pathogens such as hepatitis B, hepatitis C and cytomegalovirus should be told that it is theoretically possible to increase the risk of fetal infection via amniocentesis.

Fetal-maternal hemorrhage

If possible the placenta should be avoided due to the increased risk of fetal-to-maternal hemorrhage with transplacental amniocentesis. If avoidance is not possible, choose a relatively thin portion of the placenta for needle placement.

Rh-negative women at risk for isoimmunization should receive RhIg at the time of amniocentesis if the neonatal blood type will not be known within the next 24–48 hours. An argument could be made that in order to avoid patients 'falling through the cracks' that all Rh-negative women should receive RhIg at that time. It is important that a standard procedure is followed in this regard.

Laboratory failure

There were 16 patients among 165 reported by O'Donoghue[5] with culture failure. The risks of failure were increased if there was bloodstained fluid (66% of cases) and somewhat inexplicably in the presence of a female karyotype (14/16).

The presence of meconium in the amniotic fluid can impair biochemical analysis for pulmonary maturity testing and occurs with increasing frequency as term is approached.

Intra-amniotic blood can also compromise performance of some biochemical tests.

It is possible that the cloning efficiency of third trimester amniocytes is less than that at earlier gestations, decreasing the likelihood of being able to obtain a full karyotype. FISH analysis should be considered along with kary-otype in the third trimester in order to lessen the impact of this problem.[6]

Procedure

After discussing the possible risks of the procedure and the relative importance of the information to be gained, the patient should affirm her consent by signing a document.

- Ask the patient to empty her bladder and then an ultrasound can be performed to confirm fetal head position, localize the placenta, and identify available pockets of amniotic fluid.
- Wash the abdomen, typically with an iodine and/or alcohol-containing fluid. Cover the area wider than the skin immediately overlying the likely pocket of fluid to be targeted, as fetal movement can alter the image abruptly.
- Use ultrasound guidance for all procedures. The transducer should be covered in sonic gel and then encased in a sterile sleeve, such as a sterile glove. Confirm the absence of a latex allergy prior to using latex products.
- Place sterile sonic gel on the maternal abdomen or on the sterile covered ultrasound transducer.
- Localize the pocket of fluid, trying first to avoid pockets near the fetal face and other relatively immobile body parts, and secondarily try to avoid the placenta.
- If desired, use local anesthesia to infiltrate the skin through which the needle will pass. The patient must know that the anesthesia will not affect the discomfort associated with the needle passage through her uterus.
- Using a 20 or 22 gauge sterile needle clearly long enough to reach the selected fluid pocket, insert the needle through the skin using ultrasound guidance. If the needle placement is co-planar with the transducer (i.e., along the length of the transducer), then the needle tip should be first visible just below the skin edge. Observe the needle to the edge of the uterus and then alert the patient that she may feel some cramping. Insert the needle through the uterine wall. It can take a small wrist jab to get the needle to go through the membranes without tenting them.
- If you use ultrasound guidance transplanar (i.e., perpendicular to the transducer) you will not see the length of the needle, but rather the tip only. Do not advance the needle under either circumstance without visualizing the needle tip.
- Place the needle deeply enough into the cavity that in the event of a uter-ine contraction or movement of the needle when changing syringes the needle will not withdraw into the uterine wall or an anterior placenta.
- Once the needle is placed in the amniotic cavity, remove the stylet from the needle and withdraw the necessary amount of fluid required for the tests to be done.

- If a karyotype analysis is to be done, confirm that the appropriate syringes and tubes that are non-toxic to fibroblasts are available. If bilirubin testing is to be done, confirm that dark tubes are available to avoid light exposure of the fluid.
- If the fluid begins to flow and then stops, rotate the needle to reposition the bevel. If the flow does not restart, re-image the needle tip to confirm appropriate placement of the needle.
- After completing the withdrawal of the fluid, remove the needle with one smooth move.

Follow-up

After completing a third trimester amniocentesis, fetal monitoring for 20–30 minutes is appropriate. Antibiotic prophylaxis is not necessary. If reassuring, the patient can be discharged from the testing unit and await the results of her testing. The patient should be alerted to the fact that it is common to feel some uterine contractions following an amniocentesis. It also not unusual for there to be a small volume of vaginal fluid leaking shortly after the procedure, presumably due to fluid tracking out of the hole in the membranes immediately after the needle is removed.

She should report the loss of a large volume of fluid, the onset of fevers or chills, or uterine contractions that do not subside. An evaluation should be performed then that includes knowledge of the reason for the amniocentesis in the first place.

References

1 Gordon MC, Narula K, O'Shaughnessy R, Barth WH. Complications of third-trimester amniocentesis using continuous ultrasound guidance. *Obstet Gynecol* 2002;99:255–9.
2 Stark CM, Smith RS, Lagrandeur RM, Batton DG, Lorenz RP. Need for urgent delivery after third-trimester amniocentesis. *Obstet Gynecol* 2000;95:48–50.
3 Hodor J, Poggi S, Spong C, Goodwin K, Vink J, Pezzullo J, Ghidini A. Risk of third-trimester amniocentesis: a case-control study. *Am J Perinatol* 2006;23:177–80.
4 Zalud I, Janas S. Risks of third-trimester amniocentesis. *J Reprod Med* 2008;53:45–8.
5 O'Donoghue K, Giorgi L, Pontello V, Pasquini L, Kumar S. Amniocentesis in the third trimester of pregnancy. *Prenat Diagn* 2007;27:1000–4.
6 Gosden CM. Amniotic fluid cell types and culture. *Br Med Bull* 1983;39:348.

Suggested reading

Ghidini A. Amniocentesis: technique and complications. UpToDate (www.utdol.com).

PROTOCOL 14

Fetal Blood Sampling and Transfusion

Alessandro Ghidini

Perinatal Diagnostic Center, Inova Alexandra Hospital, Alexandria, VA, USA

Clinical significance

Fetal blood sampling (FBS) refers to three techniques used to gain access to fetal blood: cordocentesis (also known as percutaneous umbilical blood sampling); intrahepatic blood sampling; and cardiocentesis. The last two techniques are considered less preferable options because they carry a higher risk of procedure-related fetal loss; they are thus generally reserved for cases in which cordocentesis fails or cannot be performed due to fetal position.

Pathophysiology

Although fetal blood represents a rich source of cells suitable for a variety of diagnostic tests, new technologies can now provide the same information from chorionic villus sampling or amniocentesis, procedures which can be performed at an earlier gestational age and with lower rates of fetal loss than FBS. The most common indications are outlined below.

Cytogenetic diagnosis

Diagnostic FBS for karyotype analysis is indicated when results are required within a few days, such as when the time limit for legal termination is near or when delivery is imminent. In addition, FBS can be used for confirmation of fetal involvement of a true mosaicism, abnormalities at amniocentesis for trisomy 8, 9, 13, 18, 21, or sex chromosomes. However, the absence of abnormal cells in fetal blood does not exclude the possibility of a mosaic cell line in fetal tissues other than blood.

Protocols for High-Risk Pregnancies, 5th edition. Edited by J.T. Queenan, J.C. Hobbins and C.Y. Spong. © 2010 Blackwell Publishing Ltd.

Congenital infection

Fetal blood sampling has a limited role in the prenatal diagnosis of congenital infections such as toxoplasmosis, rubella, cytomegalovirus, varicella, parvovirus and syphilis. Amniocentesis is currently the primary tool used to diagnose fetal infection and guide parental counseling, since polymerase chain reaction (PCR) and traditional microbiological techniques allow isolation of the infectious agent in amniotic fluid, ascites and pleural fluid without the need to access fetal blood. FBS may still be useful in the presence of fetal hydrops following parvovirus infection, which is usually due to severe anemia.

Suspected fetal anemia

The diagnosis of fetal anemia is suspected in the presence of specific ultrasound findings (e.g., hydrops, pericardial effusions, echogenic bowel, or large chorioangiomas) or laboratory findings (e.g., positive indirect Coombs test, recent maternal parvovirus infection, unexplained high maternal serum alpha-fetoprotein, or sinusoidal fetal heart rate pattern). Peak systolic velocity at the middle cerebral artery is commonly used in such cases as an initial screening step, as it has been found to reliably detect fetal anemia in cases of hemolysis (e.g., RBC isoimmunizations), parvovirus infection, homozygous alpha-thalassemia, and feto-maternal hemorrhage. Moderate/severe anemia is diagnosed in the presence of a decrease in Hb of >5 SD below the mean or a decrease in Hb to 0.65 MoM, and it is usually an indication for delivery or fetal transfusion.

Coagulopathies

The majority of inherited hematological disorders can be diagnosed by molecular genetic testing on amniocytes or chorionic villi. FBS has a role in the prenatal diagnosis of some congenital hemostatic disorders with a risk of intrauterine or early postnatal hemorrhage, such as severe von Willebrand disease (homozygous cases) and the rare hemophilia cases in which genetic testing is not possible (i.e., the involved mutations are not identified and the family is not informative for linkage). Fresh frozen plasma should be available for fetal transfusion at the time of FBS since excessive bleeding has been reported after sampling in fetuses with coagulopathies.

Platelet disorders

Whereas FBS has been largely supplanted by DNA markers on amniocytes or chorionic cells for the diagnosis of genetic alterations in platelet count or function, FBS can still play a role in the prenatal diagnosis and management of immunological thrombocytopenias. Because exsanguination after cordocentesis has been reported in fetuses affected with alloimmune thrombocytopenia (ATP) and Glanzmann thrombasthenia, it is important to have concentrated platelets available for transfusion prior to needle withdrawal. The most common immune-mediated thrombocytopenias of importance to the obstetrician are idiopathic thrombocytopenic purpura (ITP) and ATP. The risk of neonatal intracranial hemorrhage is 1% for infants of mothers with ITP. No association between the incidence of intracranial hemorrhage and mode of delivery has been reported. Nonetheless, some physicians recommend FBS and that a fetal platelet transfusion or atraumatic cesarean delivery be performed to reduce the risk of neonatal intracranial bleeding if the fetal platelet count is less than 50×10^9/L. Neonatal ATP is a diagnosis considered after the birth of an affected infant to an immunized mother. The most serious consequence of ATP is intracranial hemorrhage in the baby, which occurs in 10% to 30% of cases (with 25% to 50% of these occurring in utero). In families with an affected fetus/infant, the rate of recurrence is in excess of 75% to 90% and the thrombocytopenia in the second affected child is always as or more severe than in the previous infant. In such cases, paternal platelet-specific antigens should be typed. Fathers homozygous for the specific platelet antigen involved in the ATP will necessarily have affected offspring. In cases of paternal heterozygosity, fetal platelet typing can be performed by PCR on amniotic fluid. Only fetuses incompatible for the relevant platelet antigen are at risk for severe thrombocytopenia from alloimmunization.

Fetal growth restriction

FBS was traditionally used in such cases to identify possible causes of early-onset severe growth restriction, such as karyotype anomalies or fetal infection. The risk of aneuploidy is higher with more severe growth disorders, earlier gestational age at diagnosis, and when growth restriction is associated with polyhydramnios, structural anomalies, or both. Availability of new diagnostic techniques on amniotic fluid (e.g., FISH analysis or PCR) has obviated much of the need for FBS. Blood gas analysis may show hypoxemia and acidemia and may possibly assist in the identification of the optimal timing for delivery. However, FBS carries a 9% to 14% risk of procedure-related loss among growth-restricted fetuses, thus its value for longitudinal assessment of fetal well-being is unproven. Moreover, it is unknown what level of acidemia can be tolerated by the fetus with little or no neurological sequelae, and the effect of gestational age on this level. Therefore, interruption of pregnancy based upon blood gas analysis appears to have a limited role below 32 weeks of gestation since the risks of preterm birth are well known, while those of acidemia are poorly understood.

Suspected fetal thyroid dysfunction

Fetal hyperthyroidism can be diagnosed by FBS in women with a history of Graves disease, high levels of thyroid-stimulating antibodies, and sonographic signs of fetal hyperthyroidism, such as tachycardia, fetal growth restriction, goiter or craniosynostosis. Serial FBS after initiation of maternal administration of PTU is needed to titrate the dose of maternal therapy. Fetal hypothyroidism can by diagnosed by FBS in the presence of fetal goiter usually with polyhydramnios. Serial FBS after initiation of fetal therapy with weekly intra-amniotic injections of levothyroxine are needed to document fetal response and titrate the dose of fetal therapy.

Technique

After ascertaining viability, FBS should be performed near an operating room since an emergency cesarean delivery may be required. Typical steps include:

- Obtain a sample of maternal blood before the procedure for quality control of the fetal samples obtained.
- Intravenous access is optional, but useful to permit administration of analgesics (e.g., Dilaudid® 0.5 mg IV, fentanyl 50–100 µg, midazolam 1–2 mg, or Phenergan 12.5 mg) and antibiotics. Broad-spectrum antibiotic prophylaxis is administered 30 to 60 minutes prior to the procedure because up to 40% of procedure-related fetal losses are associated with intrauterine infection. Antenatal corticosteroids may be given at least 24 hours prior to the procedure to enhance fetal lung maturity in fetuses at <34 weeks of gestation.
- Perform an ultrasound examination to identify either a fixed segment of the cord or the insertion site of the umbilical cord in the placenta (preferable), as these sites will be the target of most procedures.
- Clean the maternal abdomen with an antiseptic solution and drape it.
- Local anesthesia (e.g., 1% lidocaine) to needle insertion site is optional for diagnostic procedures, while it is useful for therapeutic procedures (e.g., transfusions).
- Either a 'free-hand technique' or a needle-guiding device attached to the transducer can be employed. A 20 to 22 gauge spinal needle is generally used. The length of the needle should take into account the thickness of the maternal panniculus, location of the target segment of cord, and the possibility that intervening events, such as uterine contractions, may increase the distance between the skin and target. The standard length of a spinal needle is 8.9 cm, but longer needles (15 cm) are available.
- Amniocentesis, if indicated, should be performed prior to cordocentesis to avoid blood contamination of the fluid specimen.

- The needle is imaged continuously from skin insertion to approach to the target. It is easier and safer to sample the umbilical vein than an artery (puncture of the artery has been associated with a greater incidence of bradycardia and longer post-procedural bleeding).
- Upon entering the umbilical vessel, the stylet is removed and backflow of blood is usually observed. Fetal blood is withdrawn into a syringe attached to the hub of the needle. If free blood is not obtained, the needle can be rotated by a few degrees or gently withdrawn in small increments. Proper positioning of the needle can be confirmed by injection of saline solution into the cord and observation of turbulent flow along the vessel. An initial sample should be submitted to distinguish fetal from maternal cells. Contamination with maternal blood or amniotic fluid can alter the diagnostic value of the specimen. The purity of the fetal blood sample is commonly assessed using the mean corpuscular volume of red blood cells (RBC) since fetal RBCs are larger than maternal RBCs. Dilution with amniotic fluid can be inferred by a similarly proportional decrease in the number of RBCs, white blood cells and platelets in the specimen; diluted samples are still valuable for genetic testing. Blood samples are placed into tubes containing EDTA or heparin and mixed well to prevent clotting. The maximal amount of blood removed should not exceed 6–7% of the fetoplacental blood volume for the gestational age, which can be calculated as 100 mL/kg of estimated fetal weight.
- After the sample, the needle is withdrawn and the puncture site monitored for bleeding.

Transfusion

If an intrauterine transfusion of **packed red blood cells** (PRBC) is performed after sampling, typical steps include:
- Fetal paralytic agents are rarely used (e.g., pancuronium bromide 0.1–0.3 mg/kg of estimated fetal weight IV), generally if the segment of cord sampled is prone to fetal movements and a transfusion is planned.
- Transfuse warmed, group O negative, CMV-negative, irradiated, packed red blood cells at a rate below 10 mL/kg/min. The total volume of blood transfused (mL) can be calculated using published tables or the formula:

$$\frac{\text{Estimated fetal blood volume (mL)} \times [\text{desired Hct} - \text{initial fetal Hct}]}{\text{Hct of PRBC to be transfused (usually 80\% - 90\%)}}$$

Estimated fetal blood volume is 125 mL/kg at 18–24 weeks, 100 mL/kg at 25–30 weeks, and 90 mL/kg at >30 weeks.
- If an intravascular fetal transfusion fails or is not possible, intraperitoneal transfusion can be performed by injecting PRBC into the peritoneal cavity (any ascitic fluid is aspirated before transfusion): PRBC (mL) = (weeks gestation – 20) × 10 mL.

If a transfusion of **platelets** is performed, the platelets are usually obtained from maternal thrombocytopheresis to minimize the risks of transfusion-related infections with pooled donor platelets. A transfusion of 15 to 20 mL of platelet concentrate increases the fetal platelet count by 70×10^9/L to 90×10^9/L, which is adequate to prevent cord bleeding. It is prudent to slowly transfuse the platelets while awaiting the fetal platelet count, as dislodgement of the needle before transfusion can have fatal consequences for the fetus affected.

- The fetal heart rate should be monitored intermittently by interrogating an umbilical artery near the sampling area using pulse Doppler. The fetal heart rate of a viable fetus is also monitored for 1 to 2 hours after the FBS.

Complications

Fetal complications related to FBS include:
- Bleeding from the puncture site is the most common complication of cordocentesis, occurring in up to 50% of cases.
- Cord hematoma is less common and generally asymptomatic, but can be associated with a sudden fetal bradycardia. Expectant management is recommended in the presence of reassuring fetal monitoring and a non-expanding hematoma.
- Bradycardia: usually transient; more commonly noted among growth-restricted fetuses.
- Fetal losses – an excess of 1% rate of losses before 28 weeks has been reported after FBS. The most important risk factors for procedure-related loss include operator experience, indication for the procedure (the risk of fetal loss is substantially higher in the presence of fetal growth restriction or non-immune hydrops) and presence of twins.

Suggested reading

Ghidini A, Sepulveda W, Lockwood CJ, Romero R. Complications of fetal blood sampling. *Am J Obstet Gynecol* 1993;168:1339.

Boulot P, Deschamps F, Lefort G, *et al*. Pure fetal blood samples obtained by cordocentesis: Technical aspects of 322 cases. *Prenat Diagn* 1990;10:93.

Weiner CP. Cordocentesis for diagnostic indications: two years' experience. *Obstet Gynecol* 1987;70:664.

Nicolaides KH, Clewell WH, Rodeck CH. Measurement of human fetoplacental blood volume in erythroblastosis fetalis. *Am J Obstet Gynecol* 1987;157:50.

Hogge WA, Thiagarajah S, Brenbridge AN, Harbert GM. Fetal evaluation by percutaneous blood sampling. *Am J Obstet Gynecol* 1988;158:132.

Ludomirsky A, Weiner S, Ashmead GG, *et al*. Percutaneous fetal umbilical blood sampling: procedure safety and normal fetal hematologic indices. *Am J Perinatol* 1988;5:264.

Maxwell DJ, Johnson P, Hurley P, *et al*. Fetal blood sampling and pregnancy loss in relation to indication. *Br J Obstet Gynaecol* 1991;98:892.

Tongsong T, Wanapirak C, Kunavikatikul C, *et al*. Fetal loss rate associated with cordo-centesis at midgestation. *Am J Obstet Gynecol* 2001;184:719.

Daffos F, Forestier F, Kaplan C, Cox W. Prenatal diagnosis and management of bleeding disorders with fetal blood sampling. *Am J Obstet Gynecol* 1988;158:939.

Paidas MJ, Berkowitz RL, Lynch L, Lockwood CJ, *et al*. Alloimmune thrombocytopenia: fetal and neonatal losses related to cordocentesis. *Am J Obstet Gynecol* 1995;172:475.

Volumenie JL, Polak M, Guibourdenche J, *et al*. Management of fetal thyroid goitres: a report of 11 cases in a single perinatal unit. *Prenat Diagn* 2000;20:799.

Agrawal P, Ogilvy-Stuart A, Lees C. Intrauterine diagnosis and management of congenital goitrous hypothyroidism. *Ultrasound Obstet Gynecol* 2002;19:501.

Miyata I, Abe-Gotyo N, Tajima A, *et al*. Successful intrauterine therapy for fetal goitrous hypothyroidism during late gestation. *Endocr J* 2007;54:813.

Fetal Reduction

Mark I. Evans

Comprehensive Genetics PLLC & Department of Obstetrics & Gynecology, Mt Sinai School of
Medicine, New York, NY, USA

Overview

Literally millions of previously infertile couples have been able to have
their own children because of advanced reproductive technologies. A common and potentially catastrophic side effect, however, has been an ever-
increasing proportion of multifetal pregnancies. Data from the Society of
Assisted Reproductive Technologies (SART) shows that 25% of IVF pregnancies result in twins, and 5% produce triplets or more. Over 50% of
IVF babies come from multiple gestations. High order multiples have
been reduced but not eliminated by the gradual switch from ovulation
induction to in vitro fertilization.

Since the 1980s, a limited number of groups have developed multifetal
pregnancy reduction (MFPR) in an attempt to improve the perinatal mortality and morbidity of multifetal pregnancies. It has become a 'standard'
component of infertility therapies. By convention, the term *multifetal pregnancy reduction* is used for procedures, mostly in the first trimester, that
are performed for fetal number *per se*. *Selective termination* is used for procedures, mostly in the second trimester, for diagnosed fetal abnormalities.

Diagnosis and workup

Multiple gestations, particularly in infertility couples, are commonly
diagnosed by about 7 weeks' gestation, giving couples some time to consider their options. Conversely, in non-infertility couples, the diagnosis is
commonly made later in gestation, requiring more immediate decisions
in couples not having previously considered the issues.

Workup of multifetal pregnancies includes ultrasonographic evaluation of
fetal number, gestational age, size, position and zygocity. It is best performed
at about 12 weeks in order to obtain nuchal translucency measurements.

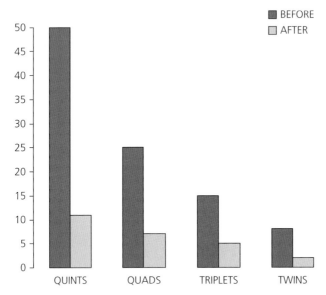

Figure 15.1 Risk reduction.

Over the years, determination of which fetuses to keep and which to reduce has become considerably more sophisticated and in our program includes, in the vast majority of cases, chorionic villus sampling to evaluate for major aneuploidies prior to reduction.

Published data reveal a lower than expected rate of congenital malformations in children in reduced pregnancies, suggesting that, to some degree, fetuses with abnormalities are more likely to be reduced. Furthermore, careful assessment for identical twins, fetuses with shared placentas, or vascular lakes, can likewise be used to reduce later complications. In an ever-increasing proportion of cases, very experienced geneticists are performing chorionic villus sampling. Molecular tests and cytogenetic analysis performed before reduction lower the risks of aneuploidy in remaining fetuses. We perform molecular testing on every chorionic villus specimen to obtain rapid answers to guide decisions as to how to proceed.

Multicenter data overwhelmingly show improvements in pregnancy outcomes with reductions. In most cases triplets or more have been reduced to twins. However, the data continue to show that perinatal morbidity and mortality are related not only to the number of remaining fetuses, but also to the starting number despite successfully performed procedures.

Counseling about expected outcomes is dependent upon exact starting and finishing numbers (Fig. 15.1). For patients presenting with triplets, counseling has become far more complex; as lowest loss rates are associated with reduction to twins, but lowest morbidity is with singletons (Fig. 15.2). Data

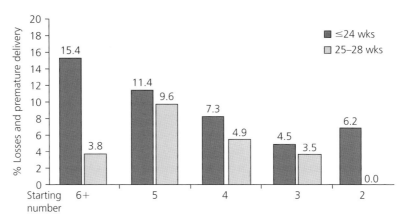

Figure 15.2 Multifetal pregnancy reduction – losses and very prematures by starting number.

from several studies (not reduction) suggest that the risk of cerebral palsy in singleton pregnancies is about 1 in 700 and for twins about 1 in 100. For triplets it is about 1 in 25–30. How patients process such complex counseling situations has also evolved, with considerable differences in how patients react as a function of their backgrounds, education and religious beliefs.

Management

First, a decision must be made as to which fetuses to keep. We carry out ultrasonography for nuchal translucency in all cases and perform chorionic villus sampling in the majority of patients. Obviously, if there is an abnormality, that is the first criterion. If not, sometimes 'suspicion' is aroused by smaller fetal size, smaller sac, questionable anatomy, poor fetal movement, or subchorionic hematoma. If nothing else matters, then – if chorionic villus sampling has been performed and the fetuses' gender is known – gender can be considered. Most patients today, if they have a preference, want one of each gender. The era of preference for males, at least in the United States, appears to be over.

Fetal reduction is now almost exclusively performed by transabdominal needle insertion of intrathoracic potassium chloride. The patient is prepared and draped, and a 22-gauge needle is inserted into the chosen amniotic sac. Once the needle is in the amniotic cavity, it is localized over the fetal thorax. In the author's experience, the needle can be best guided into the thorax using with a sharp thrust. Careful placement is necessary as poor localization may render the procedure ineffective or impossible to accomplish. Furthermore, leakage of excessive potassium chloride outside the fetus may result in weakened membranes.

In the first trimester the needle should usually be placed above the diaphragm and clearly within the thorax. The stylet is removed, a 3 mL syringe is attached, and the plunger is pulled back to check for negative pressure and to ensure that no amniotic fluid comes up the shaft. Once this has been accomplished, a 5 mL syringe filled with potassium chloride is attached, and the plunger of the syringe is slowly pushed forward. If the potassium chloride is entered too quickly, the pressure of the fluid may push the embryo off the needle. Commonly, a pleural effusion can be seen giving a pulmonary outline, which is a virtual guarantee of immediate cessation of cardiac activity. After cardiac cessation has been confirmed, the needle can be withdrawn. In most cases a separate transabdominal needle insertion per embryo is best, as significant angling of the needle through maternal tissue is actually far more painful than a separate needle insertion.

Complications

The major risk of fetal reduction is loss of the pregnancy. Loss rates are correlated with starting number, averaging 3–4% for pregnancies starting with triplet, 5–6% for quadruplets, and 8% for quintuplets or more. Survival has improved over the years as a function of both increasing experience of a small number of high-volume physicians and better ultrasound technology. Furthermore, losses have to be compared with the background loss rate for twin pregnancies known in early gestation, which is nearly 8–10%. For triplets, it is closer to 15%.

Thus the overall effect of MFPR is to significantly reduce the risks of the pregnancy. Pregnancies reduced to twins starting as triplets, quadruplets and quintuplets behave as if they started as twins. These statistics are vast improvements over unreduced higher-order multiples. There have been no known episodes of damage to surviving fetuses. Loss of one of the remaining two fetuses has been seen later in pregnancy in about 2% of cases. There have been no known episodes of coagulopathies, and testing for such was abandoned long ago. Today, most experienced operators perform the procedure at about 12 weeks to have nuchal translucency measurements and in some cases chorionic villus sampling beforehand. However, some IVF physicians have performed reduction transvaginally at 7–9 weeks but have uniformly shown much higher loss rates, approaching 25%.

An ultrasonographic examination approximately a week after the procedure is recommended to ensure that all has gone as planned, and to get a baseline to watch growth of the remaining fetuses. Rh_o (D) immune globulin (RhoGAM) is used for patients as appropriate, and the pregnancy can be managed in a generally expectant way. Alpha-fetoprotein will be useless as values will be very high. Ultrasound becomes the principal method for diagnosis of fetal well-being.

Summary

Fetal reduction has dramatically improved the outcomes in multiple pregnancies – both morbidity and mortality. Genetic testing prior to reduction improves the outcomes and allows patients' preferences to be respected. Complications are relatively rare. There will continue to be considerable societal and ethical controversy in this area.

Suggested reading

Evans MI, Berkowitz R, Wapner R, Carpenter R, *et al.* Multifetal pregnancy reduction (MFPR): improved outcomes with increased experience. *Am J Obstet Gynecol* 2001;184:97–103.

Britt DW, Risinger ST, Mans M, Evans MI. Anxiety among women who have undergone fertility therapy and who are considering multifetal pregnancy reduction: trends and implications. *J Mat-Fet Neonat Med* 2003;13(4):271–8.

Evans MI, Kaufman M, Urban AJ, Britt DW, Fletcher JC. Fetal reduction from twins to a singleton: a reasonable consideration. *Obstet Gynecol* 2004;104:102–109.

Evans MI, Britt DW. Selective reduction in multifetal pregnancies. In: Paul M, Grimes, D, Stubblefield P, Borgatta L, Lichfield S, Creinin M (eds) *Management of Unintended and Abnormal Pregnancy.* London: Wiley-Blackwell, 2009; pp. 312–18.

External Cephalic Version: Singleton Fetus

Gary D.V. Hankins

Department of Obstetrics & Gynecology, University of Texas Medical Branch at Galveston, Galveston, Texas, USA

Clinical significance

Breech presentation at term complicates 3–4% of pregnancies. Following publication of the Term Breech Trial Collaborative Group results, the American College of Obstetricians and Gynecologists concluded that a planned vaginal breech delivery may no longer be appropriate. This recommendation was based on the increased neonatal mortality, and serious morbidity associated with planned vaginal versus planned cesarean delivery of the singleton term breech. When data from this trial was adjusted to reflect practice in the United States, implementation of a policy of planned cesarean birth for breech presentation would result in seven cesarean births to avoid one infant death or serious morbidity. This was felt to be sufficient justification to alter practice and no longer perform planned vaginal breech delivery. Hence, ACOG recommended that obstetricians continue their efforts to reduce breech presentations in singleton gestations through the application of external cephalic version whenever possible.

Most groups have reported a 60–70% success rate with external cephalic version, resulting in a significant reduction in cesarean rate to 30–40% in women who present with a breech presentation at term. A meta-analysis of clinical factors to predict the outcome of external cephalic version detected 53 primary articles reporting on 10,149 women. Multiparity (OR 2.5; CI 2.3–2.8), non-engagement of the breech (OR 9.4; CI 6.3–14), a relaxed uterus (OR 18; CI 12–29), a palpable fetal head (OR 6.3; CI 4.3–9.2) and maternal weight less than 65 kg (OR 1.8; CI 1.2–2.6) were predictors for successful external cephalic version.

Protocols for High-Risk Pregnancies, 5th edition. Edited by J.T. Queenan, J.C. Hobbins and C.Y. Spong. © 2010 Blackwell Publishing Ltd.

Pathophysiology

Factors that contribute to breech presentation include gestational age, uterine relaxation associated with multiparity, multiple gestation, polyhydramnios, oligohydramnios, uterine leiomyomas, placenta previa, fetal anomalies such as hydrocephalus, and maternal uterine anomalies. When the diagnosis of breech presentation is made, the clinician should evaluate for these associated and causal factors. Finally, it is well established that breech presentation is associated with an increased risk for cerebral palsy regardless of the route of delivery.

Diagnosis

Leopold maneuvers should be performed at each clinic visit during the third trimester to determine fetal presentation. If breech presentation is suspected, an obstetric ultrasonographic examination should be carried out to confirm presentation, to estimate fetal weight, and to rule out fetal or maternal abnormalities. Exclusion criteria for external cephalic version are shown in Table 16.1.

Management

1 Schedule the external cephalic version on labor and delivery at 37 weeks or later. Intrapartum external cephalic version at term in early labor can be considered and neuraxial anesthesia may enhance success in this setting.

Table 16.1 Exclusion criteria for performing external cephalic version

Premature rupture of membranes
Third trimester bleeding
Oligohydramnios
Evidence of placental insufficiency, e.g., severe IUGR
Suspected chronic abruption
Preeclampsia
Known nuchal cord
Placenta previa
Previous uterine surgery that would contraindicate vaginal trial of labor
Fetal anomaly
Maternal uterine anomaly
Any other contraindication for vaginal delivery

IUGR, intrauterine growth restriction.

2 Anesthesia and immediate operative facilities must be available if an emergency cesarean section should become necessary. The patient should be given nil per mouth after midnight prior to the scheduled external cephalic version.

3 Obtain informed consent, including permission to proceed with emergency cesarean delivery if necessary.

4 Perform a real-time ultrasonographic examination to confirm a non-vertex presentation, adequate amniotic fluid (amniotic fluid index $\geq$ 10 cm), the absence of any gross fetal anomalies, and to determine placental location.

5 Obtain a reactive non-stress test and secure intravenous access. Type and screen for two units of packed red blood cells if the prenatal antibody screen is positive or unknown (should emergency cesarean section become necessary).

6 Consider using a uterine relaxant, which may include 250 µg of terbutaline sulfate SQ or IV injection, or ritodrine hydrochloride intravenously at 100 µg/min for 10 to 15 minutes, or magnesium sulfate as a 4 g intravenous dose given over 20 minutes. The subcutaneous terbutaline regimen is the least complex and least expensive tocolytic for this purpose.

7 Anesthesia is not recommended for the procedure unless delivery is planned if the procedure fails and the delivery will then occur in relatively close proximity.

8 Ten minutes after administration of a uterine relaxant, the external cephalic version can be attempted with two operators (Fig. 16.1) or one (Fig. 16.2). With two operators, the first operator attempts to lift the breech out of the pelvis (the critical aspect of the procedure) while the second operator attends to the head. A forward roll is usually attempted if the fetal head crosses the maternal midline. A back flip can be used if the initial method fails or if the fetus does not cross the midline. This method requires substantial teamwork to ensure that the vectors created by each attendant facilitate, rather than cancel, the forces necessary to turn the fetus. The procedure can also be attempted in a similar manner with a single operator. This author prefers the single operator method.

9 Discontinue the procedure if there is evidence of fetal intolerance, or maternal request, or if in your judgment the force required is too great.

10 Obtain real-time ultrasonography to confirm version outcome. If more than one attempt is made or if the attempt is prolonged, visualize the fetal heart rate every 30 to 60 seconds. Discontinue the procedure if fetal bradycardia is observed.

11 Even though the risk of feto-maternal hemorrhage is only 2–3%, always administer Rh immune globulin to Rh-negative unsensitized women following the procedure.

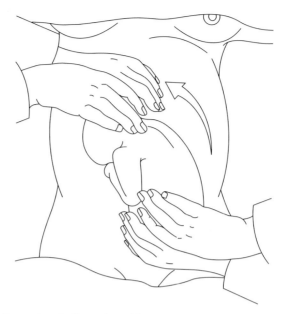

Figure 16.1 External cephalic version with two operators.

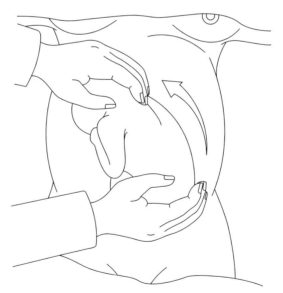

Figure 16.2 External cephalic version with a single operator.

12 Fetal heart rate monitoring should be continued post-procedure until a reactive non-stress test is obtained, or for at least 30 minutes, whichever is longer.

Complications

A meta-analysis of 84 studies reporting on 12,955 version attempts had a pooled complication rate of 6.1% (CI 4.7–7.8). Serious complications occurred in 0.24% (CI 0.17–0.34) and 35% (CI 0.26–0.47) required an emergency cesarean section. Complications did not relate to success or failure of the attempt (OR 1.2; CI 0.93–1.7).

Follow-up

In the event of failed version, the woman should be counseled on the risks and benefits of all treatment options. Most will elect a cesarean delivery which can be scheduled at 39 weeks. Persistence of the breech presentation should be confirmed ultrasonographically prior to the cesarean procedure. If external cephalic version is attempted intrapartum under conduction anesthesia, and if it fails, the woman should be counseled for timely delivery by cesarean section.

Summary

Careful assessment of fetal presentation in the third trimester is important. Otherwise, patients may be deprived of the option of external cephalic version to decrease the risk of cesarean section. External cephalic version is one tool in the armamentarium of the obstetrician when managing the term breech presentation. Before the procedure, fetal well-being and any contraindications should be determined. Informed consent and counseling with regard to the likelihood of success of the procedure should be performed. Postversion assessment for fetal presentation on subsequent encounters is vital in these patients.

Suggested reading

Hannah ME, Hannah WJ, Hewson SA, Hodnett ED, Saigal S, Willan AR. Planned cesarean section versus planned vaginal birth for breech presentation at term: a randomized multicenter trial. *Lancet* 2000;356:1375–83.

American College of Obstetricians and Gynecologists. *External Cephalic Version.* Practice Bulletin # 13 February 2000 (replaces Practice Pattern No. 4, July 1997). Washington DC: ACOG, 2000. (Reaffirmed 2008).

Committee on Obstetric Practice. ACOG Committee Opinion. Mode of term singleton breech delivery. No. 340, July 2006 (replaces Number 265, December 2001).

American College of Obstetricians and Gynecologists. *Obstet Gynecol* 2006;108:235–7. (Reaffirmed 2008).

Kok M, Cnossen J, Gravendeel L, van der Post J, Opmeer B, Mol BW. Clinical factors to predict the outcome of external cephalic version: a meta-analysis. *Am J Obstet Gynecol* 2008;199(6):630.e1.7; discussion e1–5.

Boucher M, Marquette GP, Varin J, Champagne J, Bujold E. Fetomaternal hemorrhage during external cephalic version. *Obstet Gynecol* 2008;112(1):79–84.

Grootscholten K, Kok M, Oei SG, Mol BW, van der Post JA. External cephalic version-related risks: a meta-analysis. *Obstet Gynecol* 2008;112(5):1143–51.

Induction of Labor

Deborah A. Wing

Department of Obstetrics and Gynecology, Division of Maternal-Fetal Medicine, University of California, Irvine, CA, USA

Overview

Induction of labor is the artificial stimulation of uterine contractions for the purpose of vaginal birth. It is one of the most commonly practiced procedures in obstetrics, occurring in over 20% of pregnancies.[1] Labor induction is indicated when the maternal or fetal benefits from delivery outweigh the risks of prolonging the pregnancy. Indications for induction vary in acuity and may be for medical, obstetrical or elective reasons (Table 17.1). If an elective induction for reasons such as distance from hospital or risk of precipitous labor is undertaken, the criteria for term gestation should be met including: (1) ultrasound measurements at less than 20 weeks confirms gestational age of 39 weeks or more; (2) fetal heart tones have been documented to be present for more than 30 weeks by Doppler ultrasonography; (3) it has been 36 weeks or more since a positive serum or urine human chorionic gonadotropin pregnancy test.[2]

Risks associated with labor induction include prolonged labors, uterine contractile abnormalities[3] and an increased propensity for cesarean birth. Some of these cesareans may be performed for failed inductions. There are a number of different definitions for failed induction of labor. For the most part, however, the most commonly accepted definition would involve the inability of the patient to gain entry to active labor after application of maximally accepted doses of cervical ripening agents and oxytocin infusion. The presence or absence of cervical 'ripening,' can influence the probability of induction success. An assessment of cervical readiness for labor induction can be communicated by using the modified Bishop score[4] (Table 17.2). This scoring methodology was first described

Protocols for High-Risk Pregnancies, 5th edition. Edited by J.T. Queenan, J.C. Hobbins and C.Y. Spong. © 2010 Blackwell Publishing Ltd.

Table 17.1 Selection criteria for induction of labor

Indications	Gestational hypertension
	Preeclampsia, eclampsia
	Maternal medical problems (e.g., diabetes mellitus, renal disease, chronic hypertension, antiphospholipid syndrome)
	Abruptio placentae
	Chorioamnionitis
	Post-term gestation
	Fetal compromise, (e.g., severe fetal growth restriction, isoimmunization, oligohydramnios)
	Fetal demise
	Logistic factors (e.g., risk of rapid labor, distance from hospital, psychosocial reasons)
Contraindications	Complete placenta previa or vasa previa
	Transverse fetal lie
	Umbilical cord prolapse
	Prior classical uterine incision
	Active genital herpes infection
	Previous myomectomy with entry into the endometrial cavity

Source: adapted from reference [2].

Table 17.2 Bishop pelvic scoring system

	0	1	2	3
Dilation (cm)	0	1–2	3–4	5–6
Effacement (%)	0–30	40–50	60–70	80
Station	–3	–2	–1 to 0	+1 to +2
Cervical consistency	Firm	Medium	Soft	–
Position of cervix	Posterior	Mid	Anterior	–

Source: adapted from reference [4].

to assess the likelihood of spontaneous labor following the cervical examination in multiparous women, and thus was not intended for its contemporary use. Currently, the modified Bishop score allows a systematic assessment of cervical status that facilitates choosing an induction agent (see following) and predicting induction success. A Bishop score <6 indicates an unfavorable cervix which may require a pre-labor cervical ripening agent. The higher the Bishop score, the greater is the likelihood of induction success. Choices of induction agents include some mechanical and others pharmacological. The indication for induction, modified Bishop score, and following summaries can be employed to determine appropriate management algorithms for patients.

Cervical ripening agents

Mechanical agents
Membrane stripping

Induction of labor by 'stripping' the amniotic membranes is a common practice. It is performed by manually separating the membranes from the lower uterine segment during a cervical examination, resulting in an increase in phospholipase A_2 and endogenous prostaglandin $F_{2\alpha}$ release, which are known to precede the spontaneous onset of labor.[5] Most studies have reported membrane stripping to be safe and, when performed as a general policy at term, is associated with a reduction in pregnancies extending to 41 and 42 weeks.[6] Women who undergo membrane stripping may experience discomfort, vaginal bleeding and irregular contractions after the procedure is performed.

Intracervical balloon catheter placement

Mechanical dilation of the cervix with a balloon catheter was first described in 1863. Since that time, there have been variations to this technique, including intracervical Foley balloon (14–26 F) and the Atad double balloon device. These devices work by applying local pressure on the cervix by filling the balloon (or balloons) after placement in the endocervical canal. This pressure facilitates cervical ripening most likely by stimulating the release of local prostaglandins and triggering the Ferguson reflex. Multiple studies have demonstrated efficacy of this approach to cervical ripening; however, there is a paucity of data comparing the use of intracervical balloon catheters to prostaglandin administration by which to determine whether one approach is superior to another. Moreover, variations in the size of the catheters used, duration of catheter retention and inconsistent use of extraamniotic saline infusion also limit the ability to make comparisons.[7]

Pharmacological agents
Prostaglandin E₁

Prostaglandin E_1 is a prostaglandin labeled for use by the US Food and Drug administration (FDA) for prevention of peptic ulcer disease. PGE_1 is used off-label for a variety of obstetrical and gynecological indications, including cervical ripening and labor induction. It has been found to be safe and effective in numerous clinical trials.[8] It has numerous advantages over other prostaglandin compounds including temperature stability and low cost. Misoprostol, a synthetic PGE_1, currently comes in 100 or 200 µg tablets. The dose most commonly recommended for a term pregnancy induction is 25 µg every 3–6 hours placed in the posterior fornix. Repeat dosing is not recommended if there are more than three contractions in 10 minutes. The clinical efficacy of vaginally administered misoprostol includes a decrease cesarean section rate, and higher incidence of vaginal delivery within 24 hours of initiation and a decreased need for oxytocin.[8] When used in higher doses ($\geq$50 μg), misoprostol has been reported to have a higher rate of tachysystolic uterine contractions (six or more contractions in 10 minutes averaged over 30 minutes) when compared with either placebo or PGE$_2$. An important consideration in the use of misoprostol for labor induction is the reported increased occurrence of uterine tachysystole with or without fetal heart rate abnormalities, and the potential for disruption of the uterine scar in women with a previous cesarean delivery.[9] It is recommended that, if oxytocin is necessary after misoprostol treatment for cervical ripening, it should be started no sooner than 4 hours after the last dose of misoprostol. A recently published phase II trial of two doses of misoprostol (50 μg and 100 μg) in a timed-release vaginal insert demonstrated comparable results to the dinoprostone vaginal insert, Cervidil, so continuing research efforts are under way.[10]

Other routes of misoprostol administration have been studied. Oral administration appears to be associated with less frequency of uterine tachysystole compared to vaginally administered misoprostol.[11] There is promise of comparable efficacy with titration of orally administered misoprostol solution and reductions in uterine contractile and fetal heart rate abnormalities compared to vaginal misoprostol administration.[12]

Prostaglandin E$_2$

PGE2 when applied to the female reproductive tract alters the cervical collagen milieu, which results in separation of tightly knit collagen bundles and an increase in the intervening ground substance, resulting in softening and effacement of the cervix.

There are two prostaglandin E$_2$ compounds which have been approved by the US Food and Drug Administration for cervical ripening for medically indicated inductions of labor. One is Prepidil (Pfizer, Inc.), a dinoprostone intracervical gel; the other is Cervidil (Forest Pharmaceuticals), a dinoprostone timed-release vaginal insert.

Prepidil is 0.5 mg of PGE$_2$ which is to be placed intracervically. It may be redosed as necessary again in 6 hours if regular contractions are not present and the fetal heart rate is reassuring. Intracervical placement of PGE$_2$ requires direct visualization of the cervix and may be uncomfortable for the woman. Intracervical prostaglandin application was found to be inferior to intravaginal prostaglandin application.[13]

Cervidil is 10 mg of dinoprostone in a mesh polymer; after placement in the posterior vaginal fornix, the polymer insert releases PGE$_2$ at a rate of 0.3 mg/h. The manufacturer recommends a maximum exposure of 12 hours to Cervidil.

Recommendations for fetal surveillance after prostaglandin use

Labor inductions using prostaglandin compounds should only occur in settings in which continuous uterine activity and fetal heart rate monitoring can occur for the initial observation period. Further monitoring may ensue as dictated by the clinical condition or the institutional policy. After placement of any prostaglandin, the woman should remain recumbent for 30 to 60 minutes. Thereafter, the patient should be monitored for 1 to 2 hours. There is evidence that the onset of uterine activity occurs within the first hour and peaks at 4 hours after prostaglandin administration,[14,15] so that it seems prudent in most circumstances to continue monitoring for at least this period of time. If regular contractions begin, continuous cardiotocographic monitoring should be applied as well as monitoring of the mother's vital signs.

Prostaglandins should not be used for induction of labor in the setting of frequent fetal heart rate abnormalities because of the limited ability to quickly terminate the effects on uterine contractility. If uterine tachysystole occurs, the administration of subcutaneous or intravenous terbutaline (0.25 mg) or other tocolytic may result in quiescence of uterine overactivity.

Labor-inducing procedures and agents

Amniotomy

Amniotomy can safely and effectively induce or augment labor, particularly in women with favorable Bishop scores (≥8).[16] This observation of the effect of amniotomy stems from the release of prostaglandins, which stimulate uterine contractions. The combination of oxytocin plus amniotomy for labor induction appears to shorten the time interval from start of induction to delivery compared to amniotomy alone.[17]

When performing amniotomy, care should be taken to ensure the fetal head is well applied to the cervix and the umbilical cord is not presenting. The fetal heart rate should be recorded immediately following amniotomy. Labor will usually ensue thereafter, although the timing of onset of labor may be unpredictable. If oxytocin is being used concomitantly, its dosage may need adjustment.

Oxytocin

Oxytocin is one of the most widely used medications in obstetrical practice in this country. Its original synthesis in the laboratory resulted in a Nobel Prize awarded to de Vigneaud in 1955. Oxytocin may be used for induction or augmentation of labor, although it has proven inferior as a cervical ripening agent when the cervical condition is found to be unfavorable, compared to other pharmacological approaches.[18] There are literally dozens of regimens described in the literature. The fundamental differences are based on doses and dosing intervals. The 'low-dose' regimens are considered physiological, and the 'high-dose' regimens are considered pharmacological[2] (Table 17.3). A 40-minute period is needed to reach steady-state concentrations after oxytocin initiation or dose change, and uterine response to oxytocin initiation or dose change occurs within 3–5 minutes.[19]

Recommendations for selection of a particular regimen (high dose versus low dose) vary, although in the current medical climate, which focuses on safety, some authorities have suggested standardized oxytocin dosing regimens[20,21] (Table 17.4). It should be noted that none of these dosing regimens has been tested in a scientific fashion or compared to other dosing regimens by which to demonstrate efficacy let alone safety. Multiple studies have found both protocols effective in establishing adequate labor patterns. High-dose infusion protocols have consistently demonstrated shorter time to delivery with fewer failed inductions compared to low-dose protocols. The high-dose protocols are also more often associated with uterine overactivity and fetal heart rate pattern abnormalities. Proponents of high-dose regimens have emphasized the importance of high-volume facilities and round-the-clock medical staffing. Examples of protocols for oxytocin delivery can be found in Table 17.4.

Table 17.3 Examples of low- and high-dose oxytocin infusion protocols for labor stimulation

Regimen	Starting dose (mU/min)	Incremental increase (mU/min)	Maximum dose (mU/min)
Low-dose	0.5–2.0	1–2	15–40
High-dose	6	3–6*	15–40

*The dose is reduced to 3 mU/min in the face of uterine tachysystole with fetal heart rate abnormalities, and reduced further to 1 mU/min if the uterine tachysystole with fetal heart rate abnormalities is persistent.
Source: adapted from reference [2].

Table 17.4 Oxytocin checklist example

1	Dilution: 10 U oxytocin in 1000 mL normal saline for resultant concentration of 10 mU oxytocin/mL
2	Infusion rate: 2 mU/min or 12 mL/h
3	Incremental increase: 2 mU/min or 12 mL/h every 45 minutes until contraction frequency adequate
4	Maximum dose: 16 mU/min or 96 mL/h

Source: reference [21].

Conclusion

Labor inductions have become increasingly more common. In the United States there has been a doubling of the induction rate in the past two decades, and the upward trend is continuing. Despite therapeutic advances and continued research into the initiation of human parturition, the clinical features which are most critical for determining induction management and predicting success are the cervical condition at the start of the induction, and gestational age, among other maternal demographic characteristics such as multiparity and normal weight.

References

1 Martin JA, Hilton BE, Sutton PD, Ventura SJ, Menacker F, Kirmeyer S, Mathews TJ. Births: Final data for 2006. *Natl Vit Stat Rep* 2009;57(7):1–102.
2 American College of Obstetricians and Gynecologists. *Induction of Labor.* ACOG Practice Bulletin 107. American College of Obstetricians and Gynecologists: Washington, DC, August 2009.
3 Macones GA, Hankins GDV, Spong CY, Hauth J, Moore T. The 2008 National Institute of Child Health and Human Development Workshop Report on electronic fetal monitoring. *Obstet Gynecol* 2008;11:661–6.
4 Bishop EH. Pelvic scoring for elective induction. *Obstet Gynecol* 1964;24:266–268.
5 Adair CD. Nonpharmacologic approaches to cervical priming and labor induction. *Clin Obstet Gynecol* 2000;43:447–54.
6 Boulvain M, Stan C, Irion O. Membrane sweeping for induction of labour. *Cochrane Database Syst Rev* 2005; CD000451.
7 Boulvain M, Kelly A, Lohse C, Stan C, Irion O. Mechanical methods for induction of labour. *Cochrane Database Syst Rev* 2001;(4):CD001233.
8 Hofmeyr GJ, Gulmexoglu AM. Vaginal misoprostol for cervical ripening and labour induction at term. *Cochrane Database Syst Rev* 2003;(1):CD000941.
9 Wing DA, Lovett K, Paul RH. Disruption of uterine incision following misoprostol for labor induction in women with previous cesarean delivery. *Obstet Gynecol* 1998;91:828–30.
10 Wing DA. Misoprostol Vaginal Insert Consortium. Misoprostol vaginal insert compared to dinoprostone vaginal insert: a randomized, controlled trial. *Obstet Gynecol* 2008 Oct;112(4):801–12.
11 Alfirevic Z, Weeks A. Oral misoprostol for induction of labour. *Cochrane Database Syst Rev* 2006;(2):CD001338.
12 Cheng SY, Ming H, Lee JC. Titrated oral compared with vaginal misoprostol for labor induction: A randomized controlled trial. *Obstet Gynecol* 2008;111(1):119–25.
13 Boulvain M, Kelly A, Irion O. Intracervical prostaglandins for induction of labour. *Cochrane Database Syst Rev* 2008;(1):CD006971.
14 Bernstein P. Prostaglandin E2 gel for cervical ripening and labour induction: A multicentre placebo-controlled trial. *CMAJ* 1991;145(10):1249–54.
15 Miller AM, Rayburn WF, Smith CV. Patterns of uterine activity after intravaginal prostaglandin E2 during preinduction cervical ripening. *Am J Obstet Gynecol* 1991;165(4 Pt 1):1006–9.

16 Fraser WD, Marcoux S, Moutquin JM, Christen A. Effect of early amniotomy on the risk of dystocia in nulliparous women. *N Engl J Med* 1993;324:1145–9.

17 Bricker L, Luckas M. Amniotomy alone for induction of labour. *Cochrane Database Syst Rev* 2000;(4):CD002862.

18 Kelly AJ, Tan B. Intravenous oxytocin alone for cervical ripening and induction of labour. *Cochrane Database Syst Rev* 2001;(3):CD003246.

19 Seitchik J, Amico J, Robinson AG, Castillo M. Oxytocin augmentation of dysfunctional labor. *Am J Obstet Gynecol* 1984;150:225–8.

20 Clark S, Belfort M, Saade G, *et al*. Implementation of a conservative checklist-based protocol for oxytocin administration: maternal and newborn outcomes. *Am J Obstet Gynecol* 2007;197:480.

21 Hayes EJ, Weinstein L. Improving patient safety and uniformity of care by a standardized regimen for the use of oxytocin. *Am J Obstet Gynecol* 2008;198(6):622.e1–7.

PART 4
Maternal Disease

Maternal Anemia

Alessandro Ghidini

Department of Obstetrics and Gynecology, Inova Alexandria Hospital, Alexandria, VA, USA

A comprehensive review of all causes of anemia is often intimidating for the general obstetrician. Moreover, most commonly available algorithms are not targeted to the conditions most prevalent in the obstetric population, which consists mainly of healthy young women. The current protocol aims at suggesting an initial evaluation of anemias, which will allow the identification and appropriate therapy of the majority of cases of anemia encountered in a pregnant population. The few cases which defy the algorithms outlined in this protocol are probably better managed in consultation with a hematologist.

Definition

The fall in hemoglobin level seen in healthy normal pregnancies (also known as physiological or dilutional anemia of pregnancy) is caused by a relatively greater expansion of plasma volume (50%) compared with the increase in red cell volume (25%). The fall in hematocrit reaches a nadir during the late second to early third trimester (Table 18.1). The Centers for Disease Control and Prevention defined anemia as a hemoglobin (Hb) or hematocrit (Hct) level below the fifth centile for a healthy, iron-supplemented population, i.e., Hb <11 g/dL or Hct <33% in the first trimester, and Hb <10.5 or Hct <32% afterwards (CDC 1989). Severe anemia is usually defined as Hb level <8.5 mg/dL. The two most common causes of anemia during pregnancy and the puerperium are iron deficiency and acute blood loss.

Consequences

According to the World Health Organization, severe anemia contributes to 40% of maternal deaths in underdeveloped countries.[2] In developed

Protocols for High-Risk Pregnancies, 5th edition. Edited by J.T. Queenan, J.C. Hobbins and C.Y. Spong. © 2010 Blackwell Publishing Ltd.

Table 18.1 Changes in laboratory values in pregnancy

	Non-pregnant women	Pregnant women
Hemoglobin (g/dL)	12–16	11–14
Hematocrit	36–46%	33–44%
RBC count ($\times 10^6$/mL)	4.8	4.0
MCV (fL)	80–100	=
MCHC	31–36%	=
Reticulocytes ($\times 10^9$/L)	50–150	=
Ferritin (ng/mL)	>25	>20
RDW (red cell distribution width)	11–15%	=

=, unchanged

countries anemia has been associated with increased risk of preterm birth, premature rupture of membranes, infections and fetal growth restriction.[3–6] The symptoms of mild anemia are often indistinguishable from those related to pregnancy, and include fatigue, breathlessness, palpitations, difficulty in concentration, and low intellectual and productive capacity.

Diagnostic workup and treatment

Traditionally, evaluation of anemia starts with the mean corpuscular volume (MCV), based on which anemias are defined as microcytic (<80 fL), normocytic (80–100 fL) or macrocytic (>100 fL). However, mixed nutritional deficiencies (folate and iron) often lead to normocytic anemia, and most anemias at the beginning are normocytic. The red cell distribution width (RDW) is a useful indicator of anemias due to nutritional deficiencies (i.e., it increases above 15% in the presence of iron, folate or vitamin B_{12} deficiencies).

Macrocytic anemia

Figure 18.1 shows the appropriate workup for the search of causes in the presence of macrocytic anemia. *Vitamin B12 deficiency* is rare, as most healthy individuals have 2–3 years' storage available in the liver. However, vitamin B_{12} deficiency can be encountered in individuals who have undergone bariatric surgery and are not compliant with the recommended vitamin B_{12} supplementation (350 µg/day sublingually plus 1000 µg IM every 3 months if needed), in individuals with pernicious anemia (an extremely uncommon autoimmune disease in women of reproductive age which is diagnosed by the presence of serum intrinsic

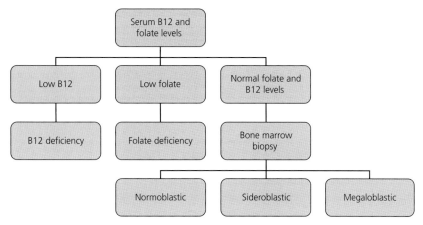

Figure 18.1 Algorithm for evaluation of macrocytic anemia.

factor antibodies), and in those with malabsorption (e.g., Crohn disease or ileal resection). *Folate deficiency* is less common nowadays given the supplementation of foods with folate. In addition to macrocytic anemia, folate deficiency often also causes thrombocytopenia. Recommended folate requirements are 400 µg/day during the pregnant state and 500 µg/day for lactating women.[7] However, higher requirements are recommended in the presence of multiple gestations, hemolytic disorders such as sickle cell anemia or thalassemia, and in patients taking antiepileptic therapies or sulfa drugs (e.g., sulfasalazine). If a diagnosis of folate deficiency is made or the woman previously had infants with neural tube defects, the recommended dose of folic acid is 4 mg/day. By 4 to 7 days after beginning treatment, the reticulocyte count is increased. In the case of macrocytic anemia with normal folate and vitamin B_{12} levels, a consultation with a hematologist is indicated for bone marrow biopsy.

Normocytic anemia
Figure 18.2 displays the pertinent laboratory workup; a reticulocyte count enables the distinguishing of cases of recent blood loss due to hemolysis (e.g., drug induced, or immune based, as witnessed by a positive direct Coombs test) or hemorrhage from the early stage of iron deficiency (see below). Low reticulocyte count with normal or high serum ferritin levels can be seen in the presence of hypothyroidism or chronic disorders, such as inflammatory bowel disease, systemic lupus erythematosus, granulomatous infections, malignant neoplasms and rheumatoid arthritis. Hematology consultation for further assessment is indicated in these circumstances.

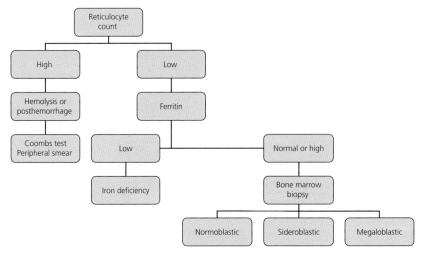

Figure 18.2 Algorithm for evaluation of normocytic anemia.

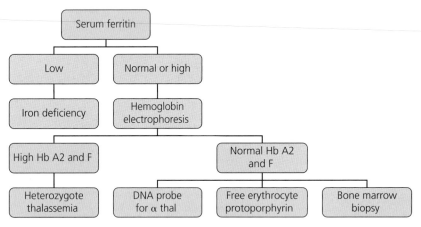

Figure 18.3 Algorithm for evaluation of microcytic anemia.

Microcytic anemia

Figure 18.3 shows the recommended flow of diagnostic workup. Because most cases of microcytic anemia in pregnancy are due to iron deficiency and because serum ferritin is an excellent indicator of body iron stores, the initial step should be assessment of serum ferritin levels. Serum ferritin is the most sensitive screening test for iron deficiency, with a level <16 ng/mL indicating depleted iron stores.[1]

Prophylaxis of iron deficiency

In a typical singleton gestation, maternal iron requirements (related to the expansion of the maternal RBC mass, fetal and placental requirements) average 1 g over the course of pregnancy. In a landmark study of healthy, non-anemic, menstruating young women who agreed to bone marrow biopsy, 66% had inadequate iron stores.[8] For the above reasons, and because gastrointestinal side effects of oral iron supplementation (constipation, nausea and diarrhea) are negligible with doses < 45–60 mg,[9] in the United States supplementation with elemental iron (30 mg/day) is recommended for all pregnant non-anemic women.[7] The prophylaxis should be continued until 3 months postpartum in areas with high prevalence of anemia. Despite such recommendations, a large study has shown that 50% of women have serum ferritin levels below 16 ng/mL by 26 weeks of pregnancy.[10] A review of randomized clinical trials (most performed in Western countries) shows that routine supplementation in non-anemic women results in higher maternal Hb levels at term and 1 month postpartum, higher serum ferritin levels, lower rates of anemia at term (RR = 0.26) and of iron deficiency anemia in particular (RR = 0.33), and higher serum ferritin levels in the infants. However no differences are noted in most clinical outcomes, such as preterm delivery, preeclampsia, or need for transfusion, birthweight, small for gestational age, perinatal mortality or need for NICU admissions.[9]

Treatment of iron deficiency anemia

Higher doses of iron are required for therapy of anemia than for prophylaxis (up to 120–150 mg/day). Table 18.2 lists the most commonly available formulations of *oral iron*. Enteric coated forms should be avoided because they are poorly absorbed; absorption is increased by intake of iron on an empty stomach and with vitamin C or orange juice. Although several trials have been conducted to compare the types of iron, it is not possible to assess the efficacy of the treatments due to the use of different drugs, doses and routes.[11] Gut absorption of iron decreases with increasing doses of iron: divide the total daily dose into 2–3 doses. A relationship is present between dose of oral iron and gastrointestinal side effects. Occurrence of such side effects leads to discontinuation of the therapy in 50% of women.[12] To ensure patients' compliance it is thus important to minimize the side effects: (1) prescribe ferric iron, which seems to have fewer side effects than ferrous fumarate or ferrous sulfate;[12] (2) increase the doses of iron gradually; (3) instruct the patient to take the large doses at bedtime. Stool softeners may be needed to prevent constipation. Serum reticulocyte count can be checked after 7–10 days of therapy to document appropriate response. The rate of increase of hematocrit is typically slow, and it increases about 1% per week. To replenish iron stores, oral therapy should be continued for 3 months after the anemia has been corrected.

Table 18.2 Oral preparations for therapy of iron deficiency anemia

Type of iron	Elemental iron (mg)	Brand
Ferrous fumarate	64–200	Femiron, Feostat, Ferrets, Fumasorb, Hemocyte, Ircon, Nephro-Fer, Vitron-C
Ferrous sulfate	40–65	Chem-Sol, Fe50, Feosol, Fergensol, Ferinsol, Ferogradumet, Ferosul, Ferratab, FerraTD, Ferrobob, Ferrospace, Ferrotime, Moliron, Slowfe, Yieronia
Ferrous gluconate	38	Fergon, Ferralet, Simron
Ferrous fumarate and ferrous asparto-glycinate	81	Replica 21/7
Ferric	50–150	Ferrimin, Fe-Tinic, Hytinic, Niferex, Nu-iron

Intravenous iron is more effective than oral therapy at improving hematological indices, with higher maternal Hb levels at 4 weeks of therapy and lower rates of gastrointestinal side effects.[11] However, randomized trials have not shown significant differences in need for maternal blood transfusion, neonatal birthweight, or neonatal anemia. Therefore IV therapy is indicated only in cases of severe anemia with intolerance to oral therapy or malabsorption.[13] Different formulations of IV iron are available: Dextran iron (INFeD®) is associated with side effects in 8.7% of cases, including delayed serum sickness reactions, fever, urticaria, and anaphylactic reactions leading to maternal death. The profile of ferric gluconate (Ferrlecit®) is safer, which has only 2% of side effects and no recorded cases of anaphylaxis.[13] Iron sucrose (Venofer®) has also been recently introduced onto the market. The required dose of IV iron can be calculated according to the formula:

IV iron dose (mg) = blood volume (dL) $\times$ Hb deficit (g/dL) $\times$ 3.3

in which the blood volume can be estimated as 65 mL $\times$ weight/100; the Hb deficit as the difference between the observed and desired Hb level (usually 12 g/dL); and 3.3 reflects the amount of iron in each gram of Hb.

Erythropoietin is not indicated in the treatment of iron deficiency anemia unless the anemia is caused by chronic renal failure or other chronic conditions, such as those outlined above among causes of normocytic anemias with low reticulocyte count and normal or high serum ferritin levels. Erythropoietin is an expensive medication with risk of side effects, ranging from flu-like illness to pure red cell aplasia.

Blood transfusion is indicated only for anemia associated with hypovolemia from blood loss or in preparation for a cesarean delivery in the presence of severe anemia.

References

1 Centers for Disease Control and Prevention. CDC criteria for anemia in children and childbearing-aged women. *MMWR* 1989;38:400.
2 Viteri FE. The consequences of iron deficiency and anemia in pregnancy. *Adv Exp Med Biol* 1994;352:127.
3 Kadyrov M, Kosanke G, Kingdom J, *et al.* Increased fetoplacental angiogenesis during first trimester in anaemic women. *Lancet* 1998;352:1747.
4 Klebanoff MA, Shiono PH, Selby JV, et al. Anemia and spontaneous preterm birth. *Am J Obstet Gynecol* 1991;164:59.
5 Lieberman E, Ryan KJ, Monson RR, *et al.* Risk factors accounting for racial differences in the rate of premature birth. *N Engl J Med* 1987;317:743.
6 Scanlon KS, Yip R, Schieve LA, *et al* High and low hemoglobin levels during pregnancy: differential risk for preterm birth and small for gestational age. *Obstet Gynecol* 2000;96:741.
7 American College of Obstetricians and Gynecologists. Clinical management guidelines for obstetrician-gynecologists. Practice Bulletin #44, July 2003. *Obstet Gynecol* 2003;102:203.
8 Scott DE, Pritchard JA. Iron deficiency in healthy young college women. *JAMA* 1967;199:147.
9 Pena-Rosas JP, Viteri FE. Effects of routine oral iron supplementation with or without folic acid for women during pregnancy. Cochrane Pregnancy and Childbirth Group. *Cochrane Database Syst Rev* 2009;(3).
10 Goldenberg RL, Tamura T, DuBard M, *et al.* Plasma ferritin and pregnancy outcome. *Am J Obstet Gynecol* 1996;175:1356.
11 Reveiz L, Gyte GML, Cuervo LG. Treatments for iron-deficiency anaemia in pregnancy. Cochrane Pregnancy and Childbirth Group. *Cochrane Database Syst Rev* 2009;(3).
12 Melamed N, Ben-Haroush A, Kaplan B, Yogev Y. Iron supplementation in pregnancy – does the preparation matter? *Arch Gynecol Obstet* 2007;276:601–4.
13 Faich G, Strobos J. Sodium ferric gluconate complex in sucrose: safer intravenous iron therapy than iron dextrans. *Am J Kidney Dis* 1999;33(3):464–70.

Sickle Cell Disease and other Hemoglobinopathies

John C. Morrison and Marc R. Parrish

Department of Obstetrics and Gynecology, University of Mississippi Medical Center, Jackson, MS, USA

Clinical significance

In the United States, sickle cell anemia affects about 70,000 people. It mainly affects African Americans but has also been observed in Hispanic Americans. It is a common genetic disease and frequently complicates pregnancy management. Patients with hemoglobin S-S (Hgb S-S), as well as with other variants, such as hemoglobin S-C (Hgb S-C) and hemoglobin S-β thalassemia (Hgb S-β Thal), are said to have sickle cell disease and this is most often responsible for adverse effects on the mother, fetus and newborn. Sickle cell disease has a significant prevalence in the African-American population, with 1 in 12 possessing the sickle cell trait. Among this same population, the frequency of sickle cell anemia (Hgb S-S) is 1 in 500, while clinically significant Hgb-SC occurs at a rate of 1 in 852. Hgb S-β Thal is somewhat less frequent, with a known prevalence of 1 in 1672.

Approximately 2 million Americans are carriers of the sickle cell trait (Hgb A-S) which has been considered to be an essentially benign condition during pregnancy, with few exceptions. However, its identification is important in offering complete genetic counseling to patients. In addition, it has been associated with twice the rate of urinary tract infections during pregnancy when compared with matched controls. More recently some have suggested that women with Hgb A-S have an increased risk for placental abnormalities resulting in stillbirth and growth restriction.

Anemia and vaso-occlusive episodes are characteristic of sickle cell diseases. Hemoglobin S-thalassemia (Hgb S-Thal) usually results in only a mild anemia, although its manifestations are variable based on the percentage of Hgb S present. Hemoglobin S-S has been associated with increased complications such as preeclampsia, preterm labor, premature preterm rupture of

Protocols for High-Risk Pregnancies, 5th edition. Edited by J.T. Queenan, J.C. Hobbins and C.Y. Spong. © 2010 Blackwell Publishing Ltd.

membranes, intrauterine growth restriction, antepartum admission, spontaneous abortion and stillbirth. Hemoglobin S-C disease has similarly been linked to intrauterine growth restriction and antepartum admission.

Pathophysiology

Both Hgb S-S and Hgb S-C are hemoglobinopathies characterized by autosomal recessive defects in the structure and function of the hemoglobin molecule. Sickle hemoglobin results from a gene mutation that substitutes a valine for glutamic acid at the sixth position in the hemoglobin beta-subunit. A missense mutation leading to the substitution of lysine in the sixth position results in hemoglobin C disease. These structurally abnormal molecules function normally in the presence of adequate oxygenation. However, in the presence of relative hypoxia, the substituted amino acid forms a hydrophobic bond with adjacent chains, forming tetramers that strand and buckle the cell wall. This structural change is responsible for the characteristic sickle shape. Hypoxia may be initiated by infection and/or exacerbated by extremes in temperature, acidosis and dehydration, all of which contribute to the abnormal, elongated sickle shape of the red blood cell. These malformed red blood cells may precipitate microvascular occlusion, resulting in further hypoxia, and ultimately tissue infarction. The hyperviscosity of pregnancy contributes to the process, and significant maternal and fetal morbidity may ensue. The life of the deformed red blood cell is only 12 days, significantly shorter than a normal circulating red cell (120 days). This results in a state of chronic anemia and increased clearance of the cells by the reticuloendothelial system.

Diagnosis

While universal screening of pregnant patients for hemoglobinopathies is not recommended, certain ethnic groups are known to carry a higher risk for these hemoglobinopathies and will benefit from testing. Individuals of African, Southeast Asian and Mediterranean descent should be offered carrier screening. In addition, any patient with a family history of a hemoglobinopathy should be tested. Cultural groups considered to be at low risk for hemoglobinopathies include the Japanese, Koreans, Native Americans and northern Europeans.

Solubility tests (Sickledex) alone are inadequate for the diagnosis of sickle cell disorders because they cannot distinguish between the heterozygous AS and homozygous SS genotypes. In addition, they fail to detect other pathological variants such as Hgb C trait, thalassemia trait, Hgb E trait,

Hgb B trait and Hgb D trait. However, solubility tests are still useful in situations when a rapid test result could alter immediate clinical management. Those patients who are considered high risk for being carriers of a hemoglobinopathy should undergo a hemoglobin electrophoresis initially. Patients with anemia and a below normal mean corpuscular volume (MCV) should also be evaluated with a hemoglobin electrophoresis in addition to serum iron studies. If a hemoglobinopathy is identified, the partner should be appropriately tested. If he is found to be affected, antenatal diagnosis may be offered in the form of DNA-based testing utilizing amniocentesis, chorionic villus sampling, or cordocentesis. These testing modalities should only be offered after counseling by the obstetrician or a genetic counselor.

There is significant variability in the course of sickle cell disease, with some experiencing frequent crises, debilitating complications and even death, while others are relatively asymptomatic. The variable clinical symptoms with which these patients present are not fully explained. There is evidence to suggest that this variability may be related to the presence of linked and unlinked genes which modify the disease expression. Another theory has been that of incomplete penetrance. The life expectancies for sickle cell anemia has also increased, approaching 42 for males and 48 for females, while those with Hgb S-C are significantly higher at 60 and 68 years, respectively.

Treatment

Maternal-fetal morbidity and mortality have decreased markedly over the last three decades because of improvements in the general medical care of sickle cell patients, improvements in transfusion medicine and advancements in neonatal care. Controversy exists concerning the role of transfusion during pregnancy. While its benefit may be questionable in the uncomplicated pregnancy, transfusions have been found to lower the incidence of painful crises in pregnancies affected by vaso-occlusive episodes. Exchange transfusions are usually reserved for women with complications such as acute chest syndrome, stroke, severe anemia, or pain crises increasing in severity or frequency. Transfusions may be beneficial in women with recurrent pregnancy losses or those with multiple gestations to maintain a hemoglobin level above 9 g/dL. Regardless, patients with sickle cell disease require more frequent prenatal evaluations, usually every 1–2 weeks. The patient should also be monitored closely for early signs of infections or the onset of a vaso-occlusive crisis. Due to a lack of sufficient evidence in women with sickle cell trait, routine

obstetrical management with monthly urinalysis is the only recommendation at this time.

Management protocol for sickle cell

1 Confirm the diagnosis and recommend testing for the partner.
2 Genetic counseling should be offered and the patient should be
   apprised of the expected course of pregnancy.
3 Discontinue hydroxyurea ideally prior to conception. While found not
   to be teratogenic in animals, little data exists on its use during human
   pregnancy.
4 Obtain a CBC every 2 weeks. Perform iron studies to determine if
   iron deficiency is a contributing factor to the anemia. Exogenous iron
   should be given only if indicated by iron studies. The patient should
   take supplemental folic acid (4 mg/day).
5 Perform a urinalysis with culture and sensitivity in each trimester and
   in the presence of clinical symptomatology.
6 Ensure patient has received a pneumoccocal vaccination in the past
   5 years (ideally prior to conception although it is safe to administer in
   pregnancy). Influenza and hepatitis vaccinations should be documented
   and updated if needed per standard protocol.
7 Initiate weekly fetal assessments in the form of NST, or biophysical profile at 34 weeks. A baseline ultrasonography at 16–20 weeks should be
   obtained, followed by repeat sonography at 24–26 weeks, then every
   3–4 weeks until delivery, specifically targeting appropriate fetal growth.
8 Consider exchange transfusion in the presence of increasing severity
   or frequency of pain crises and in those symptomatic patients who are
   unresponsive to conservative management.
9 Observe for infection or onset of pain crisis.
10 Monitor for signs of preterm delivery or onset of preeclampsia.
11 Expect routine term delivery with cesarean reserved for obstetric indications. Supplemental oxygen and laboring in the left lateral position
   should be considered, as well as adequate hydration during prolonged
   labors.
12 Epidural anesthesia and oxytocin use is not contraindicated during
   labor.
13 Postpartum contraceptive counseling is recommended.

Complications

The frequency of previous acute vaso-occlusive painful events is usually
predictive of the events during pregnancy, although some patients may

experience an increased frequency of these episodes. Infection must be excluded when a patient presents with pain, and obstetric complications including preterm labor, preeclampsia, abruption, or pyelonephritis must be evaluated. Management is similar to non-pregnant patients, including hydration, oxygen therapy and appropriate analgesia. Conside exchange transfusion or direct transfusion for patients with preeclampsia, acute chest syndrome, worsening/severe anemia and those with increasing frequency of vaso-occlusive crises during the gestation. Should infection be suspected, sources should be actively sought and empiric antibiotics used until the etiology of the infection is identified. Acute vaso-occlusive episodes and the use of opiates can cause transient, adverse affects on the fetus, which results in abnormal non-stress tests and biophysical profiles. However, antenatal assessments should normalize as the crisis subsides. Preterm delivery and intrauterine growth restriction are more common in patients with sickle cell disease. Stillbirths are also more common in this subgroup of patients. However, this devastating complication is much less likely to occur with the utilization of serial fetal assessments and appropriate interventions.

Episodic pain associated with sickle cell disease in the gravid patient is typically attributed to bouts of occlusion in the microcirculation. Many healthcare providers caring for pregnant women with sickle cell disease are not familiar with the severe, chronic pain that is associated with long-standing disease. Permanent damage to the microcirculation secondary to years of recurrent sickle injury is the likely etiology for this affliction. Fibrosis and scarring of cartilage and bone can lead to permanent damage and, in some situations, avascular necrosis. Other tissues, by inference, suffer similar insults. In addition to analgesic medications, cognitive/behavioral therapy should be considered in order to enhance coping strategies and reduce negative thoughts. Care givers must also realize that the use of opioids for acute pain relief is not addiction, regardless of the dose or duration of time that opioids are taken. An overrepresentation of a small number of patients in the healthcare system leads many providers to conclude that drug-seeking behavior is a problem for most patients with sickle cell disease. The denial of opioids to patients with sickle cell disease due to fear of addiction is unwarranted and can lead to inadequate treatment.

Many other maternal organ systems can be adversely affected by sickle cell disease, leading to other significant morbidities. These ramifications include biliary stasis, cholelithiasis, cholecystitis, osteomyelitis, high-output cardiac failure, cardiomegaly, left ventricular hypertrophy and pulmonary hypertension. A low threshold for consultation with appropriate specialists to assist in the management of these patients throughout their pregnancies is warranted.

Follow-up

Following delivery, continued surveillance for crises, thrombotic events and infection is imperative. Contraceptive options include permanent sterilization, progestin-only pills, or medroxyprogersterone (Depo-Provera). Intrauterine devices are less desirable options due to the increased risk of infection in this subgroup of patients. Randomized controlled trials do not exist to contraindicate combination oral contraceptives, but other methods are preferable.

Future directions

Research goals include improving diagnostic and treatment capabilities and a continuing search for a possible cure. Preimplantation genetic diagnosis has been successful in diagnosing affected embryos, allowing affected parents with the trait or disease the option to forego embryo implantation. Free fetal DNA found in the maternal circulation is being investigated as a source for fetal genetic testing for the defect, to replace invasive procedures such as chorionic villus sampling, amniocentesis or cordocentesis. Gene therapy is a continual source of investigation, attempting to introduce genes into the hematopoietic system capable of producing HgbA molecules. Currently bone marrow transplants are the only cure, though the complications are significant and matched donors rare. Improvements in the process of bone marrow donation and transplantation continue. These include the collection of sibling donor cord blood for stem cell transplantation, allowing marrow transplants without undergoing painful marrow harvesting. Finally, attempts to transplant hematopoietic stem cells in utero are being evaluated as a potential antenatal therapy, avoiding postnatal stem cell transplantation.

Suggested reading

American College of Obstetricians and Gynecologists. Hemoglobinopathies in pregnancy. Practice Bulletin #78. *Obstet Gynecol* 2007;109:229–37.

National Institutes of Health, National Heart, Lung, and Blood Institute. Division of Blood Diseases and Resources. *The Management of Sickle Cell Disease*. NIH Publication No. 02–2117, June 2002.

Villers MS, Jamison MG, De Castro LM, James AH. Morbidity associated with sickle cell disease in pregnancy. *Am J Obstet Gynecol* 2008;199:125.e1–5.

Sun PM, Wilburn W, Raynor D, Jamieson D. Sickle cell disease in pregnancy: twenty years of experience at Grady Memorial Hospital, Atlanta, GA. *Am J Obstet Gynecol* 2001;184:1127–30.

Rees DC, Olunjohungbe AD, Parker NE, Stephens AD, Telfer P, Wright J. Guidelines for the management of the acute painful crisis in sickle cell disease. British Committee for Standards in Haematology. General Haematology Task Force by the Sickle Cell Working Party. *Br J Haematol* 2003;120:744–52.

Benjamin LJ, Dampier CD, Jacox AK, *et al. Guideline for the Management of Acute and Chronic Pain in Sickle-Cell Disease.* Acute Pain Society Clinical Practice Guidelines Series, No. 1. Glenview, IL, 1999.

Hassell K. Pregnancy and sickle cell disease. *Hematol Oncol Clin N Am* 2005;19:903–16.

Austin H, Lally C, Benson JM, Whitsett C, Hooper C, Key NS. Hormonal contraception, sickle cell trait, and risk for venous thromboembolism among African American women. *Am J Obstet Gynecol* 2009;200:620.e1–3.

Isoimmune Thrombocytopenia

Sreedhar Gaddipati and Richard L. Berkowitz

Columbia University Medical Center, Department of Obstetrics and Gynecology, Division of Maternal Fetal Medicine, New York, NY, USA

Overview

Isoimmune or idiopathic thrombocytopenic purpura (ITP) is an autoimmune disorder where antiplatelet antibodies cause destruction of platelets by the reticuloendothelial system (RES). Acute ITP is usually self limiting and occurs predominantly in children, most often following a viral illness. The chronic form is more common in women than men and the peak incidence occurs in the third decade of life. It is estimated that ITP complicates 1 to 2 of every 1,000 pregnancies.

Pathophysiology

The autoantibodies are usually immunoglobulin G (IgG) and are directed against platelet specific membrane glycoproteins. Antigen-antibody complexes are removed from the circulation by the RES, primarily the spleen, resulting in decreased circulating platelets. The rate of platelet destruction is greater than the rate of platelet production in the bone marrow leading to thrombocytopenia.

Since platelet counts have been included in automated complete blood count (CBC) reports and since this test is routine in pregnancy, an increased incidence of thrombocytopenia has been noted in pregnant patients. Many women with mild thrombocytopenia noted late in gestation are misdiagnosed as having ITP when they actually have gestational thrombocytopenia. In this mild disorder, C3 (activated complement) rather than IgG binds to platelets. Platelet counts usually remain above 70,000/μL and normalize within 2 to 12 weeks postpartum. These patients are generally asymptomatic without a previous history of decreased platelets except perhaps in

---

Protocols for High-Risk Pregnancies, 5th edition. Edited by J.T. Queenan, J.C. Hobbins and C.Y. Spong. © 2010 Blackwell Publishing Ltd.

previous pregnancies. The recurrence risk of gestational thrombocytopenia is unknown. The risk for neonatal thrombocytopenia is negligible.

While the majority of women with ITP will have a history of easy bruising, petechiae, epistaxis, and gingival bleeding, some are asymptomatic. Maternal hemorrhage rarely occurs unless the platelet count is <10,000 to 20,000/μL. Pregnancy is not thought to increase the incidence of, or to worsen, ITP. However, ITP may have a profound impact on pregnancy as severe thrombocytopenia places the mother at risk for hemorrhage in both the antepartum and postpartum periods. ITP may also affect pregnancy as there is a small risk that it may be associated with neonatal thrombocytopenia which places the neonate at risk for poor outcomes such as intracranial hemorrhage and subsequent long-term adverse neurologic outcomes.

Maternal antiplatelet IgG antibody can cross the placenta, bind to fetal platelets, and enhance the destruction of fetal platelets resulting in transient neonatal thrombocytopenia. There is an approximately 10% risk that the neonate will have a platelet count <50,000/μL and a less than 5% risk that the neonate will have a platelet count of <20,000/μL. Neonatal platelet counts of <50,000/μL can result in minor bleeding such as purpura, ecchymoses, and melena. Rarely, fetal thrombocytopenia associated with ITP can lead to intracranial hemorrhage irrespective of mode of delivery. Serious bleeding complications are thought to be <3%, and the rate of intracranial hemorrhage is thought to be <1%, which is greater than the risk among neonates born to women without ITP. The actual incidence of neonatal thrombocytopenia and associated hemorrhage is uncertain as no large scale studies exist. The correlation between maternal and fetal platelet count is poor, and no noninvasive method is currently available to detect neonates at risk. It is thought that women with a history of splenectomy, a platelet count of <50,000/μL at some time during the pregnancy, and a previous child with neonatal thrombocytopenia are at increased risk for fetal/neonatal thrombocytopenia. Circulating antibodies also may be associated with increased fetal risk. Maternal administration of steroids and or intravenous gamma globulin has no demonstrable therapeutic effect on the fetal platelet count.

Diagnosis

ITP is a diagnosis of exclusion as there are no specific diagnostic tests or pathognomic signs or symptoms for the disorder.

Exclude other causes of decreased platelets in pregnancy such as:

1. HELLP
2. Drug reaction
3. Lab error

4. Systemic lupus erythematosus
5. Antiphospholipid antibody
6. Lymphoproliferative disorder
7. Human immunodeficiency virus infection
8. Hypersplenism
9. Disseminated intravascular coagulation
10. Thrombotic thrombocytopenic purpura
11. Hemolytic uremic syndrome
12. Congenital thrombocytopenia
13. Gestational thrombocytopenia

Diagnostic criteria include:
1. Normal CBC with the exception of persistent thrombocytopenia (platelet count <100,000/μL)
2. Peripheral smear may show decreased number of platelets, with presence of large platelets .
3. Normal coagulation studies.
4. Absence of splenomegaly.
5. No other causes of thrombocytopenia.
6. Antiplatelet antibodies may or may not be detectable.
7. Bone marrow aspirate (not essential for diagnosis) shows normal or increased number of megakaryocytes.

Antepartum Management

Pregnant women with a history of ITP require serial assessment of their platelet counts as these counts many fluctuate during pregnancy. Monthly testing is suggested for the first two trimesters. In the third trimester, patients should be tested every other week and then weekly as they approach term. Consultation with a physician who is experienced with ITP is suggested. Pregnant women with ITP and thrombocytopenia should be encouraged to restrict their activity and to avoid trauma, alcohol, aspirin, and all medications that are platelet inhibitors. They should also avoid intramuscular injections, and treat fevers with acetaminophen.

The goal of therapy in pregnant patients with ITP is to decrease the risk of bleeding complications associated with severe thrombocytopenia. Platelet function is usually normal despite decreased numbers of platelets. Thus, maintaining a normal platelet count in these patients is not necessary.

The general consensus is that treatment is not required unless the platelet count is significantly less than 50,000/μL, or if the patient is symptomatic. However, counts greater than 50,000/μL may be desired at delivery and for regional anesthesia. It is important to note that treatment is indicated for the maternal status and not for fetal indications, as these therapies have not been proven to decrease the risks of neonatal thrombocytopenia and subsequent hemorrhage. The initial treatment for ITP is prednisone 1 mg/kg orally once per day. Improvement in platelet count is usually noted within 3 to 7 days. The maximal response is usually noted within 2 to 3 weeks. The dose can be increased as necessary. Once the platelet count has increased to an acceptable level, the dosage can be tapered by 10-20% until the lowest dose required to maintain the platelet count at an acceptable level is determined.

Intravenous immune globulin (IVIG) may be warranted if the patient remains refractory to oral steroids, the platelet count is <10,000/μL, or if the platelet count is <30,000/μL and the patient is symptomatic or predelivery. A response may be noted anywhere from 6 to 72 hours following administration of IVIG. If IVIG is being considered, consultation with a physician familiar with this treatment is recommended. In cases of continued resistance, high dose IV steroids (methyl prednisolone) in conjunction with IVIG or azothioprine may be considered.

If there is no response to IVIG, splenectomy should be considered. Removal of the spleen removes the primary site of platelet destruction and antibody production. Splenectomy has been associated with complete remission of ITP, but has not consistently been found to be beneficial in patients who fail IVIG therapy. While splenectomy can be performed safely in pregnancy, the procedure should be avoided if possible as it is technically difficult and may incur fetal risks. The procedure may be warranted in pregnancy if platelet counts are <10,000/μL and the patient has failed both prednisone and IVIG therapy. The optimal timing for splenectomy is the second trimester. If deemed necessary in the third trimester, cesarean delivery followed by the splenectomy should be considered. In addition to the flu vaccine, pregnant women with a history of splenectomy should be vaccinated against pneumococcus, menigococcus, and Haemophilis influenzae.

Platelet transfusion should only be utilized as a temporizing measure for severe hemorrhage or to help prepare a patient for surgery. Donor platelets do not survive for long periods of time in women with ITP. The medications commonly used to treat ITP in non-obstetric patients such as colchicines, vinca alkaloids, cyclophosphamide, danazol and other potentially teratogenic agents are avoided in pregnancy as they are thought to have adverse effects on the fetus.

Intrapartum Management

The most significant clinical dilemma relating to ITP is the fact that the fetus may be at risk for neonatal thrombocytopenia and for severe bleeding complications. The risk is small, and unfortunately, there is no test which can accurately discern if a fetus is at risk for severe thrombocytopenia. At the present time, obtaining a fetal platelet count prior to delivery is not thought to be necessary. Scalp sampling during labor is often inaccurate and technically challenging. Cordocentesis prior to labor involves a 1–2% risk of emergent cesarean delivery secondary to complications. Vaginal delivery is not contraindicated in these patients and cesarean delivery is not thought to protect these patients from fetal bleeding complications. Thus, routine obstetric management is appropriate for pregnant women with ITP. However, fetal scalp electrodes and delivery by vacuum should be avoided. Anti-platelet medications such as nonsteroidal inflammatory drugs (NSAIDs) should not be prescribed to these patients during the postpartum period. Breast feeding is safe for women with a history of ITP.

Consultation with anesthesia is appropriate for patients with ITP. Neuraxial anesthesia (spinal or epidural) is generally safe in women with platelet counts >80,000/μL provided that coagulation studies are normal. The risk of epidural hematoma with neuraxial anesthesia is exceedingly low in patients with functional platelets and platelet counts >100,000/μL. The risk does not increase significantly until the platelet count falls below 50,000 to 75,000/μL. However, there are no good data on outcomes with these counts, and a summary of observational studies have not revealed any hemorrhagic complications due to neuraxial anesthesia with platelet counts between 50,000–100,000/μL. Generally, neuraxial anesthesia is avoided in patients with platelet counts <50,000/μL as the risk of hematoma is believed to be greater than acceptable. Stability of the platelet count weighs significantly in the decision to proceed with neuraxial anesthesia. Thromboelastogram testing is not routinely available and thus has a limited role in assessing adequate clot formation. In patients with platelet counts between 50,000 and 100,000/μL, there should be consultation between the obstetrician and anesthesiologist and a unified risk/benefit analysis should be presented to the patient

It is recommended that these women deliver in a hospital where all physicians caring for the patient including the obstetrician, anesthesiologist, and pediatrician are familiar with ITP, and where potential maternal and neonatal complications can be adequately handled. The infant's platelet count should be monitored through the first few days of life as thrombocytopenia may develop in the postpartum period. Head ultrasound should be performed if the neonate was born with, or develops thrombocytopenia.

Conclusion

In summary, ITP is a relatively rare disease in pregnancy which is a diagnosis of exclusion. For the most part, maternal and fetal outcomes are favorable. Serial platelet counts are suggested. Consultation with a physician familiar with the care of these patients is often warranted. Platelet counts significantly <50,000/μL should be considered for treatment, especially in preparation for intrapartum management. Likewise, symptomatic patients require treatment. Prednisone is the first line therapy. IVIG may be necessary for refractory cases. Splenectomy is reserved for severe cases refractory to other treatments. While up to 10% of neonates may be diagnosed with neonatal thrombocytopenia, the risk for severe complications such as neonatal intracranial hemorrhage is thought to be <1%. Delivery in a center familiar with this disorder and the potential maternal and neonatal complications is advised. Vaginal delivery is not thought to place these patients at increased risk for fetal intracranial hemorrhage and elective cesarean delivery has not been proven to be protective. As a result, routine obstetric management is appropriate for the majority of these patients. However, fetal scalp electrodes and delivery by vacuum should be avoided. The use of medications such as NSAIDs are not recommended so as to avoid interfering with the function of available platelets.

Suggested reading

American College of Obstetricians and Gynecologists. Practice Bulletin. *Thrombocytopenia in Pregnancy.* Practice Bulletin #6, September 1999. Reaffirrmed in 2009.

Burrows R, Kelton J. Low fetal risks in pregnancies associated with idiopathic thrombocytopenic purpura. *Am J Obstet Gynecol* 1990;163:1147–50.

Burrows R, Kelton J. Fetal thrombocytopenia and its relation to maternal thrombocytopenia. *N Engl J Med* 1993;329;1463–67.

Cines DB, McMillan R. Management of adult idiopathic thrombocytopenic purpura. *Annu Rev Med* 2005;56:425–42.

Choi S, Brull, R. Neuraxial techniques in obstetric and non-obstetric patients with common bleeding diatheses. *Anesth Analgesia* 2009;109:648–60.

Clark AL, Gall SA. Clinical uses of intravenous immunoglobulin in pregnancy. *Am J Obstet Gynecol* 1997;176:241–53.

Payne SD, Resnik R, Moore TR, Hedriana HL, Kelly TF. Maternal characteristics and risk of severe neonatal thrombocytopenia and intracranial hemorrhage in pregnancies complicated by autoimmune thrombocytopenia. *Am J Obstet Gynecol* 1997;177:149–55.

Samuels P, Bussel J, Baitman L, *et al.* Estimation of the risk of thrombocytopenia in the offspring of pregnant women with presumed immune thrombocytopenic purpura. *N Engl J Med* 1990;323:229–35.

Valet AS, Caulier MT, Devos P, *et al.* Relationships between severe neonatal thrombocytopenia and maternal characteristics in pregnancies associated with autoimmune thrombocytopenia. *Br J Haematol* 1998;103:397–401.

Webert KE, Mittal R, Sigouin C, *et al.* A retrospective 11-year analysis of obstetric patients with idiopathic thrombocytopenic purpura. *Blood* 2003;102:4306–11.

PROTOCOL 21

Autoimmune Disease

Charles J. Lockwood

Department of Obstetrics, Gynecology and Reproductive Sciences, Yale University School of Medicine, New Haven, CT, USA

Systemic lupus erythematosus

Overview

Systemic lupus erythematosus (SLE) complicates 1 in 2000 to 1 in 5000 pregnancies, with a five-fold increase in prevalence among African-American women. SLE is associated with multiple pregnancy complications, including spontaneous abortion, intrauterine fetal demise (IUFD), intrauterine growth restriction (IUGR), fetal distress, preeclampsia and both spontaneous or indicated preterm deliveries (PTDs).

Pathophysiology

The disease is caused by abnormal humoral antibody response that causes the production of antibodies that cross-react with a variety of tissues in genetically susceptible individuals (Fig. 21.1). It is unclear whether this overproduction of antibodies is caused by (1) the non-specific activation of B-lymphocytes (polyclonal B-cell activation) or (2) the creation of immunogenic antibodies against specific neoantigens after an environmental or infectious trigger. These antibodies cause damage by (1) forming non-specific antibody–antigen (Ab-Ag) complexes, whose resultant inflammation causes glomerulonephritides, arthritis, dermatitis, central nervous system (CNS) involvement, pericarditis, pneumonitis and hepatitis; or (2) antibodies directed against cell-specific antigens that cause isolated cell or tissue damage (e.g., autoimmune thrombocytopenia [ATP], hemolytic anemia [HA], antiphospholipid antibody syndrome [APAS], leukopenia [LPn], vasculitis and/or neonatal congenital heart block [CHB]). The risk of developing a specific manifestation is linked to a patient's HLA-DR and HLA-DQ histocompatability loci. A third theory has emerged with direct implication in pregnancy outcome, namely the activation of complement by APAS causing vascular inflammation and vascular changes within the fetus and placenta.

Protocols for High-Risk Pregnancies, 5th edition. Edited by J.T. Queenan, J.C. Hobbins and C.Y. Spong. © 2010 Blackwell Publishing Ltd.

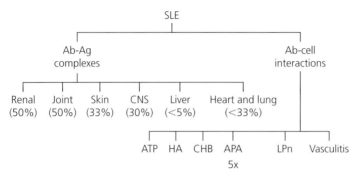

Figure 21.1 Pathogenesis of SLE primary immunoregulatory dysfunction.

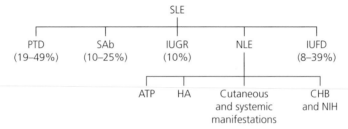

Figure 21.2 SLE effects on fetus.

Effect of SLE on pregnancy

The prognosis for a live birth depends on four factors: the activity of the disease at conception and the occurrence of subsequent flares during pregnancy, the coexistence of lupus nephritis, development of APAS, and the presence of anti-SSA (Ro) antibodies (Fig. 21.2).

1 *Lupus flares* occur in 50% of patients and are more common in the first trimester. Patients in remission for 6 months prior to conception and throughout pregnancy have a 90% live birth rate, while those undergoing a flare during pregnancy have a 65% live birth rate.

2 Clinical evidence of *glomerulonephritis* is present in 50% of SLE patients, while histological evidence is present in 90% of patients. Subtypes include (i) mesangial nephritis (better prognosis), (ii) membranous nephritis (better prognosis), (iii) focal proliferative nephritis (poor prognosis), and (iv) diffuse proliferative nephritis (poor prognosis). Clinically evident nephrotic syndrome is associated with a 60% live birth rate. However, the development of hypertension (25%) or kidney failure as evidenced by elevation in the serum creatinine to greater than 1.5 mg/dL lowers live birth rates to 50%. The presence of severe hypertension or renal failure is associated with a 20% live birth rate.

3 *APAS* (25% of SLE patients) causes second and third trimester fetal death, IUGR, preeclampsia and maternal thromboembolic phenomenon. Patients with SLE and APAS have up to a 70% risk of recurrent pregnancy loss if untreated. The diagnosis requires laboratory evidence of either lupus anticoagulant (LAC) or moderate to high concentrations of anticardiolipin antibodies (ACA; >20 GPL or MPL units) or >99th%ile anti-β-2-glycoportein-I IgG or IgM levels on two occasions, 12 weeks apart, together with a history of recurrent pregnancy loss, or history of thrombosis, or autoimmune thrombocytopenia.

4 *Anti-SSA (Ro) antibodies*, present in 25% of SLE patients, are associated with an HLA-DR3 haplotype. Anti-SSA antibodies cause 95% of all CHB in fetuses with normal cardiac anatomy; however, CHB will develop in only 2% of fetuses exposed to anti-SSA antibodies, generally between 18 weeks and term. The risk of CHB increases to 33% with a previously affected sibling. These antibodies are a marker for the development of immunoglobulin G (IgG)-mediated fetal cardiomyopathy, nonimmune hydrops (NIH), and related stillbirths. Anti-SSA antibodies are also a marker for the development of neonatal lupus [NLE], which manifests as transient lupus dermatitis, systemic and hematological abnormalities (HA and ATP), and/or CHB in the neonate. Congenital SLE is far more common in female neonates (14:1 for cutaneous and systemic involvement and 2:1 for isolated CHB). The lesions generally appear within 6 weeks of birth and persist for 1 year. Most SLE patients with anti-La/SSB antibodies will also have detectable anti-Ro/SSA antibodies; thus it is difficult to discern the independent risk attributable to SSB antibodies.

Diagnosis

Patients generally present with intermittent, unexplained fevers, malaise, arthralgias, myositis, serositis, thrombocytopenia, nephritis and/or CNS abnormalities. A positive antinuclear antibody (ANA) is found in 98% of patients (and 10–20% of uncomplicated pregnant patients). The diagnosis is established when *four or more* of the following American College of Rheumatology criteria are present:

1 Malar rash.

2 Discoid rash.

3 Photosensitivity.

4 Oral ulcers.

5 Non-erosive arthritis.

6 Pleuritis or pericarditis.

7 Renal disease manifested by proteinuria >500 mg/day, 3+ urine protein, and/or cellular casts on urinalysis.

8 Neurological abnormalities including seizures or psychosis.

9 Hematological abnormalities: including HA with reticulocytosis, ATP with platelet counts <100,000/mm³ in the absence of offending drugs, or two or more occurrences of leukopenia less than 4000 cells/mm³ or lymphopenia less than 1500/mm³.

10 Laboratory findings: including anti-dsDNA, anti-Sm, or positive finding of antiphospholipid antibodies (anticardiolipin antibody IgG or IgM, lupus anticoagulant, or a false-positive RPR) (Table 21.1).

11 Positive antinuclear antibody test in the absence of drug therapy.

Treatment

Initial visit

It is recommended that the following be obtained at the first prenatal visit:

1 CBC with differential and platelet count.

2 24-hour urine collection: evaluation of total protein and creatinine clearance.

3 Serum creatinine.

4 Hepatic transaminases (ALT, AST).

5 LAC/ACA.

6 Indices of disease activity: ANA and anti-deoxyribonucleic acid (DNA) titers, and complement factors 3 and 4.

7 Anti-SSA (Ro)/Anti-SSB (La) antibody screen, an indicator of risk for neonatal SLE and CHB.

Antepartum management

It is recommended that the following evaluations be obtained:

1 First trimester ultrasonography to establish estimated date of delivery; first trimester aneuploidy screening is also encouraged.

Table 21.1 SLE-associated laboratory findings

Antibody	HLA	Clinical feature
Anti-ds DNA	DR2	Nephritis
	DQB1	Vasculitis
Anti-SM	DR2	Nephritis
	DQw6	CNS disease
Anti-RNP	DR4	Arthritis
	DQw8	Myositis and Raynaud's
Anti-SSA (Ro)	DR3	CHB
	DQw2.1	Sjögren syndrome
Anti-SSB (La)		Negatively associated with renal disease in SSA(+) patients
Anti-centromere		CREST syndrome
Anti-U1-RNP		Mixed connective tissue disease
LAC and ACA		APAS

2 Detailed anatomy ultrasonography and, in the presence of SSB and/or SSA antibodies, echocardiography should be performed at 18 weeks and repeated monthly in patients with SSB/SSA antibodies.

3 Monthly ultrasonography to assess fetal growth from 18 weeks; ultrasonographic assessments should be more frequent if IUGR is suspected or documented sonographically; Doppler flow studies may be useful in optimizing the timing of delivery in IUGR fetuses.

4 Office visits as often as every 2 weeks may be warranted beginning at 28 weeks.

5 Non-stress tests and/or biophysical profiles, weekly beginning at 36 weeks in uncomplicated cases or at 28 weeks and beyond given the presence of IUGR, APAS, SLE flare, worsening renal function, or hypertension.

6 24-hour urine for protein and creatinine clearance every 1–2 months, or with new-onset hypertension.

7 Fetuses with CHB should be assessed antenatally with serial ultrasounds to rule-out NIH and both antenatally and intrapartum with biophysical profiles or via non-stress testing using Doppler interrogation to determine atrial rate; pediatric cardiology consultation should occur prior to delivery.

Timing of delivery
Uncomplicated SLE
In patients with SLE in the absence of SSB/SSA antibodies, APAS, worsening nephritis/hypertension, IUGR, oligohydramnios, or superimposed preeclampsia, delivery can be delayed until 40 weeks provided that the twice-weekly fetal testing initiated at 36 weeks is reassuring.

In the presence of deteriorating maternal or fetal health
Beyond 34 weeks' gestation
Patients beyond 34 weeks with worsening renal, liver, or CNS function; hypertension; IUGR with oligohydraminos, absent or reversal of diastolic Doppler flow, cessation of fetal growth, or non-reassuring fetal testing should be promptly delivered. Cesarean delivery is reserved for usual obstetric indications. Intravenous magnesium sulfate prophylaxis should be used in the presence of superimposed preeclampsia.

At 28 to 34 weeks' gestation
Patients between 28 and 34 weeks with worsening renal or liver function, development of or exacerbation of hypertension, CNS symptoms, or uteroplacental vascular compromise should be immediately hospitalized and given appropriate medical therapy (e.g., prednisone, antihypertensives) as well as a course of antenatal steroids to enhance fetal lung maturity, and daily fetal heart rate testing or biophysical profiles. Delivery is indicated

for uncontrolled maternal hypertension, the development of severe preeclampsia, or fetal distress. The cessation of fetal growth (evaluated every 2 weeks) may be an indication for delivery after 28 weeks in the presence of severe oligohydramnios, persistent reverse diastolic Doppler flow, or both. Cesarean delivery is reserved for usual obstetric indications. Intravenous magnesium sulfate prophylaxis should be used as indicated in the presence of suspected preeclampsia or for neonatal neuroprotection.

At 24 to 28 weeks' gestation

Patients between 24 and 28 weeks with deteriorating maternal or fetal health should be immediately hospitalized with daily fetal testing using non-stress testing or biophysical profile, treated with prednisone and antihypertensives if indicated, and given antenatal steroids to enhance fetal lung maturity. Delivery is indicated for deteriorating maternal renal, cardiac, liver, or CNS function unresponsive to therapy, the development of severe preeclampsia, or for fetal distress. Again, attempts at a vaginal delivery are indicated in the absence of acute fetal distress. Intravenous magnesium sulfate prophylaxis can be used as needed.

At less than 24 weeks' gestation

Patients at less than 24 weeks' gestation with a rapidly deteriorating maternal or fetal condition that is refractory to medical therapy and bed rest should be given the option of pregnancy termination since the prognosis is poor in this setting. Patients should be cautioned, however, that the maternal condition may not improve after pregnancy termination.

Postpartum care

Because some believe a lupus flare after delivery may be more likely, patients require careful monitoring during the puerperium. Patients should be counselled to promptly report any concerning symptoms. Estrogen containing contraceptives should be avoided in the presence of APAS as they may contribute to the risk of thrombosis; progestin-only contraceptives or an intrauterine device (IUD) are possible alternatives. Any prior history of thrombosis in pregnancy or while taking a combined oral contraceptive would merit prophylactic heparin or oral anticoagulation therapy for at least 12 weeks postpartum.

Specific management problems
Antiphospholipid antibody syndrome (APAS)

The presence of LAC or moderate- to high-level ACA (IgG or IgM) in a pregnant patient with SLE (30% of cases) should be an indication for treatment with low-dose aspirin (81 mg po qd) *and* prophylactic heparin (unfractionated heparin 5000–10,000 U sq bid or low molecular weight heparin (LMWH) such as enoxaparin 40 mg once a day). Therapeutic unfractionated or low molecular weight heparin should be given if the patient has a history of thromboembolic phenomenon or prior fetal loss on prophylactic heparin or LMWH. When this regimen fails in APAS patients, consideration should be given to adding intravenous gammaglobulin (IVIG). Due to an increased risk of PPROM, heparin, not prednisone, is recommended as first-line therapy.

Patients with anti-SSA (Ro) antibodies

Patients with SLE at risk for neonatal lupus or CHB on the basis of anti-SSA antibodies should have fetal echocardiography initially performed at 18 weeks and then monthly by an experienced physician. Should the fetus demonstrate evidence of incomplete heart block or early cardiomyopathy, consideration should be given to dexamethasone therapy (4 mg po qd) or plasmapheresis with IVIG therapy, or both. The former therapy should be discontinued in the presence of oligohydramnios. Pediatricians should be alerted to the risk of neonatal SLE. Infants of mothers receiving dexamethasone therapy should be observed for evidence of hypothalamic–pituitary–adrenal axis suppression.

Lupus nephritis

Patients with kidney disease are at increased risk of gestational hypertension, preeclampsia and deterioration of renal function, as well as stillbirth, IUGR and preterm delivery. While at least one-third of SLE patients who have documented proteinuria prior to the onset of pregnancy will display increases in urinary protein loss, reversible renal dysfunction occurs in only 13% and hypertension either develops or worsens in approximately 25%. The differentiation of a lupus flare from preeclampsia (Table 21.2) poses a clinical conundrum in SLE patients. Declining levels of C3, C4 and CH50 may occur in both disorders but tend to be more severe with lupus flares. Soluble FMS-like kinase (sFLT-1) has been shown to be significantly elevated in women with preeclampsia. Additional discriminators are listed in Table 21.2. It is yet to be established whether

Table 21.2 Differentiating a lupus flare from preeclampsia

Lupus flare	Superimposed PIH
Any gestational age	Third trimester
Diffuse SLE symptoms	Preeclampsia symptoms (headache, etc.)
Normal soluble FMS-like tyrosine kinase (sFLT-1)	Significantly elevated sFLT-1
Increased anti-DNA titer	Stable anti-DNA titer
Stable platelets (if no ATP or APA)	Thrombocytopenia
Normal AST, ALT	Elevations in AST, ALT
Normal plasma fibronectin	Increased plasma fibronectin
Exacerbation postpartum	Resolution postpartum

low-dose aspirin (80 mg po qd) therapy reduces the risk of superimposed preeclampsia in SLE patients without APAS.

Generalized SLE flare

The occurrence of a lupus flare should be treated with prednisone, 60 mg/day orally for 3 weeks, with gradual tapering of the dose to 10 mg/day. Patients with evidence of membranous or diffuse glomerulonephritis should be treated with even higher doses of prednisone up to 200 mg/day and/or plasmapheresis (with IVIG or fresh frozen plasma) or azathioprine. Given the osteopenic effects of glucocorticoids, patients treated with prednisone should receive calcium supplementation. In addition, they should undergo repeated glucose screens. Stress dose steroids must be given at delivery in all SLE patients treated with >20 mg/day of prednisone or its equivalent for more than three weeks during the pregnancy or for more than 1 month in the past year. Penicillamine should probably be avoided in pregnant patients because of the risk of adverse fetal sequelae. Hydroxychloroquine may be employed for women likely to experience complications from steroids, such as those with diabetes.

There are some promising attempts to modulate the immune system in SLE patients by using such treatments as anti-B cell antibodies, IVIG, DHEA, bromocriptine, zileuton, cyclosporine, anti-CD40, LJP 394, anti-C5 complement monoclonal antibody, anti-IL-10, and immunoadsorption via perfusion of patients' blood through a column of immobilized C1q. All of these therapies are considered experimental.

Serious sequelae

In general, pregnancy does not affect the natural history of SLE. However, a relapse of SLE nephritis during pregnancy can be associated with an up to 10% prevalence of irreversible renal deterioration. SLE is associated with a 1% maternal mortality; infection (secondary to leukopenia, granulocyte dysfunction, hypocomplementemia, and functional asplenia) and renal failure are the most common causes.

Rheumatoid arthritis

Overview

Rheumatoid arthritis (RA) is the most common autoimmune disease in women of childbearing age, with a prevalence of 1 per 2000 pregnancies. Its peak incidence is at 35 to 40 years of age.

Pathophysiology

RA is associated with a HLA-D4 haplotype. It is marked by specific induction of an immune response by CD4+ T-cells, with subsequent release of cytokines and recruitment of lymphocytes and monocytes into the synovia of small joints (e.g., wrist and hand) and within other tissues. An anti-IgM or IgG rheumatoid factor (RF) complex deposition is also noted in 90% of patients. The resultant joint pain and effusions are mediated by local prostaglandin generation, and result in proteolytic degradation of the cartilage via neutrophil and synovial collagenases.

Diagnosis

Rheumatoid arthritis is primarily a clinical diagnosis that may contain the following features:

1 Rheumatoid nodules: 1 to 4 cm subcutaneous lumps over the elbows, various pressure points, lungs, and heart valves.
2 Symmetric involvement that occurs simultaneously in similar joint areas on both sides of the body.
3 Radiographic findings: characteristic changes seen on posteroanterior hand and wrist radiographs.
4 Serum rheumatoid factor (RF).
5 Associated findings can include: Felty's syndrome (a rare complication seen in long-standing RA and is associated with splenomegaly and granulocytopenia), rheumatoid vasculitis, pleuritis, pericarditis and anemia.

Effect of pregnancy on rheumatoid arthritis

Seventy-four percent of patients improve, with a 90% postpartum exacerbation rate. There is controversy whether patients having significantly greater disparity in maternal-fetal HLA-DRB1 and DQA and B antigens are more likely to remit during pregnancy.

Effect of rheumatoid arthritis on pregnancy

There appears to be no increased rate of spontaneous abortion, perinatal mortality, or IUGR in the presence of RA uncomplicated by APAS or anti-SSA/SSB antibodies.

Management

Initial treatment in pregnancy should include local steroid injections into affected joints. If the response to local measures proves inadequate, begin prednisone 5 mg every morning and 2.5 mg every evening. The utility and safety of other drugs are listed below.

1 Acetominophen: analgesic of choice.
2 Nonsteroidal anti-inflammatory agents (NSAIDs): should be avoided after 20 weeks.
3 Hydroxychloroquine: useful, but may cause rare, ocular side effects in the fetus.

4 Azathioprine: can be used if the patient is refractory to steroids.
5 Intramuscular gold salts: although unconfirmed clinically, this agent may cross the placenta creating a theoretical risk; may be useful in postpartum period to reduce exacerbations.
6 Methotrexate: not recommended during pregnancy.
7 D-Penicillamine: use in RA is contraindicated given alternative therapies.
8 Cyclophosphamide (Cytoxan): this agent is teratogenic, is only used during pregnancy when disease complications pose a dire threat to the mother. Termination of pregnancy should be offered if used before 24 weeks.

New drugs for rheumatoid arthritis
Tumor necrosis factor antagonists such as etanercept, adalimumab and infliximab are being more widely used and are in Pregnancy Category B; however, they have been linked to the development of VACTERL association in some exposed infants. Thus, there is insufficient data at present to advocate their widespread use in pregnant women. The interleukin-1 antagonist, anakinra, has similar therapeutic promise and is currently without reports of teratogenicty, though data is limited. The immunomodulatory antimetabolite leflunomide is suspected to be teratogenic (Pregnancy Category X). It has an extremely long half-life, taking up to 2 years to reach undetectable levels. As a result, it should be avoided by women of childbearing age.

Scleroderma

Overview
Scleroderma is a rare autoimmune disease associated with progressive fibrosis and vasculitides that primarily affects the skin and can be further classified into diffuse cutaneous and limited cutaneous forms. When there are systemic manifestations it is called systemic sclerosis. The course of scleroderma is unaffected by pregnancy. It does not appear to cause a higher incidence of spontaneous abortion, but is associated with a modestly higher risk of stillbirth and preterm delivery, particularly in the setting of renal disease and hypertension.

Pathophysiology
Scleroderma is characterized by an autoimmune reaction causing fibroblast stimulation that coordinates the overproduction, deposition and remodeling of collagen and other extracellular matrix proteins. This excess collagen causes thickening and hardening of the skin and other organs. Important features of the tissue lesions include early microvascular damage,

mononuclear cell infiltrates into the perivascular space, and slowly developing fibrosis. Later stages of scleroderma include densely packed collagen in the dermis, loss of cells and atrophy. Clinical manifestations include:

1 Raynaud's phenomenon
2 sclerodactyly
3 telangiectasia
4 cardiomyopathy, myocardial infarctions, and cardiac conduction abnormalities
5 calcinosis
6 dysphagia
7 renal failure.

Effect of pregnancy on scleroderma

While there are reports of maternal mortality associated with scleroderma, the use of aggressive antihypertensive therapy or dialysis, or both, renders such untoward outcomes rare. The prognosis is, however, worsened by the presence of pulmonary and malignant systemic hypertension. Use of ACE inhibitors, a cornerstone of therapy in the setting of renal disease, is contraindicated in pregnancy.

Effect of scleroderma on pregnancy

Earlier reports suggested that scleroderma was associated with high rates of perinatal mortality due to preeclampsia (35%), preterm deliveries (30%) and stillbirths (30%). However, perinatal mortality appears to have lessened with the advent of improved fetal surveillance and neonatal intensive care.

Management

The progress of mothers should be followed for evidence of deteriorating renal function and worsening hypertension. The presence of coexisting APA and anti-SSA antibodies should be assessed and, if detected, managed as described for SLE patients. Fetal surveillance should follow the paradigm outlined for SLE above. The hallmarks of scleroderma management in pregnancy include:

1 Serial assessment of 24-hour urine collection for creatinine clearance and total protein.
2 Serum creatinine in each trimester.
3 Physiotherapy for hand contractures.
4 Antihypertensive therapy (calcium channel blockers) – avoid ACE inhibitors.
5 Prednisone for concomitant myositis.
6 Antacids and metoclopramide to prevent severe reflux esophagitis.

7 Dialysis in the setting of renal failure.

8 Institution of fetal surveillance as is described for patients with SLE, including early dating ultrasonography, serial scans for growth, and non-stress tests and/or biophysical profiles weekly beginning at 36 weeks in uncomplicated cases or 28 weeks and beyond given the presence of IUGR, worsening renal function, or hypertension.

Complications

The development of malignant hypertension with or without renal failure represents the most important risk factor for maternal and perinatal mortality. Renal failure mandates dialysis while the treatment of malignant hypertension includes admission to an intensive care unit with the following recommendations for management:

1 Placement of a central line/Swan Ganz catheter (if no coagulopathy): assess cardiac output, pulmonary capillary wedge pressure, pulmonary artery pressure and systemic vascular resistance.

2 Electrocardiography (ECG)/cardiac monitor.

3 Pulse oximeter/arterial line.

4 Continuous blood pressure BP monitoring.

5 Oxygen therapy.

6 Continuous fetal monitoring if undelivered and beyond 24 weeks' gestation; antenatal steroids if between 24–34 weeks gestation.

7 Hydralazine 5–10 mg q 20 minutes or labetalol load with 20 mg I.V.S.S. over 2 minutes, may give 40–80 mg at 10-minute intervals, up to 300 mg total dose; switch to oral agents when stable (e.g., labetalol 200–300 mg q 6 h), nitroglycerine drip if these measures are ineffective.

8 Placement of Foley catheter and strict hourly intake/output assessment.

9 Laboratory studies:
   • complete blood count (CBC) with platelets and prothrombin time (PT)/partial thromboplastin time (PTT)/fibrinogen;
   • AST/ALT, creatinine, uric acid, and electrolytes;
   • type and crossmatch blood.

Rarer autoimmune disorders

Juvenile rheumatoid arthritis

Juvenile rheumatoid arthritis is also associated with an HLA-DR3 haplotype. It has a variable clinical presentation, including:

1 Still's disease (fever, leukocytosis, pleurisy, rash, hepatosplenomegaly) (10%)

2 rheumatoid-like symmetric polyarthritis (50%)

3 asymptomatic arthritis of large joints (40%).

The condition is generally (70–90%) self-limited and not associated with RF IgM or IgG. In 10% of patients there will be sequelae including micrognathia and fusion of the neck, hips and knees. Pelvic contractures can lead to feto-pelvic disproportion.

Ankylosing spondylitis and seronegative arthropathy

These disorders are associated with an HLA-B27 haplotype. They present with insidious backache and stiffness that are worse in morning. Ankylosing spondylitis (AS) and seronegative arthropathy (SNA) present as a spectrum of disorders with overlapping features. In general, the course of AS/SNA is not affected by pregnancy, and vice versa.

Polyarteritis nodosa

Polyarteritis nodosa (PAN) manifests as necrotizing angiitis of small and medium muscular arteries associated with fever, myalgias, arthralgias, hypertension, abdominal pain, mononeuropathy, myocardial infarction (MI), hematuria and hepatitis.

The diagnosis can be made on the basis of:

1 clinical presentation
2 anemia
3 eosinophilia
4 greatly increased sedimentation rate
5 positive RF and ANA
6 positive hepatitis B surface antigen and antibody
7 polyclonal elevations in IgG and IgM
8 skin biopsy.

Pregnancy in patients with PAN can be associated with hypertension and renal failure, leading to a 64% maternal mortality if the disease is active at conception. However, there is no indication to terminate pregnancy since the disease tends to worsen postpartum. In general, patients should be advised to delay conception until they are in a stable period of remission. Treatment includes steroids.

Polymyositis–dermatomyositis

Polymyositis–dermatomyositis is associated with symmetric proximal muscle weakness and a dusky erythematous eruption over the face, neck and arms with a violaceous rash over the eyelids. The diagnosis is based on:

1 elevated serum muscle enzymes: creatine phosphokinase (CPK);
2 elevated ALT/AST;
3 abnormal electromyographic findings, including the triad of poly-phase shortening of small motor unit potentials, fibrillation, and high-frequency repetitive discharges;
4 biopsy: primary degeneration of muscle fibers with basophilia, necrosis, and inflammation.

While pregnancy does not seem to affect the progression of the disorder, polymyositis–dermatomyositis appears to be associated with pregnancy complications if pregnancy occurs during a period of active disease. Therapies include steroids, physical therapy and analgesia. Aggressive fetal surveillance with serial ultrasonography to assess growth as well as fetal heart rate testing and biophysical profiles initiated at 28 to 32 weeks appears warranted.

Sjögren syndrome

Sjögren syndrome is a rare autoimmune disorder often associated with prior human T-lymphotrophic virus-7 (HTLV-7) infection that results from lymphocytic infiltration of the lacrimal and salivary glands causing keratoconjunctivitis sicca. It is frequently associated with the presence of anti-SSA antibodies and the HLA-DQw2.1 haplotype. Fetuses may be at increased risk of CHB. Pregnancy outcomes are unaffected by Sjögren syndrome if unaccompanied by coexistent SLE, APAS, CHB, fetal cardiomyopathy or neonatal lupus.

Suggested reading

Doria A, Tincani A, Lockshin M. Challenges of lupus pregnancies. *Rheumatology* (Oxford). 2008 Jun;47 Suppl 3:iii9-12. Review

Gayed M, Gordon C. Pregnancy and rheumatic diseases. *Rheumatology (Oxford)* 2007;46(11):1634–40.

Keeling SO, Oswald AE. Pregnancy and rheumatic disease: "by the book" or "by the doc". *Clin Rheumatol*. 2009 Jan;28(1):1–9. Epub 2008 Nov 6. Review

Mecacci F, Pieralli A, Bianchi B, Paidas MJ. The impact of autoimmune disorders and adverse pregnancy outcome. *Semin Perinatol* 2007;31(4):223–6.

Olsen NJ, Stein CM. New drugs for rheumatoid arthritis. *N Engl J Med* 2004;350: 2167–79.

Petri M. The Hopkins Lupus Pregnancy Center: ten key issues in management. *Rheum Dis Clin North Am*. 2007 May;33(2):227–35, v. Review

PROTOCOL 22

Acquired and Inherited Thrombophilias

Charles Lockwood and Erika Werner
Department of Obstetrics, Gynecology and Reproductive Sciences, Yale University School of Medicine, New Haven, CT, USA

Pregnancy-associated physiological changes result in a prothrombotic state that increases the risk of venous thromboembolism (VTE) by five-fold when compared to age-matched non-pregnant women. In the United States, VTE complicates 1 in 1400 pregnancies and accounts for 11% of maternal deaths, most of which occur in the postpartum period. A collection of inherited and acquired thrombophilic states place pregnant women at an even higher risk for VTE. Additionally, acquired thrombophilic states may predispose women to other adverse pregnancy outcomes such as preeclampsia, abruption, fetal growth restriction and pregnancy loss. The link between inherited thrombophilias and these adverse outcomes is unproven.

Acquired thrombophilias: antiphospholipid antibody syndrome

Overview

Acquired thrombophilias occur when individuals develop antibodies that represent self-recognition immunoglobulins directed against proteins bound to negatively charged surfaces, usually anionic phospholipids. Antiphospholipid antibody (APA) syndrome occurs when these antibodies manifest pathologically, including VTE. In fact, acquired thrombophilias are found in up to 20% of individuals with VTE. Acquired thrombophilias are also associated with fetal loss after 9 weeks' gestation, abruption, severe preeclampsia, intrauterine growth restriction (IUGR) and, possibly, recurrent embryonic losses.

Pathophysiology

There are several possible pathogenic mechanisms by which APAs induce arterial and venous thrombosis, as well as adverse pregnancy

---

Protocols for High-Risk Pregnancies, 5th edition. Edited by J.T. Queenan, J.C. Hobbins and C.Y. Spong. © 2010 Blackwell Publishing Ltd.

outcomes. These include antibody-mediated impairment of endothelial thrombomodulin and activated protein C-mediated anticoagulation, induction of endothelial tissue factor expression, impairment of fibrinolysis and antithrombin activity, and augmentation of platelet activation and/or adhesion. Additional mechanisms may include impairment of the anticoagulant effects of the anionic phospholipid binding proteins β-2-glycoprotein-I and annexin V. Recently, APA-induced complement activation in the placental bed has been suggested to play a role in fetal loss. Heparin's therapeutic value rests in both its anticoagulant and anti-inflammatory effects.

Diagnosis

Diagnosis of APA syndrome requires a history of:
- thrombosis in any tissue or organ except superficial venous thrombosis;
- at least one fetal death at or beyond the tenth week of gestation;
- at least one premature birth at or before the thirty-fourth week due to preeclampsia or placental insufficiency; or
- at least three consecutive spontaneous abortions before the tenth week.

Of note, all other causes of pregnancy morbidity, such as karyotype abnormalities, must also be excluded. Patients who meet clinical criteria must also have either lupus anticoagulant (LAC) or moderate to high (>40 GPl or MPL units) levels of anticardiolipin antibodies (ACA) or >99th%-ile levels of anti-β-2-glycoprotein-1 IgG or IgM levels. In order to be diagnosed with APA syndrome, these antibodies must be present on two occasions at least 12 weeks apart. Acquired thrombophilias should not be screened for without a clinical indication as >2% of the general obstetrical population can have antibodies but no other sequelae.

Other effects of acquired thrombophilias on pregnancy outcome

Other effects include:
1 abruption
2 severe preeclampsia
3 intrauterine growth restriction (IUGR)

Antepartum management

Baseline information
- Patient education regarding the signs and symptoms of VTE.
- Maternal echocardiogram to rule out Libman-Sachs endocarditis.

- Liver function tests (APA have been linked to primary biliary cirrhosis and Budd-Chiari syndrome prior to pregnancy and HELLP syndrome <20 weeks of gestation).
- 24-hour urine collection for creatinine clearance and total protein as APA has been linked to glomerulonephritis.

Anticoagulation therapy
Low-dose aspirin plus:
- Prior VTE: therapeutic anticoagulation (enoxaparin 1 mg/kg subcutaneously every 12 hours, adjusted to achieve anti-factor Xa level at 0.6–1 U/mL 4 hours after an injection).
- APA syndrome but no prior VTE: prophylactic dose anticoagulation with low molecular weight heparin (LMWH) (e.g., enoxaparin 40 mg subcutaneously once a day) and low-dose aspirin.

Pregnancy monitoring
- Level II ultrasonography at 18 weeks.
- Fetal growth should be monitored every 4–6 weeks beginning at 20 weeks for any patient on anticoagulation; ultrasonographic assessment should be more frequent if IUGR is suspected or documented sonographically; Doppler flow studies may be useful in determining the optimal timing of delivery.
- Office visits as often as every 2 weeks beginning at 20 weeks to screen for preeclampsia.
- Non-stress tests (NST) and/or biophysical profiles (BPP) weekly beginning at 36 weeks in uncomplicated cases or earlier as clinically indicated.

Timing of delivery
If the pregnancy is complicated by IUGR or preeclampsia, antenatal testing and maternal signs and symptoms will guide the timing of delivery. If the pregnancy is not complicated by IUGR or preeclampsia, delivery can be delayed until 39 completed weeks provided that antenatal surveillance (NST/BPP) is reassuring.

Since regional anesthesia is contraindicated within 18–24 hours of LMWH administration, we recommend switching to unfractionated heparin (10,000 units subcutaneously bid for prophylaxis) at 36 weeks or earlier if preterm delivery is expected. If vaginal or cesarean delivery occurs more than 12 hours after the last dose of LMWH, patients should not experience anticoagulation-related problems with delivery. Protamine may partially reverse the anticoagulant effects of LMWH.

Postpartum

Either unfractionated heparin or LMWH can be restarted 3–6 hours after vaginal delivery or 6–8 hours after cesarean delivery. This should be continued until at least 6 weeks postpartum. If the patient has a history of VTE, long-term prophylaxis is required as there is as high as a 30% recurrence risk for VTE in an APA-positive patient with a prior VTE. In this case, warfarin can be started on postpartum day 1. It is critical to maintain these women on unfractionated heparin or LMWH for 2 additional days after the INR reaches the therapeutic range between 2.0 and 3.0.

Inherited thrombophilia

Factor V Leiden (FVL)

Overview

Present in 3% to 5% of select European populations, 3% of African-Americans and virtually absent in African Blacks, Chinese, Japanese and other Asians, FVL is the most common heritable thrombophilia. Pregnant patients who are heterozygous for the FVL gene mutation have a 0.26% risk for VTE in pregnancy in the absence of a personal or strong (first degree relative with VTE at <40 years) family history of VTE and greater than a 10% risk for VTE in pregnancy with a personal or strong family history of VTE (see Table 22.1). In addition to the VTE risk, FVL may be

Table 22.1 Inherited thrombophilias and their association with venous thromboembolism (VTE) in pregnancy

Thrombophilia	Percent of VTE in pregnancy	Relative risk [95% CI]	Probability of VTE in patients without personal or family histories during pregnancy and the puerperium
FVL (homozygous)	<1%[+]	25.4 [8.8–66]	1.5%
FVL (heterozygous)	44%	6.9 [3.3–15.2]	0.26%
PGM (homozygous)	<1%[+]	NA	2.8%
PGM (heterozygous)	17%	9.5 [2.1–66.7]	0.37%
FVL/PGM (compound heterozygous)	<1%[+]	84 [19–369]	4.7%
Antithrombin (<60% activity)	1%–8%	119	3.0%–7.2%
Protein S (<55% activity)	12%		<1%–6.6%
Protein C (<50% activity)	<14%	13.0 [1.4–123]	0.8%–1.7%

+ Calculation based on a Hardy–Weinberg equilibrium.

associated with a modest (two-fold) increase in isolated fetal loss after 10 weeks based on small case-control studies. There is no consistent evidence of a link between FVL and abruption, severe preeclampsia or IUGR.

Pathophysiology

FVL arises from a point mutation in the factor V gene causing the substitution of a glutamine for an arginine at position 506, the site of cleavage by activated protein C, thus conferring activated protein C resistance and a thrombophilic state. This abnormality is inherited in an autosomal dominant manner as the heterozygous state is also thrombogenic.

Effect on pregnancy

There is no consistent evidence of a link between FVL and embryonic losses. Among IVF patients, FVL has a 'protective' effect on early pregnancy with substantially higher implantation rates among FVL carriers than among non-carriers. However, FVL has also been associated with late first trimester pregnancy loss (10–13 weeks) and with isolated late (>19 weeks) fetal loss in multiple, but not all case-control studies but in no prospective cohort study. As noted above, FVL in associated with an increased risk of VTE in pregnancy (see Table 22.1). There is one controlled trial suggesting LMWH therapy lowers recurrence risks of fetal loss in affected FVL patients. There is contradictory evidence from case–control studies of a link between FVL and severe preeclampsia, IUGR and abruptio placenta, but no evidence from prospective cohort studies.

Diagnosis

Patients can be screened for FVL with a relatively inexpensive functional coagulation assay for activated protein C resistance. However, since pregnancy is associated with inherent resistance to activated protein C, clinical laboratories must adjust their cut-offs for such assays. Alternatively, a specific DNA assay can confirm the presence of the FVL mutation in pregnant patients. As this test is not affected by pregnancy, it is the more common method for diagnosis.

Prothrombin G20201A mutation (PGM)
Overview

Although only present in 2% to 5% of the European population, it accounts for up to 17% of VTE in pregnancy. The risk of VTE in pregnant heterozygotes without a personal or strong family history of VTE is only 0.37% to 0.5%, but with such a history the risk may be >10% (Table 22.1). Data also suggest that fetal loss and other adverse pregnancy events may be related to the PGM.

Pathophysiology

In 1996, a mutation was discovered in the promoter of the prothrombin gene (G20210A) that leads to over-expression and elevated prothrombin levels. This allows for excess conversion to thrombin and more platelet aggregation.

Effect on pregnancy

Like FVL, small case control studies have linked PGM with late first trimester pregnancy loss and second and third trimester stillbirth. By contrast a large prospective cohort showed no such association. While there are contradictory case-control studies, one of two large prospective cohort studies have linked PGM with development of later adverse pregnancy outcomes including abruption, preeclampsia and IUGR. There is one controlled trial suggesting LMWH therapy lowers recurrence risks of fetal loss in affected PGM patients.

Diagnosis

A specific DNA assay can confirm the presence of the PGM.

Antithrombin (AT) deficiency
Overview

AT deficiency is the most thrombogenic of the heritable coagulopathies. Its population prevalence ranges from 0.02% to 1.1% depending on the cut-off chosen for the AT functional activity assay. It accounts for 1%–8% of VTE episodes in non-pregnant patients (see Table 22.1). AT deficiency is strongly associated with VTE (3% to 40% depending on personal history) and increased risk of stillbirth (>28 weeks).

Pathophysiology

AT inactivates both thrombin and factor Xa. Thus, a deficiency removes a key regulatory pathway controlling both fibrin generation and platelet adhesion and aggregation. A total of 250 discrete mutations of the AT gene have been identified that lead to decreased AT levels. Two phenotypic variations are associated with these mutations. Type 1 involves a reduction in both antigen and activity. Type 2 results in normal levels of antigen but decreased activity.

Effect on pregnancy

There is a modest association with fetal loss at ≤28 weeks or spontaneous abortion, IUGR, abruption and preterm delivery. An association with preeclampsia has been difficult to prove, given the rarity of AT deficiency and the common occurrence of preeclampsia. Since affected patients always require anticoagulation therapy to prevent VTE, it is unlikely that controlled trials of anticoagulation for the prevention of AT-mediated adverse pregnancy outcomes will be performed. Affected patients should be treated with recombinant AT during the intrapartum period.

Diagnosis

Given the variety of AT mutations, deficiency is diagnosed by measuring the AT activity. While <80% activity level may indicate a slight deficiency, generally <60% is used to diagnose the disorder.

Protein C and S deficiency

Pathophysiology

Protein C deficiency results from over 160 distinct mutations which, like AT deficiency, generate a highly variable phenotype associated with either reductions in both antigen and activity (type 1 defects) or normal levels of antigen but decreased activity (type 2 defects).

Protein S deficiency results from over 130 mutations. The vast majority of patients with protein S deficiency can be characterized as having either both low total and free protein S antigen levels (type I) or as having only a low free protein S antigen level due to enhanced binding to the complement 4B binding protein (type IIa).

Effect on pregnancy

There are limited small case–control studies linking protein C deficiency to preeclampsia/eclampsia, but not stillbirth. There are insufficient studies to assess the relationship between protein C deficiency and either abruption or IUGR. Again small case-control studies have linked Protein S deficiency with recurrent late (>22 weeks) fetal loss, but not IUGR, preeclampsia/eclampsia, or abruption. Both protein C and S deficiency are modestly associated with an increase in VTE risk in pregnancy (see Table 22.1).

Diagnosis

Protein C activity levels can be ascertained by either a functional (clotting) or a chromogenic assay. Most laboratories use functional activity cut-off values of 50% to 60%.

Screening for protein S deficiency can employ an activity assay but this is associated with substantial inter-assay and intra-assay variability due in part to frequently changing physiological levels of complement 4B binding protein. Thus, detection of free protein S antigen levels of less than 55% in non-pregnant women and less than 29% in pregnant patients in the first and second trimester or less than 24% in the third trimester appear to most closely correlate with genetic defects.

Management for FVL, PGM, AT, and protein C and S deficiency

Baseline recommendations

Patient education regarding signs and symptoms of VTE.

Anticoagulation therapy (see Table 22.2)

Patients in the highly thrombogenic thrombophilia group (homozygous or compound heterozygous FVL or PGM mutations, AT deficiency with <60% activity) require antepartum and postpartum anticoagulation therapy regardless of their obstetrical history because they have a >1% risk of VTE in pregnancy. Pregnant women with less thrombogenic thrombophilias (e.g., heterozygotes for FVL or prothrombin G20210A mutations, or those with protein C and protein S deficiencies) who have no personal or strong family history of VTE have a low incidence of VTE in pregnancy (<1%) and do not need antepartum anticoagulation.

Table 22.2 Inherited thrombophilias and anticoagulation in pregnancy

Indication	Antepartum therapeutic	Antepartum prophylactic	Postpartum therapeutic	Postpartum Prophylactic
High-risk thrombophilia with no personal or strong family history of VTE				
• Factor V Leiden homozygous		X		X
• Prothrombin G20210A mutation homozygous		X		X
• Antithrombin III deficiency	X		X	X
• Compound heterozygote		X		
Any of the above with a personal history of VTE	X		X	
Low-risk thrombophilia and no personal or strong family history of VTE[2]				
• Factor V Leiden heterozygous				X[1]
• Prothrombin G20210A mutation heterozygous				X[1]
• Protein C deficiency				X[1]
• Protein S deficiency				X[1]
Any low-risk thrombophilia with a personal or strong family history of VTE		X		X

[1] Give prophylaxis if requires a caesarean delivery or has other risk factors for VTE (e.g. obesity, prolonged immobilization, fracture).

[2] Patients with less thrombogenic thrombophilias and no personal or family history of VTE should be treated prophylactically in the antepartum period only if the clinical scenario suggests a high risk for recurrence or there are other thrombotic risk factors (obesity, immobilization, etc.).

However, they should receive prophylaxis postpartum if they require a cesarean delivery since the vast majority of fatal VTEs occur during this period. Patients with these less thrombogenic thrombophilias who have a personal or strong family history of VTE require prophylactic anticoagulation during both the antepartum and postpartum periods.

- If prophylactic dose is recommended: enoxaparin 40 mg subcutaneously once a day.
- If therapeutic dose is recommended: enoxaparin 1 mg/kg subcutaneously every 12 hours titrated to anti-factor Xa level = 0.6–1 U/mL.
- Anti-factor Xa level should be obtained 4 hours after low molecular weight heparin injection 3–5 days after beginning or changing low molecular weight heparin dosing and at least once per trimester to ensure appropriate dosing.
- Consider calcium supplementation of 1500 mg/day given the osteoporosis risk associated with low molecular weight heparin.
- If on low molecular weight heparin, platelet counts should be obtained every 2 days or 3 days from day 4 to day 14, given the small risk of developing heparin-induced thrombocytopenia in the first 2 weeks on low molecular weight heparin.
- If on low molecular weight heparin, transition to unfractionated heparin at 36 weeks or earlier if preterm delivery is expected as regional anesthesia is contraindicated within 18–24 hours of taking low molecular weight heparin.
  - Prophylactic dose: 10,000 units subcutaneously bid titrated to anti-factor Xa level = 0.1–0.2 U/mL.
  - Therapeutic dose: 10,000 units subcutaneously every 8 hours titrated to aPTT 1.5–2 times control 6 hours after the injection.
- Based on Table 22.2, restart unfractionated heparin or low molecular weight heparin 3–6 hours after vaginal delivery or 6–8 eight hours after cesarean delivery. This should be continued until at least 6 weeks postpartum.

Delivery

- Consideration of a scheduled induction, or if obstetrically indicated a cesarean section, between 39 and 40 weeks' gestation so as to time the discontinuation of anticoagulation.
- Frequent ambulation or serial compression devices during labor and the immediate postpartum period.

Suggested reading

Buller HR, Girolami A, Prins MH. Frequency of pregnancy-related venous thromboembolism in anticoagulant factor-deficient women: implications for prophylaxis. *Ann Intern Med* 1996;125:955–60.

Dizon-Townson D, Miller C, Sibai B, Spong CY, Thom E, Wendel G Jr, Wenstrom K, Samuels P, Cotroneo MA, Moawad A, Sorokin Y, Meis P, Miodovnik M, O'Sullivan MJ, Conway D, Wapner RJ, Gabbe SG; National Institute of Child Health and Human Development Maternal-Fetal Medicine Units Network. The relationship of the factor V Leiden mutation and pregnancy outcomes for mother and fetus. *Obstet Gynecol.* 2005 Sep;106(3):517–24.

Galli M, Luciani D, Bertolini G, Barbui T. Anti-beta 2-glycoprotein I, antiprothrombin antibodies, and the risk of thrombosis in the antiphospholipid syndrome. *Blood* 2003;102:2717–23.

Gerhardt A, Scharf RE, Beckmann MW, Struve S, Bender HG, Pillny M, Sandmann W, Zotz RB. Prothrombin and factor V mutations in women with a history of thrombosis during pregnancy and the puerperium. *N Engl J Med* 2000;342:374–80.

Infante-Rivard C, Rivard GE, Yotov WV, Genin E, Guiguet M, Weinberg C, Gauthier R, Feoli-Fonseca JC. Absence of association of thrombophilia polymorphisms with intrauterine growth restriction. *N Engl J Med* 2002;347:19–25.

Rand JH, Wu XX, Andree HA, Lockwood CJ, Guller S, Scher J, Harpel PC. Pregnancy loss in the antiphospholipid-antibody syndrome – a possible thrombogenic mechanism. *N Engl J Med* 1997;337:154–60.

Roque H, Paidas MJ, Funai EF, Kuczynski E, Lockwood CJ. Maternal thrombophilias are not associated with early pregnancy loss. *Thromb Haemost* 2004;91:290–5.

Said JM, Higgins JR, Moses EK, Walker SP, Borg AJ, Monagle PT, Brennecke SP. Inherited thrombophilia polymorphisms and pregnancy outcomes in nulliparous women. *Obstet Gynecol.* 2010 Jan;115(1):5–13.

Silver RM, Zhao Y, Spong CY, Sibai B, Wendel G Jr, Wenstrom K, Samuels P, Caritis SN, Sorokin Y, Miodovnik M, O'Sullivan MJ, Conway D, Wapner RJ; Eunice Kennedy Shriver National Institute of Child Health and Human Development Maternal-Fetal Medicine Units (NICHD MFMU) Network. Prothrombin gene G20210A mutation and obstetric complications. *Obstet Gynecol.* 2010 Jan;115(1):14–20.

Zotz RB, Gerhardt A, Scharf RE. Inherited thrombophilia and gestational venous thromboembolism. *Best Pract Res Clin Haematol* 2003;16:243–59.

PROTOCOL 23

Cardiac Disease

Katharine D. Wenstrom
Division of Maternal-Fetal Medicine, Women & Infants' Hospital of Rhode Island and Brown Alpert Medical School, Providence, RI, USA

Overview

Cardiac disease is among the leading causes of maternal mortality during pregnancy. A thorough evaluation of the woman with preexisting heart disease is ideally initiated before pregnancy, so that she can be counseled regarding the risks of pregnancy based on her specific cardiac lesion. Counseling should include a discussion of her cardiac anomaly and baseline functional status, the possibility of optimising her cardiac status by medical or surgical means, any additional risk factors, and her risk of having a child with the same or different cardiac lesion. Perhaps most difficult, the woman's physical ability to care for a child and her life expectancy should also be addressed. During pregnancy, consultation with appropriate subspecialists as part of a team approach to antepartum and postpartum care is likely to improve both maternal and fetal outcome. Table 23.1 categorizes the risk of maternal death associated with the most common cardiac lesions.

Pathophysiology

In a normal pregnancy, the cardiovascular system undergoes significant physiological changes which may not be tolerated by the gravida with heart disease. Increases in plasma volume, oxygen demand and cardiac output may stress an already compromised cardiovascular system. As summarized in Fig. 23.1, by mid-gestation there is a 50% increase in both blood volume and cardiac output and a 20% decrease in systemic vascular resistance. By the end of the second trimester, the heart rate has increased by 20% and blood pressure has reached its nadir. Maternal position further affects these parameters (Fig. 23.2); cardiac output decreases by 20%

Protocols for High-Risk Pregnancies, 5th edition. Edited by J.T. Queenan, J.C. Hobbins and C.Y. Spong. © 2010 Blackwell Publishing Ltd.

when the woman is supine and by 16% in dorsal lithotomy position. Cardiac output increases by another 30% during labor, and further increases occur during contractions, during the Valsalva maneuver, and with pain. At delivery, central blood volume may drop as the result of blood

Table 23.1 Pregnancy-associated maternal mortality in cardiac disease

Mortality 25–50%
Coarctation of aorta (with valvular involvement)
Marfan syndrome (with aortic involvement)
Pulmonary hypertension

Mortality 5–15%
Aortic stenosis
Mitral stenosis, New York Heart Association (NYHA) classes III and IV
Mitral stenosis with atrial fibrillation
Coarctation of aorta (without valvular involvement)
Uncorrected tetralogy of Fallot
Marfan syndrome with normal aorta
Artificial valve (mechanical)
Previous myocardial infarction

Mortality less than 1%
Atrial septal defect
Ventricular septal defect
Pulmonic or tricuspid disease
Patent ductus arteriosus
Artificial valve (bioprosthetic)
Mitral stenosis, NYHA classes I and II
Corrected tetralogy of Fallot

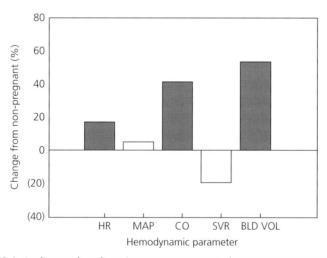

Figure 23.1 Cardiovascular adaptation to pregnancy. HR, heart rate; MAP, mean arterial pressure; CO, cardiac output; SVR, systemic vascular resistance; BLD VOL, blood volume.

loss. Immediately afterward, however, uterine contraction results in an autotransfusion from the uterine circulation, and relief of vena caval compression. With loss of the placental circulation, the peripheral resistance increases, and at the same time extravascular fluid is mobilized. All these peripartum changes lead to a high output state that may persist for up to 4 weeks. The hemodynamic effects of these pregnancy-induced changes on specific cardiac lesions, along with recommendations for management, are shown in Table 23.2.

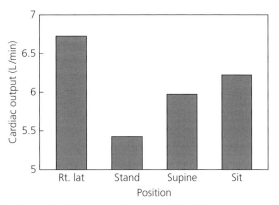

Figure 23.2   Cardiac output changes with maternal position.

Table 23.2 Management of specific cardiac lesions in pregnancy

Cardiac lesion	Hemodynamic defect	Effect on pregnancy	Management
Mitral/aortic stenosis	↓ LV filling ↑ PVR; eventual pulmonary HTN	Fixed CO; tachy- or bradycardia will ↓ LV filling and ↓ CO Left atrial dilation leading to pulmonary congestion Arrhythmias Thrombus formation	Maintain preload, but avoid ↑ central blood volume Avoid ↓ SVR Avoid tachycardia and bradycardia Beta-blocker for persistent HR >90–100 beats/min
Mitral valve insufficiency	Component of regurgitation LV hypertrophy Eventual LV failure Eventual pulmonary HTN	Complications occur late in life; generally asymptomatic during pregnancy The ↓ SVR of pregnancy improves forward flow ↑ SVR during labor increases regurgitation	Treat symptomatic prolapse with beta-blocker Avoid ↑ SVR Avoid myocardial depressants Treat arrhythmias

(Continued)

Table 23.2 (Continued)

Cardiac lesion	Hemodynamic defect	Effect on pregnancy	Management
Aortic insufficiency	LV volume overload, left heart failure, pulmonary congestion	The ↓ SVR and ↑ HR of pregnancy reduce regurgitant flow During labor, ↑ intravascular volume, ↑ SVR, and stress of labor can lead to LV dysfunction	Avoid ↑ SVR Avoid bradycardia Avoid myocardial depressants
Prosthetic valve	Component of regurgitation	Risk of embolization Valvular dysfunction Endocarditis	Full-dose anticoagulation for mechanical valve
Left-to-right shunt (septal defects)	↑ Pulmonary flow, eventual pulmonary HTN and LV failure	Small lesions: asymptomatic Large VSD associated with aortic insufficiency CHF Arrhythmia Pulmonary HTN	Avoid ↑ SVR Avoid ↑ HR If pulmonary HTN, treat as right-to-left shunt; avoid ↓ SVR
Right-to-left shunt (tetralogy of Fallot, Eisenmenger syndrome)	Blood shunted away from lungs, cyanosis	↓ SVR worsens shunt ↑ PVR during labor worsens shunt Increased hypoxia, cyanosis	Avoid hypotension Maintain preload; avoid ↓ SVR Avoid decreases in blood volume Avoid myocardial depressants Give oxygen Air filters on IV lines
Cardiomyopathy	LV dysfunction Global chamber dilation	Increased cardiac demand may lead to decompensation	↓ Afterload Careful volume administration and diuresis Inotropic support to maximize cardiac output

SVR, systemic vascular resistence; PVR, pulmonary vascular resistance; LV, left ventricle; RV, right ventricle; CO, cardiac output; HR, heart rate; VSD, ventricular septal defect; CHF, congestive heart failure; HTN, hypertension; ↓, decrease; ↑, increase.

Diagnosis and workup

Heart disease should be suspected in any pregnant woman who develops dyspnea, chest pain, palpitations, arrhythmias, or cyanosis, or who experiences a sudden limitation of activity. Particular attention should be given

Table 23.3 Functional status in cardiac disease (New York Heart Association classification)

Class I	Asymptomatic with greater than normal activity
Class II	Symptomatic* with greater than normal activity (stair climbing, etc.)
Class III	Symptomatic with normal activity (walking, etc.)
Class IV	Symptomatic at rest

*Dyspnea, chest pain, orthopnea.

to the woman who has a history of exercise intolerance, a heart murmur predating pregnancy, or a history of rheumatic fever.

Cardiac disease should be diagnosed and/or fully characterized as early in the pregnancy as possible, so that the level of maternal and fetal risk can be determined and a therapeutic plan developed. The evaluation should begin with a through history and physical examination, which allow classification of the woman's disease on a functional basis (Table 23.3). A 12-lead EKG and a transthoracic echocardiogram should be performed, and women with cyanosis should undergo percutaneous oximetry and/or arterial blood gas analysis. Any associated factors that could increase risk, such as a history of heart failure, a prosthetic valve, or a history of thromboembolism should be noted. Women determined to be at increased risk should be managed by a team that includes a maternal-fetal medicine specialist, a cardiologist, an anesthesiologist, and a pediatrician.

Management

General principles for care of the gravida with cardiac disease

Key principles in the antepartum management of heart disease center on minimizing cardiac work while optimizing perfusion of the tissues including the uteroplacental bed. Any factors that could increase cardiac work, such as anxiety, anemia, infection, arrhythmia, or non-physiologic edema should be identified and eliminated or minimized as soon as possible. Any pregnancy-induced complications such as hypertension, infection, anemia or thromboembolism should be treated promptly. Women with cardiac disease should avoid strenuous activity during pregnancy; those whose underlying cardiac lesion involves ventricular dysfunction, who are cyanotic, or who are functional class III or IV may need to significantly limit their physical activity and have specified daily rest periods. The woman's functional status should be closely monitored as pregnancy progresses. Any diminution in cardiac function or worsening of maternal functional class should prompt consideration of hospitalization. Oxygen, diuretics and inotropes such as digitalis can be used as necessary to optimize cardiac function. Fetal growth should be monitored closely and a fetal echocardiogram performed between 18–22 weeks' gestation. Depending on the maternal functional class and fetal status, weekly or biweekly evaluation of fetal well-being should be considered, beginning in the third trimester.

Route of delivery

Vaginal delivery is preferred for the patient with cardiac disease. The blood loss associated with cesarean delivery is at least twice that associated with vaginal delivery, and the hemodynamic fluctuations are significantly greater. In addition, cesarean delivery increases the risk of infection, thromboembolism and other postoperative complications. Thus, cesarean should be reserved for standard obstetric indications. Heart rate, stroke volume, cardiac output and mean arterial pressure increase further during labor and in the immediate postpartum period, and should be monitored closely. Fluid intake and output and pulse oximetry readings should also be carefully reviewed. Lateral positioning and adequate pain control can reduce maternal tachycardia and increase cardiac output (Fig. 23.2). Patients with New York Heart Association class III or IV disease should be considered candidates for intrapartum invasive hemodynamic monitoring. Operative assistance with the second stage of labor is recommended to decrease maternal cardiac work.

Anesthesia

Conduction anesthesia is the preferred method of providing intrapartum pain control for the woman with cardiac disease. However, it is important to avoid hypotension when establishing regional anesthesia. Careful administration of intravenous crystalloid before placement of the catheter and slow administration of the anesthetic agent help to prevent this complication. Ephedrine is usually the agent of choice for the treatment of hypotension associated with regional anesthesia, because it does not constrict the placental vessels. However, because ephedrine increases the maternal heart rate, phenylephrine may be more appropriate for patients in whom tachycardia and increased myocardial work must be avoided (e.g., those with mitral and aortic stenosis, left to right shunt, etc.). A single-dose spinal technique is relatively contraindicated in patients with significant cardiac disease because hypotension frequently occurs during establishment of the spinal block. A narcotic epidural is an excellent alternative method and may be particularly effective for patients in whom systemic hypotension must be avoided (e.g., those with pulmonary hypertension, etc.).

Patients receiving thromboembolic prophylaxis pose an anesthesia challenge. Because there is little data regarding the use of spinal or epidural anesthesia in such patients, it is controversial. Although some data suggest that unfractionated low dose heparin ($\leq$5000 IU twice daily) and perioperative low molecular weight heparin thromboprophylaxis appear not to pose a significant risk for spinal hematoma, the US Food and Drug Administration has reported cases in which non-pregnant patients on low molecular weight heparin had spinal or epidural anesthesia and suffered epidural or spinal hematomas, some of which caused neurological injury. The most prudent strategy is to switch patients to unfractionated heparin a few weeks before delivery, because it has a short half-life (1.5 hours) and can be readily reversed (discussed below). For patients with a normal aPTT and platelet count, epidural anesthesia is generally considered safe.

Prophylactic antibiotics

Women with a history of acute rheumatic fever and endocarditis who are taking penicillin prophylaxis should continue it throughout pregnancy. Whether women with other kinds of heart disease should receive antibiotic prophylaxis during pregnancy is controversial. Some experts have argued that the risk of bacteremia during labor and delivery is high, since even an episiotomy or insertion of a bladder catheter can result in transient bacteremia, and thus any woman with congenital heart disease should be given antibiotic prophylaxis in labor. However, the American College of Cardiology and the American Heart Association Task Force on Practice Guidelines have stated that intrapartum antibiotics are not necessary for women undergoing vaginal or caesarean delivery unless infection is suspected. Antibiotics are optional for high-risk patients such as those with mechanical heart valves, a previous history of endocarditis, complex congenital heart disease or a surgically constructed systemic-pulmonary conduit. Antibiotics should be given when bacteremia is suspected or there is an active infection (Table 23.4).

Table 23.4 Antibiotic regimens in pregnancy

Standard regimen	Ampicillin, 2 g IV or IM, plus gentamicin, 1.5 mg/kg IV (to a maximum of 120 mg) 30 min before delivery, followed by 1 g ampicillin IV or IM or 1 g amoxicillin PO 6 hours later; antibiotics should not be given for more than 6-8 hours total
Penicillin-allergic standard regimen	Substitute vancomycin, 1 g IV over 1–2 h for ampicillin
Regimen for women at moderate risk	Ampicillin, 2 g IV or IM, 30 min before delivery

Anticoagulation

Pregnancy is a hypercoagulable state, and pregnant women with mechanical heart valves or cardiac failure are at especially increased risk of thromboembolism. Unfortunately, there is little data regarding the efficacy of and best protocol for anticoagulation of such patients during pregnancy. The most effective anticoagulant, warfarin, readily crosses the placenta and has adverse fetal effects throughout pregnancy. If used in the first trimester, it increases the risk of early pregnancy loss or may result in a specific embryopathy including abnormal cartilage and hypoplastic midface; if used in the second or third trimesters, it increases the risk of pregnancy loss, growth restriction, and abnormalities caused by vascular disruption such as limb reduction defects. There is some data suggesting that these complications are less likely if the daily dose is ≤5 mg per day. The various forms of heparin do not cross the placenta, and are thus safe for the fetus, but are not completely effective in preventing thrombosis; several reports indicate a 12–30% incidence of thromboembolic complications and a 4–15% incidence of mortality for pregnant women with mechanical valves taking heparin. Heparin is also associated with an increased risk of bleeding; the increased levels of factor VIII and fibrinogen that characterize pregnancy may attenuate the aPTT response to heparin, resulting in persistent anticoagulation and hemorrhage at the time of delivery. There have been case reports suggesting that low molecular weight heparin is not any more effective than unfractionated heparin, but a general lack of data make it difficult to draw evidence-based conclusions. Antiplatelet drugs are not recommended unless the patient also has significant coronary artery disease.

The American College of Cardiology and American Heart Association recommend that all women with mechanical heart valves undergo therapeutic anticoagulation during pregnancy. Women with mechanical heart valves should be counseled about management options and should participate in creating a therapeutic plan that, ideally, achieves a balance between risks and benefits for both mother and fetus.

For women receiving therapeutic anticoagulation

1 Many women will elect to discontinue warfarin from 2 to 6 weeks after conception until 12 weeks' gestation, during which time they should receive heparin or low molecular weight heparin.
2 From 12 to 36 weeks, the patient must choose either warfarin or heparin. The risks of warfarin may be acceptable if the patient requires ≤5 mg per day. If she chooses unfractionated heparin, the aPTT should be kept at least twice the normal control value; if she chooses low molecular weight heparin, it should be given twice daily and the dose adjusted to keep the anti-Xa level between 0.7 and 1.2 U/mL, 4 to

6 hours after administration. The patient may also take low-dose aspirin in the second and third trimesters.

3 Two to three weeks prior to delivery, the patient should be switched to therapeutic unfractionated heparin, since it has a short half-life (1.5 hours) and its effects can be rapidly reversed with protamine sulphate.

4 Therapeutic heparin and warfarin should be restarted 4 to 6 hours after vaginal delivery or 12 hours after cesarean, as long as the patient has no significant bleeding. The heparin can be discontinued once the warfarin is at therapeutic level.

For women receiving prophylactic anticoagulation

1 Patients on low-dose heparin should be instructed to withhold their injections at the onset of labor.

2 For a planned labor induction or cesarean, low dose heparin given twice a day should be withheld for 8 to 12 hours prior to the procedure; low-dose heparin given once a day should be withheld for at least 18 hours.

3 After delivery, low-dose heparin may be restarted within 12 hours and low molecular weight heparin within 6 to 12 hours (see Table 23.5).

The immediate postpartum period is especially critical for the patient with cardiovascular disease. Blood loss must be minimized and blood pressure maintained, but congestive failure from fluid overload must also be avoided. For women requiring anticoagulation, heparin may be restarted 6 to12 hours after a vaginal delivery or 12 to 24 hours after a aesarean, along with warfarin. Heparin is then continued until the warfarin is therapeutic.

Table 23.5 Prophylactic heparin regimens in pregnancy

Unfractionated heparin
Low-dose prophylaxis:
1 5000–7500 U every 12 hours during the first trimester
   7500–10,000 U every 12 hours during the second trimester
   10,000 U every 12 hours during the third trimester unless the aPTT* is elevated. The aPTT may be checked near term and the heparin dose reduced if prolonged
OR
2 5000–10,000 U every 12 hours throughout pregnancy.
Adjusted-dose prophylaxis:
   ≥10,000 U twice a day to three times a day to achieve aPTT of 1.5–2.5
Low molecular weight heparin
Low-dose prophylaxis:
   Dalteparin, 5000 U once or twice daily, or enoxaparin, 40 mg once or twice daily
Adjusted-dose prophylaxis:
   Dalteparin, 5000–10,000 U every 12 hours, or enoxaparin, 30–80 mg every 12 hours
   Factor Xa = 0.7–1.2 U, 4 hours after dose

---

* Activated partial thromboplastin time.

Follow-up

Approximately 4 to 6 weeks after delivery, the cardiovascular changes of pregnancy will have resolved and the patient should be re-evaluated by a cardiologist. The infant's pediatrician can decide whether or not to perform a cardiac evaluation of the neonate, depending on the results of the targeted fetal ultrasonographic examination or echocardiogram and the newborn examination. Based on the outcome of the pregnancy and the results of the cardiac re-evaluation, the patient can be ounselled regarding the risks of subsequent pregnancy, and appropriate contraception provided if indicated.

Suggested reading

American College of Cardiology/American Heart Association Task Force on Practice Guidelines. ACC/AHA 2006 guidelines for the management of patients with valvular heart disease. *Circulation* 2006;e106:e84–231.

American College of Obstetricians and Gynecologists. *Thromboembolism in Pregnancy*. Practice Bulletin #19, August 2000.

American College of Obstetricians and Gynecologists. *Prophylactic Antibiotics in Labor and Delivery*, Practice Bulletin #47, October 2003.

Bhagwat AR, Engel PJ. Heart disease and pregnancy *Cardiol Clin* 1995;13:163–78.

Clark SL. Structural cardiac disease in pregnancy. In: Clark SL, Cotton DB, Hankins GDV, Phelan JP (eds) *Critical Care Obstetrics*. Oradell, NJ: Medical Economics, 1987; pp. 92–113.

Criteria Committee of the New York Heart Association. *Nomenclature and criteria for diagnosis of disease of the heart and great vessels*, 8th edn. Boston: Little, Brown, 1979.

Findlow D, Doyle E. Congenital heart disease in adults. *Br J Anesthesia* 1997;78: 416–30.

James AH, Brancazio LR, Gehrig TR, Wang A, Ortel TL. Low-molecular-weight heparin for thromboprophylaxis in pregnant women with mechanical heart valves. *J Mat Fet Neonat Med* 2006;19(9):543–9.

Lipscomb KJ, Smith JC, Clarke B, Donnai P. Outcome of pregnancy in women with Marfan's syndrome. *Br J Obstet Gynecol* 1997;104:201–6.

Patten DE, Lee W, Cotton DB, *et al.* Cyanotic maternal heart disease in pregnancy. *Obstet Gynecol Surv* 1990;45:594–600.

Pearson GD, Veille JC, Rahimtoola S, Hsia J, Oakley CM, Hosenpud JD, Ansari A, Boughman KL. Peripartum Cardiomyopathy: National Heart, Lung, and Blood Institute and Office of Rare Diseases (National Institutes of Health) Workshop Recommendations and Review. *JAMA* 2000;283:1183–8.

Perloff JK. Congenital heart disease and pregnancy. *Clin Cardiol* 1994;17:579–87.

Prebitero P, Somerville J, Stone S, Aruta E, Speigelhalter D, Rabajoli F. Pregnancy in cyanotic congenital heart disease: outcome of mother and fetus. *Circulation* 1994;89:2673–6.

Siu SC, Colman JM. Heart disease and pregnancy. *Heart* 2001;85:710–15.

Task Force on Management of Valvular Heart Disease of the European Society of Cardiology. Guideline on the management of valvular heart disease. *Europ Heart* 2007; doi:10.1093: 1–39.

Thorne SA. Pregnancy in heart disease. *Heart* 2004;90:450–6.

Vitale N, de Feo M, De Snato LS, Pollice A, Tedesco N, Cotrufo M. Dose-dependent fetal complications of warfarin in pregnant women with mechanical heart valves. *J Amer Coll Cardiol* 1999;33:1637–41.

Wilson NJ, Neutzs JM. Adult congenital heart disease: principles and management guidelines – Part I. *Aust NZ J Med* 1993;23:498–503.

Peripartum Cardiomyopathy

F. Gary Cunningham

Department of Obstetrics and Gynecology, University of Texas Southwestern Medical Center, Dallas, TX, USA

Clinical significance

Peripartum cardiomyopathy refers to otherwise unexplained heart failure during pregnancy following a contemporaneous evaluation that excludes known causes of cardiomyopathy such as hypertension, thyrotoxicosis or valvular heart disease. It is likely this disorder does not differ from idiopathic cardiomyopathy that is encountered in any previously healthy non-pregnant young adult, and thus it is not unique to pregnancy. Its incidence during pregnancy is inversely proportional to the diligence used to exclude known causes of cardiomyopathy. Thus, its incidence in the United States is reported to range from 1:3000 to 1:15,000 pregnancies. Its importance is underscored by its contribution to maternal mortality, viz., it is estimated to cause 10% of maternal-related deaths by the Centers for Disease Control and Prevention. Moreover, some form of cardiomyopathy accounts for 1.3 antepartum hospitalizations per 1000 pregnancies, and about a third of these are for peripartum cardiomyopathy.

Pathophysiology

The cause of peripartum cardiomyopathy is not known. Associated risk factors include gestational hypertension, multifetal pregnancy, and there is a predilection for older, obese black women. Dietary deficiencies have been implicated, but not proven. Immune activation with myocardial tissue targeted in response to fetal antigenic material is an attractive hypothesis, but this too has not been demonstrated convincingly. In at least half of cases in which endomyocardial biopsy is done, there is evidence for inflammatory myocarditis with viral genomic material identified by molecular analysis. Some of these include parvovirus B19, Epstein-Barr virus, herpesvirus 6 and

Protocols for High-Risk Pregnancies, 5th edition. Edited by J.T. Queenan, J.C. Hobbins and C.Y. Spong. © 2010 Blackwell Publishing Ltd.

cytomegalovirus. Finally, it seems likely that at least some cases will be due to cardiac gene deletions similar to those discovered in experimental animals.

Diagnosis

Because peripartum cardiomyopathy is idiopathic, it is a diagnosis of exclusion. The National Heart, Lung, and Blood Institute established the following diagnostic criteria:

1 Development of heart failure in the last month of pregnancy, or within 5 months of delivery;
2 Absence of an identifiable cause for the heart failure;
3 Absence of recognizable heart disease prior to the last months of pregnancy; and
4 Left ventricular systolic dysfunction demonstrated by typical echocardiographic findings.

Typical chest x-ray findings include impressive cardiomegaly with pulmonary edema, and there is single- to four-chamber dilatation with ventricular dysfunction evident on echocardiography.

Management

There is no specific treatment available at this time. Neither immunosuppressive agents nor corticosteroids are beneficial. Treatment of heart failure is the cornerstone of management and vigorous diuresis with drugs such as furosemide is begun promptly. Afterload reduction is accomplished with hydralazine prior to delivery and an angiotensin-converting-enzyme inhibitor given postpartum. Some use digoxin for its inotrophic properties and dangerous arrhythmias that cause rate-related dysfunction need to be controlled. There is a reportedly high concurrence of pulmonary embolism, and thus many recommend heparin prophylaxis.

Complications

Spontaneous labor commonly follows pulmonary edema and hypoxemia caused by heart failure. If hypoxemia is severe or prolonged, fetal death may ensue. There is no evidence that delivery improves the prognosis, but it may help manage heart failure. Immediate maternal mortality has been reported as high as 25%, but in large series it seldom exceeds 5%. Maternal deaths are caused by intractable heart failure, malignant arrhythmias, and pulmonary embolism. Complications of delivery – especially cesarean delivery – contribute to mortality because they may add the burden of sepsis syndrome, hemorrhage and anemia, as well as anesthetic complications.

Follow-up

The long-term prognosis following peripartum cardiomyopathy depends on the extent of residual heart muscle damage. In general, those women who regain normal ventricular function within 6 months have a good prognosis. This includes perhaps half of affected women. In the other half with ventricular dysfunction that persists there is a high incidence of chronic heart failure, including end-stage disease requiring cardiac transplantation. It follows that subsequent pregnancy outcomes also depend on residual cardiac function. Half of women with persistent ventricular dysfunction develop congestive heart failure during a subsequent pregnancy. And although women with apparent resolution of cardiomyopathy have a 20% incidence of heart failure with a subsequent pregnancy, it is usually less severe.

Prevention

There currently are no known preventive measures for peripartum cardiomyopathy. Efforts are concentrated on determining the prognosis if the woman desires a subsequent pregnancy. If there is evidence of substantively persistent ventricular dysfunction as measured by a diminished ejection fraction, or by exercise or drug-induced ventricular dysfunction, then pregnancy likely should not be undertaken. For women who choose to have a subsequent pregnancy, close follow-up with frequent assessment of cardiac function is imperative. For these women, management is the same as for heart failure of any cause.

Conclusions

In its purest form, peripartum cardiomyopathy likely represents idiopathic cardiomyopathy of young adults with at least half of cases caused by inflammatory myocarditis usually from viral infections. It is a diagnosis of exclusion. Standard treatment is given for heart failure and close observation for its complications. Evaluation is continued after delivery and persistence of ventricular dysfunction at 6 months carries a poor long-term prognosis for recovery.

Suggested reading

Cunningham FG, Pritchard JA, Hankins GDV, *et al.* Idiopathic cardiomyopathy or compounding cardiovascular events? *Obstet Gynecol* 1986;67:157–67.

Elkayam U, Akhter MW, Singh H, *et al.* Pregnancy-associated cardiomyopathy: clinical characteristics and a comparison between early and late presentation. *Circulation* 2005;111:2050–58.

Gentry MB, Dias JK, Luis A, *et al.* African-American women have a higher risk for developing peripatum cardiomyopathy. *J Am Coll Cardiol* 2010;55:654–59.

Kuklina EV, Callaghan WM. Cardiomyopathy and other myocardial disorders among hospitalizations for pregnancy in the United States: 2004–2006. *Obstet Gynecol* 2010;115:93–100.

Mielniczuk LM, Williams K, Davis DR, *et al.* Peripartum cardiomyopathy: frequency of peripartum cardiomyopathy. *Am J Cardiol* 2006;97:1765–72.

Ro A, Frishman WH. Peripartum cardiomyopathy. *Cardiol Rev* 2006;14:34–45.

Sheffield JS, Cunningham FG. Thyrotoxicosis and heart failure that complicate pregnancy. *Am J Obstet Gynecol* 2004;190:211–18.

Thromboembolism

Alan Peaceman

Division of Maternal-Fetal Medicine, Northwestern University Feinberg School of Medicine, Chicago, IL, USA

Thromboembolism remains a leading cause of obstetric morbidity and mortality, and in the United States is the leading cause of maternal death following a live birth. It is estimated that the risk of venous thrombosis is approximately five times higher during pregnancy than in the non-pregnant state due to the hypercoagulable nature of pregnancy. While previously though to be more prevalent in the third trimester, it is now recognized to occur at similar frequencies throughout pregnancy. It remains more common in the postpartum period than during pregnancy. Despite its risk, thromboembolism during pregnancy is a poorly studied area and significant controversy remains over the management of pregnant women at risk for this disorder.

Pathophysiology

Normal pregnancy is associated with an increase in the level or activity of many of the clotting factors in the blood. These increases provide a defense against hemorrhage after delivery, but they also contribute to altering the balance of procoagulant and anticoagulant factors in the circulation toward clot formation during pregnancy. Under normal circumstances, the increased levels of clotting factors do not result in thrombus formation, but some clinical situations such as trauma or vascular injury may predispose toward lower extremity clotting. Once formed, portions of the clot can embolize to the pulmonary tree, with symptoms ranging from mild hypoxia to cardiovascular collapse. Other risk factors for thrombosis during pregnancy include venous status, inactivity, obesity, prior thrombosis, antiphospholipid syndrome and thrombophilias such as factor V Leiden.

Protocols for High-Risk Pregnancies, 5th edition. Edited by J.T. Queenan, J.C. Hobbins and C.Y. Spong. © 2010 Blackwell Publishing Ltd.

Diagnosis

The diagnosis of deep venous thrombosis (DVT) is often difficult to make clinically, especially in pregnancy. Patients presenting with symmetric lower extremity swelling associated with pain and erythema should be evaluated. Assays for serum D-dimer are useful for detecting thrombosis outside of pregnancy because of its high negative predictive value, but of limited value in pregnancy because most women have increased levels by the second trimester. Venography traditionally has been the gold standard for making the diagnosis, even in pregnancy, but is performed less frequently now because of its invasive nature and its use of radiation. Several non-invasive diagnostic tests have been shown to be useful in the non-pregnant state; however, their accuracy in pregnancy is less well studied. Nonetheless, many practitioners have now moved to compression ultrasonography for pregnant women as the primary tool for evaluation of clinical symptoms in the lower extremities (Fig. 25.1). Sensitivity and specificity of ultrasonography for proximal deep venous thrombosis

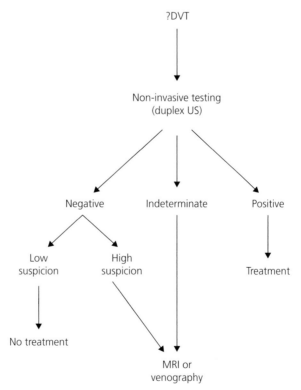

Figure 25.1 Diagnostic protocol for suspected deep venous thrombosis (DVT). IPG, impedance plethysmography; US, ultrasonography.

were both 95% in studies outside pregnancy, and use of Doppler also enables evaluation of thrombosis in the iliac veins. Ultrasonography is less sensitive for thrombosis below the knee. Venography and impedance plethysmography are used less frequently today. MRI use may become more common, especially for evaluation for pelvic vein thrombosis.

The presenting signs and symptoms suggestive of pulmonary embolism include shortness of breath, chest pain, tachypnea, tachycardia and decreased oxygen saturation by pulse oxymeter. Initial evaluation traditionally included an arterial blood gas to determine the presence of hypoxia and increased A-a gradient, both suggestive of an embolic event. However, this test is now recognized as having limited value in that many patients with pulmonary embolism are without abnormality. Ventilation-perfusion (V/Q) scanning was also an available diagnostic procedure, but more than half of V/Q scans performed in pregnancy are non-diagnostic and require further imaging. Pulmonary angiography is the gold standard for diagnosing pulmonary embolus, but is invasive and associated with a risk of significant complications. Spiral CT scanning using IV contrast is now the primary diagnostic modality for non-pregnant patients in many centers; its use in pregnancy has not been evaluated, but is likely to be of similar accuracy as in the non-pregnant state. It may also be of use in identifying other thoracic conditions that may be responsible for the patient's symptoms. Fetal radiation exposure has been estimated to be less than 1 rad, and less than that associated with ventilation-perfusion scanning. If a diagnosis of pulmonary embolism is made, a search for lower extremity thrombosis may be helpful in identifying the precipitating cause and directing therapy.

Treatment of acute thromboembolism

Because of the lack of clinical trials, all recommendations regarding treatment for or prevention of thromboembolism during pregnancy are based on expert opinion. Nonetheless, consensus does exist on some of the approaches to treatment. Acute DVT or PE should be treated with full anti-coagulation using either intravenous heparin or subcutaneous low molecular weight heparin, and it is important to achieve therapeutic doses very early to prevent extension of clot (see Table 25.1). The patient is then transitioned to either subcutaneous heparin or enoxaparin (or other forms of low molecular weight heparin) injections every 12 hours, which is continued for the remainder of the pregnancy and postpartum period to prevent recurrence. It is thought that the use of heparin injections requires monitoring to maintain the activated partial thromboplastin time (aPTT) at least 1½ times control throughout the dosing interval. However, with

Table 25.1 Management of thromboembolism

Condition	Heparin	Enoxaparin
DVT or PE during current pregnancy	IV heparin (aPTT 2–3 times control) for 5–10 days, followed by q 8–12 h injections to prolong midinterval aPTT 1½ times control for remainder of the pregnancy; warfarin can be used postpartum	Enoxaparin 1 mg/kg (up to 100 mg maximum) q 12 h; monitoring of anti-Factor Xa levels at 4–6 hours post injection
Patient who requires long-term therapeutic anticoagulation	Heparin q 8–12 h to prolong mid-interval aPTT 1½ times control	1 mg/kg (up to 100 mg maximum) q 12 h; monitoring of anti-Factor Xa levels at 4–6 hours post injection
Previous DVT or PE before current pregnancy (prophylactic treatment)	5000 units q 12 h first trimester 7500 units q 12 h second trimester 10,000 units q 12 h third trimester; monitoring unnecessary	40 mg q 12 h; monitoring unnecessary for patients under 100 kg

the more rapid metabolism of heparin during pregnancy, it is usually difficult to achieve prolongation of the aPTT throughout the dosing interval without an excessive peak level, even when administered three times a day. Enoxaparin injections are also given twice daily because of the rapid metabolism. Monitoring of enoxaparin when given outside of pregnancy is thought to be unnecessary for most patients, but its pharmacokinetics in pregnancy are incompletely studied. If monitoring is to be performed, anti-factor Xa levels are followed, with the target being 0.6 to 1.0 IU/mL. Both heparin and low molecular weight heparins do not cross the placenta, but warfarin does due to its smaller size. Warfarin is contraindicated in pregnancy due to its fetopathic effects in the first trimester (stippled epiphyses and nasal and limb hypoplasia) and the risk of fetal bleeding complications in the second and third trimesters. However, warfarin does not enter breast milk in sufficient quantities to anticoagulate the newborn, and is safe to use in the breastfeeding mother. For the patient needing full anticoagulation who prefers to take warfarin rather than frequent injections during the postpartum period, the INR is followed.

Prevention of thromboembolism

The use of anticoagulation to prevent thromboembolism is more controversial. Traditionally, chemoprophylaxis has been recommended to pregnant patients with a history of thrombosis with the idea that pregnancy significantly increases the risk of recurrence. Anticoagulant doses lower than needed to prolong the aPTT have been used (Table 25.1), unless the patient is thought to be at such increased risk that full anticoagulation is necessary. Because it is now recognized that a significant portion of these thrombotic events occur as early as the first trimester, it is prudent to start treatment soon after the pregnancy is recognized and viability confirmed, and continue until 6 weeks post delivery.

A recent study suggested that prophylactic anticoagulation may not be necessary in some patients with a history of venous thromboembolism. In this study of women with a single previous episode of thrombosis associated with a temporary risk factor (e.g., oral contraceptives, surgery, trauma), and no recognized thrombophilia, no recurrences were seen without treatment during pregnancy. However, the number of patients in this study was relatively small. Larger studies in the future may further support the idea that prophylactic treatment with anticoagulants is unnecessary for this type of patient.

Risks to the mother from heparin therapy include a rare thrombocytopenia and the possibility of heparin-induced osteoporosis. These risks are thought to be lower with the use of low molecular weight heparin. Heparin-induced thrombocytopenia occurs within the first week of treatment, so checking the platelet count 5 to 10 days after beginning therapy will provide reassurance. Up to one-third of women may demonstrate subclinical bone loss and the reversibility of this process is not assured. Significant maternal hemorrhage is a possibility in patients that are over-anticoagulated.

Special considerations

Patients with artificial heart valves are at a high risk for thromboembolism, stroke and valve failure and, therefore, must be therapeutically anticoagulated throughout pregnancy. Patients with a documented clot and also a family history of thromboembolic events should be evaluated for antithrombin-III, protein C or protein S deficiency because these traits are autosomal dominant with variable penetrance. Full-dose anticoagulation should be used when these conditions are identified. It is more difficult to diagnose protein S deficiency in pregnancy since levels normally decrease beginning in the first trimester; prophylaxis may be appropriate if protein S deficiency is suspected. Patients with a prior thromboembolic event who have been diagnosed with antiphospholipid antibody syndrome should be given heparin prophylaxis at a minimum, with consideration of full anticoagulation for those thought to be at significant risk. Screening for factor V Leiden and prothrombin mutation should not be performed in patients without a history of prior thrombosis, as patients with these mutations without prior thrombotic events do not need treatment. Patients with mutations of more than one factor (double heterozygotes or those homozygous for mutation) are thought to be at high risk for thrombosis, and treatment is warranted.

There is concern regarding the use of epidural anesthesia during labor and delivery in patients treated with anticoagulants. Some anesthesiologists suggest avoiding regional anesthesia for 12–24 hours from the last injection of low molecular weight heparin, especially if full-dose treatment is used. Because of its more rapid disappearance, a shorter waiting time is used for patients on heparin, and these patients can receive regional anesthesia when laboratory tests confirm a normal PTT result. For this reason, switching from low molecular weight to standard heparin at 36 weeks' gestation may increase the number of patients eligible for regional anesthesia.

Suggested reading

American College of Obstetricians and Gynecologists. *Thromboembolism in Pregnancy.* ACOG Practice Bulletin #19. August, 2000.

American College of Obstetricians and Gynecologists. *Prevention of Deep Vein Thrombosis and Pulmonary Embolism.* ACOG Practice Bulletin #21. October, 2000.

Barbour L, Kick S, Steiner J, *et al.* A prospective study of heparin-induced osteoporosis in pregnancy using bone densitometry. *Am J Obstet Gynecol* 1994;170:862–69.

Brill-Edwards P, Ginsberg JS, Gent M, *et al.* Safety of withholding heparin in pregnant women with a history of venous thromboembolism. *N Eng J Med* 2000;343:1439–44.

Cross JL, Kemp PM, Walsh CG, Flower CDR, Dixon AK. A randomised trial of spiral CT and ventilation perfusion scintigraphy for the diagnosis of pulmonary embolism. *Clin Radiol* 1997;53:177–82.

Dahlman TC. Osteoporotic fractures and the recurrence of thromboembolism during pregnancy and the puerperium in 184 women undergoing thromboprophylaxis with heparin. *Am J Obstet Gynecol* 1993;168:1265–70.

Dizon-Townson DS, Nelson LM, Jang H, Varner MW, Ward K. The incidence of the factor V Leiden mutation in an obstetric population and its relationship to deep vein thrombosis. *Am J Obstet Gynecol* 1997;176:883–6.

Eldor A. The treatment of thrombosis during pregnancy. *Hematology* 1999;483–90.

Maternal and Neonatal Haemostasis Working Party of the Haemostasis and Thrombosis Task. Guidelines on the presentation, investigation, and management of thrombosis associated with pregnancy. *J Clin Pathol* 1993;46:489–96.

Renal Disease

Susan Ramin

Department of Obstetrics, Gynecology and Reproductive Sciences, University of Texas Medical Center at Houston, Houston, TX, USA

Overview

Renal disease is uncommon during pregnancy, occurring in approximately 0.03–0.12% of all pregnancies. Obstetricians may encounter this patient population more frequently given the improvements in reproductive success in women with underlying renal disease. The management of pregnant women with this complication presents a challenge to obstetricians, perinatologists, nephrologists, anesthesiologists and neonatologists. Thus, it is of paramount importance that the management includes a multidisciplinary approach. As the degree of renal impairment increases there is a concomitant increase in both maternal and fetal complications. Maternal adverse effects include preeclampsia, eclampsia, worsening renal impairment, chronic hypertension, placental abruption, anemia, preterm birth and cesarean delivery, while fetal complications include prematurity, low birth weight and fetal/neonatal death.

The clinician should have a basic understanding of the normal physiology in healthy pregnant women when considering renal disorders in pregnancy. Within 1 month of conception the glomerular filtration rate (GFR) is increased by approximately 50% while renal plasma flow (RPF) is increased 50–80%. These physiological changes result in normal reduction in serum levels of creatinine and urea nitrogen to mean values of 50 μmol/L (0.6 mg/dL) and 3 mmol/L (9 mg/dL), respectively; thus, serum creatinine values of 80 μmol/L (0.9 mg/dL) and urea nitrogen values of 6 mmol/L (14 mg/dL) may represent underlying renal disease in pregnancy. During the third trimester of pregnancy, the GFR may decrease by 20% with little effect on serum creatinine. Pre-pregnancy levels are achieved within 3 months following delivery.

There is insufficient scientific data regarding the management of pregnant women with chronic renal disease. However, fertility and the ability to sustain an uncomplicated pregnancy generally relate to the degree of functional

Protocols for High-Risk Pregnancies, 5th edition. Edited by J.T. Queenan, J.C. Hobbins and C.Y. Spong. © 2010 Blackwell Publishing Ltd.

renal impairment and the presence or absence of hypertension rather than to the nature of the underlying renal disorder (Table 26.1). Pregnant women with underlying renal insufficiency are arbitrarily divided into three categories based on serum creatinine values: those with (1) preserved or only mildly impaired renal function (serum creatinine <1.4 mg/dL); (2) moderate renal insufficiency (serum creatinine 1.4 to 2.4–2.8 mg/dL); and (3) severe renal insufficiency (serum creatinine >2.4–2.8 mg/dL).

Women with mild renal impairment usually have successful obstetric outcomes and pregnancy does not appear to adversely affect their underlying disease. About half of the pregnant women with mild renal impairment experience worsening proteinuria which can progress to severe range along with nephrotic edema. Perinatal outcome is compromised by the presence of uncontrolled hypertension and nephrotic proteinuria in early pregnancy. Perinatal outcome for women with mild renal disease is minimally affected, and irreversible renal functional loss in the mother is even lower. This generalization, however, may not hold true for certain kidney diseases (Table 26.2). For instance, women with scleroderma and periarteritis nodosa, disorders often associated with hypertension, do poorly. Conception in some of these women with severe disease may be contraindicated. Women with lupus nephritis do not do as well as women with primary glomerulopathies, especially if the disease has flared within 6 months of conception. Controversy regarding adverse pregnancy effect and the effect on the natural history of the disease process exists with other diseases such as immunoglobulin A (IgA) nephritis, focal glomerular sclerosis, membranoproliferative nephritis and reflux nephropathy. However, it is generally agreed that as functional impairment progresses along with hypertension, maternal and fetal risks significantly increase.

Information on women with moderate or severe renal dysfunction who conceive is more limited. Fetal outcome is still good in the former group where 80–90% of the pregnancies succeed after exclusion of spontaneous abortions. Women with severe renal insufficiency have a

Table 26.1 Severity of renal disease and prospects for pregnancy[a]

Prospects	Mild (%)	Category[b] Moderate (%)	Severe (%)
Pregnancy complications	25	47	86
Successful obstetric outcome	96 (85)	90 (59)	25 (71)
Long-term sequelae	<3 (9)	47 (8)	53 (92)

[a]Estimates are based on 1862 women/2799 pregnancies (1973–1992) and do not include collagen diseases.

[b]Numbers in parentheses refer to prospects when complication(s) develop before 28 weeks' gestation.

Table 26.2 Specific kidney diseases and pregnancy

Renal disease	Effects and outcome
Chronic glomerulonephritis	Usually no adverse effect in the absence of hypertension. One view is that glomerulonephritis is adversely affected by the coagulation changes of pregnancy. Urinary tract infections may occur more frequently
IgA nephropathy	Risks of uncontrolled and/or sudden escalating hypertension and worsening of renal function
Pyelonephritis	Bacteriuria in pregnancy can lead to exacerbation. Multiple organ system derangements may ensue, including adult respiratory distress syndrome
Reflux nephropathy	Risks of sudden escalating hypertension and worsening of renal function
Urolithiasis	Infections can be more frequent, but ureteral dilatation and stasis do not seem to affect natural history. Limited data on lithotripsy thus best avoided
Polycystic disease	Functional impairment and hypertension usually minimal in childbearing years
Diabetic nephropathy	Usually no adverse effect on the renal lesion, but there is increased frequency of infection, edema and/or preeclampsia
Systemic lupus erythematosus (SLE)	Controversial; prognosis most favorable if disease in remission >6 months before conception. Steroid dosage should be increased postpartum
Periarteritis nodosa	Fetal prognosis is dismal and maternal death often occurs
Scleroderma (SS)	If onset during pregnancy, rapid overall deterioration can occur. Reactivation of quiescent scleroderma may occur postpartum
Previous urinary tract surgery	Might be associated with other malformations of the urogenital tract. Urinary tract infection common during pregnancy. Renal function may undergo reversible decrease. No significant obstructive problem but cesarean delivery often needed for abnormal presentation and/or to avoid disruption of the continence mechanism if artificial sphincter present
After nephrectomy, solitary kidney and pelvic kidney	Might be associated with other malformations of urogenital tract. Pregnancy well tolerated. Dystocia rarely occurs with pelvic kidney
Wegener granulomatosis	Limited information. Proteinuria (± hypertension) is common from early in pregnancy. Cytotoxic drugs should be avoided if possible
Renal artery stenosis	May present as chronic hypertension or as recurrent isolated preeclampsia. If diagnosed then transluminal angioplasty can be undertaken in pregnancy if appropriate

live birth rate of 64%. Progression of maternal renal disease is of greater concern in women with moderate or severe renal dysfunction because approximately 50% of pregnant women with an initial serum creatinine ≥1.4 mg/dL experienced an increase in serum creatinine during gestation to a mean serum creatinine of 2.5 mg/dL in the third trimester.

The greatest risk for accelerated progression to end-stage renal disease is seen in women with a serum creatinine above 2.0 mg/dL (177 μmol/L) in early pregnancy. Within 6 months postpartum, 23% of these women progressed to end-stage renal disease. Maternal problems appear greater with severe renal dysfunction even before dialysis is required. The diagnosis of 'superimposed preeclampsia' is often difficult to make because hypertension and proteinuria may be manifestations of the underlying renal disorder; however, superimposed preeclampsia may be diagnosed in up to 80% of cases. Thus, it is primarily the maternal risk in women with moderate renal insufficiency, and the added likelihood of a poor fetal outcome when renal impairment is severe, that leads the clinician to the counseling of women regarding the advisability of pregnancy.

Pre-pregnancy counseling

Serum creatinine levels above 1.5 mg/dL (132 μmol/L) and hypertension are important predisposing risk factors for permanent exacerbation of underlying renal disease, and pregnant women should be so counseled. Fertility is diminished as renal impairment progresses. Normal pregnancy is unusual when preconception serum creatinine is >3 μmol/L (GFR <25 mL/min). The reported frequency of conception among dialysis patients is 0.3–1.5% per year. Fetal wastage is markedly increased; however, recent improvements in management of these pregnant women has led to better rates of live births (approximately 50% of cases). With well-controlled blood pressure and mild renal insufficiency pregnancy outcome is similar to that of normotensive gravidas with renal disease. Ideally, diastolic blood pressure before conception should be 90 mmHg or less.

Management guidelines for pregnancy

Management is best undertaken with a multidisciplinary approach at a tertiary care center under the coordinated care of a maternal-fetal medicine specialist and a nephrologist. The initial laboratory tests should include specialized tests, which help in the early detection of renal impairment as well as superimposed preeclampsia. Thus, besides the usual prenatal screening tests, the following renal parameters should be determined.

1 Serum creatinine, its timed clearance and 24-hour protein excretion (which monitors for change in function).
2 Serum urea nitrogen, albumin and cholesterol concentrations (important in regard to nephrotic complications).

3 Electrolytes (to control for osmolar, potassium and acid–base homeostasis), urine analysis, and more frequent screening for bacterial culture.

4 Uric acid levels, aspartate and alanine aminotransferases, lactic dehydrogenase, prothrombin time, partial thromboplastin time, and platelet count (superimposed preeclampsia screening tests) should also be determined.

The number and frequency of prenatal visits should be based on the severity of renal disease and the presence of other complications such as hypertension and fetal growth restriction. In general and in most cases, women can be followed every 2 weeks until 30 to 32 weeks' gestation and weekly thereafter. Renal parameters should be tested every 4 to 6 weeks throughout pregnancy unless more frequent evaluations become necessary.

Fetal surveillance such as biophysical profile testing is best started at approximately 30 to 32 weeks' gestation, especially in nephrotic patients with hypoalbuminemia. Ultrasonographic examinations for both pregnancy dating and monitoring fetal growth are also an integral part of surveillance.

In general, diuretics should be avoided. This is especially important in nephrotic gravidas, as these women are already oligemic and further intravascular volume depletion may impair uteroplacental perfusion. Furthermore, since blood pressure normally declines during pregnancy, saliuretic therapy could conceivably precipitate circulatory collapse or thromboembolic episodes. This recommendation, however, is relative, because we have observed occasional patients whose kidneys were retaining salt so avidly that diuretics had to be cautiously used. This is especially true for women with diabetic nephropathy, in whom excessive salt retention may lead to volume-dependent hypertension during pregnancy. The use of prophylactic anticoagulation (i.e., mini-heparin) in nephrotic gravidas has been recommended by some specialists, but there is little, if any, data to prove the efficacy of such treatment.

High-protein diets were advocated in the past for women with nephrotic proteinuria, especially during pregnancy, when anabolic requirements increase, although many nephrologists currently recommend a protein-restricted diet for most patients with renal disease. Should protein be restricted in gravidas with renal dysfunction? I caution against this view, and recommend that such regimens be avoided in pregnancy until more is known regarding fetal outcome and especially brain development, first from studies in animal models and then in carefully conducted clinical trials.

Course of pregnancy and clinical decisions

Glomerular filtration rate and blood pressure are the two parameters that influence the course of the pregnancy. Pregnant women with evidence of renal functional deterioration or the appearance (or rapid worsening) of hypertension are best evaluated in the hospital, and delivery would be indicated in the case of failure to reverse these events. Since serum creatinine determinations may be quite variable in some laboratories, decisions should not be made until the direction and rate of change are very clear from repeat tests. A decrease in creatinine clearance of 15 to 20% may occur normally near term; increased proteinuria in the absence of hypertension need not cause alarm, and, therefore, such changes do not suggest a need for hospitalization.

Gravidas with preexisting renal disease or essential hypertension are more susceptible than control populations to superimposed preeclampsia, which frequently occurs in midpregnancy or early in the third trimester (see Protocol **50**). Superimposed preeclampsia, however, may be difficult to differentiate from aggravation of the underlying disease, especially in women with glomerular disease who are prone to hypertension and proteinuria. In any event, when these situations occur the patient should be hospitalized and managed as if she has superimposed preeclampsia. While there are debates on whether mild hypertension (90–100 mmHg diastolic pressure, Korotkoff V) should be treated in pregnant women without underlying renal disorders, treatment is recommended for such levels of blood pressures when known renal disease is present. The goal diastolic pressure is 80 mmHg. Detection of fetal growth restriction or fetal compromise, or both, is important (see Protocol **51**) and, regardless of maternal well-being, will influence the timing of delivery.

Suggested reading

American College of Obstetricians and Gynecologists. *Chronic Hypertension in Pregnancy.* Practice Bulletin # 29. Washington DC: ACOG, July 2001.

Cunningham FG, Cox SM, Harstad TW, Mason RA, Pritchard JA. Chronic renal disease and pregnancy outcome. *Am J Obstet Gynecol* 1990;163:453–9.

Davison JM. Pregnancy in renal allograft recipients: problems, prognosis and practicalities. *Clin Obstet Gynaecol* 1994;8:501–25.

Fischer MJ, Lehnerz SD, Hebert JR, Parikh CR. Kidney disease is an independent risk factor for adverse fetal and maternal outcomes in pregnancy. *Am J Kidney Dis* 2004;43(3):415–23.

Hou, S. Pregnancy in chronic renal insufficiency and end-stage renal disease. *Am J Kidney Dis* 1999;33:235–52.

Hou SH. Pregnancy in women on haemodialysis and peritoneal dialysis. *Clin Obstet Gynaecol* 1994;8:481–500.

Jones DC, Hayslett JP. Outcome of pregnancy in women with moderate or severe renal insufficiency [published erratum appears in *N Engl J Med* 1997;336:739]. *N Engl J Med* 1996;335:226–32.

Jungers P, Chauveau G, Choukroun G, *et al.* Pregnancy in women with impaired renal function. *Nephrology* 1997;47:281–8.

Lindheimer MD, Grunfeld JP, Davison JM. Renal disorders. In: Baron WM, Lindheimer MD (eds) *Medical Disorders During Pregnancy*, 3rd edn. St. Louis, MO: Mosby Inc, 2000; pp. 39–70.

Mastrobattista JM, Gomez-Lobo V for the Society for Maternal-Fetal Medicine. Pregnancy after solid organ transplantation. *Obstet Gynecol* 2008;112:919–32.

Pertuiset N, Grunfeld JP. Acute renal failure in pregnancy. *Clin Obstet Gynaecol* 1994;8:333–51.

Ramin SM, Vidaeff AC, Yeomans ER, Gilstrap LC III. Chronic renal disease in pregnancy. *Obstet Gynecol* 2006;108:1531–9.

Report of the National High Blood Pressure Education Program Working Group on High Blood Pressure in Pregnancy. *Am J Obstet Gynecol* 2000;183:S1–22.

Williams DJ, Davison JM. Renal disorders. In: Creasy RK, Resnik R, Iams JD, Lockwood CJ, Moore TR (eds) *Maternal-Fetal Medicine: Principles and Practice*, 6th edn. Philadelphia: Saunders, 2009; pp. 905–25.

PROTOCOL 27

Obesity

Patrick Catalano

Metrohealth Medical Center, Case Western Reserve University, Cleveland, OH, USA

Clinical significance

Obesity as defined by the WHO and the NHLBI is a significant medical problem during human pregnancy. Based on recent CDC data approximately 60% of women of reproductive age are overweight (BMI [weight/ height^2] >25). Furthermore, 30% of women are obese (BMI >30) and 8% have a BMI >40. There is an increased risk of obesity in women of low socio-economic status as well as in minority racial and ethnic groups as compared with white women. Although certain Asian populations such as women from India have a lower BMI compared with other ethnic groups, Indian women often have increased adiposity at similar BMIs. Maternal obesity in pregnancy has significant short- and long-term risk factors for both mother and fetus. Overweight and obese women have an increased risk of developing preeclampsia, gestational diabetes (GDM) and delivery complications such as deep venous thrombophlebitis. Long-term risks include the risks of type 2 diabetes, hypertension, hyperlipidemia, obstructive sleep apnea and, if not prevented or well controlled, atherosclerotic vascular disease. The fetus of the obese woman is at risk for congenital anomalies (e.g., neural tube defects), stillbirth, prematurity (secondary to maternal complications noted previously), insulin resistance and macrosomia or more specifically increased adiposity. Long-term risks are similar to that of the mother with increased risks of childhood obesity, insulin resistance, hyperlipidemia, hypertension and glucose intolerance.

Pathophysiology

The pathophysiology of obesity in pregnancy is similar to what has been observed in non-pregnant obese individuals, i.e.,metabolic dysfunction. At the core of the 'metabolic syndrome' in obese individuals is insulin

---

Protocols for High-Risk Pregnancies, 5th edition. Edited by J.T. Queenan, J.C. Hobbins and C.Y. Spong. © 2010 Blackwell Publishing Ltd.

resistance. The related conditions are manifestations of the underlying condition. For example, type 2 diabetes is a disease of increased insulin resistance and pancreatic beta-cell failure to maintain glucose homeostasis. During pregnancy obese women are at increased risk for gestational diabetes because as a population they are more insulin resistant as compared with non-obese women. Given that metabolic background, because of the 50–60% increased insulin resistance of pregnancy, the pancreatic beta-cells of obese women are less able to overcome the additional insulin resistance of pregnancy and manifest glucose intolerance which we define as GDM in pregnancy. Increased insulin resistance in pregnancy also affects lipid metabolism in that there is a decreased ability of insulin to suppress lipolysis in obese insulin-resistant women. The manifestation of this aspect of insulin resistance is hyperlipidemia, specifically increased triglyceride concentrations, which in addition to hyperglycemia have been correlated with fetal overgrowth and adiposity. The specific mechanisms accounting for these associations are not yet known with certainty but maternal inflammation and epigenetic modifications are being investigated as potential factors.

Diagnosis

Very simply, all women should have a measured height and weight on a calibrated scale at their first antenatal visit to calculate BMI. NIH has a website (http://www.nhlbisupport.com/bmi) where BMI can easily be ascertained.

Prevention and treatment

The best treatment for obesity is prevention. For the individual woman the optimal time is prior to a planned pregnancy. In the treatment of obesity, the assistance of a healthcare professional relating to lifestyle modification, i.e., diet and exercise, is not to be underestimated. These include not only physicians but nutritionists and exercise instructors. For the woman who has a BMI >40 or BMI >35 associated with medical complications and not responsive to lifestyle measures, bariatric surgery may be considered. The literature regarding the effects of bariatric surgery on pregnancy outcome are limited but preliminary data shows that weight loss associated with bariatric surgery may decrease the risk of GDM and preeclampsia, but not necessarily birthweight. For the offspring, treatment may actually begin in utero by avoiding excessive maternal weight gain.

Table 27.1 Institute of Medicine committee's recommended total and rate of weight gain during pregnancy

Pre-pregnancy BMI	BMI (kg/m²) (WHO)	Total weight gain range (lbs)	Rates of weight gain 2nd and 3rd trimester (mean range in lbs/wk)
Underweight	<18.5	28–40	1 (1–1.3)
Normal weight	18.5–24.9	25–35	1 (0.8–1)
Overweight	25.0–29.9	15–25	0.6 (0.5–0.7)
Obese (includes all classes)	≥30.0	11–20	0.5 (0.4–0.6)

While pre-pregnancy overweight and obesity are risk factors for both maternal and fetal complications, weight gain during pregnancy is a significant contributor to obesity-related morbidities during pregnancy. Recently the Institute of Medicine published a report; 'Weight Gain during Pregnancy: reexamining the Guidelines'. Based on the IOM report high maternal weight gain in pregnancy is associated with an increased risk of maternal cesarean delivery and postpartum weight retention. There was insufficient evidence to assess the association with preeclampsia or pregnancy-associated hypertension. Regarding the fetus, there is also evidence that high gestational weight gain is associated with an increased risk of large for gestational age infants, particularly in non-obese women. The evidence associating high gestational weight gain with childhood obesity was suggestive but insufficient to assess with certainty.

The IOM committee took into consideration recognition of the increase in obesity in the population as well as considering maternal and fetal risks and benefits. Based on the available data the IOM committee recommended the total and rate of weight gain during pregnancy based on maternal pre-pregnancy BMI (see Table 27.1).

Complications

1 Because there is an increased risk of spontaneous abortion and congenital anomalies in obese women, establishing viability and assessment of fetal anatomy are important. The use of vaginal probe ultrasonography in early gestation may aid in the fetal anatomic assessment of obese women and serum screening test for neural tube defects.
2 Screening for diabetes in early and late pregnancy may aid in the diagnosis of unrecognized glucose intolerance in this population and differentiate overt diabetes from gestational diabetes.

3 Assessing cardiovascular and renal function in early pregnancy in obese women with hypertension may aid in the diagnosis of underlying complications such as proteinuria and cardiac dysfunction.

4 Obese women are at increased risk of having the metabolic syndrome and the manifestation of the disorder may be mistaken for pregnancy problems. For example, decreased oxygen saturation in pregnancy may not only be a manifestation of pulmonary embolus but also obstructive sleep apnea. Elevated liver function tests may be a manifestation of severe preeclampsia but may also represent non-alcoholic fatty liver disease, the most common diagnosis for elevated liver function studies in obese non-pregnant women.

5 There is an increased risk for intrauterine fetal demise in obese women. Therefore assessment of fetal well-being using kick counts as well as other modalities may provide reassurance for the patient and healthcare provider.

6 There is an increased risk of cesarean delivery in obese women. Therefore it is important to have available support staff and equipment to address the increased risk of anesthesia complications, and postpartum complications such as wound breakdown, thrombophlebitis and endometritis.

Follow-up

During the pregnancy, encouraging breastfeeding is important for both mother and neonate. Maternal energy requirements are significantly greater when lactating as compared with pregnancy. This is an optimal means to increase energy expenditure and lose weight with the appropriate nutritional counseling. There is also the benefit of breastfeeding for the fetus regarding a potential decreased risk of obesity. Postpartum the attainment of at least pre-pregnancy body weight, if not normal BMI, is important so as not to enter a subsequent pregnancy at a greater BMI.

Conclusion

Pregnancy offers a woman a unique opportunity to affect her long-term health and that of her offspring. The ultimate treatment of obesity lies in the prevention of further obesity. This can be achieved by avoiding excessive weight gain during pregnancy and lifestyle measures to attain a more normal BMI prior to the next pregnancy. Based on preliminary evidence, achieving these measures may also have both short- and long-term benefits for the offspring.

Suggested reading

Allison DB, Fontaine KR, Manson JE, Stevens J, VanItallie TB. Annual deaths attributable to obesity in the United States. *JAMA* 1999;282:1530–8.

Catalano PM. Management of obesity in pregnancy. *Obstet Gynecol* 2007;109:419–33.

Gunderson EP. Breast-feeding and diabetes: long-term impact on mothers and their infants. *Curr Diab Rep* 2008;8:279–86.

National Research Council and Institute of Medicine. Workshop Report: *Influence of Pregnancy Weight on Maternal and Child Health*. National Academies Press, 2007.

National Research Council and Institute of Medicine. Rasmussen KM, Yaktine AL (eds) *Weight Gain During Pregnancy: Reexamining the Guidelines*. National Academies Press, 2009.

Nohr EA, Vaeth M, Baker JL, Sorensen TIA, *et al.* Combined associations of prepregnancy body mass index and gestational weight gain with the outcome of pregnancy. *Am J Clin Nutr* 2008;87:1750–9.

Ogden CL, Carroll MD, Curtin LR, McDowell MA, *et al.* Prevalence of overweight and obesity in the United States, 1999–2004. *JAMA* 2006;295:1549–55.

Ogden CL, Carroll MD, Flegal KM. High body mass index for age among US children and adolescents, 2003–2006. *JAMA* 2008;299:2401–5.

Ramos RG, Olden K. The prevalence of metabolic syndrome among US women of childbearing age. *Am J Pub Hlth* 2008;98:1122–27.

Schaefer-Graf UM, Graf K, Kulbacka I, Kjos SL, *et al.* Maternal lipids as strong determinants of fetal environment and growth in pregnancies with gestational diabetes mellitus. *Diabetes Care* 2008;31:1858–63.

PROTOCOL 28

Diabetes Mellitus

Mark B. Landon and Steven G. Gabbe

Department of Obsterics and Gynecology, The Ohio State University College of Medicine, Columbus, OH, USA

Overview

Diabetes mellitus complicates approximately 3 to 5% of all pregnancies. Gestational diabetes mellitus (GDM), or carbohydrate intolerance detected for the first time during gestation, represents about 90% of all cases, whereas pregestational diabetes mellitus, which includes both type 1 and type 2 diabetes mellitus, accounts for the remaining 10%.

Pathophysiology

The increased perinatal morbidity and mortality associated with the pregnancy complicated by diabetes mellitus can be attributed directly to maternal hyperglycemia. Glucose crosses the placenta by facilitated diffusion. Therefore, maternal hyperglycemia can produce fetal hyperglycemia. During the first trimester, maternal hyperglycemia is associated with an increased risk for abnormal fetal organogenesis. Major fetal malformations, now the leading cause of perinatal mortality in pregnancies complicated by type 1 and type 2 diabetes mellitus, occur in 6–10% of poorly controlled patients. Chronic fetal hyperglycemia in later gestation leads to fetal hyperinsulinemia, which is associated with excessive fetal growth, as well as delayed fetal pulmonary maturation. Intrauterine fetal death, which is observed in pregnancies complicated by poorly controlled diabetes mellitus, can also be attributed to fetal hyperinsulinemia that results in lactic acidosis. The likelihood that any of these complications will occur is directly related to maternal glucose control, as reflected by mean glucose levels or concentrations of glycosylated hemoglobin. The presence of diabetic vasculopathy may also affect placental function, thereby increasing the risk for fetal growth restriction and preterm delivery.

Protocols for High-Risk Pregnancies, 5th edition. Edited by J.T. Queenan, J.C. Hobbins and C.Y. Spong. © 2010 Blackwell Publishing Ltd.

Pregestational diabetes mellitus

Risk assessment
Maternal and perinatal risks are increased in the presence of:
1 vasculopathy, such as retinopathy, nephropathy, and hypertension;
2 poor glucose control;
3 prognostically bad signs of pregnancy, including ketoacidosis, pyelonephritis, pregnancy-induced hypertension, and poor clinic attendance or neglect.

Pre-pregnancy care
Objectives
1 Assess for maternal vasculopathy by an ophthalmological evaluation, electrocardiogram and 24-hour urine collection for creatinine clearance and protein excretion.
2 Improve maternal glucose control (target glycosylated hemoglobin 7% or lower with normal range 6% or lower) to reduce the risk of fetal malformations and miscarriage; assess hypoglycemic awareness.
3 Provide contraceptive counseling.
4 Educate the patient and her partner about the management plan for diabetes in pregnancy.
5 Determine rubella immune status and check thyroid function studies.
6 Begin folic acid prophylaxis to reduce risk of fetal neural tube defects.

Detection and evaluation of malformations
1 Identification of women at greatest risk: maternal glycosylated hemoglobin levels in the first trimester.
2 Quad screen at 15–20 weeks.
3 Ultrasonography at 13–14 weeks to detect anencephaly.
4 Comprehensive ultrasonography at 18–20 weeks with careful study of cardiac structure, including great vessels.

Antepartum care: regulation of maternal glycemia
Target capillary glucose levels in pregnancy are listed below:

Mean level:	100 mg/dL
Before breakfast:	<90 mg/dL
Before lunch, supper, bedtime snack:	<100 mg/dL
1 hour after meals:	<140 mg/dL
2 hours after meals:	<120 mg/dL
2 a.m. to 6 a.m:	>60 mg/dL

1 Capillary glucose monitoring with fasting, prelunch, predinner and bedtime levels daily, as well as 1-hour or 2-hour postprandial values; glycosylated hemoglobin levels in each trimester, target ≤6%.

2 Insulin therapy
- Multiple insulin injections: prandial insulin (insulin lispro or insulin aspart) with meals, snacks; basal insulin (neutral protamine Hagedorn (NPH), before breakfast (two-thirds of total NPH dose) and at bedtime (one-third of total NPH dose).
- Continuous subcutaneous insulin infusion (insulin pump): insulin lispro; continuous basal rate and boluses, in highly compliant patients.

3 Dietary recommendations
- Plan: three meals, three snacks.
- Diet: 30–35 kcal/kg normal body weight, 2000 to 2400 kcal/day.
- Composition: carbohydrate 40–50% complex, high fiber; protein 20%; fat 30–40% (<10% saturated). Weight gain: 22 to 25 lb.

4 General guidelines for insulin use and carbohydrate intake:
- 1 unit of rapid-acting insulin lowers blood glucose 30 mg/dL.
- 10 g of carbohydrate increases blood glucose 30 mg/dL.
- 1 unit of rapid-acting insulin will cover intake of 10 g of carbohydrate.

Fetal evaluation

Assessment of fetal well-being to prevent intrauterine fetal deaths and guide timing of delivery:

1 Biophysical
- Maternal assessment of fetal activity at 28 weeks.
- Non-stress test (NST), weekly at 28 to 30 weeks; twice weekly at 32 weeks and beyond; may alternate with biophysical profile (BPP).
- BPP or contraction stress test if NST nonreactive.

2 Sonographic evaluation of fetal growth during the third trimester.

3 Amniocentesis to assess fetal pulmonary maturation for elective delivery before 39 weeks.

Delivery

Timing

1 Patients at low risk for fetal death (excellent glucose control, no vasculopathy, normal fetal growth, reassuring antepartum fetal testing, no prior stillbirth): allow spontaneous labor up to 40 weeks.

2 Patients at high risk for fetal death (poor control, vasculopathy, macrosomia, hydramnios, prior stillbirth): consider delivery prior to 39 weeks. Amniocentesis may be employed to assess for lung maturity.

Method

To reduce birth trauma, counsel regarding elective cesarean delivery if estimated fetal weight is ≥4500 g. For estimated weight 4000–4500 g, mode of delivery will depend on prior obstetric history, sonographic growth characteristics, pelvic examination and patient preference.

Table 28.1 Glucose control during first stage of labor

	Insulin	Glucose
Latent phase	1 unit/hr	5 g/h
Active phase	None	10 g/h

Intrapartum glycemic control
1 Check capillary glucose hourly at the bedside; maintain below 110 mg/dL.
2 Glucose control during labor (first stage) (Table 28.1).

Contraception for the patient with type 1 or type 2 diabetes mellitus
Combination oral contraceptives
1 Low-dose pills appear safe in patients without vasculopathy.
2 Contraindicated in presence of smoking, hypertension.

Progestin-only pills
Acceptable for patients with vasculopathy.

Mechanical or barrier methods
Less effective than oral contraceptives but no effect on glucose control or vasculopathy.

Intrauterine device
Acceptable for multiparous patients.

Sterilization
Consider when family has been completed, especially for patients with significant vasculopathy.

Gestational diabetes

Definition
Gestational diabetes is defined as carbohydrate intolerance of variable severity with onset or first recognition during pregnancy. The definition applies irrespective of whether or not insulin is used for treatment or the condition persists after pregnancy. It does not exclude the possibility that unrecognized glucose intolerance may have antedated the pregnancy.

Class A_1 gestational diabetes is diet controlled; Class A_2 gestational diabetes requires diet and pharmacological treatment (insulin or glyburide).

Consequences: Why bother to screen?

1 Maternal: subsequent type 2 diabetes mellitus, shortened life expectancy.
2 Fetal and neonatal:
  • excessive fetal growth and birth trauma; neonatal hypoglycemia, hypocalcemia, hyperbilirubinemia;
  • increased perinatal mortality associated with significant maternal hyperglycemia.

Screening and diagnosis
Detection

Most practitioners continue to screen all pregnant women for glucose intolerance since selective screening based on clinical attributes or past obstetric history has been shown to be inadequate. There may be a group of women at low enough risk that screening is not necessary (see below).

According to the Fourth International Workshop Conference, Screening Strategy, risk assessment for GDM should be ascertained at the first prenatal visit.

Low risk

Blood glucose testing is not routinely required if all of the following characteristics are present:
• Member of an ethnic group with a low prevalence of GDM
• No known diabetes in first-degree relatives
• Age <25 years
• Weight normal before pregnancy
• No history of abnormal glucose metabolism
• No history of poor obstetric outcome.

Average risk

Perform blood glucose screening at 24–28 weeks using one of the following:
• Two-step procedure: 50 g GCT (glucose challenge test) followed by a diagnostic OGTT (oral glucose tolerance test) in those meeting the threshold value in GCT.
• One-step procedure: diagnostic OGTT performed on all subjects.

High risk

• Perform blood glucose testing as soon as feasible, using the procedures described above.
• If GDM is not diagnosed, blood glucose testing should be repeated at 24–28 weeks or at any time a patient has symptoms or signs suggestive of hyperglycemia.

Adapted from Fourth International Workshop Conference on GDM, *Diabetes Care*, Volume 21, Supplement 2, August 1998.

With a GCT cutoff value of 140 mg/dL, sensitivity is 90%, and 15% of patients require a GTT. With a cutoff of 130 mg/dL, sensitivity is nearly 100%, but 25% of patients require a GTT.

A plasma glucose measurement ≥200 mg/dL outside the context of a formal glucose challenge test, or a truly fasting plasma glucose ≥126 mg/dL, suggests the diabetic state and warrants further investigation.

Diagnosis

100 g oral glucose load, administered in the morning after overnight fast for at least 8 hours but not more than 14 hours, and following at least 3 days of unrestricted diet (≥150 g carbohydrate) and usual physical activity.

Venous plasma glucose is measured fasting and at 1, 2 and 3 hours. Subject should remain seated and not smoke throughout the test.

Two or more of the following venous plasma concentrations must be met or exceeded for a positive diagnosis (Table 28.2).

Future recommendations

The recently completed Hyperglycemia and Adverse Pregnancy Outcome (HAPO) study has suggested a continuous relationship between maternal glucose levels (including levels below those currently diagnostic of GDM) and perinatal outcomes. This study will be utilized to formulate new recommendations regarding screening and diagnosis of GDM.

Antepartum management
Program of care

Visits every 1 to 2 weeks until 36 weeks, then weekly.

Dietary recommendations in pregnancy

- Plan: 3 meals, bedtime snack.
- Diet: 2000 to 2200 kcal/day. Normal weight: 30 kcal/kg ideal pre-pregnancy body weight. Lean: 35 kcal/kg ideal pre-pregnancy body weight. Obese: 25 kcal/kg ideal pre-pregnancy body weight.

Table 28.2 Venous plasma concentrations for positive diagnosis of diabetes mellitus

	NDDG	Carpenter & Coustan*
Fasting	105 mg/dL	95 mg/dL
1-hour	190 mg/dL	180 mg/dL
2-hour	165 mg/dL	155 mg/dL
3-hour	145 mg/dL	140 mg/dL

*Carpenter MW, Coustan DR. Criteria for screening tests for gestational diabetes. *Am J Obstet Gynecol* 1982;144:768–73.

- Composition: carbohydrate 40–50% complex, high fiber; protein 20%; fat 30–40% (<10% saturated). Weight gain: 20 lb; 16 lb for very obese.

Note: Check morning urine for ketones if using caloric restriction in obese patients (1600–1800 kcal/day). Increase caloric intake if fasting ketonuria noted.

Exercise
Encourage regular exercise, 20–30 minutes brisk walking, 3–4 times/week.

Surveillance of maternal diabetes
1 Self-monitoring of capillary blood glucose to check fasting and 1-hour or 2-hour postprandial glucose levels daily to assess efficacy of diet.
2 If repetitive fasting plasma values are >95 mg/dL and/or 1-hour values are >140 mg/dL and/or 2-hour values are >120 mg/dL, insulin or glyburide therapy is recommended.
3 Starting insulin dose calculated based on patient's weight; 0.8 U/kg actual body weight per day in first trimester, 1.0 U/kg in second trimester, 1.2 U/kg in third trimester. Give two-thirds of total dose in fasting state: two-thirds as NPH, one-third as regular or insulin lispro; give one-third of total dose as one-half regular or insulin lispro at dinner, one-half as NPH at bedtime.
4 Glyburide can be used as alternative to insulin, although it is usually not effective if fasting glucose exceeds 115 mg/dL. Glyburide, unlike insulin, does cross the placenta and controversy exists regarding the amount of drug reaching the fetus. The usual starting dose is 2.5 mg at breakfast and 2.5 mg at dinner with doses as high as 20 mg/day employed.

Delivery
1 Women with class A_1 gestational diabetes, allow to go to term.
2 If undelivered at 40 weeks, begin fetal assessment with twice-weekly NSTs. Women with prior stillbirth or those with hypertension should be followed with twice-weekly NSTs at 32 weeks.
3 Clinical estimation of fetal size and ultrasonographic indices should be used to detect excessive fetal growth. To reduce birth trauma, counsel regarding cesarean delivery if estimated fetal weight is ≥ 4500 g. For estimated weight 4000–4500 g, consider prior obstetric history, fetal growth indices, pelvic capacity and patient preference in selecting mode of delivery.
4 Class A_2 women should be followed with twice-weekly NSTs.
5 Alert neonatal team as infant may require observation for hypoglycemia, hypocalcemia, hyperbilirubinemia.

Table 28.3 Values for venous plasma glucose

Normal	Impaired glucose tolerance	Diabetes mellitus
Fasting <100 mg/dL	100–125 mg/dL	≥126 mg/dL
2 h <140 mg/dL	140–199 mg/dL	≥200 mg/dL

Postpartum care
Evaluation for persistent carbohydrate intolerance
1 Women can continue self-blood-glucose monitoring to evaluate glucose profile although class A₁ patients generally demonstrate normoglycemia.
2 At 6 weeks postpartum, oral GTT with 75 g glucose load, administered under conditions described for 100 g oral test. Venous plasma glucose is measured fasting and at 2 hours (Table 28.3).
3 If normal, evaluate at minimum of 3-year intervals with fasting glucose; encourage exercise and, if obese, weight loss.

Effects of oral contraceptives
Deterioration of carbohydrate intolerance not reported with low-dose pills.

Recurrence risk
Approximately 60%.

Suggested reading

Type 1 and type 2 diabetes mellitus in pregnancy
American College of Obstetricians and Gynecologists. *Pregestational diabetes mellitus.* ACOG Practice Bulletin. Clinical Management Guidelines for Obstetrician-Gynecologists. Number 60, March 2005.

DeWitt DE, Hirsch IB. Outpatient insulin therapy in type 1 and type 2 diabetes mellitus. *JAMA* 2003;289(17):2254–64.

Gabbe SG, Graves CR. Management of diabetes mellitus complicating pregnancy. *Obstet Gynecol* 2003;102:4:857–68.

Kitzmiller JL, Buchanan TA, Kjos S, Combs CA, Ratner RE. Pre-conception care of diabetes, congenital malformations, and spontaneous abortions. *Diabetes Care* 1996;19:514–40.

Landon MB, Catalano PM, Gabbe SG. Diabetes mellitus complicating pregnancy. In: Gabbe SG, Neibyl JR, Simpson JL (eds) *Obstetrics: Normal and Problem Pregnancies*, 5th edn. Churchill Livingston, 2007; pp. 976–1010.

Landon MB, Gabbe, SG. Medical therapy. In: Reece EA, Coustan D, Gabbe SG (eds) *Diabetes Mellitus in Women.* Lippincott Williams & Wilkins, 2004.

Gestational diabetes mellitus
American College of Obstetricians and Gynecologists Committee on Practice Bulletins-Obstetrics, Coustan DR. *Gestational diabetes.* ACOG practice bulletin #30. Washington: American College of Obstetricians and Gynecologists, 2001.

American Diabetes Association. Gestational diabetes mellitus. *Diabetes Care* 2004; 27(Suppl.):S88–90.

Carpenter MW, Coustan DR. Criteria for screening tests for gestational diabetes. *Am J Obstet Gynecol* 1982;144:768–73.

Crowther CA, Hiller JE, Moss JR, McPhee AJ, *et al.* Australian Carbohydrate Intolerance Study in Pregnant Women (ACHOIS) Trial Group. *N Engl J Med* 2005;352(24):2477–86.

HAPO Study Cooperative Research Group. Hyperglycemia and Adverse Pregnancy Outcome (HAPO) Study: association with neonatal anthropometrics. *Diabetes* 2009;58(2):453–9.

Kjos SL, Buchanan TA, Greenspoon JS, Montoro M, Bernstein GS, Mestman JH. Gestational diabetes mellitus: the prevalence of glucose intolerance and diabetes mellitus in the first two months postpartum. *Am J Obstet Gynecol* 1990;163:93–8.

Landon MB, Spong CY, Thom E, Carpenter MW, *et al.* A Multicenter, Randomized Trial of Treatment for Mild Gestational Diabetes. *N Engl J Med* 361;14:1339–1348, 2009.

Langer O, Conway DL, Berkus MD, Xenakis EMJ, Gonzales O. A comparison of glyburide and insulin in women with gestational diabetes mellitus. *N Engl J Med* 2000; 343:1134–8.

Hyperthyroidism and Hypothyroidism in Pregnancy

Brian M. Casey
University of Texas Southwestern Medical Center, Dallas, TX, USA

Overview

Pregnancy exerts a substantial impact on maternal thyroid physiology. Changes in the structure and function of the gland sometimes cause confusion in the diagnosis of thyroid abnormalities. Serum thyrotropin levels in early pregnancy decrease due to thyroid stimulation by the weak TSH effects of human chorionic gonadotropin (hCG). Free thyroxine levels also increase slightly to suppress pituitary thyrotropin secretion. There is an intimate relationship between maternal and fetal thyroid function, and drugs that affect the maternal thyroid also affect the fetal gland. Uncontrolled thyrotoxicosis and untreated hypothyroidism are both associated with adverse pregnancy outcomes.

Hyperthyroidism

Symptomatic thyrotoxicosis or hyperthyroidism complicates about 1 in 1000 to 2000 pregnancies. The overwhelming cause of thyrotoxicosis in pregnancy is Graves disease, an organ-specific autoimmune process usually associated with thyroid-stimulating antibodies. The introduction of third-generation thyrotropin assays with analytical sensitivity of 0.002 mU/L have made it possible to identify subclinical thyroid disorders. These biochemically defined extremes usually represent normal biological variations but may also herald the earliest stages of thyroid dysfunction. Subclinical hyperthyroidism is characterized by an abnormally low serum thyrotropin concentration in concert with thyroxine hormone levels within the normal reference range. Subclinical hyperthyroidism has not been associated with adverse pregnancy outcomes. Since there is no

Protocols for High-Risk Pregnancies, 5th edition. Edited by J.T. Queenan, J.C. Hobbins and C.Y. Spong. © 2010 Blackwell Publishing Ltd.

convincing evidence that subclinical hyperthyroidism should be treated in non-pregnant individuals, treatment seems especially unwarranted in pregnancy because antithyroid drugs reach the fetus. However, women identified with subclinical hyperthyroidism may benefit from periodic surveillance.

Diagnosis

Because normal pregnancy simulates some clinical findings similar to those find with thyroxine (T_4) excess, mild thyrotoxicosis may be difficult to diagnose. Suggestive findings include tachycardia, thyromegaly, exophthalmos and failure to gain weight despite adequate food intake. Laboratory confirmation is by a markedly depressed thyrotropin (TSH) level along with an elevated serum free T_4 (fT_4) level. Rarely, hyperthyroidism is caused by abnormally high serum triiodothyronine (T_3) levels – so-called T_3 toxicosis.

Treatment

Thyrotoxicosis during pregnancy can nearly always be controlled by thionamide drugs. Propylthiouracil (PTU) partially inhibits the conversion of T_4 to T_3 and crosses the placenta less readily than methimazole. Although not definitely proven, methimazole use in early pregnancy has been associated with a rare embryopathy characterized by esophageal or choanal atresia as well as aplasia cutis. Despite the lack of evidence that PTU is safer than methimazole, PTU still is the preferred thionamide in the United States.

The initial propylthiouracil dose is empirical. In non-pregnant patients, the American Thyroid Association recommends an initial daily dose of 100 to 600 mg for PTU or 10 to 40 mg for methimazole. Thyrotoxicosis in pregnant women generally requires higher starting doses such as 300 or 450 mg of PTU daily. Serum fT_4 is a better indicator of thyroid status than TSH during the first 2 to 3 months of treatment for hyperthyroidism.

Transient leukopenia can be documented in up to 10% of women taking antithyroid drugs, but does not require cessation of therapy. In less than 1%, however, **agranulocytosis** develops suddenly and mandates discontinuance of the drug. It is not dose related and serial leukocyte counts during therapy are not helpful. Thus, if fever or sore throat develop, women should be instructed to discontinue medication immediately and report for a complete blood count.

Subtotal thyroidectomy can be performed after thyrotoxicosis is medically controlled but is seldom done during pregnancy. Ablation with therapeutic radioactive iodine is contraindicated during pregnancy. It is recommended that women avoid pregnancy for a period of 6 months after radioablative therapy.

Complications

Women with thyrotoxicosis have pregnancy outcomes that largely depend on whether metabolic control is achieved. In untreated women, or those who remain hyperthyroid despite therapy, there is a higher incidence of preeclampsia, heart failure and adverse perinatal outcomes such as intrauterine fetal growth restriction and neonatal death. Perinatal mortality rates may be as high as 10%.

Although maternal antithyroid therapy can theoretically induce fetal hypothyroidism, there is little correlation between commonly used maternal doses and fetal thyroid status. Neonatal hyperthyroidism occurs in about 2% of infants born to hyperthyroid mothers. This is due to the placental passage of maternal thyroid-stimulating immunoglobulin (TSI), which stimulates the fetal thyroid.

Fetal hyperthyroidism is a very rare event that occurs in fetuses whose mothers have been treated with ablative therapy for hyperthyroidism before pregnancy. This is presumably due to persistent high TSI levels in spite of maternal euthyroidism. Fetal tachycardia, fetal goiter and intrauterine growth restriction are suggestive of this complication. TSI should be measured in women with a history of Graves disease treated with ^{131}I and in women with a previously affected infant; its utility in other women with Graves disease is unclear. Cordocentesis may be useful in the setting of a prior affected infant, prior maternal ablative therapy with a high TSI titer or a fetus with ultrasonographic signs of fetal hyperthyroidism. Fetal thyroid function tests may then guide therapy to increase or decrease maternal antithyroid therapy.

Thyroid storm and heart failure

Thyroid storm is an acute, life-threatening, hypermetabolic state and is rare in pregnancy. In contrast, pulmonary hypertension and heart failure from cardiomyopathy caused by thyroxine is more common in hyperthyroid pregnant women. The pregnant woman with thyrotoxicosis has minimal cardiac reserve, and decompensation can be precipitated by preeclampsia, anemia, sepsis, or a combination of these.

Treatment for thyroid storm or heart failure is similar and should be carried out in an intensive care unit. Specific treatment consists of 1000 mg of PTU given orally or crushed and placed through a nasogastric tube. PTU is continued in 200 mg doses every 6 hours. An hour after initial PTU administration, iodide is given to inhibit thyroidal release of T_3 and T_4. It is given intravenously as 500 to 1000 mg of sodium iodide every 8 hours; orally as 5 drops of supersaturated solution of potassium iodide (SSKI) every 8 hours; or as Lugol solution, 10 drops orally every 8 hours. With a history of iodine-induced anaphylaxis, lithium carbonate, 300 mg every 6 hours, is given instead. Most authorities recommend dexamethasone, 2 mg intravenously every 6 hours for four doses, to further block peripheral conversion of T_4 to T_3. If a beta-blocker drug is given to control tachycardia, its effect on heart failure should be considered. Propranolol, labetalol and esmolol have all been used successfully intrapartum.

Follow-up

Women with Graves disease should be followed at regular intervals following delivery, since recurrence or aggravation of symptoms is not uncommon in the first few months postpartum. Most asymptomatic women should have a TSH and fT_4 performed about 6 weeks postpartum.

Breastfeeding is not contraindicated in mothers taking PTU or 10 to 20 mg methimazole daily. The American Academy of Pediatricians considers both drugs compatible with breastfeeding. It may be prudent to give divided doses after feeding, when possible. Periodic evaluation of the infant's thyroid function has also been suggested.

Hypothyroidism

Overt hypothyroidism complicates from 2 to 3 pregnancies per 1000. The most common cause of hypothyroidism in pregnancy is Hashimoto thyroiditis, characterized by glandular destruction from autoantibodies. Other important causes of hypothyroidism include endemic iodine deficiency and a history of either ablative radioiodine therapy or thyroidectomy. Clinical identification of hypothyroidism is particularly difficult during pregnancy because many of the signs or symptoms are also common to pregnancy itself. Thyroid testing should be performed on symptomatic women or those with a history of thyroid disease. Treatment of women with clinical hypothyroidism has been associated with improved pregnancy outcomes. Subclinical hypothyroidism is defined by an elevated serum thyrotropin level with normal serum thyroxine. It affects 2% to 3% of pregnant women and has recently been implicated in impaired neurological development in offspring. Screening and treatment of pregnant women with subclinical hypothyroidism has not been demonstrated beneficial and remains an area of controversy.

Diagnosis

Hypothyroidism is characterized by insidious nonspecific clinical findings that include fatigue, constipation, cold intolerance, muscle cramps, dry skin, hair loss and weight gain. A pathologically enlarged thyroid gland depends on the etiology of hypothyroidism and is more likely in women in areas of endemic iodine deficiency or those with Hashimoto thyroiditis. Clinical or overt hypothyroidism is diagnosed when an abnormally high serum thyrotropin level is accompanied by an abnormally low thyroxine level.

Treatment

Replacement therapy for hypothyroidism is with levothyroxine in doses of 1 to 2 μg/kg/day or approximately 100 μg daily. Serum thyrotropin levels are measured at 4- to 6-week intervals, and the thyroxine dose is adjusted by 25 to 50 μg increments until normal TSH values between 0.5 and 2.5 mU/L are reached.

Pregnancy is associated with an increase in thyroxine requirements in approximately a third of supplemented women. This is particularly true in women without thyroid reserve such as those with a previous thyroidectomy, history of radioiodine ablation, or those undergoing assisted reproductive techniques. Increasing thyroxine replacement by 25% at pregnancy confirmation will reduce this likelihood. All other women with hypothyroidism should undergo TSH testing at initiation of prenatal care.

Complications

There are excessive adverse perinatal outcomes associated with overt thyroxine deficiency. Clinical hypothyroidism complicating pregnancy has been linked to an increase in complications such as gestational hypertension, placental abruption, preterm birth and neurological dysfunction in offspring. Neurological sequelae of maternal and fetal hypothyroidism are particularly evident in iodine-deficient women. Spontaneous abortion has also been shown to be increased in women with hypothyroidism, particularly in those women with antithyroid antibodies. Finally, an increase in stillbirth, which may be related to preeclampsia and placental abruption, has been demonstrated in mothers with clinical hypothyroidism. Adequate hormone replacement during pregnancy minimizes the risk of adverse outcomes and most complications.

Follow-up

After pregnancy in women with clinical hypothyroidism, levothyroxine dose should be returned to the prepregnancy dose and a TSH should be checked 6 to 8 weeks postpartum. Periodic monitoring of hypothyroidism with an annual serum TSH concentration is advised because of the impact of changing weight and age on thyroid function. Women with subclinical hypothyroidism, particularly those with thyroid autoantibodies, are at an increased risk for developing clinical disease within 5 years. While treatment of these women remains controversial, yearly evaluation for the development of clinical disease is recommended.

Levothyroxine is excreted in breast milk in low concentrations. The American Academy of Pediatrics considers levothyroxine to be compatible with breastfeeding. Levothyroxine breast milk levels are too low to affect neonatal thyroid screening programs or to protect hypothyroid infants.

Suggested reading

Abalovich M, Amino N, Barbour L, *et al.* Management of thyroid dysfunction during pregnancy and postpartum: an Endocrine Society Clinical Practice Guideline. *J Clin Endocrinol Metab* 2007;92(8 Suppl):S1.

Alexander EK, Marquesee E, Lawrence J, *et al.* Timing and magnitude of increases in levothyroxine requirements during pregnancy in women with hypothyroidism. *N Eng J Med* 2004;351:241.

American College of Obstetricians and Gynecologists. Thyroid disease in pregnancy. Practice Bulletin # 37, August 2002.

American College of Obstetricians and Gynecologists. Subclinical hypothyroidism in pregnancy. Committee Opinion # 381, October 2007.

Brent GA: Graves' disease. *N Eng J Med* 2008;358:2594.

Casey BM, Leveno KJ. Thyroid disease in pregnancy. *Obstet Gynecol* 2006;108:1283.

Kilpatrick S. Umbilical blood sampling in women with thyroid disease in pregnancy: is it necessary? *Am J Obstet Gynecol* 2003;189:1.

Morreale De Escobar G, Obregon MJ, Escobar Del Rey F. Role of thyroid hormone during early brain development. *Eur J Endocrinol* 2004;151:U25.

Sheffield JS, Cunningham FG. Thyrotoxicosis and heart failure that complicate pregnancy. *Am J Obstet Gynecol* 2004;190:211.

Surks MI, Ortiz E, Daniels GH, *et al.* Subclinical thyroid disease: scientific review and guidelines for diagnosis and management. *JAMA* 2004;(291)2:228.

Acute and Chronic Hepatitis

Patrick Duff

Department of Obstetrics and Gynecology, University of Florida College of Medicine, Gainesville, FL, USA

Clinical significance

The principal forms of hepatitis that complicate pregnancy are hepatitis A, B, C, D and E. Hepatitis G is a relatively benign clinical disorder that does not pose a serious risk to either the pregnant woman or her baby.

Hepatitis A is the second most common cause of hepatitis in the United States, but it is relatively uncommon in pregnancy. It is caused by an RNA virus that is transmitted by fecal-oral contact. Infections in children are usually asymptomatic; infections in adults are usually symptomatic. The disease is most prevalent in areas of poor sanitation and close living. Infection does not result in a chronic carrier state, and perinatal transmission essentially never occurs.

Hepatitis B is the most common form of viral hepatitis in obstetric patients. It is caused by a DNA virus that is transmitted parenterally and via sexual contact. Acute hepatitis B occurs in approximately 1 to 2 per 1000 pregnancies in the United States. The chronic carrier stage is more frequent, occurring in 6 to 10 per 1000 pregnancies. In the United States, approximately 1.25 million persons are chronically infected.

Hepatitis C is caused by an RNA virus that is transmitted parenterally, via sexual contact, and perinatally. In some patient populations, hepatitis C is actually as common as, if not more common than, hepatitis B. Chronic hepatitis C infection now is the number one indication for liver transplantation in the United States.

Hepatitis D is an RNA virus that depends upon co-infection with hepatitis B for replication. The epidemiology of hepatitis D is essentially identical to that of Hepatitis B. Hepatitis D may cause a chronic carrier state, and perinatal transmission is possible if hepatitis B transmission occurs simultaneously.

Protocols for High-Risk Pregnancies, 5th edition. Edited by J.T. Queenan, J.C. Hobbins and C.Y. Spong. © 2010 Blackwell Publishing Ltd.

Hepatitis E is caused by an RNA virus. The epidemiology of hepatitis E is similar to that of hepatitis A. The disease is quite rare in the United States but is endemic in developing countries of the world. In these countries, maternal infection with hepatitis E often has an alarmingly high mortality, in the range of 10 to 20%. A chronic carrier state does not exist, and perinatal transmission is extremely unlikely.

Pathophysiology and clinical manifestations

Hepatitis A is transmitted by fecal-oral contact, has an incubation period of 15 to 50 days, and usually causes symptomatic infection in adults. The typical clinical manifestations include low-grade fever, malaise, poor appetite, right upper quadrant pain and tenderness, jaundice and acholic stools. Because hepatitis A does not cause a chronic carrier state, perinatal transmission virtually never occurs. The disease poses a risk only if the mother develops fulminant hepatitis and liver failure. Fortunately, such a situation is extremely rare.

Hepatitis B may be transmitted by sharing contaminated drug paraphernalia and via sexual contact and blood transfusion. Infection also can be transmitted to healthcare workers as a result of occupational exposure through needle stick or splash injuries. After exposure to the virus, approximately 90% of patients mount an effective immunological response to the virus and completely clear the infection. Less than 1% develop fulminant hepatitis and die. Approximately 10% of patients develop a chronic carrier state. These patients pose a major risk of transmission of infection to their sexual partner and their infant, and they are the patients most commonly encountered by obstetricians in clinical practice.

Hepatitis C may be transmitted parenterally, via sexual contact, perinatally and via occupational exposure. The disease usually is asymptomatic, but, unfortunately, it typically results in chronic infection which, ultimately, causes severe hepatic impairment.

Hepatitis D infection always occurs in association with hepatitis B infection. Patients may have two types of infection. Some have both acute hepatitis D and acute hepatitis B (*co-infection*). These individuals typically clear their viremia and have a favorable long-term prognosis. Other individuals have chronic hepatitis D infection superimposed upon chronic hepatitis B infection (*super-infection*). These patients are particularly likely to develop chronic liver disease.

Hepatitis E is transmitted almost entirely by fecal-oral contact. The incubation period averages 45 days, and patients typically have a symptomatic acute infection. The maternal mortality in endemic areas is high, primarily because of the associated poor nutrition, poor general health and lack of access to modern medical care within the population. Hepatitis E does not cause a chronic carrier state, and perinatal transmission is extremely rare.

Diagnosis

The best test to confirm the diagnosis of acute hepatitis A is identification of anti-hepatitis A-IgM antibody. Acutely infected patients also may have elevated liver transaminase enzymes and an elevated serum concentration of direct and indirect bilirubin. In severe cases, coagulation abnormalities may be present.

Hepatitis B virus has three distinct antigens: the surface antigen (HBsAg) which is found in serum, the core antigen (HBcAg) which is found only in hepatocytes, and the e antigen (HBeAg) which also is found in serum. Detection of the latter antigen is indicative of an extremely high rate of viral replication. Patients with *acute* hepatitis B typically have a positive serological test for the surface antigen and a positive IgM antibody directed against the core antigen. Patients with *chronic* hepatitis B infection are seropositive for the surface antigen and have positive IgG antibody directed against the core antigen. Some patients will also test positive for hepatitis B*e* antigen. The seroprevalence of hepatitis e antigen is particularly high in Asian women. Patients who are positive for both the surface antigen and e antigen have an extremely high risk of perinatal transmission of infection that approaches 90% in the absence of neonatal immunoprophylaxis.

The initial screening test for hepatitis C should be an enzyme immunoassay (EIA). The confirmatory test is a recombinant immunoblot assay (RIBA). Seroconversion may not occur for up to 16 weeks following infection. In addition, these immunological tests do not precisely distinguish between IgM and IgG antibodies. Patients who have hepatitis C infection also should be tested for hepatitis C RNA, a test that is analogous to quantitation of the viral load in patients with HIV infection. Detection of hepatitis C RNA is indicative of a high rate of viral replication.

The diagnosis of hepatitis D can be confirmed by performing a liver biopsy and identifying the delta antigen in liver tissue. However, the most useful diagnostic test for confirmation of acute infection is detection of hepatitis D IgM antibody. The corresponding test for diagnosis of chronic hepatitis D infection is identification of anti-D-IgG.

The diagnosis of acute hepatitis E can be established by using electron microscopy to identify viral particles in the stool of infected patients and by identification of IgM antibody in the serum.

Treatment

Patients with acute hepatitis A require supportive therapy. Their nutrition should be optimized. Coagulation abnormalities, if present, should be corrected, and trauma to the upper abdomen should be avoided. Of great importance, household contacts should be vaccinated with hepatitis A vaccine.

Patients with acute hepatitis B require similar supportive care. Their household contacts and sexual partners should receive hepatitis B immune globulin, followed by the hepatitis B vaccine series. Infants delivered to mothers with hepatitis B infection should immediately receive the hepatitis B immune globulin and first dose of hepatitis B vaccine while still in the hospital. These children subsequently should receive the second and third doses of the vaccine at 1 and 6 months after delivery. There is no contraindication to breastfeeding in women who have chronic hepatitis B infection.

On a long-term basis, women with hepatitis B infection should be referred to a gastroenterologist for consideration of medical treatment. Seven drugs currently are licensed for the treatment of hepatitis B infection: interferon alfa, pegylated interferon alfa-2A, lamivudine, adefovir, entecavir, telbivudine and tenofovir. The most commonly used therapy for chronic hepatitis B infection is long-acting pegylated interferon, which is injected once weekly. In patients who do not respond to interferon, the nucleoside and nucleotide analogs have been extremely effective. These agents have played a major role in reducing the need for liver transplantation in patients who have chronic hepatitis B infection.

Patients with hepatitis C, particularly those who have evidence of high viral replication and ongoing liver injury, are candidates for medical therapy. The first drug widely used for the treatment of hepatitis C was recombinant human interferon alfa. The second important advance in the therapy of hepatitis C was ribavirin, a nucleoside analog. The third major advance was the introduction of pegylated forms of interferon that allowed for once-weekly treatment. The newest agent with documented activity against hepatitis C virus is telaprevir. In a recent report, the combination of telaprevir and pegylated interferon was more effective than either drug alone in the treatment of chronic hepatitis C.

The treatment for hepatitis D parallels that described above for hepatitis B. The treatment of hepatitis E is similar to that described for hepatitis A.

Complications

The principal concern with hepatitis A infection in pregnancy is that the mother will develop fulminant hepatitis and liver failure. Fortunately, this complication is extremely rare. Hepatitis A does not cause a chronic carrier state. Perianal transmission virtually never occurs and, therefore, the infection does not pose a major risk to the baby.

Hepatitis B, particularly when associated with hepatitis D infection, may result in chronic liver disease such as chronic active hepatitis, chronic persistent hepatitis and cirrhosis. Chronic disease also predisposes to the development of hepatocellular carcinoma. Pregnant women who are infected with hepatitis B pose a significant risk of transmission to their offspring. Most neonates become infected at the time of delivery as a result of exposure to contaminated blood and genital tract secretions. Patients who are seropositive for the surface antigen alone have at least a 20% risk of transmitting infection to their neonate. Women who are seropositive for both the surface antigen and e antigen have almost a 90% risk of perinatal transmission. Neonates who become infected as a result of perinatal transmission subsequently are at risk for all the complications associated with chronic hepatic disease.

The most important sequela of hepatitis C infection is severe chronic liver disease. Infection with hepatitis C virus remains the most important indication for liver transplantation in the United States. Perinatal transmission of hepatitis C is also an important concern. In pregnant women who have a low serum concentration of hepatitis C RNA and who do not have coexisting HIV infection, the risk of perinatal transmission of hepatitis C is less than 5%. If the patient's serum concentration of hepatitis C RNA is high and/or she has concurrent HIV infection, perinatal transmission may approach 25%.

Hepatitis D virus, when superimposed upon chronic hepatitis B infection, is a major risk factor for severe chronic liver disease. Like hepatitis A, hepatitis E does not usually cause a chronic carrier state. Assuming the patient survives the acute episode, the infection usually does not have long-term sequelae. In addition, perinatal transmission of hepatitis E is exceedingly rare.

Follow-up

Patients with chronic hepatitis B (with or without co-infection with hepatitis D) and hepatitis C require long-term follow-up with a gastroenterologist. These patients are candidates for long-term treatment with either interferon or nucleoside/nucleotide analogs. Infected patients should not receive any medications that may exacerbate hepatic injury. For example, oral contraceptives should be avoided if a patient has clear evidence of ongoing hepatocellular disease. In some individuals, chronic infection progresses to such serious disease that liver transplantation will be required.

Prevention

Hepatitis A can be prevented by administration of an inactivated vaccine. Two formulations of the vaccine now are available – Vaqta® and Havrix®. Both vaccines require an initial intramuscular injection, followed by a second dose 6 to 12 months later. The vaccine should be offered to the following individuals:

- International travelers
- Children in endemic areas
- Intravenous drug users
- Individuals who have occupational exposure to hepatitis A virus, e.g., workers in a primate laboratory
- Residents and staff of chronic care institutions
- Individuals with chronic liver disease
- Homosexual men
- Individuals with clotting factor disorders.

Immunoglobulin provides reasonably effective passive immunization for hepatitis A if it is given within 2 weeks of exposure. The standard intramuscular dose of immunoglobulin is 0.02 mg/kg. However, a recent report demonstrated that hepatitis A vaccine should be the preferred method of prophylaxis both for pre-exposure and post-exposure. The principal advantage of the vaccine, compared to immune globulin, is that it provides more long-lasting protection.

There are two important immunoprophylactic agents for prevention of hepatitis B infection. The first is hepatitis B immune globulin, which can be administered immediately after an exposure to provide acute protection against a high viral inoculum. The second immunoprophylactic agent is the hepatitis B vaccine. This vaccine is prepared by recombinant technology and poses no risk of transmission of another infection such as HIV. The agent is administered intramuscularly in three separate doses and is highly effective. In healthy immunocompetent adults, seroconversion rates approach 90% after the three-dose regimen.

Immunoprophylaxis of the neonate delivered of a hepatitis B positive mother also is highly effective. In view of this high rate of effectiveness, there is no indication for cesarean delivery in women with hepatitis B infection. Interestingly, prevention of hepatitis B infection also prevents hepatitis D co-infection.

Passive and active immunization of the neonate with HBIG and HBV is approximately 90% effective in preventing perinatal transmission of hepatitis B. Presumably, some prophylaxis failure result from antenatal transmission of the virus from mother to baby. Recent evidence suggests that daily administration of oral lamivudine, 100 mg, from 28 weeks gestation until delivery, or monthly administration of intramuscular HBIG, 200 international units, at 28, 32, and 36 weeks gestation, may provide additional protection against infection of the infant.

Unfortunately, there is no hyperimmune globulin or vaccine for the prevention of hepatitis C infection. Appropriate preventive measures include adoption of universal precautions in the care of patients, intensive screening of blood donations and adherence to safe sexual practices. As a

Table 30.1 Principal features of hepatitis A, B, C, D and E

Type of hepatitis	Mechanism of transmission	Diagnostic test	Carrier state	Perinatal transmission	Prevention and treatment
A	Fecal-oral	Detection of IgM antibody	No	No	Immunoglobulin and vaccine Supportive care
B	Parenteral/ sexual	Detection of surface antigen	Yes	Yes	HBIG Hepatitis B vaccine Interferon Nucleoside/nucleotide analogs
C	Parenteral/ sexual	Detection of antibody	Yes	Yes	Interferon Nucleoside/nucleotide analogs
D	Parenteral/ sexual	Detection of antibody	Yes	Yes	Hepatitis B vaccine protects against hepatitis D
E	Fecal-oral	Detection of antibody	No	No	Supportive care

routine, cesarean delivery is not indicated in patients who have hepatitis C infection. However, there are some reports demonstrating that, in women with high HCV RNA concentrations, cesarean delivery is effective in reducing the risk of perinatal transmission of hepatitis C infection.

There is no hyperglobulin or vaccine for prevention of hepatitis E infection.

Conclusion

The key features of hepatitis in pregnancy are summarized in Table 30.1.

Suggested reading

Dienstag JL. Hepatitis B virus infection. *N Engl J Med* 2008;359:1486–500.

Duff P. Hepatitis in pregnancy. *Semin Perinatol* 1998;22:277–83.

European Pediatric Hepatitis C Virus Network. A significant sex – but not elective cesarean section – effect on mother-to-child transmission of hepatitis C virus infection. *J Infect Dis* 2005;192:1872–9.

Gibb DM, Goodall, RI, Dunn DT, *et al.* Mother-to-child transmission of hepatitis C virus: evidence for preventable peripartum transmission. *Lancet* 2000;356:904–7.

Hoofagle JH. A step forward in therapy for hepatitis C. *N Engl J Med* 2009;360:1899–901.

Poland GA, Jacobson RM. Prevention of hepatitis B with the hepatitis B vaccine. *N Engl J Med* 2004;351:2832–8.

Victor JC, Monto AS, Surdina TY, *et al.* Hepatitis A vaccine versus immune globulin for postexposure prophylaxis. *N Engl J Med* 2007;357:1685–94.

Zaretti AR, Paccagnini S, Principi N, *et al.* Mother-to-infant transmission of hepatitis C virus. *Lancet* 1995;345:289–91.

PROTOCOL 31

Asthma

Michael Schatz

Department of Allergy, Kaiser-Permanente Medical Center, San Diego, CA, USA

Overview

Asthma currently affects approximately 8% of pregnant women, making it probably the most common potentially serious medical problem to complicate pregnancy. Although data have been conflicting, the largest and most recent studies have suggested that maternal asthma increases the risk of perinatal mortality, preeclampsia, preterm birth and low birth-weight infants. More severe asthma is associated with increased risks, while better-controlled asthma is associated with decreased risks.

Pathophysiology

Asthma is an inflammatory disease of the airways that is associated with reversible airway obstruction and airway hyper-reactivity to a variety of stimuli. Although the cause of asthma is unknown, a number of clinical triggering factors can be identified, including viral infections, allergens, exercise, sinusitis, reflux, weather changes and stress.

Airway obstruction in asthma can be produced by varying degrees of mucosal edema, bronchoconstriction, mucus plugging and airway remodeling. In acute asthma, these changes can lead to ventilation perfusion imbalance and hypoxia. Although early acute asthma is typically associated with hyperventilation and hypocapnea, progressive acute asthma can cause respiratory failure with associated carbon dioxide retention and acidosis.

Diagnosis

Many patients with asthma during pregnancy will already have a physician diagnosis of asthma. A new diagnosis of asthma is usually suspected on the basis of typical symptoms – wheezing, chest tightness, cough and

Protocols for High-Risk Pregnancies, 5th edition. Edited by J.T. Queenan, J.C. Hobbins and C.Y. Spong. © 2010 Blackwell Publishing Ltd.

associated shortness of breath – which tend to be episodic or at least fluctuating in intensity and are typically worse at night. Identification of the characteristic triggers described above further supports the diagnosis. Wheezing may be present on auscultation of the lungs, but the absence of wheezing on auscultation does not exclude the diagnosis. The diagnosis is ideally confirmed by spirometry which shows a reduced FEV_1 with an increase in FEV_1 of 12% or more after an inhaled short-acting bronchodilator.

It is sometimes difficult to demonstrate reversible airway obstruction in patients with mild or intermittent asthma. Although methacholine challenge testing may be considered in non-pregnant patients with normal pulmonary function to confirm asthma, such testing is not recommended during pregnancy. Thus, therapeutic trials of asthma therapy should generally be used during pregnancy in patients with possible but unconfirmed asthma. Improvement with asthma therapy supports the diagnosis, which can then be confirmed postpartum with additional testing if necessary.

The most common differential diagnosis is dyspnea of pregnancy, which may occur in early pregnancy in approximately 70% of women. This dyspnea is differentiated from asthma by its lack of association with cough, wheezing or airway obstruction.

Another aspect of asthma diagnosis is an assessment of severity. Although more complicated severity schemes have been proposed, the most important determination is whether the patient has intermittent versus persistent asthma. This distinction has both prognostic and therapeutic significance during pregnancy. Patients with *intermittent asthma* have short episodes less than three times per week, nocturnal symptoms less than three times a month, and normal pulmonary function between episodes. Patients with more frequent symptoms or who require daily asthma medications are considered to have *persistent asthma*.

Asthma severity often changes during pregnancy; it can get either better or worse. Patients with more severe asthma prior to pregnancy are more likely to further worsen during pregnancy. Since gestational asthma course in an individual woman is unpredictable, women with asthma must be followed particularly closely during pregnancy so that any change in course can be matched with an appropriate change in therapy.

Management

General
Identifying and avoiding asthma triggers can lead to improved maternal well-being with less need for medications. In previously untested patients, in vitro (RAST, ELISA) tests should be performed to identify

relevant allergens, such as mite, animal dander, mold and cockroach, for which specific environmental control instructions can be given. Smokers must be encouraged to discontinue smoking, and all patients should try to avoid exposure to environmental tobacco smoke and other potential irritants as much as possible. Effective allergen immunotherapy can be continued during pregnancy, but benefit–risk considerations do not generally favor beginning immunotherapy during pregnancy.

Asthma medicines are classified into two types: relievers and long-term controllers. Relievers provide quick relief of bronchospasm and include short-acting beta agonists (albuterol is preferred during pregnancy, 2–4 puffs q 3–4 h prn) and the anticholinergic bronchodilator ipratropium (generally used as second-line therapy for acute asthma – see below). Long-tem control medications are described in Tables 31.1 and 31.2.

Chronic asthma

Patients with intermittent asthma do not need controller therapy. In patients with persistent asthma, controller therapy should be initiated and progressed in steps (Table 31.3) until adequate control is achieved. A classification of asthma control has been recently presented (Table 31.4). Well-controlled asthma means symptoms or rescue therapy requirement less than three times per week, nocturnal symptoms less than three times per month, no activity limitation due to asthma, and, ideally, normal pulmonary function tests. For patients with 'not well controlled' asthma (Table 31.4), one step up in therapy (Table 31.3) is recommended. For patients with 'very poorly controlled' asthma, a two-step increase, a course of oral corticosteroids, or both should be considered. Before stepping up pharmacological therapy in women whose asthma is not well controlled, adverse environmental exposures, co-morbidities, adherence and inhaler technique should be considered as targets for therapy.

Inhaled corticosteroids are the mainstay of controller therapy during pregnancy. Because it has the most published reassuring human gestational safety data, budesonide is considered the inhaled corticosteroid of choice for asthma during pregnancy. It is important to note that no data indicate that the other inhaled corticosteroid preparations are unsafe. Therefore, inhaled corticosteroids other than budesonide may be continued in patients who were well controlled by these agents prior to pregnancy, especially if it is thought that changing formulations may jeopardize asthma control. Based on longer duration of availability in the United States, salmeterol is considered the long-acting beta agonist of choice during pregnancy. As described in Table 31.1, the following drugs are considered by the National Asthma Education and Prevention Program (NAEPP) to be alternative, but not preferred, treatments for persistent asthma during pregnancy: cromolyn, due to decreased efficacy compared

Table 31.1 Long-term control medications for asthma during pregnancy (modified from NAEPP Expert Panel Report 2004 Update)

Medication	Mechanism of action	Dosage form	Adult dose	Use during pregnancy
Inhaled corticosteroids	Topical anti-inflammatory	See Table 31.2		First-line controller therapy
Systemic corticosteroids	Systemic anti-inflammatory		Short course 'burst' to achieve control: 40–60 mg/day as single or 2 divided doses for 3–10 days	Burst therapy for severe acute symptoms
Methylprednisolone		2, 4, 8, 16, 32 mg tablets		Maintenance therapy for
Prednisolone		5 mg tablets, 5 mg/mL, 15 mg/mL		severe asthma uncontrolled
Prednisone		1, 2.5, 5, 10, 20, 50 mg tablet 5 mg/mL, 5 mg/5 mL	7.5–60 mg daily in a single dose in a.m. or qod, as needed for control of severe asthma	by other means
Long-acting β agonists	β agonist mediated smooth muscle relaxation that lasts 12 hours			Add-on therapy in patients not controlled by low-medium dose inhaled corticosteroids
Salmeterol		DPI 50 μg/blister	1 blister q 12 h	
Formoterol		DPI 12 μg/single-use capsule	1 capsule q 12 h	
Cromolyn	Non-steroidal topical anti-inflammatory	MDI 1 mg/puff	2–4 puffs tid-qid	Alternative therapy for mild persistent asthma
Leukotriene receptor antagonists	Blocks activity of leukotrienes (inflammatory mediators) by means of receptor antagonism			Alternative therapy for persistent asthma in patients who have shown good response prior to pregnancy
Montelukast		10 mg tablets	10 mg q HS	
Zafirlukast		10 or 20 mg tablets	20 mg bid	
Theophylline	Bronchodilator (? anti-inflammatory effects)	Liquids, sustained-release tablets, and capsules	400–800 mg/day to achieve serum concentration of 5–12 μg/mL	Alternative therapy for persistent asthma during pregnancy

Table 31.2 Estimated comparative daily adult dosages for inhaled corticosteroids (from Expert Panel 3 2007 Report)

Drug	Low daily dose	Medium daily dose	High daily dose
Beclomethasone HFA 40 or 80 μg/puff	80–240 μg	>240–480 μg	>480 μg
Budesonide DPI 90 or 180 μg/inhalation	180–600 μg	>600–1200 μg	>1200 μg
Flunisolide 250 μg/puff CFC 80 μg/puff HFA	500–1000 μg 320 μg	>1000–2000 μg >320–640 μg	>2000 μg >640 μg
Fluticasone MDI: 44, 110, 220 μg/puff DPI: 50, 100, or 250 μg/inhalation	88–264 μg 100–300 μg	>264–440 μg >300–500 μg	>440 μg >500 μg
Mometasone DPI 200 μg/inhalation	200 μg	400 μg	>400 μg
Triamcinolone acetonide 75 μg/puff	300–750 μg	>750–1500 μg	>1500 μg

Table 31.3 Recommendations for preferred step therapy for asthma during pregnancy (modified from NAEPP 2004 and Expert Panel 3 2007 recommendations)

STEP ONE	No controller
STEP TWO	Low-dose inhaled corticosteroids*
STEP THREE	Medium-dose inhaled corticosteroids*
STEP FOUR	Medium-dose inhaled corticosteroids* + long-acting beta agonist**
STEP FIVE	High-dose inhaled corticosteroids* + long-acting beta agonist**
STEP SIX	High-dose inhaled corticosteroids* + long-acting beta agonist** + oral corticosteroids at lowest effective dose

*Budesonide is the preferred inhaled corticosteroid during pregnancy due to availability of more reassuring human gestational safety data.
**Salmeterol is the preferred long-acting beta agonist during pregnancy due to longer availability in the United States.

to inhaled corticosteroids; theophylline, due primarily to increased side effects compared to alternatives; and leukotriene receptor antagonists, due to the availability of minimal published human gestational data for these drugs. Although oral corticosteroids have been associated with possible increased risks during pregnancy (oral clefts, prematurity, lower

Table 31.4 Classification of asthma control during pregnancy*

Components of control	Well controlled	Classification of control[a] Not well controlled	Very poorly controlled
Symptoms	≤2 days/week	>2 days/week	Throughout the day
Night-time awakening	≤2 times/month	1 to 3 times/week	≥4 times/week
Interference with normal activity	None	Some limitation	Extremely limited
Short-acting beta$_2$ agonist use for symptom control	≤2 days/week	>2 days/week	Several times per day
FEV$_1$ or peak flow	>80%[b]	60 to 80%[b]	<60%[b]
Exacerbations requiring systemic corticosteroids	0–1 in past 12 months	≥2 in past 12 months	

[a] The level of control is based on the most severe category. Assess symptom frequency and impact by patient's recall of previous 2 to 4 weeks.

[b] Predicted or personal best.

*Reprinted with permission from Schatz M, Dombrowski MP. Asthma in pregnancy. *N Engl J Med* 2009;360:1862–9.

birth weight), if needed during pregnancy, they should be used because these risks are less than the potential risks of severe uncontrolled asthma (which include maternal or fetal mortality).

Acute asthma

A major goal of chronic asthma management is the prevention of acute asthmatic episodes. When acute asthma does not respond to home therapy, expeditious acute management is necessary for both the health of the mother and that of the fetus.

Due to progesterone-induced hyperventilation, normal blood gases during pregnancy reveal a higher Po_2 (100–106 mmHg) and a lower Pco_2 (28–30 mmHg) than in the non-pregnant state. The changes in blood gases that occur secondary to acute asthma during pregnancy will be superimposed on the 'normal' hyperventilation of pregnancy. Thus, a Pco_2 >35 or a Po_2 <70 associated with acute asthma will represent more severe compromise during pregnancy than will similar blood gases in the non-gravid state.

The recommended pharmacological therapy of acute asthma during pregnancy is summarized in Table 31.5. Intensive fetal monitoring as well as maternal monitoring is essential. In addition to pharmacological therapy, supplemental oxygen (initially 3 to 4 L/min by nasal cannula) should be administered, adjusting Fio_2 to maintain at Po_2 ≥70 and/or O_2 saturation by pulse oximetry > 95%. Intravenous fluids (containing

Table 31.5 Pharmacological management of acute asthma during pregnancy

1 β_2-agonist bronchodilator (nebulized or metered-dose inhaler)
  - up to 3 doses in first 60–90 minutes
  - every 1–2 hours thereafter until adequate response

2 Nebulized ipratropium (may be repeated q 6 hours)

3 Systemic corticosteroids with initial therapy in patients on regular corticosteroids and in patients with severe exacerbations (peak expiratory flow rate <40% predicted or personal best) and for those with incomplete response to initial therapy
  - 40–80 mg/day in 1 or 2 divided doses until peak expiratory flow rate reaches 70% of predicted or personal best
  - may be given orally; IV for severe exacerbation
  - taper as patient improves

4 Consider intravenous magnesium sulfate (2 grams) for women with life-threatening exacerbations (peak expiratory flow rate <25% predicted or personal best) and for those whose exacerbations remain in the severe category after 1 hour of intensive conventional therapy

glucose if the patient is not hyperglycemic) should also be administered, initially at a rate of at least 100 mL/h.

Systemic corticosteroids (40–80 mg/day in one or two divided doses) are recommended for patients who do not respond well (FEV_1 or peak expiratory flow rate [PEF] $\geq 70\%$ predicted) to the first beta agonist treatment as well as for patients who have recently taken systemic steroids and for those who present with severe exacerbations (FEV_1 or PEF <40% of predicted). Patients with good responses to emergency therapy (FEV_1 or PEF $\geq 70\%$ predicted) can be discharged home, generally on a course of oral corticosteroids. Inhaled corticosteroids should also be continued or initiated upon discharge until review at medical follow-up. Hospitalization should be considered for patients with an incomplete response (FEV_1 or PEF $\geq 40\%$ but <70% predicted). Admission to an intensive care unit should be considered for patients with persistent FEV_1 or PEF <40% predicted, Pco_2 >42 or sensorium changes. Intubation and mechanical ventilation may be required for patients whose condition deteriorates or fails to improve associated with decreasing Po_2, increasing Pco_2, progressive respiratory acidosis, declining mental status or increasing fatigue.

Follow-up

Careful follow-up by physicians experienced in managing asthma is an essential aspect of optimal gestational asthma management. Asthmatic women requiring regular medication should be evaluated at least monthly. In addition to symptomatic and auscultatory assessment, objective measures of respiratory status (optimally spirometry, minimally PEF) should be obtained on every clinic visit. In addition, patients with more severe or labile asthma should be considered for home PEF monitoring. All pregnant patients should have a written action plan for increased symptoms and facilitated access to their physician for uncontrolled symptoms.

Conclusion

Asthma is a common medical problem during pregnancy. Optimal diagnosis and management of asthma during pregnancy should maximize maternal and fetal health.

Suggested reading

American College of Obstetricians and Gynecologists. Practice Bulletin: Asthma in pregnancy. *Obstet Gynecol* 2008;111:457–64.

Breton MC, Beauchesne M-F, Lemiere C, *et al.* Risk of perinatal mortality associated with asthma during pregnancy. *Thorax* 2009;64:101–6.

Cydulka RK. Acute asthma during pregnancy. *Immunol All Clin N Am* 2006;26:103–17.

Dombrowski M. Outcomes of pregnancy in asthmatic women. *Immunol All Clin N Am* 2006;26:81–92.

Gluck JC, Gluck PA. The effect of pregnancy on the course of asthma. *Immunol All Clin N Am* 2006;26:63–80.

Kallen B, Rydhstroem H, Aberg A. Asthma during pregnancy – a population based study. *Eur J Epidem* 2000;16:167–71.

National Asthma Education and Prevention Program. Expert Panel Report 3: Guidelines for the diagnosis and management of asthma. Summary Report. *J Allergy Clin Immunol* 2007;120:S93–138.

National Asthma Education and Prevention Program. Expert Panel Report Managing Asthma During Pregnancy: Recommendations for Pharmacologic Treatment – Update 2004. *J Allergy Clin Immunol* 2005;115:34–46.

Schatz M, Dombrowski MP. Asthma in pregnancy. *N Engl J Med* 2009;360:1862–9.

Schatz M, Dombrowski MP, Wise R, *et al.* Asthma morbidity during pregnancy can be predicted by severity classification. *J Allergy Clin Immunol* 2003;112:283–8.

Epilepsy

Neil K. Kochenour

Department of Obstetrics & Gynecology, University of Utah, Salt Lake City, UT, USA

Overview

Management of the woman with epilepsy begins preconceptionally. At that time her antiepileptic drugs (AEDs) should be evaluated for their need, the minimum dose required to prevent seizures, and the teratogenic potential of the drugs. In addition, adequate folate intake should be recommended during the preconceptional period. During pregnancy the patient should be treated with the lowest effective dosage and, if possible, a single AED. After delivery vitamin K should be given to the neonates of women on AEDs during pregnancy. Studies have failed to demonstrate an increase in cesarean delivery, preeclampsia, pregnancy-induced hypertension or late pregnancy bleeding in women with epilepsy.

Pathophysiology

Epilepsy complicates approximately 0.3 to 0.5% of pregnancies. Between 14% and 32% of these patients will experience an increase in seizure frequency during pregnancy, which is most often attributable to a reduction in the plasma concentration of anticonvulsant drugs. In some, emotional stress seems significant. In general, reasons for changes in anticonvulsant drug levels include fluid retention, electrolyte changes, respiratory alkalosis and hormonal influences. Additionally, a number of physiological changes that occur during pregnancy are known to affect the pharmacokinetics of drugs. Decreased motility of the gastrointestinal tract may change the bioavailability of orally administered dosage forms. Significant increases in glomerular filtration rate influence the renal clearance rates of many drugs, and hormonal changes may affect hepatic enzyme systems responsible for drug metabolism. Women who report seizure activity within

Protocols for High-Risk Pregnancies, 5th edition. Edited by J.T. Queenan, J.C. Hobbins and C.Y. Spong. © 2010 Blackwell Publishing Ltd.

2 years of pregnancy are significantly more likely to experience antenatal, intrapartum and postpartum seizures when compared with women whose last seizure occurred more than 2 years before pregnancy.

Whatever the underlying cause of the increase in seizure frequency, potential fetal damage secondary to hypoxia and the added maternal risk due to seizures necessitate close observation and careful management. Studies to date have demonstrated no difference in the prevalence of obstetric complications, adverse neonatal outcomes, or congenital malformations in pregnancies in which the mother had one or more antepartum seizures when compared to those who had no seizures.

Teratogenicity of anticonvulsants

There is considerable controversy concerning the teratogenicity of anticonvulsant drugs. The overall rate of congenital abnormalities in association with maternal intake of AEDs is 5 to 6%. This is twice the expected rate of 2.5 to 3.0% in the general population. In addition, children of mothers with epilepsy, treated or untreated with AEDs, tend to have slightly more minor anomalies than do children of fathers with epilepsy or control subjects. Trimethadione has been shown to result in spontaneous abortions in a high percentage of pregnancies and fetal malformations in the majority of remaining pregnancies. Its use is, therefore, contraindicated during pregnancy and it probably should not be given to women of childbearing age. It is highly probable that valproate monotherapy during the first trimester of pregnancy contributes to the development of major congenital malformations (MCMs) in the offspring of women using this medication. Valproate as a part of polytherapy in the first trimester of pregnancy probably contributes to the development of MCMs when compared to polytherapy which does not include valproate. There appears to be a relationship between the dose of valproate and the risk of development of MCMs in the offspring of women with epilepsy. Carbamazepine does not appear to substantially increase the risk of MCMs when used as monotherapy and there is insufficient evidence to determine if lamotrigine increases the risk of MCMs. However, the results from a number of pregnancy registries suggest that lamotrigine probably does not significantly increase the risk of MCMs. It is highly probable that polytherapy, regardless of the medications used, contributes to MCMs in the offspring of women with epilepsy as compared to monotherapy. The incidence of MCMs increases with increasing number of anticonvulsant medications used to control seizures. Very little is known about the use of some newer anticonvulsants such as topiramate, zonisamide and oxcarbazepine during pregnancy. If possible, only one AED should be used during pregnancy.

Exposure to polytherapy and valproate during pregnancy are associated with significantly reduced verbal intelligence in the offspring. Carbamazepine monotherapy with maternal serum levels within the recommended range does not impair intelligence in prenatally exposed offspring. It should be remembered that 95% of infants born to mothers receiving AED treatment will be normal.

Serum levels

Pregnancy appears to cause an increase in clearance and a significant decrease in the levels of lamotrigine, carbamazepine and phenytoin. Sufficient data are not available to provide evidence for a change in clearance or levels during pregnancy for valproate.

Breastfeeding

Primidone probably enters breast milk in potentially clinically important amounts whereas valproate, phenytoin and carbamazepine probably do not. Lamotrigine may penetrate into breast milk in clinically important amounts. There is insufficient evidence to determine if indirect exposure to maternally ingested AEDs has symptomatic effects on the newborns.

Management

The treatment of the pregnant epileptic patient should ideally begin preconceptionally. At this time, her seizure status should be assessed to ascertain whether or not she truly needs an anticonvulsant drug. If she has been seizure-free for a long interval (at least 9 months) on minimal doses of anticonvulsant drugs and has a negative electroencephalogram (EEG), it may be reasonable to attempt anticonvulsant withdrawal before conception. Risk for relapse increases when the history includes clonic-tonic grand mal convulsions, prolonged seizures, breaking through AED treatment, or seizure control achieved with a combination of two or three drugs. One should, therefore, hesitate in withdrawing AED treatment from women who are planning pregnancy if their history includes the above risks for relapse. The current recommendation is that AEDs, if withdrawn, should be withdrawn at least 6 months prior to pregnancy. When possible, monotherapy should be used rather than polytherapy. After monotherapy is established the lowest plasma AED level that prevents seizures should be determined.

Several observations can serve as guidelines for management throughout pregnancy.

1 Steady-state plasma concentrations of most anticonvulsants decrease as pregnancy progresses.

2 These changes may be associated with a loss of seizure control, requiring an increase in anticonvulsant medications.

3 Patients appear to have a threshold concentration of drug below which seizure control is lost. In other words, seizure control may be complete in the given patient despite drug concentrations below the quoted therapeutic range.

4 The use of divided doses or slow-release preparations results in lower peak levels and may reduce the risk of malformations.

5 For valproate, the use of a single daily dose is not advisable because the adverse effects are believed to be the result of high peak serum level.

6 Total serum AED levels and, if possible, free AED fractions should be measured at regular intervals throughout pregnancy, particularly for lamotrigine, phenytoin and carbamazepine.

Treatment

Preconceptional

1 Ascertain the patient's need for anticonvulsant medications.

2 Determine the level of anticonvulsant medication at which the patient is seizure-free.

3 Attempt monotherapy wherever possible.

4 The use of divided doses or slow-release preparations results in lower peak levels and may reduce the risk of malformations.

5 Discuss the risks of anticonvulsant medications to the fetus.

6 Recommend folate supplementation (0.4 mg/day) beginning before conception.

Antenatal

1 Maintain the concentration of anticonvulsant medication(s) at the level(s) required by the patient.

2 Obtain plasma anticonvulsant levels every 3 to 4 weeks, or if a seizure occurs, if potential drug interaction is suspected, or if signs of toxicity develop.

3 Raise doses if necessary to maintain effective anticonvulsant activity. Dosage increments may need to be small (e.g., the use of 30 mg rather than 100 mg phenytoin capsules).

4 Assess drug toxicity clinically after an appropriate interval based on the estimated time to reach a steady state.

Table 32.1 Frequently prescribed anticonvulsants

For grand mal and focal psychomotor seizures	Adult daily dosage (mg)	Therapeutic level (μg/mL)	Toxicity
Carbamazepine (Tegretol)	800–1200	4–16	Ataxia, drowsiness, nystagmus, agitation
Phenytoin (Dilantin)	300–400	10–20	Ataxia, slurred speech, vertigo, nystagmus, seizures
Phenobarbital	90–120	15–40	Ataxia, drowsiness
Primidone (Mysoline)*	750–1500	5–15	Ataxia, vertigo, nystagmus

*Primidone is metabolized to phenobarbital, and combined use of phenobarbital and primidone should be avoided.

5 If seizure control is not maintained and the anticonvulsant dose has been increased until toxic effects are apparent (Table 32.1), add additional anticonvulsant medication. Prescribe supplements containing at least 0.4 mg folic acid to all patients on anticonvulsant medication and follow their complete blood counts (CBCs), since folic acid deficiency anemia is frequent in this group of patients.
6 Offer prenatal diagnosis to patients receiving AEDs.
7 Epilepsy is not usually considered an indication for the induction of labor.

First seizure during pregnancy

For the patient in whom seizures first develop during pregnancy, eclamptic seizures must be ruled out. A detailed neurological history and examination are essential. Diagnostic studies, including electroencephalography, skull x-ray films, metabolic studies including serum calcium level, and fasting and postprandial blood glucose determinations, should be performed on all patients. A lumbar puncture and computed tomography or magnetic resonance imaging are often indicated. Based on these studies and evidence of other neurological signs or symptoms angiographic studies may be appropriate.

Postpartum

1 Administer 1 mg of vitamin K intramuscularly to all newborns of patients receiving AEDs.
2 Examine the newborn carefully for signs of fetal teratogenic effects.
3 Reduction of anticonvulsant medication may be required in the postpartum period. Check the patient every 2 or 3 weeks after delivery.

Suggested reading

Management issues for women with epilepsy – focus on pregnancy (an evidence-based review): Report of the Quality Standards Subcommittee and the Therapeutics and Technology Assessment Subcommittee of the American Academy of Neurology and the American Epilepsy Society. I. Obstetrical complications and change in seizure frequency. *Epilepsia* 2009;50(5):1229–36. II. Teratogenesis and perinatal outcomes. *Epilepsia* 2009;50(5):1237–46. III. Vitamin K, folic acid, blood levels, and breast-feeding. *Epilepsia* 2009;50(5):1247–55.

Walker SP, *et al.* The management of epilepsy in pregnancy. *Br J Obstet Gynaecol* 2009; 116:758–67.

DeToledo J. Pregnancy in epilepsy: issues of concern. *Int Rev Neurobiol* 2009;83:169–80.

Shorvon SD, *et al.* The management of epilepsy during pregnancy: progress is painfully slow. *Epilepsia* 2009;50(5):973–4.

Meador KJ, *et al.* Cognitive function at 3 years of age after fetal exposure to antiepileptic drugs. *N Eng J Med* 2009;360(16):1597–605.

Richmond JR, *et al.* Epilepsy and pregnancy: an obstetric perspective. *Am J Obstet Gynecol* 2004;190:371–9.

Delgado-Escueta AV, Janz D. Consensus guidelines: preconception counseling, management, and care of the pregnant woman with epilepsy. *Neurology* 1992;42:149–60.

Meadow R. Anticonvulsant in pregnancy. *Arch Dis Child* 1991;66:62–5.

Richmond JR, *et al.* Epilepsy and pregnancy: an obstetric perspective. *Am J Obstet Gynecol* 2004;190:371–9.

Pennell PB. Antiepileptic drug pharmacokinetics during pregnancy and lactation. *Neurology* 2003;61:S35–42.

Yerby MS. Management issues for women with epilepsy. *Neurology* 2003;61:S23–6.

GlaxoSmithKline, Lamotrigine Pregnancy Registry, Interim Report, September 1992–September 2003.

Chronic Hypertension

Baha M. Sibai

Department of Obstetrics & Gynecology, University of Cincinnati College of Medicine, Cincinnati, OH, USA

Overview

According to data derived from the National Health and Nutrition Examination Survey, 1988–1991, the prevalence of chronic hypertension among women of childbearing age increases from 0.6% to 2.0% for women 18–29 years old to 4.6% to 22.3% for women 30–39 years old. The lower prevalences are for white women and higher rates are for African-Americans. Because of the current trend of child bearing at an older age, it is expected that the incidence of chronic hypertension in pregnancy will continue to rise. During the new millennium, and estimating a prevalence of chronic hypertension during pregnancy of 3%, at least 120,000 pregnant women (3% of 4 million pregnancies) with chronic hypertension will be seen in the United States each year.

Definition and diagnosis

In pregnant women chronic hypertension is defined as elevated blood pressure that is present and documented before pregnancy. In women whose pre-pregnancy blood pressure is unknown, the diagnosis is based on the presence of sustained hypertension before 20 weeks of gestation, defined as either systolic blood pressure of at least 140 mmHg or diastolic blood pressure of at least 90 mmHg on at least two occasions measured at least 4 hours apart.

Women with chronic hypertension are at increased risk of superimposed preeclampsia. The diagnosis of superimposed preeclampsia should be made in the presence of any of the following findings:

1 In women with chronic hypertension and without proteinuria early in pregnancy (<20 weeks' gestation), preeclampsia is diagnosed if there is new-onset proteinuria (≥0.5 g protein in a 24-hour specimen).

Protocols for High-Risk Pregnancies, 5th edition. Edited by J.T. Queenan, J.C. Hobbins and C.Y. Spong. © 2010 Blackwell Publishing Ltd.

2 In women with preexisting proteinuria before 20 weeks' gestation, the diagnosis is confirmed if there is an exacerbated increase in blood pressure to the severe (systolic pressure $\geq$180 mmHg or diastolic pressure $\geq$110 mmHg) range, particularly if associated with either headaches, blurred vision or epigastric pain; or if there is significant increase in liver enzymes (unrelated to methyldopa) or if the platelet count is <100,000/mm.

Etiology and classification

The etiology as well as the severity of chronic hypertension is an important consideration in the management of pregnancy. Chronic hypertension is subdivided into primary (essential) and secondary. Primary hypertension is by far the most common cause of chronic hypertension seen during pregnancy (90%). In 10% of the cases, chronic hypertension is secondary to one or more underlying disorders such as renal disease (glomerulonephritis, interstitial nephritis, polycystic kidneys, renal artery stenosis), collagen vascular disease (lupus, scleroderma), endocrine disorders (diabetes mellitus with vascular involvement, pheochromocytoma, thyrotoxicosis, Cushing disease, hyperaldosteronism), or coarctation of the aorta.

Chronic hypertension during pregnancy can be subclassified as either mild or severe, depending on the systolic and diastolic blood pressure readings. Systolic and diastolic (Korotkoff phase V) blood pressures of at least 160 mmHg and/or 110 mmHg, respectively, constitute severe hypertension.

For management and counseling purposes, chronic hypertension in pregnancy is also categorized as either low-risk or high-risk as described in Fig. 33.1. The patient is considered to be at low risk when she has mild essential hypertension without any organ involvement.

Maternal-perinatal risks

Pregnancies complicated by chronic hypertension are at increased risk for superimposed preeclampsia and abruptio placentae. The reported rates of preeclampsia in the literature in mild hypertension range from 10% to 25% (Table 33.1). The rate of preeclampsia in women with severe chronic hypertension approaches 50%. Sibai and associates studied the rate of superimposed preeclampsia among 763 women with chronic hypertension followed prospectively at several medical centers in the United States. The overall rate of superimposed preeclampsia was 25%. The rate was not affected by maternal age, race, or presence of proteinuria early in pregnancy. However, the rate was significantly greater in women who had

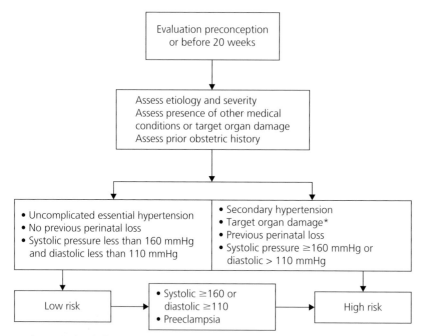

*Left ventricular dysfunction, rentinopathy, dyslipidemia, maternal age above 40 years, microvascular disease, stroke.

Figure 33.1 Initial evaluation of women with chronic hypertension.

Table 33.1 Rates of adverse pregnancy outcome in observational studies describing mild chronic hypertension in pregnancy

	Preeclampsia (%)	Abruptio placentae (%)	Delivery at <37 wk (%)	SGA (%)
Sibai *et al.* 1983 (*n* = 211)	10	1.4	12.0	8.0
Rey & Couturier 1994 (*n* = 337)	21	0.7	34.4	15.5
McCowan *et al.* 1996 (*n* = 142)	14	NR	16	11.0
Sibai *et al.* 1998 (*n* = 763)	25	1.5	33.3	11.1
Giannubilo *et al.* 2006 (*n* = 233)	28	0.5	NR	16.5
Chappell *et al.* 2008 (*n* = 822)	22	NR	22.7	27.2
Sibai *et al.* 2009 (*n* = 369)	17	2.4	29.3	15.0

SGA, small for gestational age; NR, not reported.

hypertension for at least 4 years (31% vs 22%), in those who had had preeclampsia during a previous pregnancy (32% vs 23%), and in those whose diastolic blood pressure was 100–110 mmHg when compared with those whose diastolic blood pressure was below 100 mmHg at baseline (42% vs 24%).

The reported rate of abruptio placentae, in women with mild chronic hypertension, has ranged from 0.5% to 1.5% (Table 33.1). The rate in those with severe or high-risk hypertension may be 5–10%. In a recent multicenter study that included 763 women with chronic hypertension, the overall rate of abruptio placentae was reported at 1.5% and the rate was significantly higher in those who developed superimposed preeclampsia than in those without this complication (3% vs 1%, $P = 0.04$). However, the rate was not influenced by either maternal age, race, or duration of hypertension. In addition, the results of a systematic review of nine observational studies revealed that the rate of abruptio placentae is doubled (OR, 2.1; 95% CI, 1.1–3.9) in women with chronic hypertension compared with either normotensive or general obstetric population.

Fetal and neonatal complications are also increased in women with chronic hypertension. The risk of perinatal mortality is increased 3–4 times compared with the general obstetric population. The rates of premature deliveries and small-for-gestational age infants are also increased in women with chronic hypertension (Table 33.1).

Chappell *et al.* studied 822 women with chronic hypertension that were part of patients enrolled in a randomized trial to evaluate the benefits of antioxidants (vitamin C and vitamin E) for the prevention of preeclampsia (no benefit was found). The incidence of preeclampsia was 22%. The incidence of preeclampsia was significantly higher in those with systolic blood pressure at ≥130 mmHg and/or those with diastolic blood pressure ≥80 mmHg at time of enrollment as compared to the other groups. The rate of SGA was 48% in those with superimposed preeclampsia and 21% in those without. In addition, the rate of preterm delivery at <37 weeks was 51% in those with superimposed preeclampsia as compared to 15% in those without preeclampsia.

Treatment

Most women with chronic hypertension during pregnancy have mild essential uncomplicated hypertension and are at minimal risk for cardiovascular complications within the short time frame of pregnancy. Several retrospective and prospective studies have been conducted to determine whether antihypertensive therapy in these women would improve pregnancy outcome. An overall summary of these studies revealed that, regardless of the antihypertensive therapy used, maternal cardiovascular and renal complications were minimal or absent. Based on the available data, there is no compelling evidence that short-term antihypertensive therapy is beneficial for the pregnant woman with low-risk hypertension except for a reduction in the rate of exacerbation of hypertension.

Antihypertensive therapy is necessary in women with severe hypertension to reduce the acute risk of stroke, congestive heart failure or renal failure. In addition, control of severe hypertension may also permit pregnancy prolongation and possibly improve perinatal outcome. However, there is no evidence that control of severe hypertension reduces the rates of either superimposed preeclampsia or abruptio placentae.

There are many retrospective and prospective studies examining the potential fetal-neonatal benefits of pharmacological therapy in women with mild essential uncomplicated hypertension (low-risk). Some compared treatment with no treatment or with a placebo, others compared two different antihypertensive drugs, and others used a combination of drugs. Only four of these studies were randomized trials that included women enrolled prior to 20 weeks' gestation. Only two trials had a moderate sample size to evaluate the risks of superimposed preeclampsia and abruptio placentae. Therefore, treatment of mild chronic hypertension remains controversial.

Suggested management

The primary objective in the management of pregnancies complicated with chronic hypertension is to reduce maternal risks and achieve optimal perinatal survival. This objective can be achieved by formulating a rational approach that includes preconceptual evaluation and counseling, early antenatal care, timely antepartum visits to monitor both maternal and fetal well-being, timely delivery with intensive intrapartum monitoring, and proper postpartum management.

Evaluation and classification

Management of patients with chronic hypertension should ideally begin prior to pregnancy, whereby evaluation and workup are undertaken to assess the etiology, the severity, as well as the presence of other medical illnesses, and to rule out the presence of target organ damage of long-standing hypertension. An in-depth history should delineate in particular the duration of hypertension, the use of antihypertensive medications, their type, and the response to these medications. Also, attention should be given to the presence of cardiac or renal disease, diabetes, thyroid disease, and a history of cerebrovascular accident, or congestive heart failure. A detailed obstetric history should include maternal, as well as neonatal, outcome of previous pregnancies with stresses on history of development of abruptio placentae, superimposed preeclampsia, preterm delivery, small-for-gestation infants and intrauterine fetal death.

Laboratory evaluation is obtained to assess the function of different organ systems that are likely to be affected by chronic hypertension, and as a baseline for future assessments. These should include the following for all patients: urine analysis, urine culture and sensitivity, 24-hour urine evaluations for protein, electrolytes, complete blood count and glucose tolerance test.

Low-risk hypertension

Women with low-risk chronic hypertension without superimposed preeclampsia usually have a pregnancy outcome similar to that in the general obstetric population. In addition, discontinuation of antihypertensive therapy early in pregnancy does not affect the rates of preeclampsia, abruptio placentae or preterm delivery in these women. My policy is to discontinue antihypertensive treatment at the first prenatal visit because the majority of these women will have good pregnancy outcome without such therapy. Although these women do not require pharmacological therapy, a careful management is still essential (Fig. 33.2). At the time of initial and subsequent visits, the patient is educated about nutritional requirements, weight gain and sodium intake (maximum of 2.4 g of sodium per day). During each subsequent visit they are observed very closely for early signs of preeclampsia and fetal growth restriction.

The development of severe hypertension, preeclampsia or abnormal fetal growth requires urgent fetal testing with non-stress test or biophysical profile. Women who develop severe hypertension, those with

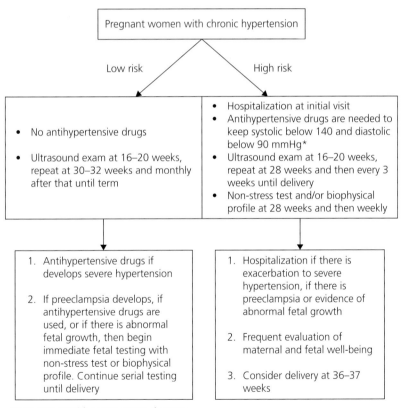

*For women with target organ damage

Figure 33.2 Antepartum management of chronic hypertension

documented fetal growth restriction by ultrasound examination and those with superimposed preeclampsia at or beyond 37 weeks require hospitalization and delivery. In the absence of these complications, the pregnancy may be continued till 40 weeks' gestation.

High-risk hypertension

Women with high-risk chronic hypertension are at increased risk for adverse maternal and perinatal complications. Women with significant renal insufficiency (serum creatinine >1.4 mg/dL), diabetes mellitus with vascular involvement (class R/F), severe collagen vascular disease, cardiomyopathy or coarctation of the aorta should receive thorough counseling regarding the adverse effects of pregnancy before conception. These women should be advised that pregnancy may exacerbate their condition with the potential for congestive heart failure, acute renal failure requiring dialysis, and even death. In addition, perinatal loss and neonatal complications are markedly increased in these women. All such women should be managed by or in consultation with a subspecialist in maternal-fetal medicine, as well as in association with other medical specialists as needed.

Women with high-risk hypertension may require hospitalization at the time of first prenatal visit for evaluation of cardiovascular and renal status and for regulation of antihypertensive medications, as well as other prescribed medications (Fig. 33.2). Women receiving atenolol, ACE inhibitors or angiotensin II receptor antagonists should have these medications discontinued under close observation. Antihypertensive therapy, with one or more of the drugs listed in Table 33.2, are subsequently used in all women with severe hypertension. In women without target organ damage, the aim of antihypertensive therapy is to keep systolic blood pressure between 140 and 150 mmHg and diastolic blood pressure between

Table 33.2 Drugs used to treat hypertension in pregnancy

Drug	Starting dose	Maximum dose
Acute treatment of severe hypertension		
Hydralazine	5–10 mg IV every 20 min	30 mg*
Labetalol**	20–40 mg IV every 10–15 min	220 mg*
Nifedipine	10–20 mg oral every 30 min	50 mg*
Long-term treatment of hypertension		
Methyldopa	250 mg bid	4 g/day
Labetalol	100 mg bid	2400 mg/day
Nifedipine	10 mg bid	120 mg/day
Thiazide diuretic	12.5 mg bid	50 mg/day

*If desired blood pressure levels are not achieved, switch to another drug.
**Avoid labetalol in women with asthma or congestive heart failure.

90 and 100 mmHg. In addition, antihypertensive therapy is indicated in women with mild hypertension plus target organ damage because there are short-term maternal benefits from lowering blood pressure in such women. In these women, I recommend keeping systolic blood pressure below 140 mmHg and diastolic blood pressure below 90 mmHg. In some women, blood pressure may be difficult to control initially demanding the use of intravenous therapy with hydralazine or labetalol or oral short-acting nifedipine with doses as described in Table 33.2. For maintenance therapy, one may choose either oral methyldopa, labetalol, slow-release nifedipine, or a diuretic. My first drug of choice for control of hypertension in pregnancy is labetalol starting at 100 mg twice daily, to be increased to a maximum of 2400 mg/day. If maternal blood pressure is not controlled with maximum doses of labetalol, a second drug such as a thiazide diuretic or nifedipine may be added. For women with diabetes mellitus and vascular disease, the preference is oral nifedipine. Oral nifedipine and/or a thiazide diuretic is the drug of choice for young African-American women with hypertension because these women often manifest a low-renin type hypertension or salt-sensitive hypertension. If maternal blood pressure is adequately controlled with these medications, the patient can continue with the same drug after delivery.

Early and frequent prenatal visits are the key for successful pregnancy outcome in women with high-risk chronic hypertension. These women need close observation throughout pregnancy and may require serial evaluation of 24-hour urine protein excretion and complete blood count with metabolic profile at least once every trimester. Further laboratory testing can be performed depending on the clinical progress of the pregnancy. Fetal evaluation should be carried out as recommended in Fig. 33.2.

The development of uncontrolled severe hypertension, preeclampsia or evidence of fetal growth restriction requires maternal hospitalization for more frequent evaluation of maternal and fetal well-being. The development of any of these complications at or beyond 34 weeks' gestation should be considered an indication for delivery. In all other women, consider delivery at 36–37 weeks' gestation after documenting fetal lung maturity.

Summary

Chronic hypertension in pregnancy is associated with increased rates of adverse maternal and fetal outcomes, both acute and long term. These adverse outcomes are particularly seen in women with uncontrolled severe hypertension, in those with target organ damage, and those who are non-compliant with prenatal visits. In addition, adverse outcomes are substantially increased in women who develop superimposed preeclampsia or abruptio placentae. Women with chronic hypertension should be evaluated either prior to conception or at time of first prenatal visit. Depending on this evaluation, they can be divided into categories of either 'high-risk' or 'low-risk' chronic hypertension. High-risk women should receive aggressive antihypertensive therapy, lifestyle changes and frequent evaluations of maternal and fetal well-being.

Suggested reading

American College of Obstetricians and Gynecologists. Chronic hypertension in pregnancy. ACOG Practice Bulletin # 29. *Obstet Gynecol* 2001;98:177–85.

Burt VL, Whetton P, Rochella EJ, Brown C, Cutler JA, Higgins M, *et al.* Prevalence of hypertension in the US adult population: results from the third national health and nutrition examination survey, 1988–1991. *Hypertension* 1995;23:305–13.

Chappell LC, Enye S, Seed P, Driley AL, *et al.* Adverse perinatal outcomes and risk factors for preeclampsia in women with chronic hypertension: a prospective study. *Hypertension* 2008;51:1002–9.

Giannubilo SR, Dell Uomo B, Tranquilli AL. Perinatal outcomes, blood pressure patterns and risk assessment of superimposed preeclampsia in mild chronic hypertensive pregnancy. *Eur J Obstet Gynecol Reprod Biol* 2006;126:63–7.

McCowan LM, Buist RG, North RA, Gamble G. Perinatal morbidity in chronic hypertension. *Br J Obstet Gynaecol* 1996;103:123–9.

Powrie RO. A 30-year-old woman with chronic hypertension trying to conceive: clinical cross roads. *JAMA* 2007;298:1548–59.

Rey E, Couturier A. The prognosis of pregnancy in women with chronic hypertension. *Am J Obstet Gynecol* 1994;171:410–16.

Sibai BM. Chronic hypertension in pregnancy. *Obstet Gynecol* 2002;100:369–77.

Sibai BM, Abdella TN, Anderson GD. Pregnancy outcome in 211 patients with mild chronic hypertension. *Obstet Gynecol* 1983;61:571–6.

Sibai BM, Anderson GD. Pregnancy outcome of intensive therapy in severe hypertension in first trimester. *Obstet Gynecol* 1986;67:517–22.

Sibai BM, Lindheimer M, Hauth J, Caritis S, Van Dorsten P, Klebanoff M, *et al.* Risk factors for preeclampsia, abruptio placentae, and adverse neonatal outcomes among women with chronic hypertension. *N Engl J Med* 1998;339:667–71.

Sibai BM, Koch M, Freire S, *et al.* The impact of a history of previous preeclampsia on the risk of superimposed preeclampsia and adverse pregnancy outcome in patients with chronic hypertension. *Am J Obstet Gynecol* 2009;201:752.

PROTOCOL 34

Immunizations

Stanley A. Gall

Department of Obsatetrics and Gynecology, University of Louisville, Louisville, KY, USA

Overview

Maternal immunization should be viewed as an opportunity to enhance the pregnant woman's protection against disease and at the same time protect the neonate with maternal passive antibodies for the first 3 to 6 months of life. Previously, immunization during pregnancy was thought to potentially cause harm to the fetus; however, if live-virus vaccines are not used during pregnancy, there are no data proving harm to the fetus from other vaccines. The appropriate attitude should be to review your patient's vaccination record and plan to administer appropriate vaccines during pregnancy which will help protect against disease based on time of year (for influenza) and immunization history. When vaccines are administered during pregnancy, the mother will generate IgG immunoglobulins, which will be transferred to the fetus, usually at a higher titer with resultant protection for the first 3 to 6 months of life.

A great opportunity exists to bring the woman's vaccines status to recommended levels when she presents for pre-conceptional counseling. At that time, both live-virus vaccines and killed or attenuated vaccines may be considered. Pregnancy should be deferred for 1 month after administration of any of the live-virus vaccines, but pregnancy may be initiated at any time with any of the attenuated vaccines. Although no risk from first trimester immunization has been proven, the risk of spontaneous abortion is greater and temporal immunization could be alleged to be the cause.

Women of childbearing age should be immunized against poliomyelitis, measles, mumps, rubella, varicella, tetanus, diphtheria and pertussis prior to becoming pregnant. Unfortunately, many women have not received the basic immunization series. This is particularly true for immigrants from third world countries where immunizations are not administered in a standardized manner nor with standardized vaccines. For these individuals, one must view them as vaccine naïve and start with basic series of vaccination.

Protocols for High-Risk Pregnancies, 5th edition. Edited by J.T. Queenan, J.C. Hobbins and C.Y. Spong. © 2010 Blackwell Publishing Ltd.

Table 34.1 Vaccination types for pregnant women

Agent	Type of agent
Hepatitis A	Killed virus
Hepatitis B	Recombinant vaccine
Influenza	Killed virus
Pneumococcal	Polysaccharide
Tetanus, diphtheria, acellular pertussis	Toxoid, antigens

The clinician has an extended period of time to administer vaccines during pregnancy. Most pregnant women are seen from 8 to 15 times for prenatal care and this presents the opportunity to discuss and administer recommended vaccines. There is little reason for the pregnant woman not to be fully immunized by the end of the pregnancy. Remember, the mother will be protected from disease and the infant will acquire IgG antibodies that will protect the neonate for 3 to 6 months depending on umbilical cord titer.

Women who are pregnant should be considered for the vaccines shown in Table 34.1.

Hepatitis A

Hepatitis A continues to be one of the most frequently reported vaccine-preventable diseases in the United States despite a vaccine being on the market since 1995. Sporadic outbreaks occur in the United States every year. Additionally, many pregnant women travel to hepatitis A endemic areas such as Mexico, Caribbean countries, South America, Africa, Eastern Europe, the Middle East and Asia.[1]

Pregnant women are at increased risk of infection with hepatitis A virus if a member of their family becomes ill with hepatitis A, if they work in an area with infected persons, if they are employed in an area with high hepatitis A infection rates such as daycare facilities or institutional facilities or have sexual contact during the incubation or clinical phase.

The Advisory Committee for Immunization Practices (ACIP) of the Centers for Disease Control recommends hepatitis A vaccine for persons at high risk for infections. These groups include:[2]

1 travelers to countries with high rates of infection (countries already mentioned);
2 men who have sex with men;
3 injecting drug users;
4 persons with clotting factor disorders;

5 persons with chronic liver disease of any type;

6 children who live in communities with high rates of disease;

7 a desire to be protected from hepatitis A virus disease;

8 prophylaxis because of a local outbreak of disease.

Fecal-oral transmission is the predominant mode of spread. Hepatitis A virus (HAV) is excreted in the stools of infected persons for 1–2 weeks before and 1 week after the onset of the illness. The viremic phases of hepatitis A infections are short and there is no chronic fecal carrier state. Because of the short viremic phase, maternal-neonatal transmission is not a recognized epidemiological entity.

The recommended regimen consists of two doses with the second dose given 6 months after the first dose.

For post-exposure prophylaxis, hepatitis A vaccine and hepatitis A immune globulin 0.02 mg/kg IM is administered. Pregnant women can safely receive both hepatitis A vaccine and hepatitis immune globulin.

Hepatitis B

Hepatitis B (HBV) infection during pregnancy can result in severe disease for the mother, fetal loss, or chronic infection for either the mother or the neonate. HBV infection results in a viremia that lasts for weeks to months and 1% to 5% of adult patients develop chronic infection and a persistent viremic carrier state with or without active liver disease. Unfortunately, neonates and children are much more susceptible to chronic infection with as many as 90% of infected neonates, 50% of infected infants and 20% of infected young children developing chronic infection.[3,4]

HBV infections have been a hazard to persons who are exposed to infected blood and blood products. HBV transmission is not limited to blood and/or blood products; sexual transmission of HBV is recognized as a major mode of spread in the United States. HBV has been found in blood, semen, cervicovaginal secretions and cells, saliva, colostrum and other body fluids. HBV is 30 times more infectious than HIV.

Maternal-fetal transmission rates depend on the presence of HBs Ag and HBe Ag. If both antigens are present the perinatal transmission rate is 90%, whereas if only HBs Ag is present the transmission rate is 10%. Since the majority of neonatal and infant HBV infections are the result of maternal-fetal transmission, the obstetrician is a critical link in the strategy to prevent perinatal transmission. All pregnant women should have routine prenatal screening for HBs Ag early in pregnancy. All patients who are HBs Ag negative but meet any of the following high-risk criteria should receive HBV vaccine during pregnancy.

1 All infants in the hospital nursery
2 All persons to age 19
3 Persons with occupational risks
   • healthcare workers
   • public service workers; police, firemen
   • laboratory workers
4 Persons with lifestyle risks
   • heterosexual persons with multiple partners (more than one partner in the preceding 6 months)
   • bisexual persons
   • diagnosis of any sexually transmitted disease
   • presentation for evaluation of a sexually transmitted disease
   • intravenous drug abusers
5 Special patient groups
   • persons with hemophilia
   • patients undergoing dialysis
   • patients with chronic liver disease
6 Environmental risk factors
   • household and sexual contacts of person with HBV
   • patients and staff of institutionalized carrier facilities
   • prison inmates
   • immigrants and refugees
   • international travelers to endemic areas.

Pregnant women who are HBs Ag negative but have any of the high-risk factors should receive the HBV vaccination series (0, 1, 6–12 months). Every pregnant woman falls into one or more high-risk group. For instance, all pregnant women are screened for not one but six STDs (chlamydia, gonorrhea, syphilis, HBV, HIV, HPV) and therefore are candidates for HBV vaccine during pregnancy. Infants born to HBs Ag negative mothers should receive a birth dose of HBV vaccine while in the hospital with the second dose 1 month later and the third dose 6–12 months later.

Infants of women who are HBs Ag positive should receive HB immunoglobulin (HBIG) 0.5 mL intramuscularly and HBV vaccine at the same time, but at a different site within 12 hours of birth. The site for injection in the neonate is the anterolateral area of the thigh. The efficacy is more than 90%.

Influenza

Influenza is an acute respiratory disease characterized by the abrupt onset of constitutional and respiratory signs and symptoms (fever, myalgia, headache, severe malaise, non-productive cough, sore throat and rhinitis).

Influenza illness typically resolves after 5–7 days for the majority of persons. However, influenza can exacerbate underlying medical conditions leading to secondary bacterial pneumonia.[5]

Pregnant women have been the victims of influenza-associated excess deaths. During the pandemics of 1918–19 and 1957–58, pregnancy-related deaths were significantly greater than for non-pregnant women. A study of 17 interpandemic influenza seasons demonstrated the relative risk for hospitalization for selected cardiorespiratory conditions among women enrolled in Medicaid increased from 1.4 during weeks 14–20 of gestation to 4.7 during weeks 37–42 in comparison with women who were 1 to 6 months postpartum.[6] Women in the third trimester of pregnancy were hospitalized at a rate (250/100,000 pregnant women) comparable to that of non-pregnant women who had high-risk conditions.

The influenza season in the northern hemisphere runs from October through March. ACIP and ACOG have advised that all pregnant women be immunized with trivalent inactivated vaccine (TIV) during the influenza season once each year. The influenza vaccine can be administered at any time during pregnancy including the first trimester. Studies have shown no adverse fetal effects associated with influenza vaccine. Recent studies have shown significant benefit to both mother and neonate from vaccination.[7] The vaccine needs to be administered yearly as new influenza strains emerge due to antigenic drift and are incorporated in the annual vaccine.

The circulation of seasonal influenza since 1976 has been mainly the H3N2 strain. In March of 2009, a new novel epidemic strain, H1N1 strain, emerged and has been designated a pandemic strain. This H1N1 strain has not been observed prior to this time and the general population is immunologically naïve. It is important to realize that in the 2009–10 influenza season, two influenza strains will be circulating at the same time (H3N2 and H1N1). ACIP recommends that all patients receive two influenza vaccines this season in order to protect against both circulating strains. The vaccines may be given at the same time in opposite arms via an intramuscular injection.

Cases of confirmed novel H1N1 influenza virus infection in pregnant women resulting in severe disease and death have been reported. Oseltamivir and zanamivir are 'pregnancy category' medications, indicating that no clinical studies have been conducted to assess safety of the medications in pregnant women. However, in pregnant women who have taken these medications, no adverse effects in the fetus have been reported. Pregnancy should not be considered a contra indication to either oseltamivir or zanamivir. Because of its systemic activity, oseltamivir is preferred for treatment of pregnant women. The choice for chemoprophylaxis is less clear. Zanamivir may be preferable because of its limited systemic absorption but respiratory complications that may be associated with zanamivir because

Table 34.2 Antiviral medication dosing for treatment and chemoprophylaxis of novel H1N1 influenza infection

Agent	Treatment	Chemoprophylaxis
Oseltamivir	75 mg capsule, bid × 5 d	75 mg capsule, once per day
Zanamivir	Two 5 mg (10 mg total) twice per day	Two 5 mg inhalations (10 mg total) once per day

Source: IDSA guidelines: http://www.journals.uchicago.edu/doi/full/10.1086/598513.

of its route of administration should be considered in women at risk for respiratory problems[8] (see Table 34.2).

Treatment for novel H1N1 influenza is recommended for:

1 all hospitalized patients with confirmed, probable or suspected novel influenza (H1N1);
2 patients who are at higher risk for seasonal influenza complications.

The following high-risk conditions are indication for influenza vaccine:[9]

1 Adults age 50 years or older.
2 Persons aged 6 months to 50 years with medical problems such as heart disease, lung disease, diabetes mellitus, renal disease, immunosuppression and persons who live in assisted care facilities.
3 All healthcare workers.
4 Pregnant women during the influenza season.
5 International travelers.
6 Anyone who wishes to reduce the likelihood of becoming ill with influenza.
7 All persons 6 months of age to 19 years of age.

Influenza vaccine does not affect the safety of mothers who are breast-feeding their infants. Breastfeeding does not adversely affect either the mother's or the infant's immune response and is not a contraindication to influenza vaccine.

Pneumococcal vaccine

Streptococcus pneumoniae infection is a major cause of pneumonia, meningitis and otitis media in young children, elderly adults and persons who are immunodeficient. *Streptococcus pneumoniae* may act as a primary pathogen or become a secondary invader following influenza or *Mycoplasma pneumoniae* infection. It is estimated that pneumococcal disease causes 3,000 cases of meningitis, 50,000 cases of bacteremia, 500,000 cases of pneumonia and 7 million cases of otitis media[10,11] in the United States annually. Approximately 150,000 persons are hospitalized with pneumococcal pneumonia with 10,000 deaths annually in the United States.

Maternal mortality is estimated to be 2% to 3% in pregnant women with severe disease, with fetal mortality approaching 30%.

Because there are no data on the increased incidence or severity of pneumococcal infection during pregnancy, ACIP does not include routine pregnancy as an indication for pneumococcal polysaccharide vaccine (PPV). However, pneumococcal polysaccharide 23-valent vaccine is recommended for individuals including pregnant women with any of the high-risk medical conditions listed below:[12,13]

1 Adults age 65 or older
2 Alaskan natives
3 American Indians
4 Organ transplant recipients
5 Smokers
6 Persons aged 2–64 with the following chronic illnesses:
   • cardiac disease pulmonary disease
   • liver disease
   • asthma
   • metabolic syndrome
   • alcoholism
   • diabetes mellitus
   • anatomic or functional asplenia
   • SC or SS disease
   • immunocompromised status
   • chronic renal disease
   • pregnant women with any of the listed high-risk conditions.

PPV can be administered at any time during pregnancy. Patients remember the PPV as the 'pneumonia shot' to differentiate it from influenza vaccine or the 'flu shot'. One-time revaccination is recommended 5 years later for persons with high-risk conditions. If the first dose is given during pregnancy, it may be repeated at age 50 and again at age 65.

There is some data to suggest that passive transfer of maternal pneumococcal antibodies to the fetus will reduce the risk of otitis media in the infant for the first 3–6 months of life. Pregnant women show good antibody response and no significant side effect of the vaccine except some soreness at the injection site. This is another example of a vaccine, which has been on the market since 1983, that is underutilized in protecting pregnant women. This vaccine has been used extensively in pregnancy.

Tetanus-diphtheria and acellular pertussis (TdaP)

Tetanus-diphtheria toxoid (Td) vaccine has been indicated routinely for pregnant women who have been previously vaccinated or who have never received Td vaccine. Td vaccine protects the mother during pregnancy and passive antibodies protect the neonate from neonatal tetanus. Neonatal tetanus kills 250,000 infants worldwide on an annual basis.[14]

Pregnant women should be routinely asked when they received their last Td vaccine. If they do not know or cannot remember then a booster dose of TdaP should be given.

Immigrants and refugees who come to the United States are infrequently fully immunized; they should receive the complete primary series. The schedule of doses is 0, 1–2 months, 6–12 months. Frequently the first two doses can be given during the prenatal period.

An adult formulation of the tetanus diphtheria (Td) containing acellular pertussis antigens was licensed by the FDA in 2005. ACIP recommended the vaccine in 2005. Since the mid 1970s the number of cases of pertussis among adults and adolescents began to rise. This rise was thought to be due to waning immunity in the adolescent and adult population. Case reports suggest that morbidity from pertussis is not increased among pregnant women as compared to non-pregnant women. However, the critical time for pertussis infection is in the neonate in the first 6 months of life.[14] Hospitalizations and complications from pertussis infection are dramatically increased in the infant less than age 1 (see Table 34.3).

The studies of the acquisition of pertussis by infants impact directly on the question of when is the best time to immunize the mother: during pregnancy or in the postpartum period? Since most of the disease is in the neonate and since infant immunization occurs at 2, 4 and 6 months of age and since the infant is not protected until 6 months of age, the logical time to immunize mother is during pregnancy. TdaP may be given in the second and third trimester. If immunization prior to pregnancy or during pregnancy is missed, the vaccine should be given in the postpartum period.

The current ACIP recommendations for routine vaccination are seen in Table 34.4.

Table 34.3 Hospitalization and complications among 16,431 infants aged <12 months with pertussis (2000–2005)

Complication	Number (% of total)
Hospitalization	8067 (61.7)
Apnea	7377 (56.3)
Pneumonia	1419 (12.8)
Seizures	169 (1.3)
Deaths	130 (0.8)

Source: CDC. National notifiable diseases surveillance system and supplemental pertussis surveillance system. 2000–2005 Atlanta, GA.

ACOG and AAP have recommended TdaP be given prior to pregnancy, during pregnancy, in the second or third trimester or postpartum.

Special vaccines

The antigens listed in Table 34.5 may be used to vaccinate pregnant women under special circumstances.

Poliomyelitis

Successful immunization programs have eliminated illness caused by wild polio-virus and the last case in the United States was reported in 1978. Worldwide eradication is a public health goal. The risk for poliomyelitis is related to international travel to areas where polio still exists. Pregnant women do not need to receive polio vaccination unless they are exposed to a risk factor for disease.[15-17]

Table 34.4 Recommendations for routine TdaP vaccination

1 Adolescents and adults should receive a single dose of tetanus, reduced diphtheria, acellular pertussis (TdaP) to replace a single dose of Td for active booster vaccination against tetanus diphtheria and pertussis if they have received their last dose of Td greater than two years ago.
2 Although previous recommendations have indicated ten year intervals for Td, the interval between Td and TdaP of two years is now recommended for a single dose of TdaP.
3 The American Academy of Pediatrics recommends that when possible women should receive TdaP in the second or third trimester of gestation to protect themselves from Pertussis and their infants with passively transferred IgG.
4 ACIP and ACOG recommend that TdaP be given postpartum but can be given during pregnancy if there is active pertussis disease in the area.
5 Lactating women may receive TdaP.
6 HealthCare workers should receive a single dose of TdaP.

Source: CDC. *MMWR* 2006;55(RR-17):1–17.

Table 34.5 Antigens for pregnant women in special circumstances

Agent or antigens	Type of agent
Poliomyelitis	Inactivated
Varicella	Live attenuated
Meningococcal	Polysaccharide
Yellow fever	Live attenuated
Measles, mumps, rubella	Live attenuated
Smallpox	Live attenuated

Two polio vaccines are available: enhanced-potency inactivated polio vaccine and oral live-virus vaccine. For pregnant women who have completed their primary series of polio vaccination more than 10 years earlier, a one-time booster of enhanced-potency inactivated polio vaccine is recommended. If less than 4 weeks are available for immunization and immediate protection is needed, a single dose of oral polio vaccine may be given.

Varicella vaccine

Varicella vaccine is a live-attenuated virus vaccine that is not recommended during pregnancy. If given to the non-pregnant woman, 30 days should elapse before pregnancy is conceived. Pregnant women should be routinely screened for varicella IgG at the first obstetric visit. If the patient is IgG seronegative she should receive her first varicella vaccination postpartum and a second dose of vaccine 4–8 weeks later. It is important to remember the second dose.[18]

Meningococcal protein conjugate vaccine

Neisseria meningitis causes rare but serious infections in pregnancy. Major manifestations of meningococcal disease are acute meningococcemia and meningitis.

Meningococcal polysaccharide vaccine is a quadrivalent vaccine against disease caused by serotypes A, C, Y and W-135. Since it is a protein conjugate vaccine, there is no risk of infectivity. The vaccine is effective in controlling epidemics.[19,20]

Meningococcal vaccine is recommended for routine administration to all adolescents, adults with terminal complement deficiencies, anatomic or functional asplenia and international travelers to countries where the disease is endemic (sub-Saharan Africa, Mecca, Saudi Arabia); college freshmen living in dormitories and military recruits are also at high risk.

Meningococcal vaccine is administered as a single 0.5 mL subcutaneous dose. This vaccine can be administered at any time during pregnancy when indicated.

Yellow fever vaccine

Yellow fever vaccine is a live-attenuated preparation made from the 17 D yellow fever strain and is grown on chick embryos. The safety of yellow fever vaccine during pregnancy has not been established and the vaccine should be administered only if travel to an endemic area is unavoidable and if an increased risk for exposure exists. Because yellow fever vaccination is a requirement for entry into certain countries, any physician who elects not to immunize a pregnant woman should provide her with a letter of explanation.[21]

Measles, mumps, rubella vaccine (MMR)

MMR vaccines are live-attenuated viruses, which are not given to pregnant women or to non-pregnant women who plan to become pregnant within 1 month of the vaccination. The immediate postpartum period is a good time to administer MMR for initiation or boosting of immunity.

All pregnant women should be screened for immunity to rubella with a rubella IgG serology. If the patient is rubella seronegative, MMR should be administered postpartum. MMR vaccination is compatible with breastfeeding.

Smallpox (vaccinia vaccine)

Smallpox vaccine is not recommended for use in pregnancy unless an outbreak of smallpox occurs. Currently, international concern is heightened regarding the potential use of smallpox (variola) as a bioterrorism agent.[22]

Currently, the only smallpox vaccine available from the Centers for Disease Control (CDC) is Dryvax, a live virus preparation using vaccinia virus. A reformulated vaccine produced by cell-culture technique is being developed.

Table 34.6 Indications for immunoglobulins in pregnancy

Infection or condition	Indication	Preparation	Dose
Rh negative	Prevent isoimmunization	Ig	250 mg IM at 28 wk & postpartum
Botulism	Treatment or prophylaxis for ingestion of botulinus toxin	Equine antibodies	Consult CDC, telephone 404-639-6370
Hepatitis A	Family contacts, sexual contacts, daycare outbreaks, international travel	Ig	0.02 mL/kg IM protects 2 mo. 0.06 mL/kg IM protects 6 mo.
Hepatitis B	Percutaneous or mucosal exposure. Sexual contacts of person with acute or chronic HBV	HBIG	0.5 mL IM at birth, vaccinate with HBV vaccine
Measles	Non-immune contacts of acute cases exposed less than 6 days previously	Ig	0.25 mL/kg IM up to 15 mL for normal; 0.5 mL/kg up to 15 mL for immunocompromised
Rabies	Persons exposed to rabid or potentially rabid animals	HRIG	20 IU/kg IM
Varicella-zoster	Immunosuppressed, pregnant or newborn contact	VZIG	125 IU/10 kg; up to 625 IU IM

Source: American College of Physicians. *Guide for Adult Immunization*, 3rd edn. Philadelphia: American College of Physicians. 1994; p. 86.

Vaccinia vaccines should not be administered to pregnant women for non-emergency indications. However, vaccinia vaccine is not known to cause congenital malformations.[23]

Immunoglobulins (Ig)

All immunoglobulin preparations are of the IgG class and may contain small amounts of other classes. Immunoglobulin for clinical use is administered intramuscularly or intravenously. Indications for use of immunoglobulin are listed in Table 34.6.[4]

Summary

Obstetricians and other healthcare workers who provide services to pregnant women should be aware of the requirements for maternal immunization:
- Non-live virus can be given at any time during pregnancy.
- Live virus vaccines should usually be deferred until the postpartum period or pre-conceptionally.
- All pregnant women should be screened for rubella varicella IgG and hepatitis Bs Ag routinely.
- All pregnant women should be asked about their last Td vaccine and whether they have ever had chickenpox.
- Hepatitis B virus and hepatitis A virus vaccines should be administered during pregnancy to women as they all have ACIP listed indications.
- Pneumococcal polysaccharide vaccine (PPV) is underutilized and should be administered at any time during pregnancy for those women who have the risk factors listed.

Contraindications to vaccination are few. They include: allergic reaction to previous vaccination with same antigen; acute illness; egg allergy for influenza and yellow fever vaccine; neomycin allergy for MMR and varicella vaccines.

References

1 Bell BP, Feinstine SM. Hepatitis A vaccine. In: Plotkin SA, Orenstein WA (eds) *Vaccines*, 4th edn. Philadelphia: Saunders, 2004: pp. 269–97.
2 Centers for Disease Control and Prevention. Prevention of Hepatitis A through active or passive immunization: Recommendations of the Advisory Committee on Immunization Practice (ACIP). *MMWR* 2006;55(RR-7).
3 Burk R D, Hwang L Y, Ho GYF. Outcome of perinatal hepatitis B virus exposure is dependent on maternal virus load. *J Infect Dis* 1994;170:14–18.
4 American College of Physicians. *Guide for Adult Immunization*, 3rd edition. Philadelphia: American College of Physicians, 1994.

5 Glezen WP. Serious morbidity and mortality associated with influenza epidemic (review). *Epidemiol Rev* 1982;4:25–44.

6 Neuzil KM, Reed GW, Mitchell EE, Simensen, L, Griffin MR. Impact of influenza on acute cardiorespiratory hospitalizations in pregnant women. *Am J. Edpidemiol* 1998;148:1094–102.

7 Zaman, K, Roy E, Arifeen SE, *et al*. Effectiveness of maternal immunization in mothers and infants. *N Engl J Med* 2008;359:1555–64.

8 Harper SA, Bradley JS, Englund JA, *et al*. Seasonal Influenza in Adults and Children – diagnosis, treatment, chemoprophylaxis, and institutional outbreak management: Clinical Practice Guidelines of the Infectious Diseases Society of America. *Clin Infect Dis* 2009;48:1003–32.

9 Prevention and control of influenza: Recommendation of the Advisory Committee on Immunization Practices (ACIP). *MMWR* 2008;57(RR-7): 1–60.

10 Kuikka A, Syrjanen J, Renkomanen OV, Valtonen V. Pneumococcal bacteremia during a recent decade. *J Infect* 1992; 24: 152–168.

11 Afessa B, Freaver Wl, Frederick WR. Pneumococcal pneumonia in adults: a 14-year experience in an inner city university hospital. *Clin Infect Dis* 1995;21:345–51.

12 Prevention of pneumococcal disease: Recommendations of the Advisory Committee on Immunization Procedures (ACIP). *MMWR* 1997;46(RR-8):1–24.

13 Nuorti JP, Butler JC, Farley CC. Cigarette smoking and invasive pneumococcal disease. *N Engl J Med* 2000;342:681–9.

14 Centers for Disease Control and Prevention. Preventing tetanus, diphtheria and pertussis among adults: use of tetanus toxoids, reduced diphtheria toxoids and acellular pertussis vaccine (TdaP). Recommendation of the Advisory Committee on Immunization Practice (ACIP). *MMWR* 2006:55(RR-17):1–37.

15 Centers for Disease Control and Prevention. Poliomyelitis Prevention in the United States: Updated Recommendations of the Advisory Committee on Immunization Practices (ACIP). *MMWR* 2000;49(RR-5):1–22.

16 Centers for Disease Control and Prevention. Poliomyelitis Prevention in the United States: Updated Recommendations of the Advisory Committee on Immunization Practices (ACIP). *MMWR* 1999;48(RR-6):1–5.

17 Centers for Disease Control and Prevention. Poliomyelitis Prevention in the United States: Updated Recommendations of the Advisory Committee on Immunization Practices (ACIP). *MMWR* 2002;51(RR-17):1–11.

18 Shields KE, Galil K, Seward J, Shanac RG, Cordero JF Slater E. Varicella exposure during pregnancy; data from first five years of the pregnancy registry. *Obstet Gynecol* 2001;98:14–19.

19 Jackson LA, Baxter R, Reisinger K, *et al*. Phase III comparison of an investigational quadrivalent meningococcal conjugate vaccine with the licensed meningococcal ACWY conjugate vaccine in adolescents. *Clin Infect Dis* 2009;49(1):e1–10.

20 Jackson LA, Wenger JD. Laboratory-based surveillance for meningococcal disease in selected areas, United States 1998–1991. *MMWR* 1993;42:21.

21 Marfin AA, Barwick ER, Monath TP. Yellow fever. In: Guerrant RL, Walker DH, Weller PF (eds) *Tropical Infectious Diseases: Principles, Pathogens and Practice*, 2nd edn. Philadelphia: Elsevier, 2006; pp. 797–812.

22 Henderson DA. Looming threat of bioterrorism. *Science* 1999;283:1279–82.

23 Greenberg M, Uankauer A, Krugman S, Osborn JJ, Ward RD, Dancis J. Effect of smallpox vaccination during pregnancy on the incidence of congenital malformations. *Pediatrics* 1949;3:456.

PROTOCOL 35

Cytomegalovirus, Genital Herpes, Rubella, Syphilis and Toxoplasmosis

George D. Wendel

Department of Obstetrics & Gynecology, University of Texas Southwestern Medical Center, Dallas, TX, USA

Cytomegalovirus

Perinatal cytomegalovirus (CMV) infection can occur in utero, intrapartum and through breast milk. Maternal primary CMV infection results in 30% to 40% of infants with congenital infection, while less than 1% of infants born to mothers with recurrent CMV infection will have perinatal infection. Overall approximately 1% to 2% of all newborns are CMV infected, about half due to primary infection during pregnancy and the other half due to reactivation of a prior infection.

Women with primary CMV infection are usually asymptomatic, but about 10% of women can have an infectious mononucleosis-like disease (but with a negative heterophile antibody test). Primary infection during any trimester can lead to intrauterine infection, but the first half of pregnancy carries the highest risk. Between 85% and 90% of congenitally infected infants are clinically asymptomatic; and only 5% to 10% of these at birth asymptomatic infants will later have abnormal development, most commonly unilateral or bilateral hearing impairment. Infants who are symptomatic at birth, however, can present with thrombocytopenia, hepatosplenomegaly, chorioretinitis, deafness, microcephaly, cerebral calcification, mental retardation or early death, often due to disseminated intravascular coagulation, hepatic failure and sepsis.

It has been estimated that among the 1 to 2% of infected newborns, as many as 10 to 20% may ultimately develop some impairment due to CMV infection. Postnatal CMV infection of the infant through breast milk, however, does not lead to visceral or neurological sequelae.

Protocols for High-Risk Pregnancies, 5th edition. Edited by J.T. Queenan, J.C. Hobbins and C.Y. Spong. © 2010 Blackwell Publishing Ltd.

Diagnosis

The great majority of CMV infections in women are asymptomatic and can be identified only by prospective antibody testing. After primary CMV infection, virus replication may persist for many months and can be reactivated months or years later, with intermittent CMV shedding from the cervix and other sites. The presence of IgM-specific CMV antibody correlates quite well with infection. Immunoglobulin M antibody is detected with about 90% of primary infections; however, it may also appear with recurrent infections. CMV IgG avidity testing may be of value in assessing a patient's likelihood of recent infection too.

Management

If a woman has primary infection with CMV, there is a 30% chance her child will be infected and thus, approximately a 6 to 7% chance her child will have some damage due to this infection. In about half of the cases the damage will be evident at birth. Therapeutic abortion can be considered. There can be a role for amniocentesis and amniotic fluid polymerase chain reaction (PCR) for CMV to assess for *in utero* infection. A negative test should rule out fetal infection; however, a positive test would not necessarily indicate that the fetus is damaged.

Recent studies suggest that there may be role for anti-CMV-specific hyperimmune globulin as prophylaxis to reduce the risk of fetal infection after maternal infection and as treatment to prevent fetal sequelae after in utero infection. However, prospective randomized studies are needed in larger groups of infected women to examine the efficacy and safety of this therapy, before this strategy can be recommended.

Women who have antibody (IgG) to CMV before being pregnant can be assured that it is very unlikely that subsequent children will have sequelae due to congenital CMV infection.

Genital herpes simplex virus

Both HSV-1 and HSV-2 cause clinical maternal and neonatal disease. Most orolabial lesions are secondary to HSV-1, and genital lesions may be caused by either virus.

The majority of neonatal herpes cases are born to women who have subclinical viral shedding at delivery and who often have no history of disease, making transmission prevention difficult. In utero infection occurs in approximately 5% of neonatal HSV cases. The risk of transmission from asymptomatic shedding in a woman with recurrent HSV is much lower, approximately 1 in 10,000 deliveries. The duration of rupture of membranes, the use of fetal scalp electrodes and the mode of delivery also influence neonatal transmission. Two-thirds of neonatal HSV infection is due to HSV-2 and the remaining one-third to HSV-1 infection.

Diagnosis

The diagnosis of HSV infection is often made clinically. Isolation of virus by cell culture is the most sensitive test widely available. PCR is highly sensitive but not as widely available. Antibodies begin to develop within 2 to 3 weeks of infection. Serological tests now available are based on antibodies formed to type-specific G-glycoproteins. These tests allow specific typing for HSV-1 and HSV-2 and are useful for counseling.

Management

Antepartum management

Late pregnancy primary HSV has the highest likelihood for neonatal transmission. Counseling the woman who is HSV serology negative about safe sexual practices may lead to a decrease in acquisition of genital herpes in late pregnancy. Though some experts recommend screening, at this time universal screening of all pregnant women with type-specific serology is not recommended.

An active lesion in the antepartum period should be cultured to confirm the clinical diagnosis. If this is an initial episode, type-specific serology should be performed to determine if this is a primary or non-primary infection. Systemic antivirals may be used to attenuate signs and symptoms of HSV, especially if this is a primary infection. However, these will not eradicate latent virus.

Antiviral suppression therapy in the latter part of pregnancy (36 weeks until delivery) has been shown to decrease the rate of clinical HSV recurrences at delivery and the rate of asymptomatic shedding at delivery.

Intrapartum management

A woman with a history of HSV should be asked about prodromal symptoms and recent HSV lesions. A careful vulvar, vaginal and cervical examination should be performed. Suspicious lesions should be cultured. Currently, cesarean delivery is indicated if the woman has an active lesion or prodromal symptoms. However, a cesarean delivery does not eliminate the risk. Ten to fifteen percent of infants with HSV are born to women who have had a cesarean delivery. If a lesion is present distant from the vulva, vagina or cervix, the risk of neonatal transmission is lower. The non-genital lesions may be covered with an occlusive dressing and a vaginal delivery allowed. Cesarean delivery should not be performed in a woman solely for a history of HSV.

The management of the woman presenting with an active HSV lesion and ruptured membranes is controversial. At term, cesarean delivery should be offered regardless of how long the membranes have been ruptured. In the setting of preterm PROM, especially remote from term, expectant management should be considered; as the risk of prematurity complications may outweigh the benefit of immediate delivery.

Rubella

Rubella virus infection is acquired via the upper respiratory tract through inhalation. Infection during the first 5 months of pregnancy can result in severe fetal damage or death. The mother with rubella may have no symptoms (30%) or a mild 3-day rash with posterior auricular adenopathy.

The child, however, may have severe congenital heart damage, cataracts, deafness, damage to major blood vessels, microcephaly, mental retardation or other abnormalities. In addition there may be severe disease during the newborn period, including thrombocytopenia, bleeding, hepatosplenomegaly, pneumonitis or myocarditis. The risk of major fetal damage varies with the time of maternal infection: 80 to 90% in the first 3 months of pregnancy; 10% in the fourth month; and 6% in the fifth month, often as isolated hearing impairment. There is probably no risk after the fifth month.

Diagnosis
After exposure, a woman will develop infection in 2 to 3 weeks, and antibody shortly thereafter. To document the infection, collect paired sera and test them for antibody. The first specimen should have no antibody; the second specimen, taken about 4 weeks after exposure, would have significant antibody. Immunoglobulin M rubella antibody can also be used to document recent rubella following exposure or subclinical rubella when only a late serum specimen is available. This test becomes positive shortly after the onset of rash and remains positive for about 4 weeks.

Management
Routine use of immune globulin (IG) for post-exposure prophylaxis in pregnant susceptible women is not recommended. IG has been shown to suppress symptoms; however, it does not prevent viremia. Congenital rubella infections have occurred despite immediate post-exposure use of IG. It may be considered for exposed women when termination of the pregnancy is not an option.

The primary approach to the prevention of rubella is immunization (in the United States the RA 27/3 vaccine). Vaccine for measles, mumps and rubella (MMR) should be given to all children between 12 and 15 months of age and repeated at school age. Also, all women of childbearing age should be tested for antibody to rubella. If a non-pregnant woman does not have antibody, the vaccine should be given.

If the woman is pregnant, she should not receive the vaccine. Non-pregnant vaccine recipients should be instructed not to become pregnant for 3 months. These reservations are based on the hypothetic possibility that the vaccine virus might damage the developing fetus early in pregnancy. However data from the Centers for Disease Control (CDC) for over 800 susceptible pregnant women who inadvertently received the rubella vaccine during early pregnancy showed no evidence of rubella-related fetal damage. Two children, however, had immunoglobulin M (IgM) rubella antibody, indicating that fetal infection had occurred. The maximum theoretical risk for fetal damage could be about 2%; the currently observed risk is zero.

Women who are to be immunized may experience transient rash and arthralgia. Members of a household who have received rubella vaccine may have vaccine virus isolated from their pharynx, but do not transmit to others, likely due to the low quantity of rubella virus shedding.

Syphilis

The most common clinical findings in congenital syphilis are hepatosplenomegaly, osteochondritis or periostitis, jaundice or hyperbilirubinemia, petechiae, purpura, lymphadenopathy and ascites or hydrops. There appears to be a continuum of fetal syphilis as it progresses in utero (Fig. 35.1).

Diagnosis
The majority of pregnant women with syphilis are asymptomatic, and the diagnosis is frequently made by serological testing, which is recommended at the first prenatal care visit, during the third trimester and at delivery. Of infected fetuses, 40 to 50% will die in utero. The most common cause of fetal death is placental infection and overwhelming fetal infection. *Treponema pallidum* can be identified in infected amniotic fluid using PCR testing; however prenatal diagnosis is not recommended prior to maternal treatment.

Management
Patients with early syphilis (primary, secondary and early latent syphilis of less than 1 year's duration) should receive a single intramuscular dose of 2.4 million units of benzathine penicillin G. Some specialists also recommend a second dose of benzathine penicillin G one week after the initial dose for pregnant women who have early syphilis. After treatment of early disease, more than 60% of women will have the Jarisch-Herxheimer

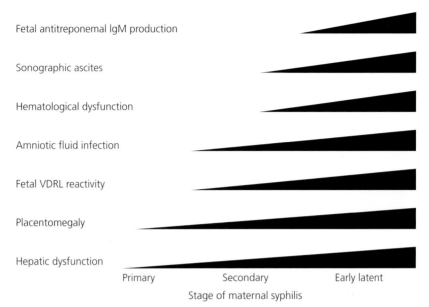

Figure 35.1 Continuum of fetal syphilis in utero with stages of maternal syphilis. Adapted from Hollier LM, Harstad TW, Sanchez PJ, *et al*. Fetal syphilis: clinical and laboratory characteristics. *Obstet Gynecol* 2001:97:947–53.

reaction. Pregnant patients should be warned to watch for fever, decreases in fetal activity and signs of preterm labor.

For pregnant women with late latent syphilis of more than 1 year's duration or of unknown duration, or with cardiovascular syphilis, benzathine penicillin G, 2.4 million units intramuscularly, should be given weekly for three doses (7.2 million units total). Pregnant women with neurosyphilis should receive aqueous crystalline penicillin G intravenously or intramuscular procaine penicillin plus oral probenecid for 10 to 14 days.

Serological tests should be repeated at the previously recommended times of during the third trimester and at delivery. It is expected that there will be a fourfold drop in serological test titers over a 6- to 12-month period in women treated for early syphilis. However, it is not unusual for pregnant women to have insufficient time to be evaluated for serological evidence of cure of their syphilis by delivery.

Treatment before 20 weeks is uniformly effective in preventing congenital syphilis, barring re-infection. Treatment failures occur in 1 to 2% of patients because of advanced, irreversible fetal infection. These failures are seen more frequently with maternal high-titer early latent syphilis, secondary syphilis or treatment after 30 weeks' gestation. In adults, HIV infection may affect the clinical presentation of syphilis, the serologies and the response to recommended therapy.

Treatment after 20 weeks should be preceded by ultrasonography to look for evidence of fetal infection. In the case of an abnormal sonogram (hydrops, ascites, skin edema, hepatomegaly), antepartum fetal heart rate testing is useful prior to treatment. Spontaneous late decelerations and non-reactive fetal heart rate patterns have been associated with an infected fetus. When sonographic abnormalities are found and antepartum testing is abnormal, a neonatologist and maternal fetal medicine specialist should be consulted.

The pregnant woman with syphilis who is allergic to penicillin presents a therapeutic challenge. Because of reported treatment failures, resistance concerns and the lack of clinical data in pregnancy, azithromycin is not recommended for routine use in pregnant patients. Skin testing and referral for penicillin desensitization for the pregnant patient who has been proved to be allergic to penicillin is recommended. Desensitization can be accomplished either orally or intravenously.

Toxoplasmosis

The sequelae of congenital toxoplasmosis may be severe and include fetal death, blindness, deafness and mental retardation. At birth, infected children may have a maculopapular rash, hepatosplenomegaly, seizures or hydrocephalus. The overall risk of having an affected child is approximately 2% in the first trimester, nearly 10% around 28 weeks, and about 4% at term. At this time, antepartum screening, optimal methods for prenatal diagnosis of congenital toxoplasmosis, and treatment are controversial.

Diagnosis

The most common clinical sign is bilateral, non-tender lymphadenopathy that often involves the posterior cervical nodes. Additional symptoms include generalized fatigue, myalgias, fevers and headaches.

Serological tests for immunoglobulins (Ig) G and M antibodies should be obtained in patients who have suggestive symptoms. IgG antibodies generally appear within 1 to 2 weeks of infection, and will peak between 6 and 8 weeks. IgM antibodies appear within the first week of infection and then will usually decline over several months. Immunoglobulin M antibodies may persist for years, and their presence is not necessarily indicative of an active or recent infection. At reference laboratories, a combination of tests, including IgG avidity testing, is helpful in determining a recent or distant infection. One such laboratory is the Palo Alto Medical Foundation Research Institute's Toxoplasma Serology Laboratory. Table 35.1 illustrates the potential antibody test results and their interpretation and management.

Table 35.1 Maternal serum antibody results and interpretation

Maternal serum antibodies	Interpretation/action
IgG – / IgM –	No evidence of infection
IgG – / IgM +	Possible current/recent infection. Send serum for confirmation to reference laboratory
IgG + / IgM –	Probable past infection, unless known to be IgG negative previously
IgG + / IgM +	Possible current/recent infection. Send serum for confirmation to reference laboratory

PCR testing of the amniotic fluid is the most accurate method for diagnosing fetal infection. This is generally performed in the second trimester or 4 weeks after an acute maternal infection. There are multiple sonographic abnormalities that may be seen with congenital toxoplasmosis; however, these are only suggestive of fetal infection. Some of these abnormalities include the following:

• ventricular dilation
• intracranial calcifications
• increased placental thickness
• hepatomegaly and/or intrahepatic calcifications
• fetal ascites
• pericardial or pleural effusions.

Treatment

The rationale for treatment of women with *Toxoplasma* infection during pregnancy is that it has been shown to reduce the incidence of severe sequelae and that the shorter the interval between diagnosis and treatment, the lower the incidence of sequelae. Neither the time between diagnosis and treatment with antibiotics nor the actual administration of maternal antibiotics appears to affect the rate of transmission to the fetus. Randomized trials in this area are currently lacking.

Once maternal infection is confirmed, treatment is started with spiramycin. This antibiotic is similar to erythromycin and concentrates in the placenta. This drug is not available commercially in the United States; however, it can be obtained with the permission of the US Food and Drug Administration. If there is evidence of fetal infection, as diagnosed by amniocentesis and PCR, additional treatment is given. If the PCR is negative for fetal infection, spiramycin is generally continued until delivery.

When fetal infection is confirmed, treatment is changed in favour of medications that cross the placenta and penetrate the fetal brain and cerebrospinal fluid. This includes both pyrimethamine and sulfadiazine. Pyrimethamine and sulfadiazine are both folic acid antagonists that work synergistically against the *T. gondii* parasite. These are generally administered after the second trimester and with supplementation with folinic acid. Of note, when a woman becomes infected after 32 weeks, some will begin treatment with pyrimethamine and sulfadiazine immediately rather than spiramycin because of the increased risk for fetal transmission.

Suggested reading

Cytomegalovirus

Bhide A, Papageorghiou AT. Managing primary CMV infection in pregnancy. *Br J Obstet Gynaecol* 2008;115:805–7.

Adler SP, Nigro G. Findings and conclusions from CMV hyperimmune globulin treatment trials. *J Clin Virol* 2009;46S:S54–7.

Guerra B, Simonazzi G, Puccetti C, Lanari M, Farina A, Lazzarotto T, Rizzo N. Ultrasound prediction of symptomatic congenital cytomegalovirus infection. *Am J Obstet Gynecol* 2008;198:380.e1–7.

Genital herpes simplex virus

Wald A, Corey L. Maternal and neonatal herpes simplex virus infections. *N Engl J Med* 2009;361:1376–85.

Hollier LM, Wendel GD. Third trimester antiviral prophylaxis for preventing maternal genital herpes simplex virus (HSV) recurrences and neonatal infection. *Cochrane Database Syst Rev* 2008;(1):CD004946. Review.

American College of Obstetricians and Gynecologists. ACOG Practice Bulletin # 82, June 2007. Management of herpes in pregnancy. *Obstet Gynecol* 2007;109:1489–98.

Rubella

Best JM. Rubella. *Semin Fetal Neonatal Med* 2007;12:182–92.

Dontigny L, Arsenault MY, Martel MJ, Biringer A, Cormier J, Delaney M, Gleason T, Leduc D, Martel MJ, Penava D, Polsky J, Roggensack A, Rowntree C, Wilson AK; Society of Obstetricians and Gynaecologists of Canada. Rubella in pregnancy. *J Obstet Gynaecol Can* 2008;30:152–68.

Haas DM, Flowers CA, Congdon CL. Rubella, rubeola, and mumps in pregnant women: susceptibilities and strategies for testing and vaccinating. *Obstet Gynecol* 2005;106:295–300.

Syphilis

Centers for Disease Control and Prevention, Workowski KA, Berman SM. Sexually transmitted diseases treatment guidelines, 2006. *MMWR Recomm Rep* 2006; 55(RR-11):1–94.

Hollier LM, Harstad TW, Sanchez PJ, Twickler DM, Wendel GD Jr. Fetal syphilis: clinical and laboratory characteristics. *Obstet Gynecol* 2001:97:947–53.

Wendel GD Jr, Sheffield JS, Hollier LM, Hill JB, Ramsey PS, Sánchez PJ. Treatment of syphilis in pregnancy and prevention of congenital syphilis. *Am J Obstet Gynecol* 2003; 189:1178–83.

Zhou P, Qian Y, Xu J, Gu Z, Liao K. Occurrence of congenital syphilis after maternal treatment with azithromycin during pregnancy. *Sex Transm Dis* 2007;34:472–4.

Toxoplasmosis

Gilbert R, Gras L, European Multicentre Study on Congenital Toxoplasmosis. Effect of timing and type of treatment on the risk of mother to child transmission of *Toxoplasma gondii. Br J Obstet Gynaecol* 2003;110:112–20.

Montoya JG, Remington JS. Management of *Toxoplasma gondii* infection during pregnancy. *Clin Infect Dis* 2008;47:554–66.

SYROCOT (Systematic Review on Congenital Toxoplasmosis) study group, Thiébaut R, Leproust S, Chêne G, Gilbert R. Effectiveness of prenatal treatment for congenital toxoplasmosis: a meta-analysis of individual patients' data. *Lancet* 2007;369:115–22.

Influenza, West Nile Virus, Varicella-Zoster and Tuberculosis

Jeanne S. Sheffield
Division of Maternal-Fetal Medicine, University of Texas Southwestern Medical Center, Dallas, TX, USA

Influenza

Influenza infection, while clinically recognized for centuries, remains a significant contributor to morbidity and mortality from febrile respiratory illness. Occurring annually, this viral infection affects all age groups and has caused approximately 36,000 deaths per year in the United States from 1990 to 1999. While children and adults aged 65 and older are at highest risk for serious complications and death, other high-risk groups have been identified, including pregnant women.

The data regarding influenza infection and pregnancy are limited. Early studies from the 1918 and 1957 influenza pandemics reported higher risks of complications such as abortion, stillbirth, low birth weight, congenital anomalies, and mortality rates (as high as 30%) in pregnant women compared to the general population. However, recent studies over the last two decades have contradicted the frequency of these early findings. It is now thought that a small increase in overall complication rates and congenital anomalies is associated with influenza. Though the virus can cross the placenta, fetal infection is rare.

Pathophysiology

Influenza is a myxovirus with three antigenic types – A, B and C. Only influenza A and B cause clinically significant disease. Influenza A is further subtyped using two surface glycoproteins, hemagglutinin (H) and neuraminidase (N). Hemagglutinin is a viral attachment protein and mediates viral entry. The neuraminidase enzyme facilitates viral spread. The annual antigenic variation noted worldwide is secondary to either antigenic drift or shift. Antigenic drift occurs when mutations accumulate in the N or H antigen. It is a slow, often subtle, process and the mutations

---

Protocols for High-Risk Pregnancies, 5th edition. Edited by J.T. Queenan, J.C. Hobbins and C.Y. Spong. © 2010 Blackwell Publishing Ltd.

directly affect vaccine efficacy. Antigenic shift, seen only in influenza A, involves replacement of the current either H or N antigen with a new subtype. This shift to a novel antigen subtype is responsible for the intermittent worldwide influenza pandemics.

The influenza virus is spread through respiratory droplets and direct contact with recently contaminated articles. The incubation period ranges from 1 to 4 days. Adults often shed virus the day before symptoms develop until 5 days after symptom onset. Though many cases of influenza are asymptomatic, adults present with a sudden onset of fever and rigors, diffuse myalgias, malaise, headache and a non-productive cough. Sore throat, rhinitis, abdominal pain, nausea and vomiting may also be present. Tachycardia and tachypnea are common, especially in pregnant women. Though most symptoms resolve within a few days, the cough and malaise may persist for longer than 2 weeks.

Diagnosis
During the influenza 'season', the diagnosis is usually made using clinical features. Diagnostic tests are best performed within 72 hours of onset of illness, as viral shedding is greatest at this time. Viral culture of throat washings and nasopharyngeal secretions allow subtyping of the virus, important for epidemiological evaluation and vaccine development. Serology, polymerase chain reaction and immunofluorescence testing is also available. Finally, rapid antigen tests, though of lower sensitivity than the viral culture, are readily available and allow rapid viral detection of nasopharyngeal secretions.

Treatment
Hospitalization of the pregnant woman with influenza depends on the severity of symptoms and any associated complications. The patient should be evaluated for evidence of pneumonia and other complications as the clinical findings dictate. If influenza is suspected, initiate respiratory and contact isolation procedures along with strict hand hygiene.

Four antiviral medications are currently marketed for use during influenza outbreaks. Amantadine and ramantadine are adamantanes with activity against influenza A only. Their use in pregnancy has been reported with no adverse outcomes to date. The second class of antiviral medications, the neuraminidase inhibitors, include zanamivir and oseltamivir, both highly effective for influenza A and B. Secondary to early variations in resistance patterns, the Centers for Disease Control and Prevention publish treatment guidelines every year based on the influenza subtypes and antiviral sensitivity patterns (www.cdc.gov). Optimally, treatment should begin within 48 hours of symptom onset.

Complications

Physiological changes in pregnancy such as an elevated diaphragm, increased oxygen consumption and decreased functional residual capacity may worsen the pulmonary complications of influenza (i.e., pneumonia). Secondary bacterial infections, particularly pneumonia, are not uncommon. Myocarditis has also been reported. Death, though rare, usually complicates influenza in patients with underlying chronic disease. There is no evidence that influenza A or B cause congenital malformations.

Prevention

Vaccination is the primary method to prevent influenza and its severe complications. Each year, a new vaccine formulation consisting of two influenza A subtypes and one influenza B virus is determined based on typing of current virus worldwide. The efficacy of the vaccine is variable depending on how well the vaccine antigens correlate with the virus circulating in a specific community. Pregnant women respond to vaccination with increases in antibody titers similar to non-pregnant women. Only the inactivated influenza vaccine is recommended in pregnancy and can be used in any trimester. Secondary prevention strategies such as hand hygiene, respiratory and contact isolation should be implemented.

H1N1 influenza virus

The emergence of the novel influenza A virus, subtype A/H1N1 in 2008/2009 has been associated with significant febrile illness worldwide – the World Health Organization declared a pandemic on June 11, 2009. A recent review of 34 confirmed or probable cases of pandemic H1N1 in pregnant women was conducted by the Centers for Disease Control and Prevention. Pregnant women were more likely to require hospitalization. Six maternal deaths in the pregnant women were reported, each in women with pneumonia and subsequent acute respiratory distress syndrome.

   At press, the diagnostic techniques, management strategies and preventive measures are evolving. The rapid influenza tests available have a lower sensitivity and specificity for the novel A/H1N1 virus compared to seasonal influenza test results. Polymerase chain reaction tests are being optimized for the A/H1N1 virus and are becoming more widely available. As pregnant women are at higher risk for severe complications of death, treatment with oseltamivir or zanamivir is recommended for any pregnant woman with confirmed or suspected influenza regardless of trimester. Dosing recommendations for treatment are oseltamivir 75 mg orally twice a day for 5 days or zanamivir two 5 mg inhalations twice a day for 5 days.

Treatment should be initiated as early as possible and should not be delayed to wait on laboratory confirmation. Post-exposure chemoprophylaxis may decrease but not eliminate the risk of novel A/H1N1 in pregnant women exposed to someone with influenza. Oseltamivir 75 mg once daily for 10 days or zanamivir two 5 mg inhalations once daily may be used.

A vaccine for the novel A/H1N1 is currently undergoing safety and efficacy trials and has been available for use during the 2009–2010 season. It currently is a separate vaccine from the seasonal influenza vaccine – both are recommended for pregnant women. The up-to-date treatment and prevention strategies are available at www.cdc.gov/H$_1$N1flu.

West Nile virus

West Nile virus, originally isolated in 1937 in Uganda and endemic in Africa, Asia and the Middle East, was first reported in North America in 1999. By 2003, there were 9,858 reported cases with 2,864 cases of neuroinvasive disease. Subsequent years have noted a decrease in numbers. In 2008, there were 1,356 cases with 44 deaths; 51% reported had meningitis or encephalitis (neuroinvasive) and 46% had West Nile fever (milder disease). The high number of neuroinvasive disease likely reflects surveillance reporting bias. In population-based surveys, neuroinvasive disease will develop in less than 1% of cases.

Pathophysiology
West Nile virus is an anthropod-borne flavivirus, a member of the Japanese encephalitis virus antigenic complex. It is maintained in nature through biological transmission involving bird reservoirs and mosquitoes, with humans an incidental host via a bite of an infected mosquito. Human transmission occurs mainly in the late summer months and there is no documented animal-to-human (except mosquitoes) or human-to-human transmission. The incubation period is 2 to 14 days.

Diagnosis
Most human West Nile virus infections are subclinical – only 1 in 5 develop a mild febrile illness with symptoms lasting 3 to 6 days. Pregnant women with symptoms may present with fever, headache, fatigue, rare truncal skin rash, lymphadenopathy and eye pain. CNS involvement or neuroinvasive disease is diagnosed in <1% of adult cases. The diagnosis of West Nile virus is based on clinical symptoms and serology. West Nile virus serum IgM and IgG and cerebrospinal fluid IgM are used for laboratory confirmation, though cross-reaction to

other flaviviruses have been reported. Polymerase chain reaction testing is limited secondary to transient and low viremia. Amniotic fluid, chorionic villi, fetal serum or products of conception can be tested for evidence of fetal West Nile virus infection though the sensitivity and specificity are not known.

Treatment

There is no known effective antiviral treatment – management is supportive based on the severity of the disease. Clinical trials are ongoing.

Complications

Patients with neuroinvasive disease often have long-term sequelae including fatigue, memory loss, difficulty walking, muscle weakness and depression. Fetal infection has been reported complicating pregnancy. A CDC West Nile Virus Pregnancy Registry found a small rate of neonatal infection (3/72 liveborn infants) though it could not be established conclusively that the infection was acquired congenitally. One case of transmission through breast milk has been reported.

Prevention

The primary strategy for preventing exposure in pregnancy is the use of mosquito repellent. Avoid outdoor activity around stagnant water and wear protective clothing from dusk to dawn. A vaccine is not currently available.

Varicella-zoster

Varicella-zoster virus (VZV) is a double-stranded DNA herpes virus acquired predominantly during childhood – in the United States, 95% of adults have serological evidence of immunity. Primary infection with VZV manifests as varicella (chickenpox). Herpes zoster (shingles) is an eruption that results from reactivation of latent VZV infection of dorsal root ganglia.

Pathophysiology

Humans are the only source of infection with VZV. The virus is highly contagious and transmission occurs primarily through direct contact with an infected individual, although airborne spread from respiratory tract secretions have been reported. The incubation period is 10–21 days and a susceptible woman has a 60–95% risk of becoming infected with exposure. The patients are contagious from 1–2 days prior to the onset of rash until the lesions are crusted.

Diagnosis

Varicella is usually diagnosed clinically. A 1- to 2-day prodrome of fever, malaise, myalgias and headache is followed by a rash on the head and trunk which then spreads to the extremities and abdomen. The rash occurs in 'crops' of maculopapular lesions which rapidly form vesicles. It is intensely pruritic and slowly crusts over several days. Herpes zoster presents as painful skin lesions over sensory nerve root distributions (dermatomes).

Laboratory diagnosis is occasionally helpful. The virus may be isolated by scraping the vesicles and performing a tissue culture, Tzank smear or direct fluorescent antibody testing. Nucleic acid amplification tests are available and are very sensitive and specific. Serological testing is commonly available – the enzyme-linked immunosorbent assay (ELISA) is the most popular though useful mainly to confirm prior infection.

Treatment

Pregnant women with uncomplicated varicella who are immunocompetent require only supportive care. Acyclovir (500 mg/m^2 or 10–15 mg/kg every 8 hours) is reserved for pregnant women with complicated varicella infection (e.g., varicella pneumonia) or who are immunocompromised.

Complications

Primary varicella infection in adults has higher complication rates than in children and is most pronounced in pregnant women. The increased morbidity is primarily respiratory. Pneumonitis is diagnosed in 5–14% of pregnant women with varicella, especially in smokers and women with ≥100 skin lesions; mortality has decreased to <2%. VZV encephalitis and other neurological complications are rare. Bacterial super-infection can lead to cellulitis, abscess formation or rarely necrotizing fasciitis.

Congenital varicella syndrome among infants born to mothers with varicella is approximately 2% when infection occurs before 20 weeks of gestation. Children exposed to varicella-zoster virus in utero during the second 20 weeks of pregnancy can develop inapparent varicella and subsequent zoster early in life without having had extrauterine varicella. Fetal infection after maternal varicella during the first or early second trimester of pregnancy occasionally results in varicella embryopathy, characterized by cutaneous scars, denuded skin, limb hypoplasia, muscle atrophy and rudimentary digits. Other more frequent abnormalities are microcephaly, intracranial calcifications, cortical atrophy, cataracts, chorioretinitis, microphthalmia and psychomotor retardation. Fetal exposure just before or during delivery results in neonatal VZV infection in 25–50% of cases. The case fatality rate approaches 25% as there is no protective transplacental passage of maternal VZV-specific IgG. Varicella-zoster immune globulin should be given to neonates whose mothers developed varicella 5 days before and up to 2 days post-delivery.

Prevention

Pregnant women exposed to VZV who deny prior infection should have a VZV lgG titer performed –70% of individuals with no history of VZV are actually immune. Seronegative women should be given varicella-zoster immune globulin (VariZIG) available currently through an expanded access protocol. Contact information is available on the Centers for Disease Control and Prevention website (www.cdc.gov). It is most effective when given early but may be given up to 96 hours post-exposure. A live virus vaccine (Varivax©) is available in the United States but is not recommended for pregnant women.

Tuberculosis

While tuberculosis (TB) remains a serious health problem worldwide, TB has been steadily declining in the United States, to a lowest recorded rate in 2007 of 4.4 cases per 100,000 persons. The tuberculosis rate in foreign-born persons was 10 times greater than that of US-born persons, with almost three-fifths of all TB cases in the United States occurring in immigrants. The majority of cases in the United States are latent tuberculosis infection (LTI).

Pathophysiology

Tuberculosis is a chronic bacterial infection caused by *Mycobacterium tuberculosis* or *M. bovis*, which is transmitted by respiratory droplet and spread from person to person via air. Transmission of TB is dependent on the number and/or viability of bacilli in expelled air, susceptible host factors, environment/shared air, and duration and/or frequency of exposure. In over 90% of patients, infection is dormant for long periods and remains localized to the respiratory tract.

Primary tuberculosis infection can be asymptomatic, can produce a typical primary complex, or result in typical chronic pulmonary TB without a demonstrable primary complex. Early pulmonary TB is usually asymptomatic, and does not produce symptoms until the bacillary population has reached a certain size. When symptoms occur they range from non-specific constitutional symptoms such as anorexia, fatigue, weight loss, chills, afternoon fever, and when this subsides, night sweats. A productive cough is usually present, and hemoptysis can occur. In some women, extrapulmonary disease may occur – the greatest risk is in the immunocompromised patient. Pregnancy does not appear to increase the risk for developing active TB.

Children born to women with active TB have an increased risk of morbidity and mortality in the neonatal period, with an increase in prematurity, perinatal death and low birth weight. However, when adequate therapy is initiated, TB appears to have no adverse effect on the pregnancy. Most perinatal infections occur when a mother with active TB handles her infant, and the risk of the child contracting TB from a mother with active disease during the first year of life may be as high as 50%. Transplacental passage of TB is extremely rare.

Diagnosis

The Centers for Disease Control and Prevention recommend skin testing of pregnant women in high-risk groups (Fig. 36.1). Most pregnant women

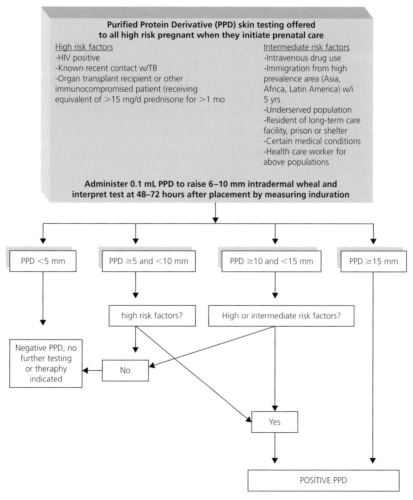

Figure 36.1 Screening and diagnosis of tuberculosis during pregnancy.

diagnosed with TB are asymptomatic and are only detected secondary to PPD screening. Pregnancy does not increase the risk for anergy – an anergy panel is unnecessary in the HIV non-infected pregnant woman. False-positive reactions may be caused by cross-reaction with other mycobacteria or prior vaccination with BCG (bacille Calmette-Guérin). Patients with a positive PPD skin test should be evaluated regardless of history of BCG vaccination. The in vitro Quantiferon-TB Gold test and the T-spot TB test are also used to identify patients with latent disease as well as to distinguish between immune responses from BCG vaccination and responses secondary to actual infection.

The definitive diagnosis of TB is based on identifying *M. tuberculosis* by culture or acid-fast stain of the sputum. First morning sputum specimens obtained on 3 consecutive days are usually the best source for detecting TB and should be undertaken in those with symptoms of active TB and those with a positive PPD and abnormal chest x-ray (Fig. 36.2).

Treatment

A positive PPD only means that the patient has been previously exposed to tuberculosis and that there are latent organisms present. Less than 10% of patients with a positive PPD and an intact immune system will progress to active disease. However, targeted tuberculin skin testing for LTI is a strategic component of TB control to identify persons at high risk for developing TB who would benefit by treatment of LTI, if detected. Persons with increased risk for developing active TB include those who have recent infection with *M. tuberculosis* and those who have clinical conditions that are associated with an increased risk for progression of LTI to active TB, such as HIV infection, injection drug use, chest radiograph evidence or prior TB or chronic illness.

Latent infection

Individuals with LTI who are at high risk for progression to TB disease should be given high priority for treatment of LTI regardless of age. Asymptomatic pregnant women with a negative chest x-ray should start isoniazid preventive therapy as soon as possible if they have one of the following factors: HIV infection; close contact to infectious TB disease; recent (within 2 years) skin test conversion; high-risk medical conditions. Isoniazid 300 mg daily for 6–9 months is the preferred regimen for treatment of LTI. Asymptomatic women with a negative chest x-ray and none of the risk factors listed above may elect to delay therapy until after delivery. Pyridoxine (vitamin B_6) 50 mg daily should be given with isoniazid to prevent peripheral neuropathy. Isoniazid is not contraindicated in breastfeeding women. Isoniazid for LTI is contraindicated in those with active hepatitis or end-stage liver disease. All patients should be assessed for isoniazid-induced hepatitis.

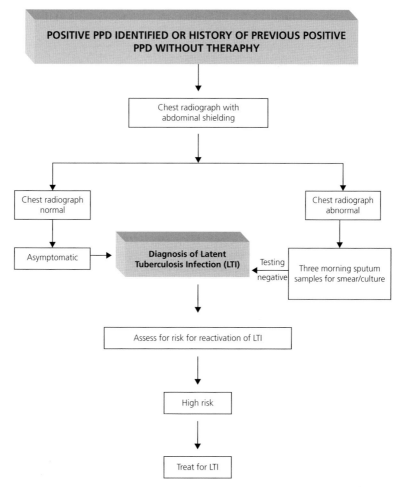

Figure 36.2 Evaluation of postive PPD during pregnancy.

Active tuberculosis infection

Untreated TB in pregnancy poses a significant threat to the mother and fetus. Current recommendations for active disease in pregnancy is a three-drug regimen with isoniazid, ethambutol and rifampin. In areas of high isoniazid resistance, pyrazinamide is added until susceptibility testing is available. Streptomycin should be avoided secondary to possible congenital ototoxicity. For HIV-infected women, rifampin may be an issue secondary to interactions with certain protease inhibitors.

Complications

Congenital and neonatal tuberculosis are fortunately uncommon. It presents with hepatosplenomegaly, fever, respiratory disease and lymphadenopathy.

Neonatal infection is unlikely if the mother is adequately treated. Isolation of the uninfected newborn until the mother has a negative sputum culture is recommended.

Suggested reading

http://www.cdc.gov/ncidod/dvbid/westnile/surv&controlCaseCount08_detailed.htm

Mostashari F, Bunning ML, Kitsutani PT, *et al.* Epidemic West Nile Encephalitis, New York, 1999; Results of a household-based seroepidemiological survey. *Lancet* 2001;358:261–4.

Granwehr BP, Lillibridge KM, Higgs S, *et al.* West Nile Virus; where are we now? *Lancet Infect Dis* 2004;4:547–56.

O'Leary DR, Kuhn S, Kniss KL, *et al.* Birth outcomes following West Nile Virus infection of pregnant women, United States, 2003–2004. *Pediatrics* 2006;117(3):e537–45.

Harger JH, Ernest JM, Thurnau GR, *et al.* Frequency of congenital Varicella syndrome in a prospective cohort of 347 pregnant women. *Obstet Gynecol* 2002;100(2):260–5.

Chandra PC, Patel H, Schiavello HJ, Briggs SL. Successful pregnancy outcome after complicated Varicella pneumonia. *Obstet Gynecol* 1998;92:680–2.

http://www.cdc.gov/mmwr. MMWR Weekly March 3, 2006/55(08);209–10. *A New Product (VariZIG^{TM}) for Postexposure Prophylaxis of Varicella Available Under an Investigational New Drug Application Expanded Access Protocol.*

www.cdc.gov/tb October 2008. *Trends in Tuberculosis, 2007.*

Harper SA, Fukuda K, Uyeki TM, Cox NJ, Bridges CB. Prevention and control of influenza. *MMWR* 2004;53:1–40.

www.cdc.gov/H1N1flu/pregnancy/antiviral September 17, 2009. *Updated Interim Recommendations for Obstetric Health Care Providers Related to Use of Antiviral Medications in the Treatment and Prevention of Influenza for the 2009–2010 Season.*

Jamieson DJ, Honein MA, Rasmussen SA, Williams JL, *et al.* H1N1 2009 influenza virus infection during pregnancy in the USA. *Lancet* 2009;374:451–58.

Malaria in Pregnancy

Richard M.K. Adanu

Department of Obstetrics and Gynaecology, University of Ghana Medical School, Ghana

Overview

Malaria is a parasitic infestation caused by the protozoan *Plasmodium* which is transmitted through the bite of the female *Anopheles* mosquito. The four species of *Plasmodium* responsible for malaria are *P. falciparum*, *P. vivax*, *P. ovale* and *P. malariae*. *P. falciparum* is responsible for most of the cases of malaria worldwide. It has been reported that, worldwide, there are about 350 to 500 million cases of malaria annually with one to three million deaths. Malaria in pregnancy is responsible for 5 to 12% of all low birth-weight (LBW) babies and for 35% of all preventable LBW deliveries resulting in 75,000 to 200,000 infant deaths per year. Over 90% of malaria cases occur in sub-Saharan Africa.

Clinical significance

Pregnancy results in a reduction in cell-mediated immunity. This decreased immunity makes pregnant women more susceptible to malaria than non-pregnant women. Among pregnant women it has been shown that primigravidae are at increased risk from malaria than are multigravid women. Even in places that are holoendemic for malaria, where people have an acquired immunity to malaria, pregnant women tend to have more severe episodes of malaria and are more likely to die from the complications of malaria than other adults. The presentation and effects of malaria are more severe and results in higher case fatality when the sufferer, being from an area where the disease is not common, does not have any acquired immunity. Immunocompromised people such as those suffering from human immunodeficiency virus (HIV) infection also tend to suffer more severe malaria with a higher mortality rate.

Protocols for High-Risk Pregnancies, 5th edition. Edited by J.T. Queenan, J.C. Hobbins and C.Y. Spong. © 2010 Blackwell Publishing Ltd.

Anemia in pregnancy is estimated to occur in about 56% of all pregnancies in low-income countries. Figures for Africa give a prevalence ranging from 35% in Southern Africa to 56% in West Africa. Untreated anemia leads to several complications in pregnancy and anemia-related causes play a major role in maternal mortality. Malaria in pregnancy is a major cause of anemia and this is one of the routes through which malaria causes maternal deaths.

Pathophysiology

Malaria starts with the bite of an infected female *Anopheles* mosquito. These mosquitoes usually bite between dusk and dawn. When a person is bitten by an infected mosquito the sporozoite of the *Plasmodium* parasite is introduced into the bloodstream. In the bloodstream, the sporozoites move into the hepatocytes, where they mature and develop into the hepatic schizonts. This process takes between 7 and 30 days. These schizonts then burst within the hepatocytes resulting in the release of merozoites into the circulation. The merozoites enter the red blood cells and go through another stage of development to become trophozoites within the red blood cells. The trophozoites in the red blood cells develop into erythrocytic stage schizonts which later rupture and release merozoites into the bloodstream. This erythrocytic stage of the life cycle is repeated several times resulting in the destruction of the red blood cells. Some of the trophozites later develop into the sexual form of the *Plasmodium* parasite known as gametocytes. These gametocytes are taken up by the female *Anopheles* mosquito when it bites an infected person. In the gut of the female *Anopheles* mosquito, the gametocytes develop into gametes which then fuse and develop into sporozoites. The sporozoites migrate to the salivary glands of the mosquito from where they are transmitted to an uninfected person to restart the life cycle of the parasite.

Clinical features

Infestation with *P. falciparum* initially causes a non-specific flu-like reaction. This presents as a fever, headaches and general malaise. Among people in holoendemic areas with acquired immunity, this stage of the disease might pass unnoticed. It is more severe in people without acquired immunity and in the immunocompromised resulting in mild jaundice and hepatosplenomegaly.

Malaria is characterized by febrile paroxysms which occur with the periodic release of merozoites from the red blood cells. The febrile episodes last for between 6 to 10 hours and are characterized by three stages.

There is first a cold stage which causes intense shivering. This is followed by the development of a high-grade fever which later breaks and brings on the sweating stage. After the resolution of these stages, symptoms subside for a time and then recur within 36 to 48 hours.

The repeated destruction of red blood cells during the erythrocytic stage of the life cycle results in anemia. The destruction of the red blood cells is also responsible for the jaundice that occurs during the disease. This is from the breakdown of the heme portion of the hemoglobin. There is also splenomegaly as the spleen works to remove the destroyed red blood cells from the circulation.

These clinical features are most severe in pregnant women without acquired immunity. Pregnant women with acquired immunity could be either less symptomatic or asymptomatic despite having *P. falciparum* infestation.

Pregnancy-associated malaria results in placental malaria, which occurs even when the pregnant woman is asymptomatic. In placental malaria, the *Plasmodium*-infected red blood cells accumulate in the intervillous spaces of the placenta leading to damage of the trophoblastic basement membrane. The infected red blood cells bind to receptors in the placenta and so affect oxygen and nutrient transport across the placenta. Placental malaria is responsible for the effects of malaria seen in the fetus. Placental malaria is more severe in primigravidae. Immunity to placental malaria has been shown to develop over successive pregnancies.

Diagnosis

Diagnosis of malaria in pregnancy is made by a combination of the clinical features and laboratory investigations. In holoendemic areas, there is a tendency to overdiagnose malaria because of over-reliance on symptomatology and because it is known that the complete clinical picture is rare among those with acquired immunity.

Suspicion of malaria should be followed by performing a thick or thin peripheral blood film for microscopic examination. The thick blood film is used for low parasitemias and the thin blood film for high parasitemias. The level of parasitemia as well as the species of *Plasmodium* present can be determined by microscopic examination. Microscopy is the gold standard for routine laboratory diagnosis of malaria and is very reliable when performed by a laboratory technologist with experience in malaria diagnosis.

In places where medical laboratories do not usually deal with malaria, polymerase chain reaction (PCR) procedures are more accurate for making the diagnosis even though the PCR-based diagnostic testing is more expensive and takes longer to arrive at a diagnosis. Where laboratory facilities and microscopy expertise are limited, rapid diagnostic tests which are able to determine the presence of plasmodial antigens can be used for diagnosis.

Treatment

The treatment of malaria in pregnancy is determined by the stage of pregnancy at which the disease is diagnosed.

The recommended treatment for malaria diagnosed in the first trimester is a combination of quinine and clindamycin. Quinine alone can be used if clindamycin in unavailable or unaffordable.

Malaria in the second and third trimesters is treated using artemisin-based combination therapy (ACT). The recommended forms of ACT are artemether-lumefantrine, artesunate plus amodiaquine, artesunate plus mefloquine and atesunate plus sulfadoxine-pyremethamine.

The use of ACT in the first trimester is not recommended because of limited availability of data on its effects. It is however recommended that in cases where ACT is the only available treatment it can be used in early pregnancy. In holoendemic areas ACT is recommended as the standard preferred treatment in order to improve efficacy and to limit drug resistance.

Antiemetics and analgesics which are recommended for use in pregnancy are employed to manage severe vomiting, headaches and myalgia associated with malaria in pregnancy.

Complications

Malaria has effects on both the mother as well as the fetus. Malaria can result in severe anemia leading to cardiac failure. Malaria has been known to result in acute renal failure as a result of infected red blood cells causing endothelial damage and resultant reduced blood flow to the kidneys. It also causes hypoglycemia and could lead to central nervous complications of cerebral malaria characterized by seizures and loss of consciousness. These complications of malaria could result in maternal mortality.

Malaria causes miscarriages when it occurs in the first trimester. The reduction in oxygen and nutrient delivery due to placental malaria leads to intrauterine growth restriction and intrauterine fetal death. Malaria has been shown to be a cause of low birth-weight babies because of the associated maternal anemia and the intrauterine growth restriction. Placental malaria can also lead to intrauterine infection of the fetus with malaria – congenital malaria. The febrile paroxysms due to malaria are associated with preterm labor and prematurity.

Prevention

To prevent malaria in pregnancy, the World Health Organization (WHO) recommends three interventions in holoendemic areas. The interventions are:

- intermittent preventive treatment
- use of insecticide treated nets
- effective case management of malaria and anemia.

Intermitted preventive treatment is the use of antimalarial medications at defined intervals during the pregnancy regardless of the presence or absence of confirmed malaria. The WHO recommends that all pregnant women in holoendemic areas should receive three doses of sulfadoxine-pyrimethamine at 1-month intervals after quickening. The first dose should not be administered before 16 weeks and the last dose should not be after 36 weeks.

It is recommended that pregnant women in holoendemic areas should sleep under insecticide-treated bed-nets in order to reduce the frequency of mosquito bites during pregnancy.

Effective diagnosis and treatment of malaria helps prevent the occurrence of maternal and fetal complications of malaria.

Conclusion

Malaria in pregnancy is a leading cause of maternal morbidity and mortality with as many as 10,000 maternal deaths in sub-Saharan Africa being reported due to malaria-related anemia. It is very important for both obstetricians and pregnant women to be aware of the disease so that proven methods of malaria prevention can be employed, there will be early reporting when symptoms of malaria are noticed and recommended effective therapy is employed when the diagnosis is established.

Suggested reading

Bardaji A, Sigauque B, Bruni L, Romagosa C, Sanz S, Mabunda S, *et al*. Clinical malaria in African pregnant women. *Malar J* 2008;7:27.

Brooks MI, Singh N, Hamer DH. Control measures for malaria in pregnancy in India. *Ind J Med Res* 2008;128(3):246–53.

Kabanywanyi AM, Macarthur JR, Stolk WA, Habbema JD, Mshinda H, Bloland PB, *et al*. Malaria in pregnant women in an area with sustained high coverage of insecticide-treated bed nets. *Malar J* 2008;7:133.

Lagerberg RE. Malaria in pregnancy: a literature review. *J Midwif Women's Hlth* 2008; 53(3):209–15.

Savage EJ, Msyamboza K, Gies S, D'Alessandro U, Brabin BJ. Maternal anaemia as an indicator for monitoring malaria control in pregnancy in sub-Saharan Africa. *Br J Obstet Gynaecol* 2007;114(10):1222–31.

World Health Organization. *Role of laboratory diagnosis to support malaria disease management.* Report of a WHO consultation. Geneva: World Health Organization, 2006.

World Health Organization. *The Use of Malaria Rapid Diagnostic Tests,* 2nd edn. Geneva: World Health Organization, 2006.

World Health Organization. *Guidelines for the Treatment of Malaria.* Geneva: World Health Organization, 2006.

World Health Organization. *Malaria in Pregnancy: Guidelines for measuring key monitoring and evaluation indicators.* Geneva: World Health Organization, 2007.

World Health Organization. *World Malaria Report 2008.* Geneva: World Health Organization, 2008.

Human Immunodeficiency Virus Infection in Pregnancy

Howard Minkoff

Department of Obstetrics and Gynecology, Maimonides Medical Center and State University of New York (SUNY), Brooklyn, NY, USA

Overview

The remarkable pace of antiretroviral drug development, starting in the 1990s, has transformed human immunodeficiency virus (HIV) disease from a uniquely dreaded and rapidly fatal illness to one that can be controlled for increasingly long periods of time, perhaps decades. Those advances, once accessible almost exclusively in the developed world, have now started to become available in less advantaged countries as well. The same agents that have been used to treat HIV can also prevent the overwhelming majority of pediatric HIV infections. However, maintaining women's health and preventing the mother-to-child transmission of HIV can only be assured if women's healthcare providers are comfortable and rigorous in their efforts to identify HIV-infected women, assess the status of their illness, implement appropriate drug therapy and monitor the success and toxicities that may be associated with the chosen agents.

Epidemiology

Approximately 1.2 million people in the United States are HIV-infected and over 56,000 were infected in 2006 alone. Over 500,000 Americans have died from acquired immunodeficiency syndrome (AIDS). The number of people living with HIV infection worldwide is now estimated to be over to 30 million.

In the United States, 49% of the HIV/AIDS cases diagnosed in 2005 among adults and adolescents were attributed to male-to-male sexual contact. Heterosexual contact accounted for another 32%. Worldwide, the most common mode of infection, particularly in developing countries, is

Protocols for High-Risk Pregnancies, 5th edition. Edited by J.T. Queenan, J.C. Hobbins and C.Y. Spong. © 2010 Blackwell Publishing Ltd.

clearly heterosexual transmission. Circumcision has been shown to lower the risk of transmission to men. In the United States the yearly incidence of new cases of AIDS attributed to heterosexual transmission is steadily increasing, mainly among minorities, particularly women. However, it also continues to be spread by the sharing of contaminated needles. Exposure in the healthcare setting, of the patient by the doctor or vice versa, if universal precautions are utilized, is a rare event. Transmission from mother to child may occur in the antepartum, intrapartum or, via breast milk, in the postpartum period. Perinatal transmission occurs primarily (perhaps two-thirds to three-quarters of transmissions) in the intrapartum period. If a mother breastfeeds there may be an ongoing transmission rate of 0.5% per month. Breast milk transmission occurs at the greatest rate during the first months of breastfeeding. Breast only (not mixed breast-bottle) and ongoing antiretroviral treatment of mothers may reduce rates of breast milk transmission.

Risks for transmission include:
- advanced disease (low CD4 count, high viral load, clinical illness);
- delivery after ruptured membranes, particularly if there is chorioamnionitis;
- cigarette smoking, illicit drug use and unprotected sexual intercourse with multiple partners during pregnancy may increase risk;
- preterm birth;
- vaginal delivery.

Pathophysiology

The most common cause of HIV disease throughout the world, and certainly in the United States, is HIV-1. HIV-2 was originally confined to West Africa. However, a number of cases have now been identified throughout the world. Both HIV-1 and HIV-2 are zoonotic infections, i.e., they can be transmitted to humans from other animals. A species of chimpanzee is the natural reservoir of HIV-1 while HIV-2 is more closely related to the simian immunodeficiency virus (SIV).

HIV is a single-stranded ribonucleic acid (RNA)-enveloped virus that has the ability to become incorporated into cellular deoxyribonucleic acid (DNA). HIV preferentially infects cells with the CD4 antigen, particularly helper lymphocytes and macrophages. At least two cell surface molecules, CXCR4 and CCR5, which are cytokine receptors, help HIV to enter the cells. After the virus enters the cell its RNA is released from the nucleocapsid and is reverse-transcribed into proviral DNA. The provirus is inserted into the genome and then transcribed into RNA that is translated leading to the assembly of virions that are extruded from the cell membrane by budding.

Virions have a plasma half-life of about 6 hours. In moderate to heavy HIV infection, about 10^8 to 10^9 virions are created and removed daily. The high volume of HIV replication and high frequency of transcription errors by HIV reverse transcriptase result in many mutations, increasing the chance of producing strains resistant to host immunity and drugs.

The virus is composed of core (p18, p24 and p27) and surface (gp120 outer membrane and transmembrane gp41) proteins, genomic RNA and the reverse transcriptase enzyme surrounded by a lipid bilayer envelope. The virion contains three structural genes (*gag, pol* and *env*) and a complex set of regulatory genes, including *tat, vif, nef, vpu* and *ref,* that control the rate of virion production. Each point in the replication cycle of HIV is a potential target for therapeutic intervention and the reverse transcriptase, protease and integrase enzymes as well as the process of virus–target cell binding and fusion have already been shown to be susceptible to pharmacological interventions.

At the time of initial infection, there may be no symptoms or an acute mononucleosis-like syndrome, sometimes accompanied by aseptic meningitis, may develop. There is an immediate, dramatic viremia (up to a billion viral particles turned over per day) and a rapid immune response with similar levels of T-cell turnover. After the initial viremia, the level of virus returns to a set point after about 6 months at values that vary widely but average 30,000 to 100,000/mL. The level of virus in the plasma at the time a set point is established correlates with long-term survival. The higher the set point, the more quickly the CD4 count decreases to a level that seriously impairs immunity (<200/mL) and results in the opportunistic infections (e.g., *Pneumocystis carinii* pneumonia and central nervous system toxoplasmosis) and neoplasias (e.g., Kaposi sarcoma) that define AIDS. A CD4 count drop below 200 lymphocytes/mm^3 also makes the diagnosis of AIDS. Studies in the pre-HAART era found that the incidence rate of AIDS after seroconversion was over 2.5 per 100 person-years and was directly related to age (AIDS developed in younger individuals at a slower rate). Antibodies are usually detectable 1 month after infection and are almost always detectable within 3 months.

Diagnosis and management

Early diagnosis improves prognosis. Over 40% of patients are diagnosed 'late' (when CD4 counts are less than 200 cells/µL).

Diagnosis
- Recommend the HIV test to all prenatal patients as well as gynecology patients. The American College of Obstetricians and Gynecologists and

the Centers for Disease Control recommend a policy of routine testing with an informed 'right of refusal' (opt-out testing).

- Patients should be tested at their first prenatal visit and, if from a high prevalence area or engaged in risky behaviors, should be retested later in pregnancy.
- The standard approaches to the diagnosis of HIV (ELISA and confirmatory Western blot) remain among the most reliable diagnostic tools used by obstetricians. Most turn positive 2–12 weeks after infection.
- Recently these tests have been supplemented by rapid tests, including a saliva-based test, that allow obstetricians to treat patients whose status was not known prior to the intrapartum period. These tests are reliable in ruling out infection, but must be followed by a definitive test to prove infection. Treatment to prevent transmission can begin prior to the confirmatory test.

Management
- Refer the patient to social service for case management.
- Obtain a baseline evaluation with complete blood cell count and renal and liver function testing.
- Assess the patient's immune status by determining a CD4 count at baseline and then each trimester.
- Assess HIV RNA levels at the initial visit, 2 to 6 weeks after initiating (or changing) antiretroviral therapy, monthly until RNA levels are undetectable, and then at least every 3 months thereafter.
- HIV RNA levels should also be assessed at approximately 34 to 36 weeks' gestation for decisions on mode of delivery.
- Screen for other sexually transmitted diseases, such as syphilis, gonorrhea, chlamydia, and hepatitis B, as well as hepatitis C.
- Provide appropriate vaccinations.
- Papanicolaou (Pap) smears should be performed with liberal recourse to colposcopy because of high HPV carriage and dysplasia rates.
- First trimester ultrasonography is recommended for confirmation of gestational age and potential timing for scheduled cesarean delivery, if needed.

Antiretroviral therapy
- Before starting therapy discuss:
  - the risks of these drugs during pregnancy as well as benefits both for the infected woman and for reducing the risk for HIV-1 transmission to her infant;
  - a long-term treatment plan;
  - the importance of adherence to any prescribed antiretroviral regimen;

Table 38.1 Antiretroviral drug use in pregnant HIV-infected women: pharmacokinetic and toxicity data in human pregnancy and recommendations for use in pregnancy. The reference is www.AIDSinfo.nih.giv

Antiretroviral drug	Pharmacokinetics in pregnancy	Concerns in pregnancy	Recommendations for use in pregnancy
Recommended agents			
Lamivudine	Pharmacokinetics not significantly altered in pregnancy; no change in dose indicated	No evidence of human teratogenicity. Well-tolerated, short-term safety demonstrated for mother and infant	Because of extensive experience with lamivudine in pregnancy in combination with zidovudine, lamivudine plus zidovudine is the recommended dual NRTI backbone for pregnant women
Zidovudine	Pharmacokinetics not significantly altered in pregnancy; no change in dose indicated	No evidence of human teratogenicity. Well-tolerated, short-term safety demonstrated for mother and infant	Preferred NRTI for use in combination antiretroviral regimens in pregnancy based on efficacy studies and extensive experience; should be included in the antenatal antiretroviral regimen unless there is severe toxicity, stavudine use, documented resistance, or the woman is already on a fully suppressive regimen
Alternate agents			
Abacavir	Pharmacokinetics not significantly altered in pregnancy; no change in dose indicated	No evidence of human teratogenicity. Hypersensitivity reactions occur in ~ 5%–8% of non-pregnant persons; a much smaller percentage are fatal and are usually associated with rechallenge. Rate in pregnancy unknown. Testing for HLA-B*5701 identifies patients at risk of reactions, and should be done and documented as negative before starting abacavir. Patient should be educated regarding symptoms of hypersensitivity reaction	Alternate NRTI for dual nucleoside backbone of combination regimens

(Continued)

Table 38.1 (Continued)

Antiretroviral drug	Pharmacokinetics in pregnancy	Concerns in pregnancy	Recommendations for use in pregnancy
Didanosine	Pharmacokinetics not significantly altered in pregnancy; no change in dose indicated	Cases of lactic acidosis, some fatal, have been reported in pregnant women receiving didanosine and stavudine together	Alternate NRTI for dual nucleoside backbone of combination regimens. Didanosine should be used with stavudine only if no other alternatives are available
Emtricitabine	Pharmacokinetic study shows slightly lower levels in third trimester compared to postpartum. No clear need to increase dose	No evidence of human teratogenicity	Alternate NRTI for dual nucleoside backbone of combination regimens
Stavudine	Pharmacokinetics not significantly altered in pregnancy; no change in dose indicated	No evidence of human teratogenicity. Cases of lactic acidosis, some fatal, have been reported in pregnant women receiving didanosine and stavudine together	Alternate NRTI for dual nucleoside backbone of combination regimens. Stavudine should be used with didanosine only if no other alternatives are available. Do not use with zidovudine due to potential for antagonism
Use in special circumstances			
Tenofovir	Limited studies in human pregnancy; data indicate AUC lower in third trimester than postpartum but trough levels similar. Phase I study in late pregnancy in progress	No evidence of human teratogenicity. Studies in monkeys at doses approximately 2-fold higher than that for human therapeutic use show decreased fetal growth and reduction in fetal bone porosity within 2 months of starting maternal therapy. Clinical studies in humans (particularly children) show bone demineralization with chronic use; clinical significance unknown. Significant placental passage in humans	Because of limited data on use in human pregnancy and concern regarding potential fetal bone effects, tenofovir should be used as a component of a maternal combination regimen only after careful consideration of other alternatives. Because of potential for renal toxicity, renal function should be monitored

NNRTIs

Recommended agents

Nevirapine	Pharmacokinetics not significantly altered in pregnancy; no change in dose indicated	No evidence of human teratogenicity. Increased risk of symptomatic, often rash-associated, and potentially fatal liver toxicity among women with CD4 counts >250/mm³ when first initiating therapy; unclear if pregnancy increases risk	Nevirapine should be initiated in pregnant women with CD4 counts >250 cells/mm³ only if benefit clearly outweighs risk, due to the increased risk of potentially life-threatening hepatotoxicity in women with high CD4 counts. Women who enter pregnancy on nevirapine regimens and are tolerating them well may continue therapy, regardless of CD4 count

Use in special circumstances

Efavirenz	In small study of 600 mg once daily, third trimester peak levels were 61% higher than in non-pregnant individuals	FDA Pregnancy Class D; significant malformations (anencephaly, anophthalmia, cleft palate) were observed in 3 (15%) of 20 infants born to cynomolgus monkeys receiving efavirenz during the first trimester at a dose giving plasma levels comparable to systemic human therapeutic exposure; there are 5 retrospective case reports and 1 prospective case report of neural tube defects in humans with first trimester exposure	Use of efavirenz should be avoided in the first trimester. Use after the first trimester can be considered if, after consideration of other alternatives, this is the best choice for a specific woman. If efavirenz is to be continued postpartum, adequate contraception must be assured. Women of childbearing potential must be counseled regarding risks and avoidance of pregnancy. Because of the known failure rates of contraception, alternate regimens should be strongly considered in women of childbearing potential

Insufficient data to recommend use

Etravirine	No pharmacokinetic studies in human pregnancy	No experience in human pregnancy	Safety and pharmacokinetics in pregnancy data are insufficient to recommend use during pregnancy

(Continued)

Table 38.1 (Continued)

Antiretroviral drug	Pharmacokinetics in pregnancy	Concerns in pregnancy	Recommendations for use in pregnancy
Protease inhibitors			
Recommended agents			
Lopinavir/ritonavir	Pharmacokinetic studies of the new lopinavir/ritonavir tablet formulation are under way, but data are not yet available	No evidence of human teratogenicity. Well-tolerated, short-term safety demonstrated in phase I/II studies	Some experts would administer standard dosing (2 tablets twice daily) throughout pregnancy and monitor virologic response and lopinavir drug levels, if available. Other experts, extrapolating from the capsule formulation pharmacokinetic data, would increase the dose of the tablet formulation during the third trimester (from 2 tablets to 3 tablets twice daily), returning to standard dosing postpartum. Once daily lopinavir/ritonavir dosing is not recommended during pregnancy because there are no data to address whether drug levels are adequate with such administration
Alternate agents			
Atazanavir (recommended to be combined with low-dose ritonavir boosting)	Two of three intensive pharmacokinetic studies of atazanavir with ritonavir boosting during pregnancy suggest that standard dosing results in decreased plasma concentrations compared to non-pregnant adults. Atazanavir concentrations further reduced ~25% with concomitant tenofovir use	No evidence of human teratogenicity. Transplacental passage is low. Theoretical concern re: increased indirect bilirubin levels exacerbating physiologic hyperbilirubinemia in the neonate not observed in clinical trials to date.	Alternative PI for use in combination regimens in pregnancy. Should give as low-dose ritonavir-boosted regimen, may use once daily dosing. In naïve patients unable to tolerate ritonavir, 400 mg once daily dosing without ritonavir boosting may be considered, although there are no data describing atazanavir concentrations or efficacy under these circumstances. If coadministered with tenofovir, atazanavir must be given with low-dose ritonavir boosting

Indinavir (combined with low-dose ritonavir boosting)	Two studies of women receiving indinavir 800 mg three times daily showed markedly lower levels during pregnancy compared to postpartum, although suppression of HIV RNA was seen. In a study of ritonavir-boosted indinavir (400 mg indinavir/100 mg ritonavir twice daily), 82% of women met the target trough level	No evidence of human teratogenicity. Theoretical concern re: increased indirect bilirubin levels, which may exacerbate physiological hyperbilirubinemia in the neonate, but minimal placental passage. Use of unboosted indinavir during pregnancy is not recommended	Alternate PI for use in combination regimens in pregnancy. Must give as low-dose ritonavir-boosted regimen
Nelfinavir	Adequate drug levels are achieved in pregnant women with nelfinavir 1250 mg, given twice daily although levels are variable in late pregnancy. In a similar study of pregnant women in their second and third trimester dosed at 1250 mg given twice daily, women in the third trimester had lower concentration of nelfinavir than women in their second trimester	No evidence of human teratogenicity. Well-tolerated, short-term safety demonstrated for mother and infant	Given pharmacokinetic data and extensive experience with use in pregnancy, nelfinavir is an alternative PI for combination regimens in pregnant women receiving HAART only for perinatal prophylaxis. In clinical trials of initial therapy in non-pregnant adults, nelfinavir-based regimens had a lower rate of viral response compared to lopinavir-ritonavir or efavirenz-based regimens, but similar viral response to atazanavir or nevirapine-based regimens
Ritonavir	Phase I/II study in pregnancy showed lower levels during pregnancy compared to postpartum	Limited experience at full dose in human pregnancy; has been used as low-dose ritonavir boosting with other PIs	Given low levels in pregnant women when used alone, recommended for use in combination with second PI as low-dose ritonavir 'boost' to increase levels of second PI
Saquinavir-hard gel capsule [HGC] (Invirase®) (combined with low-dose ritonavir boosting)	Limited pharmacokinetic data on saquinavir-hard gel capsule (HGC), and the new 500 mg tablet formulation, suggest that 1000 mg saquinavir-HGC/100 mg ritonavir given twice daily achieves adequate saquinavir drug levels in pregnant women	Well-tolerated, short-term safety demonstrated for mother and infant for saquinavir in combination with low-dose ritonavir	There are only limited pharmacokinetic data on saquinavir-HGC and the new tablet formulation in pregnancy. Ritonavir-boosted saquinavir-HGC or saquinavir tablets are alternative PIs for combination regimens in pregnancy, and are alternative initial antiretroviral recommendations for non-pregnant adults. Must give as low-dose ritonavir-boosted regimen

(Continued)

Table 38.1 (Continued)

Antiretroviral drug	Pharmacokinetics in pregnancy	Concerns in pregnancy	Recommendations for use in pregnancy
Insufficient data to recommend use			
Darunavir (combined with low-dose ritonavir boosting)	No pharmacokinetic studies in human pregnancy	No experience in human pregnancy	Safety and pharmacokinetics in pregnancy data are insufficient to recommend use during pregnancy. Must give as low-dose ritonavir-boosted regimen
Fosamprenavir (recommended to be combined with low-dose ritonavir boosting)	No pharmacokinetic studies in human pregnancy	Limited experience in human pregnancy	Safety and pharmacokinetics in pregnancy data are insufficient to recommend use during pregnancy. Recommended to be given as low-dose ritonavir-boosted regimen
Tipranavir (combined with low-dose ritonavir boosting)	No pharmacokinetic studies in human pregnancy	No experience in human pregnancy	Safety and pharmacokinetics in pregnancy data are insufficient to recommend use during pregnancy. Must give as low-dose ritonavir-boosted regimen
Entry inhibitors			
Insufficient data to recommend use			
Enfuvirtide	No pharmacokinetic studies in human pregnancy	Minimal data in human pregnancy	Safety and pharmacokinetics in pregnancy data are insufficient to recommend use during pregnancy
Maraviroc	No pharmacokinetic studies in human pregnancy	No experience in human pregnancy	Safety and pharmacokinetics in pregnancy data are insufficient to recommend use during pregnancy
Integrase inhibitors			
Insufficient data to recommend use			
Raltegravir	No pharmacokinetic studies in human pregnancy	No experience in human pregnancy	Safety and pharmacokinetics in pregnancy data are insufficient to recommend use during pregnancy

- availability of support services, mental health services and drug abuse treatment that may be required.
- To reduce the potential for emergence of resistance, if therapy requires temporary discontinuation for any reason during pregnancy, all drugs should be stopped and reintroduced simultaneously. Similarly women who must temporarily discontinue therapy because of pregnancy-related hyperemesis should not resume therapy until sufficient time has elapsed to ensure that the drugs will be tolerated.
- In considering treatment, the first consideration is the treatment of maternal disease.
- If on therapy before pregnancy, continue the antiretroviral treatment regimen if it is effective in suppressing viral replication; however, avoid use of EFV in the first trimester of pregnancy.
- If not yet on therapy, apply non-obstetrical standards for starting HAART, i.e., start if the CD4 count drops to 350/μL. If above that level consider therapy if there is active hepatitis B needing treatment or HIV-associated nephropathy. Many experts are now recommending starting therapy sooner, at CD4 counts of 350/μl–500/μl, and some at even higher levels.
- If a woman doesn't reach traditional criteria for starting HAART (noted above) but has a detectable viral load (some providers use a threshold of greater than 1000 copies), there is still a role for HAART during pregnancy in order to decrease transmission and reduce the need for cesarean delivery.
  - Women who are in the first trimester of pregnancy may consider delaying initiation of therapy until after 10–12 weeks' gestation. However if a woman needs immediate initiation of therapy drug for her own health there should be no delay.
- HAART is any regimen that results in maximal and durable reduction in viral load.
  - Commonly used regimens consist of two nucleoside reverse transcriptase inhibitors (including ZDV) and either a protease inhibitor (ritonovir boosted) or a non-nucleoside reverse transcriptase inhibitor.
  - In pregnancy include ZDV when feasible.
  - First regimens should be 'class sparing,' i.e., should not use both non-nucleosides and protease inhibitors.
- Results of therapy are evaluated through plasma HIV RNA levels.
  - Expected to indicate a 1.0 $\log_{10}$ decrease at 2–8 weeks and no detectable virus (<50 copies/mL) at 4–6 months after.
  - Failure of therapy at 4–6 months might be ascribed to non-adherence, inadequate potency of drugs or suboptimal levels of antiretroviral agents, viral resistance, and other factors that are poorly understood.
  - Patients whose therapy fails in spite of a high level of adherence to the regimen should have their regimen changed; this change should

be guided by a thorough drug treatment history and the results of drug resistance testing in collaboration with an HIV expert.
- If no detectable virus is found (some providers would use a threshold of 1000 copies of virus) the ACTG 076 regimen alone can be used:
  - 300 mg two times a day (or 200 mg three times a day), beginning at 14 weeks, given until labor;
  - Intrapartum: loading – 2 mg/kg over the first hour; maintenance – 1 mg/kg/hr until delivery;
  - Neonatal: oral ZDV syrup, 2 mg/kg orally four times a day for 6 weeks per protocol supervised by pediatricians;
  - Monitoring: complete blood count (CBC) every 2 weeks two times; then every month; liver function test each month; creatinine each month.

For a woman not treated prior to labor
- Intrapartum intravenous ZDV followed by 6 weeks of ZDV for the newborn is recommended.
- Some experts would combine this with single-dose intrapartum/newborn nevirapine.
- If using nevirapine note that since data raises concerns about failure rates of single doses of nevirapine, if it is given (alone or in combination with ZDV), consideration should be given to adding 3TC during labor and maternal ZDV/3TC for 7 days postpartum, which may reduce development of NVP resistance in the woman.
- In the immediate postpartum period, the woman should have appropriate assessments (e.g., CD4+ count and HIV-1 RNA copy number) to determine whether antiretroviral therapy is recommended for her own health.

Resistance testing
- Recommended for all pregnant women not currently receiving antiretrovirals, before starting treatment or prophylaxis.
  - For optimal prevention of perinatal transmission, empiric initiation of antiretroviral therapy before results of resistance testing are available may be warranted, with adjustment as needed after the results are available.
- Additional recommendations are the same as for resistance testing of all other individuals:
  - Failing regimen, suboptimal suppression, high likelihood of exposure to resistant strain based on community prevalence of knowledge of source.
- Obtain blood *before* switching from a failing regimen.
- Resistance testing is useful to rule a drug out, but cannot guarantee success of a new regimen.

Risks from drug exposure in pregnancy

- Nevirapine (Viramune): should be used with caution in pregnant women with CD4+ lymphocyte counts >250/mm^3 who are starting combination therapy for preventing perinatal transmission but do not require therapy for own health. There is a significant risk of rash and hepatotoxicity. If used, monitor closely for liver toxicity in first 18 weeks of therapy. Women who enter pregnancy on nevirapine regimens and are tolerating well may continue therapy, regardless of CD4+ lymphocyte count.
- Efavirenz (Sustiva): animal teratogenicity studies reveal anencephaly, anophthalmia, microophthalmia in the cynomolgus monkey.
- Some studies suggest a heightened risk of preterm birth or low birth weight associated with HAART, but many other studies do not.
- Mitochondrial toxicity: pregnant women receiving nucleoside analog drugs should have hepatic enzymes and electrolytes assessed more frequently during the last trimester of pregnancy, and any new symptoms should be evaluated thoroughly.
  - The combination of ddI and d4T should be avoided because of reports of several maternal deaths secondary to lactic acidosis with prolonged use.
- Diabetes: new-onset hyperglycemia has been reported in association with protease inhibitors.
- Tenofovir: has been associated with osteomalacia.
- Abacavir: use HLA-B*5701 screening to identify patients at risk of abacavir-associated hypersensitivity reaction.

Prophylaxis for opportunistic infections

Pneumocystis carinii pneumonia

- Offered to women with CD4+ lymphocyte counts below 200/μL, unexplained fever (greater than 100°F) for 2 weeks or more, or a history of oropharyngeal candidiasis.
- Prophylaxis may be discontinued for women on highly active antiretroviral therapy with sustained elevations in their CD4+ lymphocyte count above 200/μL.
- Trimethoprim-sulfamethoxazole (TMP-SMZ) one double-strength tablet daily, is the first choice for prophylaxis in pregnancy. Alternatives include Atovaquone 1500 mg po daily or oral dapsone 100 mg daily. Atovaquone, a class C drug, should only be given during pregnancy when benefit outweighs risk.

Mycobacterium avium complex

- Prophylaxis for CD4 lymphocyte counts less than 50/μL or previous documented MAC infection.
- Azithromycin, 1200 mg once weekly, is first choice for therapy. Clarithromycin should be avoided in pregnancy because of teratogenicity in animals.

Toxoplasma

- TMP-SMZ will also provide prophylaxis against toxoplasma encephalitis in women who are seropositive for antibodies to *Toxoplasma gondii.*
- For women with previous toxoplasma encephalitis, an appropriate prophylaxis regimen should be offered throughout pregnancy.

Obstetrical management

- Cesarean delivery will lower transmission if virus is detectable.
  - Evidence unclear regarding any benefit when viral load is less than 1000 copies.
  - Procedure is performed at 38 weeks with no amniocentesis for lung maturity.
  - Use prophylactic antibiotics.
- If patient is allowed to labor, avoid scalp electrodes and scalp pH if possible.
- Delay amniotomy. Some data suggest a relationship between the duration of ruptured membranes and the vertical transmission rate of HIV.
- Universal precautions.
- Counsel against breastfeeding.

Conclusions

This protocol provides a very brief summary of a very complex topic. There are now more than 20 approved antiretroviral agents from which to craft drug regimens. The choice of regimen and the starting point for initiating therapy should be tailored to the individual patient's needs and should be decided upon in collaboration with an HIV expert who will assume the ongoing care of the patient in the postpartum period. That same expert should be called upon to provide guidance in those cases in which adequate response to a first course of therapy is not obtained or the need for prophylaxis or treatment of opportunistic infections arises. Obstetricians have made a remarkable contribution to the rapid advances in the field of HIV, including improved survival and reduced rates of mother-to-child transmission. However, challenges remain and the price of progress has been complexity. By assisting women to learn their serostatus, to get optimal therapy and to be adherent to treatment, obstetricians will continue to earn their reputation as the principal advocates for the health of all pregnant women.

Suggested reading

American College of Obstetricians and Gynecologists. Scheduled Cesarean delivery and the prevention of vertical transmission of HIV infection. Committee Opinion # 234, May 2000 (replaces # 219, August 1999). *Int J Gynaecol Obstet* 2001;73(3):279–81.

American College of Obstetricians and Gynecologists. *Human Immunodeficiency Virus Infection.* Technical Bulletin (revised). 1992;162:1–11.

Centers for Disease Control and Prevention. Rapid HIV-1 antibody testing during labor and delivery for women of unknown HIV status: a practical guide and model protocol. 2004. (www.cdc.gov/hiv/topics/testing/resources/guidelines/pdf/Labor&Delivery RapidTesting.pdf)

Connor EM, Sperling RS, Gelber R, *et al.* Reduction of maternal-infant transmission of human immunodeficiency virus type 1 with zidovudine treatment. *N Engl J Med* 1994;331(18):1173–80.

Cooper ER, Charurat M, Mofenson L, *et al.* Combination antiretroviral strategies for the treatment of pregnant HIV-1 infected women and prevention of perinatal HIV-1 transmission. *J Acquir Immune Defic Syndr Hum Retrovirol* 2002;29(5):484–94.

Culnane M, Fowler MG, Lee SS, *et al.* Lack of long-term effects of *in utero* exposure to zidovudine among uninfected children born to HIV-infected women. *JAMA* 1999;281(2):151–7.

Fauci AS, Lane HC. Protocol 182. Human immunodeficiency virus disease: aids and related disorders. In: *Harrison's Principles of Internal Medicine*, 17th edn. New York, London: McGraw-Hill, 2008.

Garcia PM, Kalish LA, Pitt J, *et al.* Maternal levels of plasma human immunodeficiency virus type 1 RNA and the risk of perinatal transmission. *N Engl J Med* 1999;341(6):394–402.

Guay LA, Musoke P, Fleming T, *et al.* Intrapartum and neonatal single-dose nevirapine compared with zidovudine for prevention of mother-to-child transmission of HIV-1 in Kampala, Uganda: HIVNET 012 randomised trial. *Lancet* 1999;354(9181):795–802.

Hammer SM, Enron JJ, Reiss P, Schooley RT, Thompson MA, Cahn P, *et al.* Antiretroviral treatment of adult HIV infection: 2008 Recommendations of the International AIDS Society–USA Panel. *JAMA* 2008;300(5):555–70.

International Perinatal HIV Group. The mode of delivery and the risk of vertical transmission of human immunodeficiency virus type 1: a meta-analysis of 15 prospective cohort studies. *N Engl J Med* 1999;340(13):977–87.

Ioannidis JPA, Abrams EJ, Ammann A, *et al.* Perinatal transmission of human immunodeficiency virus type 1 by pregnant women with RNA virus loads <1000 copies/mL. *J Infect Dis* 2001;183(4):539–45.

Mandelbrot L, Jasseron C, Ekoukou D, Batallan A, Bongain A, Pannier E, Blanche S, Tubiana R, Rouzioux C, Warszawski J; ANRS French Perinatal Cohort (EPF). Amniocentesis and mother-to-child human immunodeficiency virus transmission in the Agence Nationale de Recherches sur le SIDA et les Hépatites Virales French Perinatal Cohort. *Am J Obstet Gynecol* 2009;200(2):160.e1–9. Epub 2008 Nov 4.

Masur H, Kaplan JE. New guidelines for the management of HIV-related opportunistic infections. *JAMA* 2009;301:2378–80.

Tai JH, Udoji MA, Barkanic G, Byrne DW, Rebeiro PF, *et al.* Pregnancy and HIV disease progression during the era of highly active antiretroviral therapy. *J Infect Dis* 2007;196:1044–52.

Tuomala RE, Shapiro D, Mofenson LM, *et al.* Antiretroviral therapy during pregnancy and the risk of adverse outcome. *N Engl J Med* 2002;346:1863–70.

Wade NA, Birkhead GS, Warren BL, *et al.* Abbreviated regimens of zidovudine prophylaxis and perinatal transmission of the human immunodeficiency virus. *N Engl J Med* 1998;339(20):1409–14.

www.aidsinfo.nih.gov

Parvovirus B19 Infection

Maureen P. Malee

Division of Maternal-Fetal Medicine, Bryan LGH Medical Center, Lincoln, NE, USA

Overview

The spectrum of clinical manifestations caused by parvovirus B19 infection, a single-stranded DNA virus, is unlikely completely described. In the normal host, B19 infection can be manifest as an asymptomatic or subclinical infection, erythema infectiosum (EI) or fifth disease, or as an arthropathy. In patients with thalassemia or sickle cell disease, B19 infection can cause a severe transient red cell aplasia (transient aplastic crisis; TAC). In the immunocompromised population, B19 infection can persist and manifest as chronic anemia. In the fetus, B19 infection is associated with anemia, non-immune hydrops and death.

Pathophysiology

The rash of EI and B19 arthralgias are thought to be secondary to an immunological phenomenon. The hematological manifestations of B19 infection result from selective infection and lysis of erythroid precursor cells with interruption of normal red blood cell production. In the otherwise healthy but infected host, this infection produces a limited and clinically unapparent red cell aplasia. However, in the patient with chronic red cell destruction, dependent upon the ability to increase red blood cell production, B19 infection may lead to aplastic crisis.

The pathogenesis of fetal and congenital disease is fairly well understood. Infection of the fetus occurs through transplacental passage of the virus. The red cell aplasia is particularly devastating for the fetus, given the dramatic increase in red cell mass necessary to promote accelerated growth, as well as the shortened life span of the fetal red cell. Transient pleural or pericardial effusions may reflect direct pleural or myocardial

Protocols for High-Risk Pregnancies, 5th edition. Edited by J.T. Queenan, J.C. Hobbins and C.Y. Spong. © 2010 Blackwell Publishing Ltd.

inflammation. The pathogenic mechanism of hydrops is associated with severe fetal anemia, which may result in tissue hypoxia and increased capillary permeability, as well as increased cardiac output and increased umbilical venous pressure. High output cardiac failure results, is associated with increased hydrostatic pressure and decreased venous return, and as a result of ascites and/or organomegaly, leads to further cardiac decompensation. Compromised hepatic function and placental hydrops likely play a role as well.

Epidemiology

B19 is presumably transmitted person-to-person through direct contact with respiratory secretions, vertically from mother to fetus, and via transfusion with contaminated blood products or needles.

Cases of EI occur sporadically and as part of school outbreaks. The peak incidence of B19 infection occurs among school-aged children, with reported attack rates amongst susceptible students between 34 and 72%. Patients with EI are likely most contagious before the onset of the rash, and may remain contagious for a few days after appearance of the rash. During school outbreaks, reported attack rates amongst employees vary from 12% to 84%, with the highest rates in elementary school teachers, reflecting exposure to greater numbers of children or a greater likelihood of contacting respiratory secretions of younger children. When serological criteria are used, the frequency of asymptomatic infection was greater than 50% in most studies. Healthcare workers are another susceptible population, with over 30% demonstrating seroconversion following exposure to children with TAC.

Diagnosis

Seroprevalence
The seroprevalence of specific IgG antibodies increases with age, and is below 5% in those less than 5 years of age. The greatest increase in seroprevalence occurs between 5 and 20 years of age, increasing from 5% to 40%. Seroprevalence then increases more slowly, exceeding 75% by 50 years of age.

Specific IgM antibodies can be detected 10 days after inoculation, and IgG is detectable 2–3 days thereafter. Rash/arthropathy may develop about 18 days after inoculation. IgM antibodies persist typically for months, and IgG antibodies persist for years. Antibodies are detected by enzyme-linked immunoabsorbent assay (ELISA) or radioimmunoassay (RIA) and viral DNA by polymerase chain reaction.

An individual is susceptible in the absence of documented IgM and IgG. The presence of only IgG denotes an immune individual, who may have been infected as recently as 4 months previously. The presence of only IgM denotes a very recent infection, whereas the presence of both IgM and IgG is typical of a patient with recent (typically 7 days to 4 months) exposure.

Fifth disease

The most frequently recognized manifestation of B19 infection is the rash illness, EI. The most distinctive feature of EI, or slapped cheek disease, is an erythematous maculopapular rash that affects the cheeks and typically spares the remainder of the face. The trunk and extremities are also affected, and the rash may be pruritic. The rash occurs coincidentally with the production of specific antibodies, suggesting that it is an immune-mediated phenomenon.

Arthralgias, sometimes accompanied by inflammatory changes in affected joints, are a manifestation of acute B19 infection and can accompany EI, particularly in adults. Arthropathy, most often affecting wrists, hands and knees, can also be the sole manifestation of B19 infection. As with the rash, onset of arthropathy is accompanied by a rise in anti-B19 antibodies, suggesting an immunological phenomenon.

Fifth disease and pregnancy
Sequelae

Many pregnant women are susceptible to B19 infection, as the reported seroprevalence in reproductive-aged and pregnant women is between 35% and 55%. The infection rate during pregnancy is estimated at 1.1%. Transplacental transmission of B19 to the fetus may be common after maternal infection, but the frequency with which infection occurs is uncertain, and whether efficiency of transmission varies with gestational age is unknown. Many infants infected in utero are asymptomatic at birth.

Adverse pregnancy outcomes following B19 infection include non-immune hydrops and fetal death. It is difficult to say with certainty the proportion of all deaths attributable to B19 infection. At present, it appears that the primary mechanism leading to fetal death is anemia and hydrops, in those gestations before 20 weeks, with demise usually in the second trimester. The crude fetal death rate is less than 10%. In the United States, it is likely that less than 1% of all demises result from B19 infection. Although infection with B19 may be a common cause of non-immune hydrops especially during community outbreaks of EI, it does not follow that intrauterine B19 infection frequently causes hydrops. The most common outcome is normal seronegative newborns, followed by liveborn seropositive babies and finally hydrops in less than 1%. Although there are case reports which support a link between B19 infection and congenital malformations, the relationship is not supported by epidemiological studies.

Management

Our knowledge of optimal management of B19 infection in pregnancy lags behind our understanding of the potential adverse consequences. As a result, there are considerable resources devoted to the pregnancy with this diagnosis, even though there are little data demonstrating efficacy of any particular therapeutic approach or intervention.

In the event that a pregnant patient presents with complaints potentially consistent with B19 infection, such as arthralgias, exposure to someone with EI, hydropic changes or a death on ultrsonography, for example, maternal blood should be sent for determination of anti-B19 IgM and IgG antibodies to determine immunity or risk. In the event of a school outbreak of EI, the decision to limit presumptive exposure of a pregnant schoolteacher should be individualized, as the risk of that teacher becoming infected and suffering a fetal demise is less than 1.5%. Intrauterine B19 infection can be determined by polymerase chain reaction DNA detection of viral B19 in amniotic fluid or fetal blood. An amniocentesis is the method of choice for fetal diagnosis, as cordocentesis carries a 1% loss rate.

There are no studies to identify the optimal management of a pregnant patient with an acute B19 infection. As the spectrum of fetal response is no effect vs hydrops vs demise, and the only treatment for hydropic changes is transfusion, which cannot be accomplished before 20 weeks, many question the utility of serial surveillance before 20 weeks. Serial ultrasonography is often advocated when infection is thought to have occurred before 20 weeks, as the peak in fetal morbidity and mortality is 4–6 weeks post-exposure, and as late as 3 months following onset of symptoms. However, the yield of such intensive observation is low. Serial determinations of fetal middle cerebral artery (MCA) Doppler velocimetry for detection of anemia has utility in the management of a B19-infected fetus, as increasing anemia may precede hydropic changes. If the MCA doppler peak systolic velocity (PSV) (done after 18 weeks) is greater than 1.5 MOMs for gestational age, a periumbilical blood sampling (PUBs) can be offered to determine the fetal hematocrit, would be the suggested plan for the overtly hydropic fetus. If anemia is detected, a transfusion to replace half of the RBC volume is accomplished during the same procedure, and the remainder in the next 48 hours. This strategy can be followed until the fetus recovers from the infection. However, this intervention is not without its own inherent risk of fetal morbidity and mortality (1% fetal loss). Two retrospective series demonstrate that transfusion confers a survival advantage to fetuses with B19-associated hydrops. There are no B19 vaccines for B19 immunization available at this time, and the role of hyperimmune serum globulin in the prevention or modification of B19 infection is unclear.

Summary

Intrauterine B19 infection is a cause of fetal anemia, hydrops and death, but unlikely of congenital anomalies. The best strategy for surveillance of the infected pregnant patient is unclear, as are strategies to decrease infection rate and untoward outcomes.

Suggested reading

Adler SP, Manganelio AA, Koch WC, *et al*. Risk of human parvovirus B19 infections among school and hospital employees during endemic periods. *J Infect Dis* 1993;168:361.

Al-Khan A, Caligiuri A, Apuzzio J. Parvovirus B19 infection during pregnancy. *Inf Dis Obstet Gynecol* 2003;11:175–9.

American College of Obstetricians and Gynecologists. Perinatal viral and parasitic infections. ACOG Practice Bulletin, # 20, 2000.

Centers for Disease Control. Risks associated with human parvovirus B19 infection. *MMWR* 1989;38:81–8.

Cosmi E, Mari G, Chiaie LD, Detti L, *et al*. Noninvasive diagnosis by Doppler ultrasonography of fetal anemia resulting from parvovirus infection. *Am J Obstet Gynecol* 2002;187:1290–3.

Crane J. Parvovirus B19 infection in pregnancy. *J Obstet Gynecol Can* 2002;24:727–43.

Dembinski J, Haverkamp F, Maara H, Hansmann M, Eis-Hubinger AM, Bartmann P. Neurodevelopmental outcome after intrauterine red cell transfusion for parvovirus B-19-induced fetal hydrops. *Br J Obstet Gynecol* 2002;109:1232–4.

Divakaran TG, Waugh J, Clark, TJ, Khan KS, Whittle MJ, Kilby MD. Noninvasive techniques to detect fetal anemia due to red blood cell alloimmunization: a systematic review. *Obstet Gynecol* 2001;98:509–17.

Goldenberg RL, Thompson C. The infectious origins of stillbirth. *Am J Obstet Gynecol* 2003;189:861–73.

Harger JH, Adler SP, Koch WC, Harger GF. Prospective evaluation of 618 pregnant women exposed to parvovirus B19: risks and symptoms. *Obstet Gynecol* 1998; 91:413–20.

Hernandez-Andrade E, Scheier M, Dezerega V, Carmo A, Nicolaides KH. Fetal middle cerebral artery peak systolic velocity in the investigation of nonimmune hydrops. *Ultrasound Obstet Gynecol* 2004;23:442–5.

Kinney J, Anderson L, Farrar J, *et al.* Risk of adverse outcomes of pregnancy after human parvovirus B19 infection. *J Infect Dis* 1988;157:663.

Miller E, Fairley CK, Cohen BJ, Seng C. Immediate and long-term outcome of human parvovirus B19 infection in pregnancy. *Br J Obstet Gynecol* 1998;105:174–8.

Parilla BV, Tamura RK, Ginsberg NA. Association of parvovirus infection with isolated fetal effusions. *Am J Perinatol* 1997;14:357.

Pickering LK, Reves RR. Occupational risks for chil-care providers and teachers. *JAMA* 1990;263:2096.

Tolfvenstam T, Papadogiannakis N, Norbeck O, Petersson K, Broliden K. Frequency of human parvovirus B19 infection in intrauterine fetal death. *Lancet* 2001;357:1494–7.

Torok TJ. Human Parvovirus B19. In: Remington JS, Klein JO (eds) *Infectious Diseases of the Fetus and Newborn Infant.* Philadelphia: Saunders, 2001; pp. 770–811.

Group B Streptococcus

Mara J. Dinsmoor

Department of Obstetrics and Gynecology, NorthShore University Health System, Evanston, IL
and Department of Obstetrics and Gynecology, Pritzker School of Medicine, University of Chicago,
Chicago, IL, USA

Clinical significance

Between 10 and 30% of pregnant women are colonized with group B
streptococcus (GBS), formally known as *Streptococcus agalactiae*. Colonization
may result in symptomatic infection in some women, most commonly
manifested as chorioamnionitis, postpartum endometritis, or urinary tract
infections. Intrapartum and postpartum bacteremia may also occur in
the face of maternal infection. Neonates may be colonized and develop
symptomatic infections via transmission from the mother or by contact
transmission in the nursery. These neonatal infections, including localized
infections, meningitis, or septicemia, carry a high risk of sequelae and are
potentially fatal.

Pathophysiology

Carriage of GBS may be intermittent, and risk factors for maternal GBS
colonization have been inconsistent in prior reports, although African-
American women and non-smokers appear to be at higher risk. However,
risk factors for transmission to, and subsequent infection of, the neonate
are well characterized. They include prematurity (<37 weeks' gestation),
prolonged membrane rupture (>18 hours), and fever in labor (>100.5°F).
The increased risk with prematurity is thought to be a result of incomplete GBS antibody transfer across the immature placenta. The latter two
risk factors are probably related to prolonged contact with the organism and increased colony counts in the presence of infection. Having a
prior infected neonate is also a risk factor for having subsequent infected

Protocols for High-Risk Pregnancies, 5th edition. Edited by J.T. Queenan, J.C. Hobbins and
C.Y. Spong. © 2010 Blackwell Publishing Ltd.

Table 40.1 Rate of early-onset neonatal group B streptococcus sepsis in the presence of maternal colonization and/or risk factors (prematurity, prolonged membrane rupture, fever in labor)

Maternal colonization	Risk factor(s)	Rate per 1000 births
Present	Present	40.8
Present	Absent	5.1
Absent	Present	0.9
Absent	Absent	0.3

Adapted from Boyer and Gotoff, 1985.

babies. Overall, the risk of neonatal colonization following delivery to a colonized mother, in the absence of treatment, is approximately 50%. Up to 2% of these infants will develop symptomatic disease, so that the overall risk of neonatal disease following delivery to a colonized mother is less than 10 per 1000 exposed births, and is as low as 1–2 per thousand in term neonates (Table 40.1).

There are five major serotypes of GBS (Ia, Ib, II, III and V), and all appear capable of causing both maternal and neonatal disease. Serotype III is found in most cases of late-onset disease. Babies born to mothers who do not have antibodies to types II and III GBS appear to be at increased risk for developing GBS disease. Because of its predominance in neonatal infections, efforts at creating an effective vaccine have focused on serotype III.

Diagnosis

The most accurate mode of diagnosis of GBS is by means of a culture. Although GBS will grow on ordinary blood agar, use of selective media will increase the detection of GBS by about 50%. For this reason, it is currently recommended that all GBS cultures be performed on sheep blood agar following incubation in selective broth medium. Examples include Todd-Hewitt broth supplemented with antibiotics and the commercially available medium, Trans-Vag broth, supplemented with 5% defibrinated sheep blood or LIM broth.

Most GBS cultures are done in the setting of late pregnancy (35–37 weeks), in an attempt to identify colonized women, so that they may be offered intrapartum antibiotic prophylaxis. The highest yield is obtained when the culture is obtained from the distal vagina and the rectum. Swabbing only the cervix or vaginal fornix will fail to detect approximately 50% of colonized women. To guide intrapartum therapy, antibiotic susceptibility testing should be performed on all isolates from penicillin-allergic women. GBS is also frequently isolated from amniotic fluid cultures obtained during the evaluation of patients with suspected subclinical or clinical intraamniotic infection.

In the postpartum period, GBS is commonly found in endometrial cultures from patients with postpartum endometritis. Some patients with uterine infections with GBS will also have bacteremia with the same organism. GBS rarely causes endocarditis in immunocompetent patients, but there have been case reports of endocarditis due to GBS.

Although a number of rapid tests for the detection of GBS have been evaluated, none have proven adequately sensitive for clinical use. A new polymerase chain reaction (PCR)-based test is currently under review, but is not widely available and is prohibitively expensive even in those institutions with PCR technology available.

Treatment

The recommended treatment regimens for intrapartum GBS prophylaxis are outlined in Table 40.2.

The treatment of clinically evident GBS infection depends somewhat on the clinical context in which it is identified. Appropriate antibiotic choices include penicillin, ampicillin and first-generation cephalosporins. Because there has been increasing resistance of GBS strains to clindamycin and erythromycin, treatment of the penicillin-allergic patient should be based, if at all possible, on the results of sensitivity testing of the

Table 40.2 Recommended regimens for intrapartum antibiotic prophylaxis* (adapted from the CDC, *MWWR*, 2002)

Recommended	Penicillin G: 5 million units IV followed by 2.5 million units IV q 4 h
Alternative	Ampicillin: 2 g IV followed by 1 g IV q 4 h
Penicillin allergy: not high risk for anaphylaxis	Cefazolin: 2 g IV followed by 1 g IV q 8 h
Penicillin allergy: high risk for anaphylaxis[†]	Clindamycin: 900 mg IV q 8 h OR erythromycin 500 mg IV q 6 h
Penicillin allergy: GBS resistant to clindamycin or erythromycin, or sensitivities unknown	Vancomycin: 1 g IV q 12 h

*All antibiotics to be discontinued following delivery, in the absence of the clinical diagnosis of maternal infection.

[†]History of immediate hypersensitivity or history of anaphylaxis; underlying medical problems such as asthma that would make anaphylaxis potentially more dangerous or difficult to treat.

isolate. Up to 20% of GBS strains may be resistant to either clindamycin or erythromycin. The practitioner should also be mindful of the poor placental transfer of erythromycin when choosing this drug to treat any maternal infection that may potentially be transmitted to the fetus in utero. Vancomycin is another appropriate antibiotic choice for the penicillin-allergic patient, although concerns regarding the selection of vancomycin-resistant enterococcus and maternal side effects should temper its use.

The Centers for Disease Control and Prevention currently recommend obtaining vaginal/rectal cultures in pregnant women between 35 and 37 weeks' gestation. Mothers who are colonized should be offered intrapartum antibiotic prophylaxis (IPAP), with penicillin being the preferred agent, as outlined in Table 40.3. Patients with unknown GBS colonization status who are less than 37 weeks' gestation should also be offered IPAP. All mothers who have previously delivered a baby infected with invasive GBS disease should be offered IPAP, and the antepartum GBS culture may be eliminated. Although IPAP is not indicated in women undergoing planned cesarean delivery prior to labor or membrane rupture, the CDC recommends obtaining antepartum cultures from these patients so that IPAP may be offered in the event of membrane rupture prior to scheduled cesarean. Cesarean delivery should not be delayed, however, to complete 4 hours of IPAP. Given that it is also recommended that women undergoing cesarean delivery be given perioperative antibiotic prophylaxis, usually a cephalosporin given prior to skin incision, many practitioners choose not to perform the antepartum culture, with the understanding that the administration of prophylactic antibiotics also serves to reduce GBS in the newborn.

Table 40.3 Suggested treatment of the asymptomatic colonized mother

Site of GBS isolation	Treatment	Rationale
Urine	Ampicillin 500 mg tid × 7 days	Reduction in PTB
Vagina/rectum – antepartum	None	No benefit of treatment
Vagina/rectum – intrapartum	Intravenous antibiotics (IPAP)	Reduces neonatal colonization and infection
Vagina/rectum – preterm rupture of the membranes – antepartum	Intravenous broad-spectrum antibiotics with gram-positive coverage	Prolongs latency period
Vagina/rectum – preterm rupture of the membranes – intrapartum	Intravenous antibiotics (IPAP)	Reduces neonatal colonization and infection

IPAP, intrapartum antibiotic prophylaxis.

In laboring patients *at term* for whom antepartum GBS culture results are not available, patients should be offered IPAP in the presence of risk factors for invasive GBS disease, i.e. prolonged membrane rupture (>18 hours) or fever in labor. Ideally, women with a fever in labor should be treated for clinical chorioamnionitis, with a broad-spectrum antibiotic regimen that includes coverage for GBS, such as ampicillin and gentamicin.

Prevention

Although the CDC algorithm outlined above has reduced the incidence of early onset neonatal GBS sepsis by 50–80%, there are persistent cases that still occur. Some are a result of a false-negative maternal antepartum culture, while others are a result of 'protocol violations', i.e., the failure to administer appropriate or adequate antibiotic prophylaxis. Lastly, some babies will develop GBS sepsis despite appropriate and timely intrapartum antibiotic treatment. Although prevention of GBS sepsis appears to be effective, whether or not the overall incidence of early-onset neonatal sepsis is decreasing is somewhat controversial. Some institutions are reporting increases in neonatal infections with gram-negative organisms, particularly *Escherichia coli*, and particularly in low birth-weight babies.

Conclusion

GBS is commonly isolated in maternal and neonatal infections, and can potentially lead to mortality and serious morbidity. However, since 1994, when the initial draft of the CDC guidelines for the prevention of GBS disease was released, the incidence of neonatal early onset GBS sepsis has been declining. Although not well studied, maternal GBS disease may also be reduced by prenatal screening and intrapartum treatment. The long-term effects of such widespread antibiotic use remain unclear, however.

Suggested reading

American College of Obstetricians and Gynecologists. Prevention of early onset group B streptococcal disease in newborns. ACOG Committee Opinion #279. *Obstet Gynecol* 2002;100:1405–12.

Boyer KM, Gotoff SP. Strategies for chemoprophylaxis of GBS early-onset infections. *Antibiot Chemother* 1985;35:267–80.

Boyer KM, Gotoff SP. Prevention of early-onset neonatal group B streptococcal disease with selective intrapartum chemoprophylaxis. *N Engl J Med* 1986;314:1665–9.

Centers for Disease Control and Prevention. Prevention of perinatal group B streptococcal disease. *MMWR Recomm Rep* 2002;51:1–22.

Honest H, Sharma S, Khan K. Rapid tests for group B streptococcus colonization in laboring women: a systematic review. *Pediatrics* 2006;117:1055–66.

Schrag SJ, Zell ER, Lynfield R, *et al.* A population-based comparison of strategies to prevent early-onset group B streptococcal disease in neonates. *N Engl J Med* 2002;347:233–9.

Stoll BJ, Hansen N, Fanaroff AA, *et al.* Changes in pathogens causing early-onset sepsis in very-low-birth-weight infants. *N Engl J Med* 2002;347:240–7.

Van Dyke MK, Phares CR, Lynfield R, *et al.* Evaluation of universal screening for group B streptococcus. *N Engl J Med* 2009;360:2626–36.

Urinary Tract Infections

F. Gary Cunningham

Department of Obstetrics and Gynecology, University of Texas Southwestern Medical Center, Dallas, TX, USA

Overview

Urinary infections are the most common bacterial infections encountered during pregnancy. They are of three types: one is asymptomatic bacteriuria, which has a prevalence of 2% to 7% depending on the population studied; and two symptomatic infections that include cystitis and pyelonephritis. The latter is the most common serious infection during pregnancy with up to 4% of women hospitalized antepartum.

Pathophysiology

Under certain conditions, covert bacteriuria can cause symptomatic cystitis or pyelonephritis. Normal pregnancy-induced urinary stasis and vesicoureteral reflux predispose to these infections. The invading organisms are those from the normal perineal flora, and about 10% of women have perineal colonization with strains of *E. coli* that have adhesins such as S- or P-fimbriae. These appendages enhance bacterial virulence, and indeed, 90% of *E. coli* isolates from women with acute pyelonephritis have these fimbriae.

Diagnosis

Because one-fourth of pregnant women with untreated asymptomatic bacteriuria go on to develop acute pyelonephritis, early prenatal screening and eradication is recommended by most, including the American College of Obstetricians and Gynecologists. When the prevalence is low, standard urine cultures may not be cost effective and other test systems such as the dipstick culture technique have been reported to be accurate.

Protocols for High-Risk Pregnancies, 5th edition. Edited by J.T. Queenan, J.C. Hobbins and C.Y. Spong. © 2010 Blackwell Publishing Ltd.

Cystitis typically is characterized by dysuria, urgency and frequency with minimal manifestations. Infection is confirmed by pyuria, hematuria and bacteriuria. The upper urinary tract may also become involved by ascending infection, either with or without concomitant cystitis. The incidence of acute pyelonephritis during pregnancy is reported to be as high as 4%. Because of this, renal infection is a leading cause of sepsis syndrome (see Protocol **26**). Pyelonephritis is more common after mid-pregnancy and it is right-sided in about half of cases and bilateral in another fourth. The onset is usually abrupt with fever, shaking chills and pain in one or both lumbar regions. There may be anorexia, nausea and vomiting. Tenderness usually can be elicited by percussion in one or both costovertebral angles. The urinary sediment usually contains many leukocytes, frequently in clumps, and numerous bacteria. *E. coli* strains are isolated from urine cultures in 75 to 80% of women with pyelonephritis. The other isolates include *Klebsiella*, *Enterobacter* or *Proteus* species or group B streptococci. Women with acute pyelonephritis usually appear quite ill, and bacteremia is confirmed in 15 to 20%.

Treatment

Bacteriuria or cystitis are treated empirically with any of several antimicrobial regimens that include single-dose or 3-day treatment with ampicillin or amoxicillin; one of the cephalosporins or quinolones; nitrofurantoin; or trimethoprim-sulfamethoxazole. Regardless of the regimen chosen, the recurrence rate is about 30% after completion of any of these regimens. For women with a recurrent infection, a second course with the same or another one of these agents is given. For women with persistent bacteriuria, or those with frequent recurrences, suppressive therapy for the remainder of pregnancy can be given with nitrofurantoin, 100 mg at bedtime.

Complications

Most major complications encountered with antepartum pyelonephritis are caused by the sepsis syndrome. Between 5 and 20% of women will manifest reversible acute kidney injury manifest by elevated serum creatinine levels. In some of these, it may be necessary to modify dosing with potentially nephrotoxic antimicrobials such as amnioglycosides. Up to 5 to 10% of women with acute pyelonephritis develop varying degrees of acute respiratory distress syndrome. In some of these, tracheal intubation with mechanical ventilation is lifesaving. After midpregnancy, septicemia may cause uterine activity, but caution is urged for co-administration of tocolytics that may increase the risk of permeability pulmonary edema. Finally, persistence of the sepsis syndrome should prompt a search for ureteral obstruction as well as for a perinephric phlegmon or abscess. Endotoxin-induced hemolysis causes anemia in about a third of women.

Management

A scheme for management of acute pyelonephritis during pregnancy is shown in Table 41.1. Hydration with intravenous crystalloid solutions and antimicrobials is the cornerstone of therapy and is begun promptly at diagnosis. Therapy is empirical, and ampicillin plus gentamicin; cefazolin or ceftriaxone; or an extended-spectrum beta-lactam have been found to be 95% effective in randomized trials. Ongoing surveillance in an acute care unit is recommended in order to recognize worsening of sepsis syndrome. To do so, frequent determinations of vital signs and urinary output are monitored. Clinical response is usually relatively prompt and clinical symptoms usually resolve within 2 days and 95% of women are afebrile by 72 hours. As discussed, for those who do not respond promptly and appropriately, consideration is given for urinary tract obstruction, usually from stone disease, and imaging studies may be indicated. At discharge, oral antimicrobial therapy is given for 7 to 10 days.

Follow-up

Recurrent covert bacteriuria develops in about a third of women following treatment for pyelonephritis. Because a third of these will again develop recurrent symptomatic infection, then asymptomatic bacteriuria is treated again as

Table 41.1 Management of the pregnant woman with acute pyelonephritis

1   Hospitalization
2   Urine culture; blood culture if overtly septic
3   Hemogram, serum creatinine and electrolytes
4   Monitor vital signs frequently, including urinary output with indwelling bladder catheter
5   Intravenous crystalloid to establish urinary output to ≥50 mL/h
6   Intravenous antimicrobial therapy
7   Chest x-ray if there is dyspnea or tachypnea
8   Repeat hemogram and creatinine in 48 hours
9   Switch to oral antimicrobials when afebrile
10   Discharge when afebrile 24 hours, give antimicrobial therapy for 7 to 10 days
11   Urine culture 1 to 2 weeks after antimicrobial therapy completed

described above. Unless urine culture surveillance is performed to ensure urine sterility, then nitrofurantoin, 100 mg at bedtime, is given for the remainder of the pregnancy.

Suggested reading

Berg CJ, MacKay AP, Qin C, Callaghan WM. Overview of maternal morbidity during hospitalization for labor and delivery in the United States. 1993–1997 and 2001–2005. *Obstet Gynecol* 2009;113:1075.

Butler EL, Cox SM, Eberts E, *et al.* Symptomatic nephrolithiasis complicating pregnancy. *Obstet Gynecol* 2000;96:753.

Cunningham FG, Lucas MJ, Hankins GDV. Pulmonary injury complicating antepartum pyelonephritis. *Am J Obstet Gynecol* 1987;156:797.

Dodson KW, Pinkner JS, Rose T, *et al.* Structural basis of the interaction of the pyelonephritic E. coli adhesin to its human kidney receptor. *Cell* 2001;1105:733.

Fihn SD. Acute uncomplicated urinary tract infection in women. *N Engl J Med* 2003;349:259.

Hooton TM, Scholes D, Stapleton AE, *et al.* A prospective study of asymptomatic bacteriuria in sexually active young women. *N Engl J Med* 2000;343:992.

Migini L, Carroli G, Abalos E, *et al.* Accuracy of diagnostic tests to detect asymptomatic bacteriuria during pregnancy. *Obstet Gynecol* 2009;113:346.

Raz R, Sakran W, Chazan B, *et al.* Long-term follow-up of women hospitalized for acute pyelonephritis. *Clin Infect Dis* 2003;37:1014.

Sheffield JS, Cunningham FG. Urinary tract infection in women. *Obstet Gynecol* 2005;106:1085.

Vasquez JC, Villar J. Treatments for symptomatic urinary tract infections during pregnancy. *Cochrane Database Syst Rev* 2006;(3):CD002256.

Wing DA, Hendershott CM, Debuque L, *et al.* Outpatient treatment of acute pyelonephritis in pregnancy after 24 weeks. *Obstet Gynecol* 1999;94:683.

Acute Abdominal Pain Due to Non-obstetric Causes

Fred M. Howard

Department of Obstetrics and Gynecology, University of Rochester School of Medicine and Dentistry, Rochester, NY, USA

Overview

Evaluation and treatment of the pregnant woman with acute abdominal pain represents a challenging clinical dilemma that demands great care and judgment. Common pregnancy symptoms such as nausea, vomiting and urinary frequency are similar to those of many non-obstetrical illnesses that cause acute abdominal pain. The etiology of acute abdominal pain in pregnancy can be separated into obstetric and non-obstetric causes; only non-obstetric causes will be discussed in this protocol. The most common etiologies for non-obstetric causes of acute abdominal pain in the pregnant patient are appendicitis, cholecystitis, pyelonephritis, hepatitis, pancreatitis and degenerating uterine leiomyomata. Management is also more difficult, as interventions may adversely affect the pregnancy and concerns about harming the fetus may delay treatment. It is important to develop the clinical acumen to identify patients with problems that demand immediate intervention.

Pathophysiology

Maternal physiological and anatomic changes may modify symptoms and clinical responses from those normally seen in non-pregnant patients. The physical examination of the abdomen and pelvis are altered by the pregnant state. By 12 weeks of gestation the uterine fundus rises from the pelvis and become an abdominal organ, as do the adnexal structures. The intestines and omentum are displaced superiorly and laterally with the appendix more likely to be closer to the gallbladder than to the McBurney point by late pregnancy (see Fig. 42.1). Routine laboratory

Protocols for High-Risk Pregnancies, 5th edition. Edited by J.T. Queenan, J.C. Hobbins and C.Y. Spong. © 2010 Blackwell Publishing Ltd.

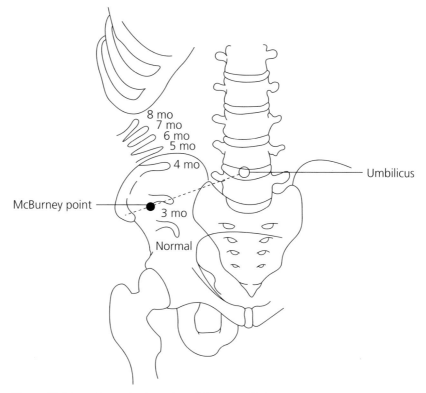

Figure 42.1 Location and orientation of the appendix in pregnancy.

measures may also be altered in the pregnant state. For instance, the leukocyte count varies considerably during normal pregnancy with elevations up to 12,000 to 16,000/mL, levels that overlap with intraabdominal inflammatory conditions, such as appendicitis.

Diagnosis and treatment

History and physical examination

A systematic and detailed history and physical examination are paramount. Having the most common diagnoses in mind during evaluation is essential to formulating a differential diagnosis, yet the clinician must remain sufficiently open-minded and unhurried to avoid missing important information. Acute abdominal crises should be recognized in an expedient manner. They may present with pain as the sole symptom but often will also involve vomiting, muscular rigidity, abdominal distention or shock. In early pregnancy, excluding the possibility of ectopic pregnancy is often the first priority.

Location is crucial to potential diagnoses. Table 42.1 summarizes the location of pain associated with many of the causes of acute abdominal pain. Differentiating uterine from non-uterine pain can be difficult. One possible way to do so is to have the patient lie supine and then roll to the left or the right. If the pain shifts when she lies on her side, it is more likely to of uterine origin. If it remains in the same location, consider an intraabdominal or retroperitoneal process.

Acute abdominal pain exacerbated by movement and coughing is generally consistent with peritoneal inflammation or irritation due to an infectious process or visceral rupture. Colicky pain refers to pain that is wavelike, with spasms that crescendo and decrescendo in a somewhat

Table 42.1 Differential diagnosis of acute non-obstetric abdominopelvic pain by location (*the more common causes are in italic*)

Right upper quadrant

- *Cholecystitis/cholelithiasis*
- Diaphragmatic pleuritis/abscess
- *Hepatitis*
- *Pancreatitis*
- Pneumonia/pneumonitis
- *Appendicitis* (later gestation)

Epigastric

- *Cholecystitis/cholelithiasis*
- Early acute *appendicitis*
- Early small bowel obstruction
- *Gastroenteritis*/gastric ulcer
- *Gastroesophageal reflux*
- Mesenteric thrombosis/ischemia
- Myocardial infarction
- *Pancreatitis*
- Pericarditis
- Ruptured aortic aneurysm

Left upper quadrant

- *Gastroenteritis/gastric ulcer*
- Myocardial infarction
- *Pancreatitis*
- Pericarditis
- Pnuemonia/pneumonitis
- Splenic rupture/abscess/infarction

Periumbilical

- All early-stage visceral diseases
- Abdominal trauma

- Abdominal wall hernias
- Bowel obstruction

Diffuse or generalized

- All late-stage visceral diseases
- Bowel obstruction
- Diabetic ketoacidosis
- Irritable bowel syndrome
- Mesenteric ischemia
- Metabolic disorders
- Peritonitis/perforated viscera
- Muscular strain/sprain

Lower quadrants

- *Adnexal torsion*
- *Appendicitis* (right lower quadrant)
- *Constipation*
- *Diverticulitis*
- *Endometriosis*
- Inflammatory bowel disease
- Inguinal hernia
- Irritable bowel syndrome
- *Leiomyomata*
- *Ovarian cyst/ruptured cyst*
- *Pelvic inflammatory disease*
- *Pyelonephritis*
- *Urinary calculi*

Suprapubic

- *Cystitis/urethritis*
- Obstruction of the urinary bladder
- *Urinary calculi*

rhythmic pattern. This type of pain is characteristic of intestinal disorders, especially small bowel obstruction. It may also be consistent with adnexal torsion. Steady or constant pain is characteristic of a distended gallbladder or kidney.

The nature of the onset of the pain, chronological sequence of events in the patient's history and duration of the pain are important diagnostic elements. Associated symptoms may narrow the diagnosis. Fever and chills may suggest an infectious etiology. Pain followed by nausea and emesis is more characteristic of appendicitis while viral or bacterial enteritis may present with gastrointestinal complaints followed by pain.

Severity of pain does not necessarily correlate with the severity of disease and is not always useful in diagnosis. In most patients it is appropriate to give analgesia while the evaluation of acute pain is ongoing. A history of radiation of pain may also be helpful. For instance, acute obstruction of the intravesicular portion of the ureter is characterized by severe suprapubic and flank pain that radiates to the labia or inner aspect of the upper thigh. Pain referred to the abdomen from the thorax can be a difficult diagnostic problem and an intrathoracic etiology should be considered in every patient with acute abdominal pain.

Physical examination of the abdomen, pelvis and rectum are critical components of evaluation of the pregnant woman with abdominal pain. The examination should be gentle but thorough. Examination begins with observation of the patient's appearance and activity. The patient with peritoneal inflammation may minimize motion and lie with hips flexed to reduce pain. Patients with urinary colic from calculi usually move around. Vital signs are essential. Hypotension and tachycardia suggest hypovolemia, which may be due to dehydration or blood loss. Fever suggests an infectious process.

The fetal status should also be determined at this point in a manner appropriate for gestational age. The uterus should be monitored for contractions with a tocodynamometer because preterm labor may occur in this clinical setting. If viable, the fetus should be assessed by means of a non-stress test (NST) followed by a biophysical profile if the NST is not reactive. Fetal tachycardia due to a maternal fever may resolve with fever reduction measures.

Gentle examination of the abdomen may reveal tenderness, involuntary guarding and rebound tenderness, which are characteristic of peritoneal inflammation of any etiology. Abdominal distention may occur with peritoneal inflammation or bowel obstruction. Palpation should be directed to the detection of possible abdominal masses as well as tenderness. Auscultation may reveal decreased or absent bowel sounds consistent with peritonitis or ileus. High-pitched bowel sounds and rushes may be heard if obstruction is present. Patients with findings consistent with generalized peritonitis, with guarding and rebound tenderness in all four quadrants of the abdomen, are commonly said to have a 'surgical abdomen' and may require operative evaluation to arrive at a clear diagnosis.

Pelvic examination is often of limited value after the first trimester. Ultrasound is usually essential to rule out a pelvic mass in acute abdominal pain during pregnancy. The rectal examination may be helpful in further clarifying pelvic pathology and testing for occult blood at the time of the examination may help recognize gastrointestinal bleeding.

Laboratory and imaging evaluation

Table 42.2 lists many of the laboratory and imaging studies generally useful in evaluating the gravid woman with acute abdominal pain. Laboratory examinations may be of great value, but rarely establish a definitive diagnosis. Not all are indicated in all women and their use should be predicated by the differential diagnosis determined from the history and physical examination. Studies that are usually indicated include complete blood count, urinalysis, urine culture, electrolytes and pregnancy test (when gestational age uncertain).

Imaging may be helpful. MR and ultrasound scans are considered safe in pregnancy and can be used without reservations. In general, examinations with ionizing radiation exposure are avoided, particularly in the first trimester. As a general rule, no single imaging study provides enough radiation exposure to the fetus to cause damage. Accumulative doses

Table 42.2 Studies that may be useful in acute abdominal pain in the gravid patient

Laboratory testing
Serum quantitative β-hCG
Urinalysis: assess for pyuria, hematuria, glucosuria, ketones
Urine culture and sensitivity: assess for urinary tract infection
Cervical cultures: assess for gonorrhea, chlamydia infection
Complete blood count and differential: assess for leukocytosis, anemia
Glucose
Serum ketones: assess in patients who may have diabetic keoacidosis
Liver function tests, total and direct bilirubin: assess for liver, gallbladder disease
Amylase, lipase: assess for pancreatic disease
Electrolytes, BUN, creatinine: assess metabolic state, renal function
Other specific tests when indicated (e.g., hemoglobin electrophoresis, ANA)
Imaging (scans with radiation exposure are generally second-line)
Pelvic ultrasound: assess pregnancy, adnexa, uterus
Abdominal ultrasound: assess gallbladder, appendix, liver, free fluid
Renal ultrasound: assess kidneys for hydronephrosis, calculi
Chest radiograph: assess lungs, heart silhouette
Abdominal x-ray series: assess bowels if perforation, obstruction suspected
CT or MR scans as indicated

should not exceed 5 rad. Radioactive isotopes should also be avoided in pregnancy. It should be kept in mind that if the pregnant woman requires abdominal imaging such as a CT scan, this might be an indication of severity of disease and need to proceed with operative exploration.

Treatment

Appropriate treatment of acute abdominal pain in the pregnant patient will be dictated by the differential diagnosis. In most cases, management will be unchanged from that employed in non-pregnant patients.

Acute appendicitis

About 2% of women require a non-obstetrical surgical procedure during pregnancy and acute appendicitis is the most common reason. Appendicitis occurs more often in the middle trimester and perforation of the appendix is skewed toward later pregnancy. This probably reflects both the difficulty and delay of diagnosis in later pregnancy. The clinical presentation of appendicitis during pregnancy is not greatly different from that in the non-pregnant woman. Most patients will complain of abdominal pain, nausea or vomiting. Anorexia is not a consistent finding in pregnancy and diarrhea may be present. The presence of fever may be less common in pregnancy and white blood counts may be just mildly elevated although the majority of women will have a left shift. Treatment is expedient appendectomy. Tolerance of a significant rate of normal appendixes is necessary to prevent the serious maternal and fetal morbidity associated with perforation. Antibiotics are generally administered prior to and after surgery. Tocolysis may be indicated.

Ovarian cysts and adnexal torsion

Ovarian cysts may case acute abdominal pain due to rupture. Adnexal torsion may occur with normal adnexae, but more often occurs with adnexal cystic lesions, neoplastic lesions or hyperstimulated ovaries. The majority of torsions occur in the first half of the pregnancy. Ovarian torsion usually presents with unilateral pelvic pain possibly with vomiting. Ultrasound may demonstrate a pelvic mass and absent flow on Doppler evaluation. Adnexal torsion represents a surgical emergency due to the potential danger of permanent destruction of the organs involved, peritonitis, or even death. The traditional approach has been surgical removal of the adnexa. However, untwisting and preservation of the ovary is usually successful even with an apparently necrotic ovary or tube.

Cholecystitis/cholelithiasis

Asymptomatic cholelithiasis occurs in 3–4% of pregnant women and is the cause of over 90% of cases of cholecystitis in pregnancy. Cholecystitis during pregnancy is uncommon, with 5–10 cases per 10,000 births. Steady and severe right upper quadrant pain is often the presenting symptom. Fever, leukocytosis, nausea, vomiting and anorexia may also be present. Ultrasonography will show gallstones in almost all cases. Medical treatment is preferred in pregnancy. Initial treatment consists of no oral intake, intravenous hydration, bed-rest, pain relief and antibiotics if febrile. Most women respond to this approach and avoid surgical treatment during pregnancy. Surgery, if needed for failed medical management, is best performed in the second trimester.

Urinary tract infection

Acute cystitis is very common in gravid women. It may occur alone or in conjunction with pyelonephritis. Acute uncomplicated cystitis is manifested primarily by dysuria, with associated frequency, urgency, suprapubic pain and/or hematuria. Fever, flank pain, costovertebral angle tenderness and nausea or vomiting suggest pyelonephritis and warrant more aggressive diagnostic and therapeutic measures. Pyenolonephritis is identified in 1–2% of all pregnancies. Treatment includes parenteral antibiotics and intravenous hydration. Close monitoring for complications such as renal impairment, hematological abnormalities, septic shock and pulmonary dysfunction, is critical in the pregnant patient. Prophylatic antibiotics may be indicated for the remainder of the pregnancy.

Urinary calculi

Stones or calculi of the urinary tract usually case severe abdominal pain associated with nausea, but sometimes present with milder symptoms during pregnancy. With ureteral obstruction, flank pain is present which may radiate to the ipsilateral groin and percussion may elicit tenderness over the costovertebral angle. Hematuria is usually present. Ultrasonographic examination may demonstrate hydroureter, hydronephrosis or calculi. In most cases of renal or ureteral calculus, the stone eventually passes, thus supportive treatment with intravenous hydration and pain control is usually sufficient. Lithotripsy is contraindicated in pregnancy.

Pancreatitis

Acute pancreatitis complicates 1 in 1,000 to 10,000 pregnancies. Gallbladder disease is the most common cause; medications, infection and hyperlipidemia are less frequent causes. Signs and symptoms are similar to those in the non-pregnant woman. Medical management includes bowel rest, pain relief and correction of fluid and electrolyte imbalances. Patients with pancreatic abscess, ruptured pseudocyst or hemorrhagic pancreatitis may require surgery while they are still pregnant.

Hepatitis

Viral hepatitis is the most common serious, non-obstetrical liver disease in pregnant women. Although pregnancy has little influence on the presentation or course of hepatitis, hepatitis carries significant implications to the pregnancy, fetus and neonate depending on the type and gestational age. Management is generally unchanged during pregnancy.

Uterine leiomyomata

Acute pain from myomata during pregnancy is usually due to degeneration secondary to inadequacy of blood supply to the myoma. Pain and tenderness are generally localized and can be severe. Low-grade fever and leukocytosis can occur. Preterm labor may be initiated due to irritation of adjacent myometrium. Ultrasonography is helpful in making the diagnosis. Management is non-surgical with use of analgesics and observation for preterm labor.

Intraabdominal hemorrhage

Acute abdominal hemorrhage, other than from ectopic pregnancy, is uncommon during pregnancy, but may rarely occur. It has been reported with rupture of the aorta, splenic artery and endometriotic lesions. Evaluation with imaging studies usually demonstrate the presence of a hemoperitoneum. Management is almost always acute surgical intervention.

Pelvic inflammatory disease

Acute endometritis, salpingitis and/or oophoritis are not common in pregnancy, but do occasionally occur, even with the development of tubo-ovarian abscesses. Findings with cervical cultures of gonorrhea or Chlamydia or with imaging studies of tubo-ovarian complexes or pyosalpinges supports the clinical diagnosis. Many clinicians think that PID is not possible during pregnancy, but this is incorrect and may lead to missed diagnoses and inappropriate treatment.

Conclusion

The ability to distinguish an acute process that requires surgical intervention or referral to a specialist is based on the clinical skills of the provider. This requires a complete history, careful physical examination, judicious use of laboratory and radiological studies, and frequent reevaluation until a firm diagnosis is reached. The primary care clinician should have a low threshold for seeking advice from a surgeon, obstetrician or other specialist. The difficulties of diagnosing abdominal pain in pregnancy are well known. Prompt clinical diagnosis and surgical intervention when indicated are necessary to minimize maternal and fetal morbidity and mortality.

Suggested reading

Hasiakos D, Papakonstantinou K, Kontoravdis A, Gogas L, Aravantinos L, Vitoratos N. Adnexal torsion during pregnancy: report of four cases and review of the literature. *J Obstet Gynaecol Res* 2008;34(4 Pt 2):683–7.

Kilpatrick CC, Orejuela FJ. Management of the acute abdomen in pregnancy: a review. *Curr Opin Obstet Gynecol* 2008;20(6):534–9.

Oto A, Ernst RD, Ghulmiyyah LM, Nishino TK, Hughes D, Chaljub G, Saade G. MR imaging in the triage of pregnant patients with acute abdominal and pelvic pain. *Abdom Imag* 2009;34(2):243–50.

Upadhyay A, Stanten S, Kazantsev G, Horoupian R, Stanten A. Laparoscopic management of a nonobstetric emergency in the third trimester of pregnancy. *Surg Endosc* 2007;21(8):1344–8.

PROTOCOL 43

Gallbladder, Fatty Liver and Pancreatic Disease

Jeffrey R. Johnson
Dartmouth Hitchcock Medical Center, Lebanon and Manchester, NH, USA

Clinical significance

Disorders of the gallbladder are common during pregnancy. Cholestasis affects about 1 in 500 pregnancies, can recur during subsequent pregnancies, and there appears to be a mother–daughter correlation in disease incidence. It is related to a history of oral contraceptive use as well. Gallstones are seen in up to 4% of pregnancies, the majority being asymptomatic. Pigmented stones comprise 15% and mixed pigmented and cholesterol also comprise about 15% of stones. Increased formation of gallstones is associated with being female (four times more likely than in males), increasing age, obesity, a diet high in fat, diabetes, high parity and exogenous hormone administration, particularly estrogen. About 90% of cases of cholecystitis are associated with stones while 10% are acalculous and are due to trauma, obstruction, tuberculosis or parasitic infections.

Acute fatty liver of pregnancy (AFLP) is rare, affecting 1 in 15,000 pregnancies. It is a particularly aggressive form of liver dysfunction: maternal mortality is 25%, and perinatal morbidity and mortality are related to gestational age at delivery. It is seen more commonly with a male fetus or multiple gestations. Its typical presentation is the third trimester or within 48 hours postpartum. AFLP has been associated with preeclampsia, although whether AFLP represents a variant of severe preeclampsia remains debatable.

Acute pancreatitis is a rare complication in pregnancy, occurring in between 1 per 1,000 and 1 per 3,000 pregnancies. Most are due to gallstones, which is different than in non-pregnant cases which are primarily alcohol. Hypertriglyceridemia is a rare but important cause of pancreatitis

Protocols for High-Risk Pregnancies, 5th edition. Edited by J.T. Queenan, J.C. Hobbins and C.Y. Spong. © 2010 Blackwell Publishing Ltd.

in pregnancy, and can be difficult to treat. It is more common in 20- to 30 year-old primigravidas in the third trimester. Pancreatitis due to hyper-triglyceridemia carries a 10% mortality rate for both mother and fetus. There has also been shown to be an association of AFLP and pancreatitis, and the prognosis is especially poor in these patients.

Pathophysiology

Cholestasis results from a decrease in excretion of bile acids, causing hepatic canalicular plugging without evidence of necrosis. The bile acids are hydrophobic, resulting in deposition of bile salts in the dermal layer of the skin, leading to extreme pruritis. Due to the hydrophobic nature of bile acids, they also readily cross the placenta and blood–brain barrier, and may result in fetal complications.

Seventy percent of gallstones are comprised of cholesterol, and gall-stones form from supersaturation of cholesterol and lipids. Pregnancy is associated with stone formation, due to high levels of circulating sex hormones, as well as increasing progesterone. As progesterone levels rise through the first half of gestation there is an overall decrease in motil-ity of smooth muscle, including the gallbladder. This results in decreased emptying and an increase in biliary sludge, which forms a nidus for stone formation.

The exact etiology of AFLP is not clear, but in some cases it may be related to preeclampsia. A mother who is heterozygous for an autosomal recessive mutation in the long chain 3-hydroxyacyl-coenzyme A dehy-drogenase (LCHAD) in mitochondria, and has a fetus that is homozygous for the same LCHAD mutation, has a significantly higher incidence of AFLP. These pregnancies are also affected with IUGR and poor overall neonatal outcomes, although whether this may be a result of concomi-tant severe preeclampsia or represents a truly separate entity remains to be elucidated. The risk of recurrence is less than 5%, but if it is recurrent, then testing for the LCHAD defect is warranted.

The majority (80%) of cases of pancreatitis in pregnancy are due to cholelithiasis. Increasing rates of obesity among females, as well as higher levels of steroid synthesis and breakdown during pregnancy, are both etiologic factors contributing to the development of cholelithiasis. Other causes of pancreatitis in decreasing order of frequency are: alcohol, infec-tions (mumps, coxsackie B, tuberculosis), drugs (corticosteroids, acetami-nophen, nitrofurantoin and flagyl), trauma, post-surgical iatrogenic, and idiopathic.

Hypertriglyceridemia is recognized as a rare but important cause of pancreatitis. It is thought that the decreased activity of lipoprotein lipase, which initiates catabolism of triglyceride-rich proteins, plays the major role in development of pancreatitis in this group of patients. The decreased activity of lipoprotein lipase is related to the increased insulin resistance seen in the second and third trimesters. This decrease in lipoprotein lipase activity can make treatment in these patients particularly problematic.

Diagnosis

Cholestasis is most commonly diagnosed with extreme, unrelenting, miserable pruritis that does not respond to any of the usual antihistamine or topical steroid therapy. There is occasionally a nonspecific rash on the trunk, face and legs. There is no liver dysfunction, and the liver enzymes are normal, with a normal to minimally elevated total bilirubin. There is an elevation in bile acid levels when tested. Although not recommended during pregnancy, hepatic biopsy will show deposition of bile in the canaliculi, without surrounding hepatic necrosis. Ultrasonography of the right upper quadrant is not helpful.

Cholelithiasis is usually asymptomatic; however, there may be right upper quadrant pain, particularly after a fatty meal. Severe symptoms occur when a stone enters the cystic or common bile duct. There is a sudden onset of right upper quadrant pain, which may radiate to the mid-epigastrium or right scapula; there is nausea with rapid progression to vomiting and anorexia. The serum alkaline phosphatase is an excellent predictor of obstructive cholelithiasis in the non-pregnant patient, but is less useful during pregnancy due to placental production of alkaline phosphatase. However, an elevated hepatic alkaline phosphatase can be determined by exposing the sample to heat in the laboratory, as the placental fraction of alkaline phosphatase is heat-stable.Ultrasonography is sensitive and specific for cholelithiasis, detecting more than 95% of gallstones. It is also useful to find evidence of obstruction of the cystic or common bile duct by looking for ductal dilatation. Ultrasonography will detect gallbladder wall thickening or pericystic fluid collections, which are evidence for cholecystitis. The risk of preterm labor with cholecystitis is increased. The fetal loss rates are less than 5% in appropriately treated cases.

AFLP can initially present with vomiting, followed by a rapid progression in sequence of right upper quadrant pain, coma, hepatic failure with disseminated intravascular coagulation, and death. Hepatomegaly is not a feature of AFLP. A severe coagulopathy is nearly always present, with an abnormal INR due to absence of vitamin K dependent clotting factors. An elevated INR will differentiate AFLP from HELLP syndrome, which may also have an associated coagulopathy, but does not result in an elevation in INR. Patients may develop hepatorenal syndrome or diabetes insipidus. Liver enzymes are elevated but less than 500 U/L. There is hypoglycemia and also increased serum ammonia levels. The ammonia testing is for academic purposes as it may take many hours to days to obtain a result, and should not be the initial laboratory test to make the diagnosis. Ultrasonography of the liver will demonstrate fatty infiltration of the liver. Computed tomography scanning is neither sensitive nor specific for AFLP, and is not recommended. Magnetic resonance imaging which is T_2 weighted is very sensitive for fatty infiltration of the liver, but not specific to AFLP.

Pancreatitis may present with nausea and vomiting, low-grade fever and leukocytosis. Abdominal examination usually reveals tenderness in the epigastric area, occasionally radiating to the flank or shoulders. There is rarely guarding or rebound tenderness. Computed tomography scanning is best avoided during the second and third trimester due to the concerns of radiation exposure. Ultrasonography may be performed, but the gravid uterus may interfere with adequate visualization of the pancreas. Ultrasonography may demonstrate a large pancreatic cyst or pseudocyst. Magnetic resonance imaging may reveal cystic changes in the pancreas, as well as obstruction of the common bile duct by a stone. Ileus is a frequent clinical and radiological finding. Elevated amylase, especially three times the normal range, is the most common laboratory abnormality. Other abnormalities may include elevated lipase and liver enzymes, particularly if obstruction due to a gallstone is present. Serum alkaline phosphatase may be elevated in cases of cholelithiasis, and differentiation between placental and hepatic alkaline phosphatase can be made by determining the heat-stable versus total alkaline phosphatase.

Treatment

The majority of pregnancies affected with cholestasis are uncomplicated. There is a marginally increased rate of premature labor and postpartum hemorrhage, and stillbirth. Maternal therapy should be directed both at alleviating the pruritic symptoms and decreasing bile acids. An effective therapy in most cases is with ursodeoxycholic acid which allows binding of the bile acids into salts, so that they may be excreted in the feces. Relief may take 48 to 72 hours after initiating therapy. Cholestyramine is marginally effective, and is best used as an adjuvant therapy if ursodeoxycholic acid is not completely effective. Corticosteroids have been shown to be an effective second agent in cases that are otherwise refractory. Antihistamines provide some symptomatic relief, as does hydroxyzine. The limitations for both these therapies are their side effects, particularly sedation.

Cholelithiasis is treated with intravenous hydration and withholding oral nutrition for several days. A low-fat diet, once feedings are reestablished, is essential. Pain medications are given parenterally initially, and meperidine is the drug of choice. Morphine should be avoided as it precipitates spasms of the sphincter of Oddi, and can exacerbate symptoms. Antibiotics are indicated if there is concomitant cholecystitis. The risk of preterm labor in is significantly elevated, and antipyretics and tocolytics are indicated. Surgical intervention is indicated after 48 hours of antibiotics. Non-pregnant patients are often managed conservatively with antibiotics for first episode cholecystitis. However, sepsis and acute respiratory distress syndrome are increased during pregnancy from cholecystitis, and surgical intervention is recommended for first episode cholecystitis in pregnancy. Non-surgical medical therapy (bile acid therapy, dissolution with methyl terbutyl ether, or lithotripsy) is not recommended in pregnancy. Laparoscopic cholecystectomy has been shown to be safe in multiple reports, and may often be the primary mode of treatment. Seventy percent of patients with significant stones will have a relapse of symptoms. Laparoscopic cholecystectomy is preferred for initial management if there is a high probability of recurrence, if the episodes are repeated, or for evidence of perforation. The laparoscopic approach is best used through about 24 weeks' gestation, with the open approach after 24 weeks. Laparoscopic cholecystectomy is the second most common non-obstetric surgical procedure performed during pregnancy, after appendectomy. If there is obstruction of the common bile duct, endoscopic retrograde cholangiopancreatography (ERCP) may also be safely performed in pregnancy. There is no increased rate of prematurity seen with ERCP performed in the second or third trimesters, although the loss rate may be elevated with first trimester ERCP. The rate of post-ERCP pancreatitis is higher (15%) than in the non-pregnant population.

Treatment for AFLP is directed towards immediate recognition and delivery. Vaginal delivery is preferred due to the risks of bleeding with abdominal delivery, although cesarean delivery may be preferred if the induction were to be prolonged. Regional anesthesia is preferable due to both the potential for hepatotoxicity with inhaled agents, and also the ability to monitor maternal levels of consciousness. These patients are best served in an intensive care setting in a tertiary medical center. Clotting factor replacement is essential to survival, as disseminated intravascular coagulation is the cause for mortality in the majority of patients. Hepatic failure is also a potential concern. Careful monitoring of serum glucose and electrolytes is essential. Liver transplantation has been used in some cases, although with intensive support these patients do recover without transplantation.

Most cases of acute pancreatitis resolve spontaneously. Approximately 10% of patients may be critically ill and require treatment in an intensive care unit. The general management is bowel rest, and nasogastric suction in cases associated with ileus. Adequate intravenous hydration and electrolyte monitoring is essential due to fluid and electrolyte loss associated with large pancreatic cysts or prolonged vomiting. A low-fat elemental enteral nutrition program is essential in the treatment of pancreatitis regardless of etiology with meperidine, as morphine may cause spasm of the sphincter of Oddi, and exacerbate symptoms of biliary colic. Antibiotics are indicated only if infection is suspected. Cases associated with large or a high number of stones may not respond to conservative management. The rate of relapse can be as high as 70%. In 68 ERCPs performed between 2000 and 2006, indications were recurrent biliary colic, abnormal liver function testing and dilated bile duct. The median fluoroscopy time was 1.45 minutes, and there were no complications related to the procedure (perforation, post-spincterotomy bleeding, cholangitis, or maternal or fetal loss). However, 11 patients (16%) developed post-ERCP pancreatitis. All were managed successfully with conservative therapy. The term pregnancy rate was 90% overall, although patients who underwent ERCP in the first trimester had the highest loss rate of 20%. ERCP in pregnancy was associated with a higher rate of post-procedure pancreatitis than in the general population. Cases due to hypertriglyceridemia are best managed with enteral feeding of a low-lipid diet, and generally do not respond to routine nasogastric suctioning and intravenous fluids alone. Careful attention to glucose is mandated due to an increase in glycemic indices. Plasmapheresis has been reported, but is considered largely investigational, and should not be routinely performed. In general, pregnancy does not have an adverse effect on pancreatitis, and delivery does not improve the clinical course in most cases. Fetal monitoring is suggested, particularly in the third trimester.

Complications

Pregnancies complicated by cholestasis have an increased rate of stillbirth, thus monitoring for fetal well-being in the third trimester is recommended. The bile acids may have a direct depressive or toxic effect on the fetal myocardium, and twice-weekly non-stress testing after 32 weeks is advocated. Cholestasis is one of the few obstetric indications for early amniocentesis at 37 to 38 weeks for fetal lung maturity determination, and delivery if mature. Cesarean delivery is reserved for the usual obstetric indications.

The primary complications associated with pancreatitis in pregnancy are maternal, due to fluid and electrolyte imbalances. Complications due to obstruction are no higher than in the non-pregnant complication, but may include perforation by the stone in rare cases. There is a slightly higher rate of preterm labor and delivery as with any peritoneal inflammatory response which can cause increased uterine irritability.

Conclusion

Gallbladder disorders may occur more frequently during pregnancy. Cholestasis presents with maternal symptoms and is associated with increased stillbirth and pregnancy complications. Monitoring and therapy are guided both to decreasing maternal symptoms and preventing perinatal complications.

Cholelithiasis is more commonly seen due to increasing obesity as well as diets high in fats. It is best treated during pregnancy surgically, and evaluation for concomitant cholecystitis is required for optimal management. Surgical interventions during pregnancy have been shown to be safe, and should not be withheld if it is the appropriate management.

Acute fatty liver of pregnancy (AFLP) presents an unusual and rare constellation of findings, and can be life-threatening. Optimal and early treatment is essential for maternal survival, but fortunately is rare and tends not to recur.

Pancreatitis is an unusual obstetric complication, and is commonly due to stone obstruction of the cystic or common bile duct. Diagnosis is usually made by a combination of clinical findings, and radiological studies such as ultrasound or magnetic resonance imaging. Treatment is conservative in the majority of cases, although surgical intervention is warranted in some cases. ERCP has been shown to be safe in pregnancy, and used when appropriate. Pancreatitis due to hypertriglyceridemia is rare and should be treated with low-lipid enteral feeding. Morbidity and mortality due to hypertriglyceridemic pancreatitis is elevated for both mother and fetus if inappropriately diagnosed or treated.

Suggested reading

American College of Obstetricians and Gynecologists. *Acute fatty liver of pregnancy in multiple gestation: complicated twin, triplet, and high order multifetal pregnancy.* ACOG Practice Bulletin #56, October 2004.

Crisan LS, Steidl ET, Rivera-Alsina ME. Acute hyperlipidemic pancreatitis in pregnancy. *Am J Obstet Gynecol* 2008;198:e1–3.

Glantz A, Marschall HU, Lammert F, Mattsson LA. Intrahepatic cholestasis of pregnancy: a randomized controlled trial comparing dexamethasone and ursodeoxycholic acid. *Hepatology* 2005;42:1399–405.

Guntupalli SR, Steingrub J. Hepatic disease and pregnancy: an overview of diagnosis and management. *Crit Care Med* 2005;33(10 Supple):S332–9.

Kayatas SE, Eser M, Cam C, *et al.* Acute pancreatitis associated with hypertriglyceridemia: a life-threatening complication. *Arch Gynecol Obstet* 2009 Aug 6. [Epub ahead of print]

Ko H, Yoshida EM. Acute fatty liver of pregnancy. *Can J Gastroenterol* 2006;20(1):25–30.

Moldenhauer JS, O'Brien JM, Barton JR, *et al.* Acute fatty liver of pregnancy associated with pancreatitis: a life-threatening complication. *Am JObstet Gynecol* 2004;190:502–5.

Petrov MS, Zagainov VE. Influence of enteral versus parenteral nutrition on blood glucose control in acute pancreatitis: a systematic review. *Clin Nutr* 2007;26:514–23.

Tang SJ, Mayo MJ, Rodriguez-Frias E, *et al.* Safety and utility of ERCP during pregnancy. *Gastrointest Endosc* 2009;69(3):453–61.

PROTOCOL 44

Mastitis

Wendy F. Hansen

Department of Obstetrics and Gynecology, University of Kentucky, Lexington, KY, USA

Clinical significance

Lactation is the secretion of immunologically active, high-energy milk from the mammary glands and is one of the defining characteristics of all mammals. The last decade has seen a significant increase in the number of women choosing to breastfeed their infants. This has largely been the result of a growing body of evidence and an increased awareness of the benefits of breastfeeding for an infant. Healthy People 2010, a national prevention initiative to improve the health of all Americans, had set the national goal for the percentage of women breastfeeding early post-partum to 75% (1998 baseline 64%).[1] In October 2008 the Centers for Disease Control, using data from the National Immunization Survey, published statistics describing breastfeeding practices in the United States.[2] Of children born in 2005, 74% were initially breastfed, whereas 43% were breastfed at 6 months (32% exclusive) and 21% at 12 months (12% exclusive). Another CDC report using data from the Pediatric Nutrition Surveillance System published their 2007 statistics on breastfeeding of nearly 8 million low-income children.[3] Their report on breastfeeding is not as optimistic, showing 59.8% ever breastfed, 25.4% at least 6 months and 17.6% for at least 12 months. Although short of the Healthy People 2010 goal, both reports show significant increases for all indicators of breastfeeding. Accompanying this increase in breastfeeding is a natural increase in the number of women presenting to healthcare providers with symptoms and signs of mastitis.

Although mastitis can occur at any time, the incidence of mastitis is highest in the first few weeks postpartum with 74–95% of cases occurring in the first 3 months. Recent data from two large prospective cohorts of breastfeeding women suggest that the incidence rates range from 9.5% to 20%. The first study followed 1075 breastfeeding women

Protocols for High-Risk Pregnancies, 5th edition. Edited by J.T. Queenan, J.C. Hobbins and C.Y. Spong. © 2010 Blackwell Publishing Ltd.

in New Zealand for 6 months and found a 20% incidence.[4] The second study followed 946 women from Michigan and Nebraska until they stopped breastfeeding. Mastitis occurred in 9.5%.[5] The two-fold difference in incidence can be accounted for in part by differences in case definition.

These same studies found a history of mastitis with a previous child to be the most significant risk factor for development of mastitis, challenging the long-held belief that primiparity and inexperience are actual risk factors. Other identified risk factors include: blocked duct, cracked nipples, use of creams on nipples (papaya cream in New Zealand and an antifungal nipple cream in the United States), and the use of a manual breast pump. (Women with sore or cracked nipples would more likely use creams.) Sociodemographic factors do not seem to play a significant role in the risk for mastitis. The role of mother/infant skin and nasal bacterial colonization in the development of mastitis has not been well studied.

Pathophysiology

Mastitis is an acute inflammation of the connective tissue of the mammary gland: a mammary cellulitis. Traditional teaching holds that nipple trauma allows the portal of entry for microorganisms and that inadequate emptying causes milk stasis, allowing a medium for bacterial growth.

The microbiology of mastitis is changing. Although mastitis is a connective tissue infection, cultured breast milk has been used in identifying the pathogenic microorganism. *Staphylococcus aureus* accounts for most commonly identified pathogens (35–50% of isolates), along with coagulase-negative staphylococci, followed by group A and B hemolytic streptococci, *Escherchia coli*, *Hemophilus influenzae*, *Klebsiella* and *Bacteroides*. More recent experience has shown an emergence of community-acquired methicilin-resistant *S. aureus* (MRSA) in postpartum mastitis infections. A single-center case–control study from 1998 to 2005 found an increase in MRSA with 81% of MRSA cases occurring in 2005.[6] A second study from a single center from 1997 to 2005 found that community-acquired MRSA was most commonly associated with breast abscess and did not see the increase over time.[7] Interestingly, in the latter study, women with a breast abscess and MRSA-positive culture improved clinically with drainage and antibiotics not directed against MRSA (before culture results were known) suggesting that drainage of the abscess and emptying of the breast are essential to complete resolution. A case of toxic shock syndrome secondary to mastitis caused by MRSA was reported in Japan in 2001.[8]

Diagnosis

The diagnosis of mastitis is a clinical one. It most commonly presents with unilateral breast tenderness or pain, redness in an area that often demarcates the underlying lobe involved, fever (often greater than 38.9°C, 102°F), and flu-like symptoms.

Mastitis needs to be differentiated from other conditions. Simple breast engorgement usually presents gradually with bilateral generalized warmth, swelling and very firm breasts. There is no erythema or fever. With a plugged duct, a breast segment is swollen, firm and tender, but there is no evidence of infection. These patients should continue nursing frequently.

Treatment

Treatment goals include resolution of infection, amelioration of symptoms, prevention of complications and the continuation of breastfeeding. First-line clinical treatment for uncomplicated postpartum mastitis relies on an antibiotic with sensitivity to staphylococcal/streptococcal organisms along with continued emptying of the breast and supportive care.

There is widespread agreement that breastfeeding should be continued, and that proper drainage of the breast is essential to prevent complications. Mastitic milk is associated with increased concentrations of immune components and inflammatory molecules that resolve within 1 week of proper treatment.[9] Mastitic milk poses no risk to the infant.

Penicillinase-resistant penicillins and cephalosporins are commonly used: dicloxacillin 125 to 250 mg q 6 h, or cephalexin (Keflex®) 500 mg po q 6 h. In penicillin-allergic patients, erythromycin 250 mg q 6 h is another alternative. There are no data on duration but most prescribe for 7–10 days of treatment. Resolution of symptoms within 2 days was seen in 96% of women when treated with antibiotics and breast emptying in a Danish study.[10]

Symptoms can be treated with non-steroidal analgesics, fluids and rest. Follow-up is not necessary unless the mastitis persists longer than 48 hours or worsens despite treatment. Weaning should be delayed until the infection has cleared. For severely cracked or damaged nipples the use of a topical antibiotic ointment can aid healing and prevent mastitis (e.g., mupirocin/Bactroban® ointment).

Complications and follow-up

If mastitis signs and symptoms do not improve in 48 hours, the woman should be reexamined. A culture of the milk should be done and strong consideration should be given to the addition of an antibiotic for MRSA while awaiting culture results. Intravenous therapy (inpatient or outpatient) should be considered. If the physical examination is suggestive of an abscess (5–11% incidence), ultrasonography of the breast can be performed for confirmation. Traditionally, incision and drainage has been the recommended treatment. Recently, successful ultrasonographic guidance with percutaneous catheter drainage has been described. Culture of the abscess material can potentially guide antibiotic treatment. Episodes of recurrent mastitis warrant repeated therapy and continuation of nursing/pumping (emptying) the breast. A referral to a lactation consultant can be beneficial.

Conclusion

Mastitis is a common complication of breastfeeding and one that virtually all healthcare providers will encounter. The diagnosis is clinical and most will respond promptly to penicillinase-resistant penicillin or cephalosporin. If the clinical response is not prompt, reexamination is necessary with concern for MRSA or development of a breast abscess. Abscess requires incision and drainage and continued emptying of the breast by either suckling or pumping. Consultation should be strongly considered for complicated cases.

References

1 Centers for Disease Control and Prevention and Health Resources and Services Administration. *Healthy People 2010*, Protocol 16: Maternal, infant, and child health (http://healthypeople.gov/).

2 Centers for Disease Control and Prevention Department of Health and Human Services. Breastfeeding among US children born 1999–2005. *CDC National Immunization Survey. 2008* (http://www.cdc.gov/breastfeeding/data/NIS_data/index.htm).

3 Polhamus B, Dalenius K, Borland E, Smith B, Grummer-Strawn L. *Pediatric Nutrition Surveillance 2006 Report*. Atlanta: US Department of Health and Human Services, Centers for Disease Control and Prevention; 2007. (http://www.cdc.gov/nccdphp/dnpa/pednss.htm).

4 Kinlay J, O'Connell D, Kinlay S. Risk factors for mastitis in breastfeeding women: results of a prospective cohort study. *Aust NZ J Publ Hlth* 2001;25:115–20.

5 Foxman B, D'arcy H, Gillespie B, Bobo J, Schwartz K. Lactation mastitis: occurrence and medical management among 946 breastfeeding women in the United States. *Am J Epidemiol* 2002;155:103–14.

6 Reddy P, Qi C, Zembower T, Noskin GA, Bolon M. Postpartum mastitis and community acquired methicillin-resistant *Staphylococcus aureus*. *Emerg Infect Dis* 2007; 13(2):298–301.

7 Stafford I, Hernandez J, Laibl V, Sheffield J, Roberts S, Wendel G. Community-acquired methicillin-resistant *Staphylococcus aureus* among patients with puerperal mastitis requiring hospitalization. *Obstet Gynecol* 2008;112:533–7.

8 Fujiwara Y, Endo S. A case of toxic shock syndrome secondary to mastitis caused by methicillin-resistant *Staphylococcus aureus*. *Kansenshogaku Zasshi* 2001;75:898–903.

9 Buescher E, Hair P. Human milk anti-inflammatory component contents during acute mastitis. *Cell Immunol* 2001;210:87–95.

10 Thomsen AC, Espersen T, Maigaard S. Course and treatment of milk stasis, non-infectious inflammation of the breast, and infectious mastitis in nursing women. *Am J Obstet Gynecol* 1984;149:492–5.

PART 5
Obstetric Problems

PROTOCOL 45

First Trimester Vaginal Bleeding

Marsha Wheeler

Department of Obstetrics & Gynecology, University of Colorado Denver, Health Sciences Center, Denver, CO, USA

The most common emergency in the first trimester is vaginal bleeding. It accounts for 1–2% of all emergency room visits. As many as 15–25% of pregnant women have vaginal bleeding. Half will have a pregnancy loss and half will have a normal pregnancy; 50–60% of early losses are from chromosomal abnormalities. The differential diagnosis of first trimester vaginal bleeding includes spontaneous abortions, ectopic pregnancies and gestational trophoblastic disease. It is important to make a diagnosis because ectopic pregnancy is a leading cause of maternal mortality.

Evaluation of the pregnant patient with vaginal bleeding

When a reproductive-age female presents with vaginal bleeding, the following evaluation should be performed.

1 Obtain vital signs.

2 Obtain a menstrual, gynecological, sexual and birth control history.

3 Perform a physical examination including a speculum examination to evaluate for lacerations, cervical lesions, uterine size, adnexal masses, abdominal tenderness and peritoneal signs.

4 If the patient has amenorrhea then a pregnancy test should be obtained starting with a urine test and proceeding to a quantitative serum hCG if indicated.

5 If the pregnancy test is positive and you are concerned about an ectopic pregnancy, pelvic ultrasonography should be performed including a transvaginal examination. The ultrasound is to determine the location and type of the pregnancy.

6 If the pregnancy test is positive and the findings are consistent with a threatened abortion of at least 6 weeks' gestational age in a Rh-negative patient, give Rh immune globulin (Rhogam).

Protocols for High-Risk Pregnancies, 5th edition. Edited by J.T. Queenan, J.C. Hobbins and C.Y. Spong. © 2010 Blackwell Publishing Ltd.

Diagnosis

When a patient presents with vaginal bleeding, the history and physical examination along with an hCG test and ultrasonography will help differentiate between an intrauterine pregnancy, pregnancy failure, ectopic pregnancy or a hydatidiform mole.

Viable intrauterine pregnancy

The most common diagnosis in a patient with a positive pregnancy test and vaginal bleeding is a threatened abortion. Once a positive pregnancy test is obtained, ultrasonography and serial HCG values can be used to make a diagnosis of an intrauterine pregnancy. If a patient on post-conception day of 33–36 has a fetal heart rate, gestational sac size of greater than equal to 12, or a yolk sac of 2 to 6 mm, the odds of an ongoing pregnancy are over 90%. An older study gave a likelihood of continuing the pregnancy of between 90% and 97% if ultrasonography shows an intrauterine pregnancy over 7 weeks with a heart rate over 90. Prognosis improves with increasing gestational age, but is worse with increasing maternal age, subchorionic hematomas, low fetal heart rate and the increasing severity of the vaginal bleeding. Subchorionic hematomas are associated with operative vaginal deliveries, cesarean deliveries, hypertension, preeclampia, abruptions, preterm deliveries, growth restriction, fetal distress and neonatal intensive care unit admissions. Table 45.1 outlines the adverse pregnancy outcomes with first trimester vaginal bleeding.

Management should be conservative. Bed rest is usually recommended but poorly supported by the literature. Vaginal progestin therapy has not been shown to improve outcomes. A Cochrane review in 2007 included two trials that looked at vaginal progesterone compared to placebo in reducing the risk of miscarriage. The meta-analysis showed no improvement with

Table 45.1 Adverse pregnancy outcomes with first trimester vaginal bleeding

Vaginal bleeding	Heavy Odds ratio	Light Odds ratio
Spontaneous loss <24 weeks	4.2	2.5
Cesarean delivery	1.4	1.1
Preeclampsia	1.1	1.5
Preterm delivery	3.0	1.3
Placental abruption	3.6	1.6
Premature rupture of membranes	3.2	1.3
Fetal growth restriction	2.6	1.4

threatened abortions (relative risk 0.49; 95% confidence interval 0.17–1.30). The safety of progestins in the first trimester is not known.

Early pregnancy failure

The diagnosis of pregnancy failure is made when a normal pregnancy cannot be demonstrated. Several parameters are used to identify a pregnancy that is not progressing normally. These parameters involve ultrasonography, dating and hCG levels.

1 95% of the time a gestational sac should be visualized at 33.5 days with transvaginal ultrasonography.
2 95% of the time fetal cardiac activity should be seen at 44.5 days with transvaginal ultrasonography.
3 In a normal pregnancy the serum hCG levels increase by 66% in 48 hours.
4 An intrauterine gestational sac should be visualized by transvaginal ultrasonography between 1,000 and 2,000 mIU/mL IRP.
5 Embryonic cardiac activity should be seen with a crown rump of 5 mm.
6 A mean gestational sac diameter (MSD) of 8 mm or more without a yolk sac and MSD of 16 mm or more without an embryo are predictors of a non-viable pregnancy.
7 A difference of <5 mm of the MSD and the CRL carries an 80% risk of a spontaneous abortion.
8 A normal gestational sac grows 1 mm/day.

These landmarks can be used with the serial hCG measurements to determine if a pregnancy is non-viable. Once the diagnosis is made a management plan can be discussed. It could involve a surgical dilation and curettage, expectant management, or medical management involving misoprostol. The differences in these three management approaches have been studied. Medical management with misoprotol is felt to be effective, safe and cost effective.

Ectopic pregnancy

Ectopic pregnancies account for 2% of all pregnancies, but are the most common cause of pregnancy-related death in the first trimester. Transvaginal ultrasonography is very helpful in patients with a concern for an ectopic pregnancy. The failure to visualize an intrauterine gestational sac on transvaginal ultrasonography with an hCG >1,000 mIU/mL has a positive predictive value of 86% and specificity of 93% for ectopic pregnancy. Other helpful ultrasonographic findings are abnormal complex adnexal masses and adnexal gestational sacs with or without embryos. A false-negative diagnosis can result from a thick decidual reaction called a pseudogestational sac that mimics an intrauterine pregnancy.

If diagnosis cannot be made by ultrasonography then a repeat hCG in 48 hours can be used. The hCG level should increase by 66%. If the serum hCG is rising and an intrauterine pregnancy cannot be identified, then a ectopic pregnancy is likely. The diagnosis of an intrauterine pregnancy and extrauterine pregnancy (heterotopic pregnancy) is very rare except with artificial reproductive technologies (ART). Patients with heterotropic pregnancies are at greater risk for hypovolemic shock and requiring blood transfusions, so this diagnosis should be considered in patients who have had ART. Treatment of an ectopic pregnancy can be done medically with methotrexate, or surgically, usually via laparoscopy.

Molar pregnancy

The diagnosis of a complete mole can be made by identifying a characteristic ultrasonographic pattern. The typical mole is an echogenic mass (commonly called a snowstorm) in the uterine cavity without evidence of an embryo. The ultrasonographic image in the first trimester may be atypical and more similar to a non-viable pregnancy. HCG levels may be helpful. The diagnosis of a partial mole can be a challenge since a gestational sac and embryo are present. The placenta is usually abnormal with multiple cystic spaces and the fetus is growth restricted. A karyotype analysis may reveal a triploid conception. Management involves evacuation of the uterus after staging has been evaluated.

Conclusion

Using a physical examination, history, hCG level and ultrasonography, a physician can determine the etiology of first trimester vaginal bleeding. The appropriate management plan can be started and the patient's care can be tailored to her needs. The complications associated with first trimester bleeding that impact maternal mortality and morbidity can be minimized.

PROTOCOL 46

Cervical Insufficiency

John Owen

Department of Obstetrics and Gynecology, Division of Maternal-Fetal Medicine, University of Alabama at Birmingham, Birmingham, AL, USA

Introduction

Traditional teaching depicted the cervix as competent or incompetent; however, current evidence suggests that, analogous to other biological processes, cervical competence functions on a continuum of reproductive performance.[1] Although some women whose history suggests a cervical factor actually have tangible evidence of poor cervical integrity, most women with a clinical diagnosis of cervical insufficiency have ostensibly normal cervical anatomy. In a biological model of cervical competence as a continuum, a poor obstetric history from a primary cervical component more likely results from a process of *premature cervical ripening* (in the absence of clinical labor or chorioamnion rupture) due to one or a combination of underlying factors, including subclinical infection, local inflammation, hormonal effects or genetic predisposition. If and when the mechanical (and secondarily, the immunological) integrity of the cervix is compromised, other pathways to prematurity may be stimulated, appearing clinically as the preterm birth syndrome.[2]

The term 'cervical insufficiency' first appeared in the *Lancet* in 1865; however, because of the pejorative connotations, 'insufficiency' has now replaced 'incompetence'. Yet, the contemporary concept was not widely accepted until nearly a century later when two investigators (McDonald and Shirodkar) independently described interval repair of anatomic cervical defects associated with an obstetric history of recurrent spontaneous mid-trimester birth. In spite of its wide application, the literature on cerclage for the treatment of cervical insufficiency has largely been a story of surgical techniques to correct anatomic disruption of the internal os in women who had experienced recurrent painless dilation and mid-trimester birth. Evidence-based guidelines for many aspects of the

Protocols for High-Risk Pregnancies, 5th edition. Edited by J.T. Queenan, J.C. Hobbins and C.Y. Spong. © 2010 Blackwell Publishing Ltd.

diagnosis and management are still lacking; randomized trials were rarely performed prior to the 1980s. Cervical insufficiency is customarily a clinical diagnosis, made retrospectively after poor obstetric outcomes have occurred (or occasionally are in acute evolution). Reasonably, obstetricians have sought prospective and more objective diagnostic criteria, coupled with an effective intervention.

Diagnosis of cervical insufficiency

A clinical diagnosis

Clinical diagnosis of cervical insufficiency is considered in women with recurrent painless dilation and spontaneous mid-trimester birth, often of a live-born who quickly succumbs to extreme prematurity. Since there are few, if any, proven or even practical objective criteria (other than the rare gross cervical malformation), a careful review of the history and past obstetric records is essential. In many instances the records are unavailable or incomplete, and many women are unable to provide an accurate history. Even with excellent records and a reliable history, clinicians might have divergent opinions about the diagnosis, save for the most classic circumstances. Confounding factors in the history or physical examination might either support or refute the diagnosis, depending on their perceived importance. Clearly the physician managing a patient who has a spontaneous mid-trimester birth is in the optimal position to document the events and findings and to further assess whether clinical criteria for cervical insufficiency were present (e.g. hour-glassing membranes). However, because the preterm birth syndrome may involve other anatomic components, namely the chorioamnion and uterus, it should not be surprising that some women with cervical insufficiency have antecedent chorioamnion rupture or clinically apparent uterine activity. Vaginal bleeding may occur with cervical dilation, although the diagnosis of placental abruption should direct one away from cervical insufficiency. Acute chorioamnionitis might also contraindicate the diagnosis of insufficiency; however, if premature cervical ripening and subacute dilation caused loss of the mucus plug and compromised the normal immunological barrier between the vaginal flora and chorioamnion, intrauterine infection may simply be the culminating clinical event.[3] Other causes of mid-trimester loss may be sought, and some consider cervical insufficiency to be a diagnosis of exclusion. The extent to which other causes should be ruled out has never been completely defined; however, antiphospholipid syndrome and fetal aneuploidy, for example, are well-characterized causes of mid-trimester fetal loss.

Physical examination

Physical examination criteria are based primarily on case series and comparative studies of women who present with 'silent' cervical dilation of at least 2 cm with visible membranes at or beyond the internal os on a speculum examination. In most cases appreciable cervical length has been maintained and little effacement is recognized. At times clinicians may choose to follow selected patients with serial pelvic examinations hoping to detect earlier changes on palpation which may also suggest the diagnosis. Common accompanying symptoms may include a sensation of pelvic pressure, vaginal discharge, urinary frequency and the absence of regular painful contractions. Termed *acute cervical insufficiency* by most investigators, it provides insight into the natural history of this condition.

Sonography

Numerous investigators have suggested that cervical insufficiency may be diagnosed with vaginal sonography, and clearly there is a relationship between cervical length, as determined with a vaginal probe and reproductive performance.[4] These investigations have supported the concept of cervical *competence* as a continuum. Various sonographic findings, including shortened cervical length, 'funneling' at the internal os and dynamic responses to fundal pressure (or spontaneously occurring dynamic changes) have been used to support the diagnosis of cervical insufficiency and to select patients for treatment, usually cerclage. Since the possible additive effects of funneling and dynamic changes have been shown to be equivocal (when cervical length is accounted for), the most commonly cited criterion is a mid-trimester cervical length <25mm, likely chosen because it represented the lower 10th percentile in a large population of United States gravidas.[4] That this finding was actually a poor predictor of preterm birth (only 18% of low-risk, unselected women delivered <35weeks) and also implied that as many as 10% of the gravid population might be given a diagnosis of insufficiency, was largely overlooked.

However, it is also well documented that women with progressively shorter cervical lengths have correspondingly higher rates of preterm birth, but rarely develop complete cervical dilation as described in the next section. Even more compelling is the relationship between obstetric history and cervical length, for the predictive accuracy of cervical length assessment for spontaneous preterm birth is appreciably higher in women with a history of a prior spontaneous preterm birth, especially an early birth <34weeks.[5] Thus, defining appropriate diagnostic criteria for the sonographic diagnosis of insufficiency (and application of an effective intervention) has been extremely problematic, and it is likely that many women have inappropriately been given this diagnosis and received an ineffective therapy.

Patient selection for cerclage

History-indicated (prophylactic) cerclage

Women who meet criteria for the clinical diagnosis of cervical insufficiency should be counseled regarding the risks and benefits of cerclage. Although no randomized trials have been performed in women with a typical history, numerous case series using historic control populations have been summarized[6,7] and suggest that, prior to cerclage, perinatal survival ranged from 7% to 50% but that, with cerclage, survival increased to a range of from 63% to 89%. Since older series used a metric of perinatal survival and not birth gestational age, the effect on pregnancy prolongation and neonatal morbidities was never properly assessed. Associated risks appear to be low, but include those associated with anesthesia; generally a regional technique is chosen. Contraindications include active cervicitis, certain fetal problems (e.g., anomaly, oligohydramnios) and hemorrhage. Appropriately selected candidates generally undergo surgery at around 14 weeks after sonographic confirmation of a normal fetus and confirmation of negative screening results for known cervical pathogens (e.g., gonorrhea, Chlamydia).

Physical-examination-indicated (emergent) cerclage

The use of cerclage in the clinical setting of acute cervical insufficiency has been investigated through the use of both case series (absent control populations) and retrospective cohort studies where pregnancy outcomes following the uncontrolled use of cerclage were compared to the outcomes of women with similar examination findings who did not undergo surgery and were usually managed expectantly with bed rest. Only one small randomized trial of cerclage for acute cervical insufficiency has been published comprising 23 patients. Collectively, these reports demonstrate a measurable benefit from the use of emergent cerclage using pregnancy prolongation and neonatal morbidity outcomes.

Women who present with prolapsing membranes at or beyond the external os represent an extraordinarily high-risk and surgically challenging group. Various techniques have been suggested to reduce the membranes at surgery and include combinations of Trendelenberg positioning, therapeutic amnioreduction, uterine relaxants and bladder filling as well as manual replacement and intraoperative support using a 30–60 mL Foley catheter balloon. These techniques are used empirically and have not been systematically compared to determine the best strategy. As expected, increasing amounts of dilation and effacement greatly increase the surgical complexity and may even cause the obstetrician to abandon the surgery; iatrogenic membrane rupture is the most common serious complication. Many clinicians also recommend a preoperative observation period of 12–24 hours to rule out active clinical infection and preterm labor, well-known contraindications to cerclage. Recently the potential utility of analyzing amniotic fluid harvested in women with acute cervical insufficiency has been investigated. It is clear that a subgroup of these women will have biochemical evidence of inflammation and infection, but whether these results can be used to improve perinatal outcomes has not been demonstrated. Thus, amniotic fluid analysis remains largely investigational.

Ultrasound-indicated (rescue or urgent) cerclage

As of this writing, five randomized trials of cerclage in women with shortened cervical length have been published. These were performed after cohort series investigated cerclage in similar populations; clinicians hoping to derive guidance in this area were understandably puzzled by contradictory findings of efficacy. The first was a small trial from the Netherlands comprising only 35 women.[8] Enrollment was limited to gravidas whose history or symptoms suggested cervical insufficiency and who had a cervical length <25mm. Such patients are uncommonly encountered in clinical practice. The investigators showed a marked reduction in preterm birth <35 weeks' gestation with McDonald cerclage: 0% vs 44% in the no-cerclage group. A large multinational European trial[9] studied unselected, but generally low-risk women with a cervical length ≤15mm and found a small, but insignificant reduction in preterm birth <33 weeks following Shirodkar cerclage. Finally, two trials in the United States[10,11] enrolled women with various risk factors and shortened cervical length <25mm or a funnel size >25% of the canal length. These investigators observed no benefit from McDonald cerclage and nearly equivalent rates of preterm birth in the cerclage and no-cerclage groups.

Of appreciable interest was a subsequent patient-level meta-analysis of these four trials which demonstrated that cerclage benefit was concentrated in women with singletons and a prior preterm birth.[12] These findings corroborate the conclusions of a multinational trial performed from 1983 to 1988 and published in 1993;[13] herein, nearly 1300 women whose managing physicians were 'uncertain' if cerclage was indicated on the basis of their history were recruited. This study predated the use of high-resolution vaginal sonography and cervical length assessment. While the study population was inevitably heterogeneous, secondary analysis demonstrated that only the subgroup of women with at least three prior preterm births or mid-trimester losses had a significant benefit from cerclage: the rate of preterm birth was approximately 50% lower in the cerclage group. Thus, the clinical significance of obstetric history in selecting women for cerclage clearly required additional investigation.

In the fifth, recently completed[14] investigators sought to confirm the importance of obstetric history. This was the largest trial to date of (McDonald) cerclage for shortened cervical length and included 302 women with singletons and the risk factor of at least one prior spontaneous preterm birth <34 weeks. Using a cervical length cutoff <25mm, preterm birth <35 weeks was lower in the cerclage group, 32% vs 42% in the no-cerclage group. While this difference was not statistically significant, previable birth and perinatal mortality were significantly lower in the cerclage group. Importantly, there was significant interaction between cervical length at randomization and cerclage efficacy: women whose cervical length was <15mm enjoyed a marked benefit from cerclage. Thus, the 'optimal' cervical length to consider cerclage could not be strictly defined, but like the continuum of cervical competence, it is not surprising that a continuum of cerclage *efficacy* was demonstrated. In summary, the clinical significance of obstetric history in selecting women for cerclage seems irrefutable, and cervical ultrasound can now be recommended to follow high-risk women who have had a prior spontaneous preterm birth <34 weeks.

Can cervical ultrasonography be used to avoid cerclage?

In a systematic review of studies that included women with suspected cervical insufficiency, pregnancy outcomes of ultrasound-indicated versus history-indicated cerclage were compared.[15] Five of the six reports selected for the review showed similar pregnancy outcomes (spontaneous preterm birth <24 weeks' gestation) between the ultrasound-indicated and the history-indicated cerclage groups. However, in one prospective cohort study, preterm birth was significantly *lower* in the ultrasound-indicated group. The authors concluded that using ultrasound-measured shortened cervical length to select women with suspected cervical insufficiency for cerclage reduces cerclage rates, but yields pregnancy outcomes similar to cases where cerclage was placed on the basis of clinical suspicion alone. Based on this systematic review, women with suspected, but non-classic cervical insufficiency may undergo mid-trimester transvaginal cervical length assessment to optimize surgical candidate selection.

Cerclage technique

McDonald cerclage is favored by many obstetricians because of its simplicity in placement (and removal in anticipation of vaginal birth). Under regional anesthesia and with adequate visualization of the cervix, a non-absorbable suture is placed in a circumferential pattern as close as possible to the bladder reflection anterior and just below the reflection of rectum posterior.

Though originally described with but four needle insertions, the actual number of penetrations may vary depending on the size of the ectocervix and the penetration depth of the curved needle. Our practice is to leave as little suture as possible exposed on the ectocervix and take the next bite of tissue close to the exit point of the previous. Choice of suture varies but includes Mersilene and Prolene. Some prefer Mersilene 0.5 mm tape, which is technically more difficult to place, but is felt to have some theoretic advantages. Others recommend two separate sutures to spread the tension over a wider area. No comparative studies of these preferences have been performed. We generally place one suture of #1 Merseline, followed by another, if it is believed that the second stitch can be placed above the first, expanding the supported length of the canal. Knot placement is not important, but anterior knots are easier to grasp and remove, particularly if the suture above the knot is cut long.

The Shirodkar cerclage also has strong proponents, although comparative studies have not confirmed its superiority. This technique has the theoretic advantage of placing the Mersilene tape higher along the cervical canal. Special training and experience are required. The initial step is similar to one used in vaginal hysterectomy whereby the bladder and rectum are dissected off the cervix and displaced upward. An Allis clamp grasps and stabilizes the cervical tissue at 3 and 6 o'clock. Then the tape, threaded on an aneurysm needle, is placed medial to the clamp and buried with its securing knot with a separate line of suture under the mucosal edges left from the anterior and posterior dissection. Not surprisingly, removal of a Shirodkar stitch can be challenging and has been associated with an increased risk of cesarean delivery.

Benson originally described an abdominal technique for women whose anatomy prohibited a vaginal approach. Women with cervical hypoplasia, prior cone or large LEEP biopsies or extensive cervical damage from failed cerclage or birth trauma may be selected for this procedure. An evolving indication is prior failed transvaginal cerclage.[16] Originally placed via laparotomy, these have been successfully placed and removed with laparoscopy. Similarly, most have been placed in the first trimester, after viability has been established, although interval placement has also been reported. Appropriate candidate selection and placement are generally relegated to specialty centers.

Cerclage removal

In the absence of urgent indications, transvaginal cerclage is removed at term, generally 37 weeks' gestation in anticipation of vaginal birth. The McDonald stitch can generally be removed as an outpatient, but some bleeding may occur and can generally be managed with local pressure. Removal of a Shirodkar stitch usually involves tissue dissection and appreciable risk for bleeding; thus removal as an inpatient is preferred.

Urgent indications for preterm removal include labor, bleeding, non-reassuring fetal status and membrane rupture. Cervical change in the setting of painful contractions with cerclage in place may be more difficult to appreciate, but serial examination should confirm labor. If tocolytics are prescribed and ineffective, the suture should be removed to avoid cervical laceration. Bleeding at the suture line should in itself prompt removal with suspected labor.

Since many women who undergo cerclage are also at risk for developing other components of the preterm birth syndrome, in addition to spontaneous labor, premature membrane rupture (PROM) may also occur. Several series have confirmed that when the cerclage is removed on admission for preterm PROM, the risk of adverse perinatal outcomes is not higher than for those women with preterm PROM and no cerclage. Studies comparing cerclage retention and removal after preterm PROM have shown trends towards increased perinatal infection with retained cerclage; however, no individual study has had conclusive findings. Importantly, no study has found a significant benefit from cerclage retention, and one study documented increased neonatal death (largely due to infection) with cerclage retention. Thus, the weight of available evidence favors cerclage removal after preterm PROM. Whether cerclage should be empirically retained during corticosteroid administration to enhance fetal maturation with concurrent broad-spectrum antibiotic administration has been considered, but if this plan is chosen, the stitch should be removed after 24–48 hours.

Adjunctive therapies

Commonly recommended are perioperative *prophylactic* antibiotics and tocolytics, since active genital infection and labor are contraindications. Published series and trial suggest that investigators are increasingly likely to prescribe prophylaxis in women undergoing ultrasound-indicated and especially physical-examination indicated procedures, as compared to history-indicated cases. Lack of clinical evidence confirming that these pharmacological adjuncts improve perinatal outcomes suggests that these recommendations are largely empiric. We do recommend screening for and treating known cervical pathogens prior to placing history-indicated and ultrasound-indicated stitches. A short course of indomethacin is also used in women with postoperative uterine activity.

The use of progesterone congeners, most commonly 17α-hydroxy-progesterone caproate has been widely investigated for the prevention of recurrent preterm birth. Since many women who are candidates for cerclage have delivered a prior preterm infant, adjunctive administration of progesterone may be recommended. Less clear and in need of further investigation is whether there is an interaction between progesterone and cerclage in selected patients, rendering progesterone ineffective or possibly heightening its efficacy. Also in need of further investigation is the use of vaginal pessary for preterm birth prevention in women with suspected cervical insufficiency.

Widely recommended, bed rest has not been demonstrated to improve pregnancy outcomes for numerous types of pregnancy conditions. Yet it continues to be empirically used in women with cervical insufficiency. Some clinicians have even justified cerclage placement by suggesting that this mechanical support permits women to expand their physical activities; evidence for this is also absent. The recommendation for post-cerclage pelvic rest seems more practical, leaving activity recommendations individualized and based on maternal symptoms and pelvic findings.

Summary

Contemporary lines of evidence tell us that cervical insufficiency is a poorly defined entity, lacking objective and reproducible criteria. It may be more effectively conceptualized as one factor in the complex syndrome of spontaneous preterm birth. Deciding whether an individual patient has a significant (and treatable) component of insufficiency requires significant clinical judgment. Herein we have presented (as currently available) evidence-based guidelines for the selection of patients who would reasonably benefit from cerclage.

References

1 Iams JD, Johnson FF, Sonek J, Sachs L, Gebauer C, Samuels P. Cervical competence as a continuum: A study of ultrasonographic cervical length and obstetric performance. *Am J Obstet Gynecol* 1995;172:1097–106.
2 Romero R, Espinoza J, Kusanovic JP, *et al.* The preterm parturition syndrome. *BJOG*. 2006 Dec;113 Suppl 3:17–42.
3 Jones G. The weak cervix: failing to keep the baby in or infection out? *Br J Obstet Gynaecol* 1998;105:1214–15.
4 Iams JD, Goldenberg RL, Meis PJ, Mercer BM, Moawad A, Das A, Thom E, McNellis D, Copper RL, Johnson F, Roberts JM for the National Institute of Child Health and Human Development Maternal Fetal Medicine Unit Network. The length of the cervix and the risk of spontaneous premature delivery. *N Engl J Med* 1996;334:567–72.
5 Owen J, Yost N, Berghella V, Thom E, Swain M, Dildy GA, Miodovnik M, Langer D, Sibai BM, McNellis D for the National Institute for Child Health and Human

Development Maternal Fetal Medicine Unit Network. Mid-trimester endovaginal sonography in women at high risk for spontaneous preterm birth. *JAMA* 2001;286:1340–8.

6 Cousins LM. Cervical incompetence 1980: a time for reappraisal. *Clin Obstet Gynecol* 1980;23:467–79.

7 Branch DW. Operations for cervical incompetence. *Clin Obstet Gynecol* 1986; 29:240–54.

8 Althuisius SM, Dekker GA, Hummel P, Bekedam DJ, van Geijn HP. Final results of the cervical incompetence prevention randomized cerclage trial (CIPRACT): therapeutic cerclage with bed rest versus bed rest alone. *Am J Obstet Gynecol* 2001;185:1106–12.

9 To MS, Alfirevic Z, Heath VCF, Cicero S, Cacho AM, Williamson PR, Nicolaides KH on behalf of the Fetal Medicine Foundation Second Trimester Screening Group. Cervical cerclage for prevention of preterm delivery in women with short cervix: randomised controlled trial. *Lancet* 2004;363:1849–53.

10 Rust OA, Atlas RO, Reed J, van Gaalen J, Balducci J. Revisiting the short cervix detected by transvaginal ultrasound in the second trimester: Why cerclage may not help. *Am J Obstet Gynecol* 2001;185:1098–105.

11 Berghella V, Odibo AO, Tolosa JE. Cerclage for prevention of preterm birth in women with a short cervix found on transvaginal ultrasound: a randomized trial. *Am J Obstet Gynecol* 2004;191:1311–17.

12 Berghella V, Odibo AO, To MS, Rust OA, Althuisius SM. cerclage for short cervix on ultrasonography, meta-analysis of trials using individual patient-level data. *Obstet Gynecol* 2005;106(1):181–9.

13 Anonymous. Final report of the Medical Research Council/Royal College of Obstetrics and Gynecology multicentre randomized trial of cervical cerclage. *Br J Obstet Gynaecol* 1993;100:516–23.

14 Owen J, Hankins G, Iams JD, *et al.* Multicenter randomized trial of cerclage for preterm birth prevention in high-risk women with shortened midtrimester cervical length. *Am J Obstet Gynecol* 2009;201:375.e1–8.

15 Blikman MJC, Le T, Bruinse HW, van der Heijden GJMG. Ultrasound-predicated versus history-predicated cerclage in women at risk of cervical insufficiency: a systematic review. *Obstet Gynecol Surv* 2008;63:803–12.

16 Debbs RH, Guilleremo ADV, Pearson S, Sehdev H, Marchiano D, Ludmir J. Transabdominal cerclage after comprehensive evaluation of women with previous unsuccessful transvaginal cerclage. *Am J Obstet Gynecol* 2007;197:317.e1–4.

PROTOCOL 47

Nausea and Vomiting

Gayle Olson
University of Texas Medical Branch, Galveston, TX, USA

Clinical significance

Approximately 75% of women experience some degree of nausea and vomiting during pregnancy. In addition, approximately 35% of gravidas with nausea and vomiting will consider their symptoms severe enough to limit activities of daily living. This disruption in quality of life further extends to loss of time at work, ineffectiveness at home or on the job and deterioration in relationships. The economic impact alone has been estimated in the $3000–17,000 range for women with mild to severe symptoms of nausea and vomiting of pregnancy (NVP) respectively.[1] Hyperemesis gravidarum (HG), typically described as vomiting, dehydration, acid–base disturbance, weight loss due to vomiting, ketonuria and electrolyte disturbances, is seen in no more than 2% of cases. Unfortunately, because NVP can be so common, symptoms and therefore treatment risk being minimized by both patients and healthcare providers, resulting in progression to more severe levels before therapy is initiated.[2]

Pathophysiology

A single etiology responsible for the pathophysiology of NVP has not been identified but many hypotheses have been proposed which include psychological factors, evolutionary adaptation, hormone alterations, infection and gastrointestinal tract dysfunction.[2] To date, data does not link a psychological alteration as a causal factor in NVP; however, women in the throes of severe NVP may experience anxiety or demoralization as a result of their infirmity.[3] Adaptive mechanisms preventing a woman from eating foods that could harm the fetus are as difficult to conceptualize as they would be to verify. Gastrointestinal motility is diminished by pregnancy, and gastric emptying time is prolonged. Further, *Helicobacter pylori* has

Protocols for High-Risk Pregnancies, 5th edition. Edited by J.T. Queenan, J.C. Hobbins and C.Y. Spong. © 2010 Blackwell Publishing Ltd.

been suggested as a factor in the etiology of NVP. Goldberg *et al.* reviewed 14 studies investigating the association between *H. pylori* and hyperemesis and though *H. pylori* did not appear to have a causal association with NVP/HG, when the organism was present the symptoms of NVP were more severe. In limited examples, treatment for *H. pylori* during pregnancy has hastened resolution of symptoms.[4]

Finally, increased estrogen and human chorionic gonadotropin (hCG) concentrations during pregnancy have been shown to be associated with nausea and vomiting in a dose-dependent fashion.[2]

Risk factors for NVP include an increased placental mass as seen with molar gestation or multiple gestations, a family history or personal history of hyperemesis gravidarum, and a history of motion sickness or migraines. BMI had also been investigated as a risk factor for NVP. In a retrospective study, Cedergren *et al.* were able to demonstrate that women with BMI <20 (kg/m^2) were at increased risk for requiring the use of antiemetic drugs and hospitalization for NVP/HG compared to normal weight and obese women.[5]

Diagnosis

It is common for nausea to be most severe on arising; hence the term *morning sickness*. However, a number of pregnant women experience their most severe symptoms at other times of the day, and the failure of nausea to be restricted to the morning in no way invalidates the complaint.

In addition, other underlying conditions (Table 47.1) should be considered and excluded when symptoms of nausea and vomiting begin before 5 weeks, persist after 12 weeks, are accompanied by other complaints and are persistently severe in spite of adequate treatment. Symptoms and findings not associated with simple NVP include abdominal or epigastric pain, fever, headache, cough, goiter and an abnormal neurological examination.[2]

The disease along the entire spectrum of its presentation has been categorized according to severity, duration and early manifestations. The condition may be considered mild when nausea and vomiting occurs for less than 1 hour during the day and the vomiting and retching occurs only up to twice daily. When the symptoms persist for 6 hours or more with five or more episodes of vomiting and retching NVP may be considered severe. Hyperemesis gravidarum is at the most severe end of this spectrum and, in addition to nausea and vomiting, is further characterized by weight loss (≥5% of body weight), ketonuria, electrolyte disturbances, especially hypokalemia, and dehydration.

Scoring systems have been developed and validated by various investigators to assess the severity of nausea and vomiting (Rhodes score,

Table 47.1 Differential diagnosis of nausea and vomiting of pregnancy

Gastrointestinal conditions	Gastroenteritis
	Biliary tract disease
	Hepatitis
	Peptic ulcer disease
	Pancreatitis
	Appendicitis
Genitourinary tract conditions	Pyelonephritis
	Ovarian torsion
	Kidney stones
Metabolic disease	Diabetic ketoacidosis
	Hyperthyroidism
Neurological disorders	Pseudotumor cerebri
	Vestibular lesions
	Migraines
	Tumors of the central nervous system
	Drug toxicity or intolerance
	Psychological condition

Source: ACOG Practice Bulletin #52 *Nausea and Vomiting of Pregnancy.*

pregnancy-unique quantification of emesis and nausea (PUQE) and modified-PUQE). The PUQE and modified-PUQE were designed for use during pregnancy and are simplified when compared to the older 'gold standard' Rhodes system. All scoring systems were designed to provide objective measures to quantify symptoms to guide and compare drug therapy.[6,7]

In addition to assessing symptoms, the laboratory tests in Table 47.2 could be considered. This battery of tests may identify medical conditions confused with NVP but in most cases no cause other than pregnancy will be found. Thyroid function testing has not been included in this battery of tests. The structural homology of hCG and TSH contribute to the appearance of transient hyperthyroidism in early pregnancy. The transient hyperthyroidism of early pregnancy usually subsides by 18 weeks' gestation without further sequelae. Symptoms and/or laboratory testing suggestive of hyperthyroidism that predate the pregnancy are more likely to identify true thyroid disease; therefore, review of symptoms in these cases is most helpful in making the diagnosis.[8]

As mentioned above, women may experience anxiety and demoralization due to NVP. Demoralization, a normal response to illness, is characterized by sadness, fear, irritability, passive aggressive behavior and an active struggle with illness and should be distinguished from depression. An in-depth discussion with the patient can usually determine this distinction.[3]

Table 47.2 Laboratory evaluation

- Complete blood count
- Urinalysis or urine culture, or both
- Urine specific gravity, acetone, ketones
- Serology for hepatitis A, B and C
- Hepatic transaminases
- Serum acetone
- Serum electrolytes

Treatment

Treatment of NVP varies with the severity of the disease and can range between dietary/lifestyle modification, vitamin/herbal supplementation, antiemetic drug therapy and hospitalization. The initial therapy is generally non-pharmacological and includes increased rest and avoidance of foods or odors that trigger symptoms (perfumes, smoke, petroleum products). Adjustment in eating habits may include small, frequent snacks with a focus on bland and dry foods or foods high in protein. Spicy, fatty and acidic foods may need to be eliminated. High-protein meals have been shown to alleviate nausea and vomiting better than carbohydrate or fatty meals.

Acupressure has been used to alleviate symptoms of nausea and vomiting by applying pressure at the Neguian P6 acupoint. This point is located approximately 2 inches proximal to the wrist crease between the flexor carpi radialis and palmaris longus tendons.[9] Trials evaluating the efficacy of P6 acupressure for NVP have been difficult to blind, are underpowered by small sample size and thus unable to show benefit. Though benefit is difficult to demonstrate, acupressure continues to be low cost and no adverse effects have been documented.[10] Women with mild degrees of NVP who are highly motivated to try acupressure may possibly benefit without adverse effects.

Ginger root, a common spice and flavorer, has also been used for the treatment of NVP. Several randomized trials are now available suggesting benefit from the ingestion of ginger root for the reduction of nausea and vomiting. Most recently, Ozgoli *et al.* randomized women to ginger 250 mg four times a day for 4 days versus placebo. The groups were comparable for estimated gestational age, parity and degree of nausea and vomiting at the onset of the trial. Ginger users demonstrated an improvement in nausea (85% v 56%; $P < 0.01$) and a decrease in vomiting (50% versus 9%; $p < 0.05$). compared to the placebo group. No complications were reported.[11]

Vitamin therapy, specifically vitamin B_6 (pyridoxine) has been demonstrated as effective in randomized controlled trials, using the dosing schedule 10–25 mg orally every 8 hours.[10,12] Historically, vitamin B_6 when combined with the antihistamine doxylamine succinate proved a successful antiemetic. A single pill combining both of these medicines is no longer available in the United States; however, the separate products can be obtained over the counter.

Pharmacological agents (see Table 47.3) have also been used for successful treatment of NVP/hyperemesis. The most common categories for use are antihistamines, dopamine antagonists, phenothiazines and serotonin antagonists.

Treatment decisions for NVP must be based on numerous factors, including symptom severity, clinical consequences of treatment versus lack of treatment, and fetal safety. Treatment decisions must be individually based;

Table 47.3 Pharmacological agents for use in nausea and vomiting in pregnancy

Agent	Risk factor category
H₁ blockers	
Doxylamine (Unisom)	Unlisted
Dimenhydrinate (Dramamine)	B
Cetirizine (Zyrtec)	B
Meclizine (Antivert)	B
Hydroxyzine (Vistaril, Atarax)	C
Diphenhydramine (Benadryl)	B
Promethazine (Phenergan)	C
Anticholinergics	
Scopolamine	C
Dopamine antagonists	
Trimethobenzamide (Tigan)(Benzacot)	C
Metoclopramide (Reglan)	B
Butyrophenones	
Droperidol (Inapsine)	C
Haloperidol (Haldol)	C
Phenothiazines	
Prochlorperazine (Compazine)	C
Chlorpromazine (Thorazine)	C
Perphenazine (Trilafon)	C
Serotonin antagonist	
Ondansetron (Zofran)	B
Steroids	
Methylprednisolone	C

Adapted from ACOG Practice Bulletin # 52 *Nausea and Vomiting of Pregnancy*. Briggs GG, Freeman RK, Yaffe SJ (eds) *Drugs in Pregnancy and Lactation*, 6th edn. Baltimore, MD: Lippincott Williams & Wilkins, 2001.

however, treatment algorithms have been proposed to facilitate rational use of medicines (Fig. 47.1). For example, a general approach to treatment for NVP could follow this or a similar sequential pathway: Diet and lifestyle modification; vitamin B, 25 mg, three or four times daily plus doxylamine 12.5 mg three or four times a day; diphenhydramine 25–50 mg four times a day or meclizine 25 mg four times a day; prochlorperazine 10 mg

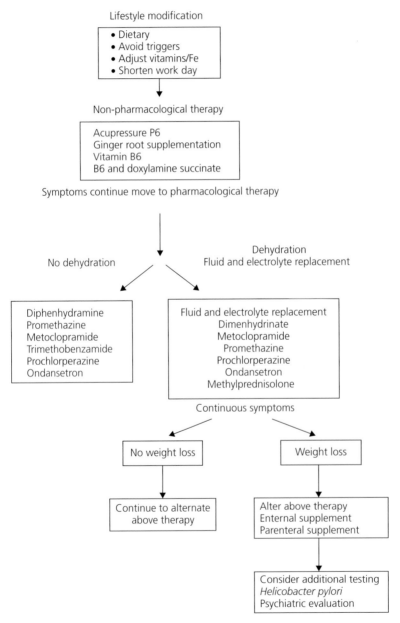

Figure 47.1 Treatment algorithm for nausea and vomiting in pregnancy.

four times a day or metoclopramide 10 mg three times a day; ondansetron 4–8 mg every 8 hours; methylprednisolone 16 mg every 8 hours for 3 days followed by a 2-week taper.[13,14]

Complications

Though rare, persistent vomiting over several weeks may result in a deficiency of vitamin B_1 (thiamin). Severe thiamin deficiency can further lead to Wernicke encephalopathy characterized by the classic triad of ophthalmoplegia, gait ataxia and mental confusion. Therefore, in the severest cases of NVP or HG, thiamin levels should be considered and treated if needed.[15]

In a population-based retrospective cohort study, Dodds *et al.* have shown that women who are diagnosed with HG and gain less than 7 kg during their pregnancy are more likely to have infants who are low birthweight, premature and have 5-minute Apgar scores less than 7 compared to women without HG or who gain more than 7 kg.[16]

Prevention

Women with previous NVP and/or hyperemesis may be at risk for similar occurrences in subsequent pregnancies. Studies suggest that multivitamin use at the time of conception may be associated with a reduction of pregnancy-related nausea and vomiting. It is reasonable, therefore, to advise a woman with a history of NVP to begin multiple vitamin supplementations prior to conception.

Conclusion

Nausea and vomiting during pregnancy affects up to 75% of pregnant women, becoming severe enough to inhibit activities of daily living and result in poor neonatal outcome. If treated early, there are a wide variety of modalities that can be successfully utilized to ameliorate this condition.

References

1 Attard CL, Kohli MA, Coleman SK, *et al.* The burden of illness of severe nausea and vomiting of pregnancy in the United States. *Am J Obstet Gynecol* 2002;186:S220–7.
2 American College of Obstetricians and Gynecologists. Nausea and vomiting of pregnancy. ACOG Practice Bulletin # 52. *Obstet Gynecol* 2004;103:803–15.

3 Kim DR, Connolly KR, Cristancho P, Zappone M, Weinrieb RM. Psychiatric consultation of patients with hyperemesis gravidarum. *Arch Women's Mental Hlth* 2009; 12:61–7.

4 Golberg D, Szilagyi A, Graves L. Hyperemesis gravidarum and *Helicobacter pylori* infection. *Obstet Gynecol* 2007;110:695–703.

5 Cedergren M, Brynhildsen J, Josefsson A, Sydsjö G. Hyperemesis gravidarum that requires hospitalization and the use of antiemetic drugs in relation to maternal body composition. *Am J Obstet Gynecol* 2008;198:412.e1–412.e5.

6 Koren G, Boskovic R, Hard M, Maltepe C, Navioz Y, Einarson A. Motherisk PUQE (pregnancy-unique quantification of emesis and nausea) scoring system for nausea and vomiting of pregnancy. *Am J Obstet Gynecol* 2002;186:228–31.

7 Lacasse A, Rey E, Ferreira E, Morin C, Bérard A. Validity of a modified pregnancy-unique quantification of emesis and nausea (PUQE). *J Obstet Gynaecol* 2008;198:71.e1–71.e7.

8 Caffrey TJ. Transient hyperthyroidism of hyperemesis gravidarum: a sheep in wolf's clothing. *J Am Bd Fam Pract* 2000;13:35–8.

9 Chen E, Flower A (eds). *Cross-Sectional Anatomy of Acupoints.* Edinburgh: Churchill Livingstone, 1995.

10 Jewell D, Young G. Interventions for nausea and vomiting in early pregnancy. Cochrane Database. 4: Available at: http://www.mrw.interscience.wiley.com/cochrane/clsysrev/articles/CD000145/frame.html.

11 Ozgoli G, Goli M, Simbar M. Effects of ginger capsules on pregnancy, nausea, and vomiting. *J Altern Complem Med* 2009;15:243–6.

12 Sahakian V, Rouse D, Sipes S, Rose N, Niebyl J. Vitamin B_6 is effective therapy for nausea and vomiting of pregnancy: a randomized, double-blind placebo-controlled study. *Obstet Gynecol* 1991;78:33–6.

13 Goodwin TM. Hyperemesis gravidarum. *Obstet Gynecol N Am* 2008;35:401–17.

14 Badell ML, Ramin SM, Smith JA. Treatment option for nausea and vomiting during pregnancy. *Pharmacol Ther* 2006;26:1273–87.

15 Gárdián G, Vörös E, Járdánházy T, Ungureán A, Vécsei L. Wernicke's encephalopathy induced by hyperemesis gravidarum. *Acta Neurol Scand* 1999;99:196–8.

16 Dodds L, Fell DB, Joseph KS, Allen VM, Butler B. Outcomes of pregnancies complicated by hyperemesis gravidarum. *Obstet Gynecol* 2006;107:285–92.

Missed Abortion and Antepartum Fetal Death

Robert M. Silver

Departement of Obstetrics & Gynecology, Division of Maternal-Fetal Medicine, University of Utah Health Sciences Center, Salt Lake City, UT, USA

Overview

The death of an advanced pregnancy is an extremely difficult medical and emotional challenge for clinicians and families. The problem is common, as pregnancy loss occurs in about 12% of clinically recognized pregnancies. Most of these are spontaneous abortions that happen early in gestation. However, approximately 3% of pregnancies result in fetal death. Thus, obstetric providers will care for many women with the condition. Missed abortion is a general term which refers to the presence of a non-viable pregnancy in utero prior to 20 weeks' gestation. Non-viable pregnancies after 20 weeks' gestation are traditionally referred to as stillbirths. It is more useful to distinguish between anembryonic pregnancy loss (gestational sac without an embryo – previously referred to as 'blighted ovum'), embryonic demise (embryo without cardiac activity at less than 10 weeks' gestation) and fetal demise (fetus without cardiac activity after 10 weeks' gestation). These terms refer to fetal loss that occurs prior to the onset of labor. Fetal death or stillbirth that occurs during the labor process is referred to as intrapartum fetal death.

Pathophysiology and etiology

There is no single pathophysiological mechanism that explains all cases of missed abortion and fetal death. There are a myriad of causes and in many cases an etiology is never determined. Causes and risk factors of fetal loss include genetic problems such as chromosomal abnormalities, syndromes and single gene mutations, birth defects, bacterial infections, viral infections, fetal-maternal hemorrhage, red cell alloimmunization,

---

Protocols for High-Risk Pregnancies, 5th edition. Edited by J.T. Queenan, J.C. Hobbins and C.Y. Spong. © 2010 Blackwell Publishing Ltd.

hypertension, diabetes, renal disease, thyroid disease, antiphospholipid syndrome, substance abuse, disorders unique to multiple gestation, abruption, and uterine anomalies such as uterine septum. Umbilical cord accidents are often attributed as the cause of fetal death, but this is difficult to prove. Common features of some of these conditions include placental insufficiency, fetal anemia, cardiac insufficiency and hypoxia. The frequency of these disorders varies among populations and also with gestational age. For example, chromosomal abnormalities are more common in pregnancy loss during the first trimester, while antiphospholipid syndrome is more strongly associated with second or third trimester losses. A majority of women in the United States with fetal deaths have incomplete or inadequate evaluations for possible causes (see below; 'follow-up').

Diagnosis

Women may note the cessation of signs and symptoms associated with pregnancy or absence of previously perceived fetal movements. On physical examination, the uterus may be smaller than expected, and fetal heart tones are inaudible. After 10 weeks' gestation, the hand-held Doppler to detect fetal heart tones may further assist in the diagnosis. Real-time ultrasonography confirms the absence of fetal movements and/or absence of fetal heart or aortic pulsations. In cases of anembryonic loss, there are specific sonographic criteria that can be used to confirm that the pregnancy is not viable. In cases of very early anembryonic loss, serial sonograms may be required to make a definitive diagnosis. Vaginal bleeding or uterine cramping will only occur in a subset of women with pregnancy loss. It is unclear why some, but not all, cases of pregnancy loss will present with bleeding or labor. Also, fetal death may precede bleeding or cramping by an extended and variable period of time.

Treatment

A significant part of the treatment of families with pregnancy loss is dealing with their (almost universal) feelings of failure and personal guilt. It is crucial to provide reassurance that there was nothing they did to cause the loss, nor anything they could have done to prevent it. They should be offered bereavement services, counseling, support groups, etc. Making every effort to determine an etiology (see below; 'follow-up') is also very important for most couples. If a cause of pregnancy loss is determined it facilitates grieving and helps to bring 'emotional closure' for the couple. It is also critical for counseling regarding subsequent pregnancies.

In all cases of pregnancy loss, the couple should be offered the options of uterine evacuation (either surgical or medical) or expectant management. Both of these options are medically safe for most women, and the decision may be made on an emotional basis. Many women have strong feelings about wanting to proceed immediately, while others desire as natural a process as possible. Most women will eventually miscarry or labor after a period of expectant management. In general, the later in gestation, the less likely patients are to elect expectant management.

Expectant management

There are some theoretical risks of expectant management including intra-uterine infection and maternal coagulopathy. These risks have prompted some authorities to advise delivery within 2 weeks of the demise and to institute surveillance for infection and coagulopathy. Examples of such surveillance include weekly visits for counseling and support and examination for evidence of rupture of membranes, infection, cervical dilation and/or bleeding. Determination of weekly complete blood count, platelet count, and fibrinogen level after 3 weeks of expectant therapy also has been advised. This latter recommendation is based on a reported 25% chance of consumptive coagulopathy if a dead fetus remains in utero for longer than 4 weeks. However, the risk appears to be less than originally reported and is limited to stillbirths. The vast majority of women with fetal deaths after 20 weeks' gestation do not choose prolonged expectant management. Although the aforementioned surveillance is not medically harmful, it is of unproven efficacy and is not required in the absence of symptoms, especially in cases less than 20 weeks' gestation. Patients should be advised to report symptoms associated with infection or bleeding.

Dilation and curettage (uterus 12 weeks' size or less)

1 Admit to the hospital, day operating room, office, or clinic.
2 Obtain baseline hematocrit if there is concern for baseline anemia. Obtain blood type if unavailable.
3 Administer misoprostol 4 hours prior to the procedure in order to facilitate cervical instrumentation. A typical dose is 200 μg placed in the posterior fornix (may be placed by patient) or taken orally as a lozenge.
4 Perform dilation and evacuation.
5 Discharge home after conscious sedation/anesthesia has worn off and the patient exhibits minimal vaginal bleeding.
6 Administer RhD immune globulin if the patient is RhD negative.
7 Schedule a follow-up visit in 2 weeks.
8 Prescribe NSAIDs or mild narcotics.

Dilation and evacuation (uterus between 13 and 22 weeks' size)

1 Admit to the hospital, day operating room, office, or clinic.
2 Obtain baseline hematocrit and blood type and screen.
3 Administer misoprostol 4 hours prior to the procedure in order to facilitate cervical instrumentation. A typical dose is 200 μg placed in the posterior fornix (may be placed by patient) or taken orally as a lozenge.
4 Perform dilation and evacuation.
5 Discharge to home after conscious sedation/anesthesia has won off and the patient exhibits minimal vaginal bleeding.
6 Administer RhD immune globulin if the patient is RhD negative.
7 Schedule a follow-up visit in 2 weeks.
8 Prescribe NSAIDs or mild narcotics.

Dilation and evacuation at gestations beyond 22 weeks' gestation may be safely performed by a small number of experienced practitioners. Modifications to this protocol may be required for gestations beyond 22 weeks.

Induction of labor

Many patients wish to proceed with induction of labor rather than dilation and evacuation. This may be due to a late gestational age or a desire to deliver an intact fetus. The availability of prostaglandins has greatly improved our ability to successfully induce labor at early gestational ages. The appropriate dosing of prostaglandins is determined by (1) whether the fetus is viable and (2) the size of the uterus. Even in the presence of a non-viable fetus, lower dosing is required when the uterus is greater than 28 weeks' size due to the potential for uterine rupture. Prostaglandin $E_{2\alpha}$ has been the most commonly used drug for the induction of labor during the past 30 years. However, misoprostol has become the prostaglandin of choice for induction of labor in cases of fetal demise due to similar efficacy (compared with prostaglandin $E_{2\alpha}$) with fewer side effects. Misoprostol may be placed in the vaginal fornix or taken orally as a lozenge. The interval to delivery is shorter on average when the drug is administered vaginally. Adverse effects of prostaglandins include nausea, vomiting, diarrhea, or pyrexia. There may be only minimal changes in cervical dilation with strong uterine contractions. Delivery often occurs suddenly, after only minimal cervical dilation. Contraindications to the use of misoprostol include active cardiac, pulmonary or renal disease, and glaucoma. Also, the drug (or any prostaglandin product) should not be used for labor induction in cases of prior uterine scar if the uterus is greater than 26 weeks' size.

Fetal demise (uterus less than 28 weeks' size)

1 Admit the patient to the hospital.
2 Obtain baseline laboratory values of complete blood cell count (CBC) and type and screen. Consider assessment of platelet count and fibrinogen level if the fetus has been dead for over 4 weeks duration.
3 Misoprostol is administered at a dose of 200 μg placed in the posterior fornix. This is repeated every 4 hours until delivery of the fetus and placenta. Up to 400 μg given every 2 hours may be safely used at this gestation. However, it does not shorten the interval to delivery compared with 200 μg given every 4 hours. The misoprostol also may be given orally (taken as a lozenge) at a dose of 200 to 400 μg every 2–4 hours. This route of administration requires (on average) a few hours longer to cause delivery compared with vaginal administration. However, it is preferred by some patients or providers. There is substantial risk for retained placenta, especially prior to 20 weeks' gestation. This risk can be diminished by allowing the placenta to spontaneously deliver. Patience and the avoidance of pulling on the cord are essential. Additional doses of misoprostol can be administered (at appropriate intervals) to promote uterine contractility between delivery of the fetus and placenta.
4 Vital signs should be assessed per routine for labor and delivery.
5 Epidural anesthesia can be utilized.
6 Narcotics, antiemetics and antipyretics should be used as needed.
7 If vital signs are stable and the patient is not bleeding excessively, she may be discharged from the hospital in 6 to 24 hours. Many women wish to leave the hospital as soon as it is medically safe so as to avoid emotional duress. If possible, patients suffering fetal demise should receive postpartum care on a non-maternity ward.
8 Parents should be encouraged to spend time with their infant and offered pictures, hand and foot prints, casts, etc.
9 Administer RhD immune globulin to RhD-negative mothers.
10 A follow-up visit (2 to 6 weeks) and bereavement services should be offered.

Fetal demise (uterus greater than 28 weeks' size)

1 Admit the patient to the hospital.
2 Obtain baseline laboratory values of complete blood cell count (CBC) and type and screen. Consider assessment of platelet count and fibrinogen level if the fetus has been dead for over 4 weeks duration.
3 Misoprostol is administered at a dose of 25 μg placed in the posterior fornix. This is repeated (at a dose of 25–50 μg) every 4 hours until delivery of the fetus and placenta. The misoprostol also may be given orally

(taken as a lozenge) at a dose of 25 µg every 4 hours. This route of administration requires (on average) a few hours longer to cause delivery compared with vaginal administration. There is substantial risk for retained placenta, especially prior to 20 weeks' gestation. This risk can be diminished by allowing the placenta to spontaneously deliver. Patience and the avoidance of pulling on the cord are essential. Additional doses of misoprostol can be administered (at appropriate intervals) to promote uterine contractility between delivery of the fetus and placenta.

4 In the presence of a favorable cervix (Bishop score of 6 or more), either before or after the administration of one or more doses of misoprostol, oxytocin may be infused per usual protocol for induction of labor.

5 Vital signs should be assessed per routine for labor and delivery.

6 Epidural anesthesia can be utilized.

7 Narcotics, antiemetics and antipyretics should be used as needed.

8 If vital signs are stable and the patient is not bleeding excessively, she may be discharged from the hospital in 12 to 24 hours. Many women wish to leave the hospital as soon as it is medically safe so as to avoid emotional duress. If possible, patients suffering fetal demise should receive postpartum care on a non-maternity ward.

9 The parents should be encouraged to spend time with their infant and offered pictures, hand and foot prints, casts, etc.

10 Administer RhD immune globulin to RhD-negative mothers.

11 A follow-up visit (2 to 6 weeks) and bereavement services should be offered.

If the duration of fetal death is more than 4 weeks or is unknown, obtain blood fibrinogen levels and complete blood and platelet counts. Because fibrinogen levels are elevated up to 450 mg/dL in pregnancy, normal blood fibrinogen level (300 mg/dL) may be an early signs of consumptive coagulopathy. Significant coagulopathy does not occur until fibrinogen levels fall to less than 100 mg/dL. Subsequent tests showing elevated prothrombin time and thromboplastin time, decreased fibrinogen and platelet count, and the presence of fibrin degradation products confirm the diagnosis of a consumptive coagulopathy. Manifestations of the coagulopathy are variable and may include localized bleeding, petechiae, or minor generalized bleeding or no evidence of bleeding. Upon diagnosis of a clotting deficit, continue monitoring clotting mechanisms and deliver the patient by the most appropriate means. If the clotting defect is severe or there is evidence of bleeding, replenish blood volume and depleted clotting factors with blood component therapy before inducing labor and delivery. Again, this complication of fetal demise is extremely rare. Thus, it is unnecessary to order extensive and serial laboratory studies in the absence of clinical bleeding and if an initial coagulation screen is normal.

Diagnostic evaluation

1 Obtain a Kleihauer-Betke to assess for feto-maternal hemorrhage. Ideally this should be accomplished soon after the diagnosis of fetal demise. In addition to determining a potential cause for the demise, excessive feto-maternal hemorrhage may require additional dosing of RhD immune globulin in RhD-negative individuals.

2 The placenta should undergo gross and microscopic evaluation.

3 Autopsy should be offered and encouraged. If the family does not consent to autopsy, consider magnetic resonance imaging, x-ray and/or gross evaluation by a trained dysmorphologist (typically a pediatric geneticist). This can provide valuable information in lieu of autopsy.

4 Clinical data should be assessed for evidence of hypertension, renal disease, infection, occult rupture of membranes, cervical insufficiency, abruption, etc.

5 Antibody screen should be obtained (if unavailable from the prenatal record).

6 Serological screen for syphilis should be assessed.

7 Toxicology screen should be assessed.

8 Although cost may be an issue, fetal karyotype should be considered. This may be of greater emotional value in patients with recurrent pregnancy loss, or with second or third trimester losses. Although abnormal karyotypes are common in first trimester losses (relative to losses later in gestation), they are usually due to *de novo* non-disjunctional events that do not tend to recur. Tissues that remain alive despite in utero death (either placental tissue or tissues that remain alive at low oxygen tension) are most likely to provide cells for chromosome analysis. Examples include chorionic plate (near the insertion of the umbilical cord), fascia lata and the nape of the neck. Techniques such as comparative genomic hybridization (CGH) may allow for the assessment of chromosomal abnormalities, even in cases wherein cells will not grow in culture.

9 Consider testing for antiphospholipid syndrome with lupus anticoagulant screen and testing for anticardiolipin antibodies if there is evidence of placental insufficiency, and/or the patient has recurrent pregnancy loss, thromboembolism, or autoimmune disease.

10 TORCH titers are recommended by some authorities. However, clinical utility is uncertain. Careful autopsy and placental evaluation may be more valuable in the diagnosis of fetal infection.

11 Clinically overt diabetes and thyroid disease are associated with fetal death. However, the utility of screening for asymptomatic disease with glycosylated hemoglobin and/or TSH is uncertain and is not routinely advised.

12 Several investigators report an association between heritable thrombophilias such as the factor V Leiden mutation, the 2010A prothrombin

gene mutation, hyperhomocysteinemia, protein C deficiency, protein S deficiency and antithrombin III deficiency and fetal death. However, the association is controversial and routine screening is not currently advised for isolated cases of fetal demise. Consider testing in cases of recurrent fetal death or thromboembolism.

13 Consideration should be given to assessment of the uterine cavity after the patient fully recovers (3 months postpartum). Clinical evidence of cervical insufficiency, second trimester losses and evidence of placental insufficiency increase the likelihood of finding a uterine abnormality.

Follow-up

The patient should be offered a postpartum visit at 1–2 weeks to assess emotional well-being and to offer support and psychological counseling. Another visit should be scheduled at 6 weeks postpartum. At this time, data should be available from diagnostic testing so that obstetric counseling may be accomplished. In some cases, further evaluation may be appropriate.

The risk of recurrent fetal death is estimated to be 2–10-fold increased over baseline. Also, there is an increased rate of obstetric complications such as preeclampsia, fetal growth impairment and preterm birth in subsequent pregnancies. No interventions are proven to improve obstetric outcome. However, antenatal surveillance and/or elective delivery at term may provide emotional benefit and have the potential to reduce subsequent complications.

Suggested reading

American College of Obstetricians and Gynecologists. Practice Bulletin #102, Management of stillbirth. *Obstet Gynecol* 2009;113:748–61.

American College of Obstetricians and Gynecologists. Committee Opinion #383, Committee on Genetics. Evaluation of stillbirths and neonatal deaths. *Obstet Gynecol* 2007;110:963–6.

American College of Obstetricians and Gynecologists. Committee Opinion #283, May 2003. New US Food and Drug Administration labeling on Cytotec (misoprostol) use and pregnancy. *Obstet Gynecol* 2003;101:1049–50.

Fretts RC. Etiology and prevention of stillbirth. *Am J Obstet Gynecol* 2005;193:1923–35.

Pauli RM, Reiser CA. Wisconsin Stillbirth Service Program II. Analysis of diagnoses and diagnostic categories in the first 1,000 referrals. *Am J Med Genet* 1994;50:135–53.

Reddy UM. Prediction and prevention of recurrent stillbirth. *Obstet Gynecol* 2007;110:1151–64.

Silver RM, Varner MV, Reddy UM, *et al.* Work-up of stillbirth: a review of the evidence. *Am J Obstet Gynecol* 2007;196:433–44.

Silver RM. Fetal death. *Obstet Gynecol* 2007;109:153–67.

Abnormal Amniotic Fluid Volume

Thomas R. Moore

Department of Reproductive Medicine, Division of Perinatal Medicine, University of California at San Diego, CA, USA

Overview

Adequate amniotic fluid volume is necessary for proper fetal growth and development. Severe and longstanding oligohydramnios, especially prior to 22 weeks of gestation, inhibits lung growth and promotes limb positional defects such as club foot and arm contractures. Thick meconium, deep variable fetal heart rate decelerations, and low birth-weight centile are common findings in the term or post-term gestation complicated by low amniotic fluid. Perinatal mortality has been reported to be increased 13–47-fold in the presence of marginal to severe oligohydramnios, respectively. Presence of oligohydramnios in the second trimester carries a 43% perinatal mortality rate. Table 49.1[1] contains some figures for oligohydramnios and perinatal morbidity. When amniotic fluid is essentially absent (anhydramnios), lethal outcomes are as high as 88%.[2] Similarly, excessive amniotic fluid, polyhydramnios, has a 2–5-fold increase in perinatal mortality.[3]

Table 49.1 Correlation of oligohydramnios and perinatal morbidity

Antepartum AFI <5.0 cm	Relative risk*	95% confidence interval
Risk of cesarean delivery for fetal distress	2.22	1.47–3.37
Risk of Apgar score <7 at 5 minutes	5.16	2.36–11.29

AFI, amniotic fluid index.
*Pooled relative risks from meta-analysis.
Adapted from Chauhan *et al. Am J Obstet Gynecol* 1999;81:1473–8.[1]

Protocols for High-Risk Pregnancies, 5th edition. Edited by J.T. Queenan, J.C. Hobbins and C.Y. Spong. © 2010 Blackwell Publishing Ltd.

Physiology of normal amniotic fluid volume

Amniotic fluid volume is normally regulated within a surprisingly narrow range. Studies of normal human pregnancies have shown that the amniotic fluid volume rises linearly from early gestation up to 32 weeks, whereupon it remain constant in the range of 700–800 mL until term. After 40 weeks of gestation, the volume declines at a rate of 8% per week. By 42 weeks, this volume decreases to about 400 mL (Fig. 49.1).[4]

Factors influencing amniotic fluid volume
Amniotic fluid production
Fetal urination is the predominant source of amniotic fluid after fetal kidney function begins at 10–12 weeks. This notion is confirmed by the almost complete absence of amniotic fluid with fetal renal obstruction or agenesis. Estimates of human fetal urine output from sonographic bladder measurements indicate urine production rate of 1000–1200 mL/day

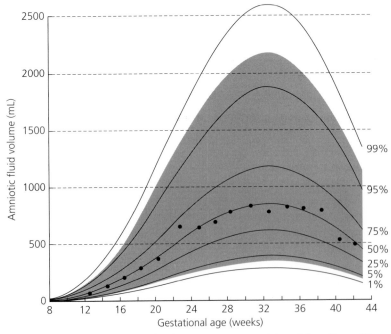

Figure 49.1 Normal amniotic fluid volume in pregnancy. Adapted from Brace RA, Wolf EJ. Normal amniotic fluid volume changes throughout pregnancy. *Am J Obstet Gynecol* 1989;161(2):382–8.[4]

near term. Thus changes in fetal urine production has a major impact on amniotic fluid volume. Fetal lung fluid is an additional contributor to amniotic fluid volume, but comprises less than half of urine flow. Fetal urinary flow rates are reduced in conditions of placental insufficiency and hypoxia, and increased in the setting of fetal hydrops (e.g., twin transfusion syndrome, fetal anemias). Thus sonographic assessment of placental and fetal cardiac function is an important adjunct to the workup of abnormal amniotic fluid volume.

Amniotic fluid removal

Fetal swallowing is the major mechanism by which fluid leaves the amniotic cavity and has been estimated at 500 mL/day from radio-labeled erythrocytes injected into the amniotic cavity, a rate considerably less than the volume flowing into the amniotic space from urinary output. Thus other paths must exist to balance amniotic fluid volume and these are *transmembranous fluid movement* across the amniotic membranes into the maternal circulation and *intramembranous movement* into the fetal circulation via the vessels on the fetal surface of the placenta. Unfortunately these pathways, well demonstrated in non-human species, cannot be measured or manipulated clinically. When evaluating cases of apparently high amniotic fluid volume, therefore, sonographic evaluation of fetal swallowing function is important. Problems with fetal swallowing can be inferred by failing to visualize a normal-sized stomach, noting anatomic anomalies of the fetal face and neck, potential esophageal obstruction due to a thoracic mass, or intestinal obstruction due to gastroschisis or segmental atresia.[5]

Amniotic fluid volume changes with gestational age

Figure 49.1 demonstrates the changes in amniotic fluid volumes during gestation. Important features of this curve include (1) amniotic fluid volume rises progressively during gestation until approximately 32 weeks; (2) from 32 to 39 weeks, the mean amniotic fluid volume is relatively constant in the range of 700–800 mL; (3) from 40 to 44 weeks there is a progressive decline in amniotic fluid volume at a rate of 8% per week, averaging only 400 mL at 42 weeks; (4) the variation in 'normal' fluid volume below the mean value is modest. 'Oligohydramnios' (the 5th percentile) is approximately 300 mL. However, variation in the upper range is almost threefold greater, with 'hydramnios' (>95th percentile) varying from 1700 to 1900 mL. Thus 'abnormal' amniotic fluid volume should be determined after reference to a curve or table which includes gestational age as a variable (see Fig. 49.2).[6]

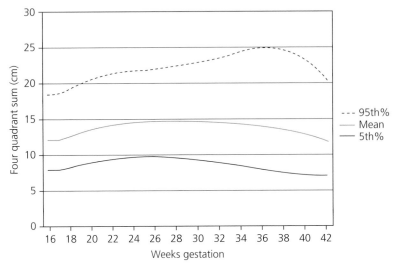

Figure 49.2 Amniotic fluid index percentiles during pregnancy. Adapted from Moore TR, Cayle JE. The amniotic fluid index in normal human pregnancy. *Am J Obstet Gynecol* 1990;162:1168–73.[6]

Oligohydramnios

Diagnosis

Effective management of oligohydramnios begins with accurate diagnosis. Unfortunately, sonographic methods for determining amniotic fluid volume such as amniotic fluid index (AFI) and maximal vertical pocket (MVP) perform best for the identifying normal amniotic fluid volumes, while sonographic methods for identifying oligohydramnios or hydramnios are much less than optimal.

The AFI is calculated by summing the vertical amniotic fluid pocket depth in each of four quadrants of the uterus.[7] Mild oligohydramnios should be suspected with an AFI of less than 7 cm. Amniotic fluid index values less than 5 cm are distinctly abnormal (<2% of normal pregnancies at term; Fig. 49.2). However, it should be noted that the lower 5th centile boundary for the AFI varies significantly with gestational age. At term, an AFI of <5 cm has been used as a common cut-off value to define oligohydramnios.[8] Particular care should be taken in measuring the AFI when amniotic fluid volume appears to be low. Intraobserver and interobserver errors have been shown to average between 5 and 10 mm, respectively, or approximately 3 to 7% overall but the error can be as high as ±30% for an AFI below 7 cm. To minimize this error in patients with decreased amniotic fluid, the AFI measurements should be done in triplicate and averaged. It is also important to avoid measuring into narrow, slit-like amniotic fluid pockets. All amniotic fluid pockets should have a width of at least 1 cm and no intervening structures should be visible (e.g., umbilical cord, fetal limbs

Table 49.2 Comparison of use of amniotic fluid index (AFI) or maximum vertical pocket (MVP) in antepartum testing

AFI vs MVP	Relative risk	95% confidence interval
NICU admission	1.04	0.85–1.26
Umbilical artery pH < 7.1	1.1	0.74–1.65
Diagnosis of oligohydramnios	2.39	1.73–3.28
Induction of labor	1.92	1.5–2.46
Cesarean delivery	1.09	0.92–1.29
Cesarean delivery for fetal distress	1.46	1.08–1.96

Source: Nabhan AF, Abdelmoula YA. Amniotic fluid index versus single deepest vertical pocket as a screening test for preventing adverse pregnancy outcome. *Cochrane Database Syst Rev* 2008;(3): CD006593.[9]

or digits). Similar conventions apply to measuring the MVP: care must be taken to survey the entire uterus and visualize the deepest pocket at least 1 cm in width. For the diagnosis of oligohydramnios, the absence of an MVP of 2 cm in depth is typically diagnostic.

For documentation of relative amniotic fluid volume at the time of diagnostic sonography, the AFI is most commonly used and referenced to the values in Fig. 49.2. However, for determining the presence or absence of oligohydramnios as part of antepartum testing, a significant body of evidence suggests that the maximal vertical pocket (MVP) can be used with equivalent or even superior effectiveness. A recent systematic review of five randomized controlled trials comparing AFI and MVP by Nabhan and Abdelmoula (2008)[9] determined that MVP measurement during fetal biophysical surveillance seems a better choice since the use of the amniotic fluid index increases the rate of diagnosis of oligohydramnios and the rate of induction of labor with equivalent results in peripartum outcomes (Table 49.2).

Table 49.3 is a tabulation of the average and upper/lower 5% boundary values for both the AFI and MVP during gestation reported by Magann et al.[10]

Evaluation

Rule out ruptured membranes

The workup of oligohydramnios is generally initiated by careful sonography and physical examination. Near term, ruptured membranes as the cause of oligohydramnios can reliably be confirmed by examination of the fluid in the vaginal fornix. However, chronic leakage of amniotic fluid may be difficult to detect especially in the second trimester. If a normal-sized fetal bladder is observed in the presence of oligohydramnios, the most likely cause is preterm rupture of membranes (PROM). Prior to

Table 49.3 Diagnostic categories of ultrasonographic amniotic fluid volume assessment

Week of gestation	20	21	22	23	24	25	26	27	28	29	30	31	32	33	34	35	36	37	38	39	40	41
Maximum vertical pocket (cm)																						
5th percentile	3	3	3	3	3	3	3	3	3	3	3	3	3	3	3	3	3	2	2	2	2	
50th percentile	4	5	5	5	5	5	5	5	5	5	5	5	5	5	5	5	5	4	4	4	4	
95th percentile	7	7	7	7	7	7	7	7	7	7	7	7	7	7	7	7	7	7	7	6	6	
Amniotic fluid index (cm)																						
5th percentile	5	5	6	6	6	7	7	7	8	8	8	8	8	7	7	7	6	6	6	5	5	4
50th percentile	8	9	9	10	11	11	12	13	13	13	14	14	14	13	13	12	12	11	10	9	9	8
95th percentile	11	12	13	14	15	16	17	18	19	19	20	20	21	21	20	20	19	19	18	17	16	15

Adapted from Magann EF, Sanderson M, Martin JN, Chauhan S. The amniotic fluid index, single deepest pocket, and two-diameter pocket in normal human pregnancy. *Am J Obstet Gynecol* 2000; 182:1581–8.[10]

20 weeks of gestation, sterile speculum tests may be negative or equivocal, and the patient may not be sure whether vaginal moisture represents amniotic fluid or cervical mucus. Although instillation of a dye such as indigo carmine may provide unequivocal proof of PROM, such invasive procedures rarely affect management except in cases of previable PROM (<23 weeks).

Assess fetal urinary tract anatomy and function

If there is no evidence of PROM, detailed assessment of fetal urinary tract anatomy is in order since renal and ureteral anomalies are the most common causes of severe oligohydramnios. Sonographic evaluation should include the renal dimensions and morphology of the parenchyma, dimensions of the renal pelvis and morphology of the urinary bladder. Bilateral renal agenesis is typically associated with severe oligohydramnios and is usually detectable after 16 weeks of gestation. However, unilateral or bilateral ureteropelvic junction obstruction or polycystic kidney disease may not be detectable until late in the second trimester and is usually associated with less severe oligohydramnios. Unilateral urinary obstruction rarely causes measurable decrement in amniotic fluid volume. Since urinary tract defects are commonly found in aneuploid fetuses, amniocentesis should be offered if these findings are present.[2]

Assess fetal growth and placental function

In the absence of PROM and urinary tract anomalies, uteroplacental insufficiency should be considered. Oligohydramnios may result from poor placental function associated with maternal hypertension, chronic placental abruption and autoimmune states such as systemic lupus and antiphospholipid syndrome. In such cases, fetal abdominal circumference growth typically lags that of the head. Increased placental vascular resistance evident on umbilical artery Doppler studies may help corroborate the diagnosis of oligohydramnios due to placental insufficiency.[11] The risk of fetal asphyxia and death is high when severe oligohydramnios accompanies intrauterine growth restriction (IUGR). Intensive fetal testing and hospitalization should be considered in cases diagnosed after the point of fetal viability. After 32 weeks, severe oligohydramnios and fetal growth restriction should generally lead to evaluation for delivery.

Assess likelihood of pulmonary hypoplasia

Longstanding oligohydramnios predisposes to pulmonary hypoplasia. Although the mechanism of this potentially lethal complication is not clear, inhibition of fetal breathing, loss of lung liquid because of reduction in amniotic pressure, and simple mechanical compression of the chest have been proposed.[12] The end result is restricted lung growth leading to alveolar volume inadequate to support postnatal respiration. It appears that the risk of pulmonary hypoplasia is greatest when severe oligohydramnios is present from 16 to 24 weeks of gestation, the period of alveolar proliferation.

Though several methods have been proposed to predict pulmonary hypoplasia, no single criterion has adequate sensitivity and specificity for clinical decision-making. Measurement of chest circumference, use of thoracic–head circumference ratio, calculating the lung area ratio [(chest area–cardiac area)/chest area] and thin-slice three-dimensional fetal lung volume/fetal body weight ratios have been proposed to assess the presence of pulmonary hypoplasia.[13] Recently, magnetic resonance imaging and Doppler assessment of fetal pulmonary tissues have also been utilized for prediction of pulmonary hypoplasia. In a recent small study, use of MRI-based abnormal lung volume/fetal weight ratio gave a sensitivity of 88% with a false positive diagnosis of pulmonary hypoplasia of 12%.[14] When chest development appears markedly compromised in a pre-viable fetus with severe oligohydramnios, the option of termination of pregnancy should be discussed.

Treatment options

Delivery

Although the outcome of severe, longstanding oligohydramnios is at best guarded, lesser degrees of fluid restriction may be amenable to intervention. Data suggests that most of the perinatal morbidity associated with postdate pregnancy is confined to cases with an AFI of less than 5 cm and, particularly, those that lack a MVP of at least 2×1 cm. In such cases, continued expectant management and antepartum testing is likely to result in higher rates of meconium staining, fetal distress, low Apgar scores and cesarean delivery.[15]

Amnioinfusion

At term, induction of labor in patients with severe oligohydramnios is associated with decreased perinatal morbidity but carries risk of prolonged labor and failed induction. One meta-analysis indicates that, in women with PROM and oligohydramnios, prophylactic transcervical saline infusion significantly improves neonatal outcome and lessens the rate of cesarean delivery, without increasing the rate of postpartum endometritis.[16] Potential complications associated with amnio-infusion include inadvertent overdistention of the uterus, increased uterine contractions during the infusion, and the theoretical possibility of amniotic fluid embolus.

Theoretically in the preterm pregnancy with intact membranes, the adverse consequences of prolonged oligohydramnios could be reduced or eliminated by transabdominal amnioinfusion.[17] While such amnio-infusions are controversial, at least one trial,[18] which compared outcomes of women with intact membranes and AFI <9 cm who received 250 mL Ringer solution instilled transabdominally to a group of control women. Transabdominal amnio-infusion resulted in a mean increase in AFI of 4 cm and a reduction in cesarean delivery (18% of case patients vs 46% of controls). The perinatal mortality rate was 18% among controls and 4% among case patients. These findings aside, however, a systematic review of trials reporting an impact of amnio-infusion on stillbirths (9 trials, $n = 1681$ women) and perinatal mortality (10 trials, $n = 3656$ women) revealed a non-significant reduction in risk associated with amnio-infusion.[19]

Maternal hydration

The interrelationship between amniotic fluid and maternal intravascular volumes has been demonstrated experimentally and clinically. Oosterhof et al.[20] demonstrated increased fetal urine output following rehydration of pregnant women. In hypertensive patients with decreased maternal intravascular volume, amniotic fluid volumes are lower than those with normal intravascular volume.[21] In a systematic review of randomized trials of maternal hydration by Hofmeyr and Gülmezoglu,[22] the amniotic fluid index was significantly increased in women with oligohydramnios undergoing hydration vs controls (mean difference 2.01, 95% CI 1.43–2.60).[23] Doi (1998)[24] compared intravenous isotonic and hypotonic fluid infusions as well as oral hydration and found that hypotonic but not isotonic infusion increased the amniotic fluid volume at a level similar to that of oral hydration. Thus in cases of isolated oligohydramnios (lacking evidence of coexisting fetal hypoxia or urinary tract anomalies), a trial of maternal oral hydration with 2 liters of water, allowing at least 2 hours before reassessing amniotic fluid volume, may be effective.

Summary

Mild oligohydramnios (AFI 5–8 cm, MVP 2–3 cm) near term should be managed conservatively with frequent fetal surveillance and emphasis on maternal hydration as long as a 2 × 1 cm pocket of amniotic fluid is demonstrable. Labor induction for significant oligohydramnios (absence of 2 × 1 cm pocket) at term is appropriate. Remote from term with oligohydramnios, fetal structural and chromosomal anomalies should be ruled out. If intrauterine growth restriction is present with oligohydramnios, the risk of fetal asphyxia and death is high. Such pregnancies should be managed aggressively with early delivery unless lethal anomalies are present.

Polyhydramnios

Overview

Polyhydramnios is the pathological accumulation of excessive quantities of amniotic fluid. When polyhydramnios is diagnosed, a thorough examination for underlying abnormalities is indicated and the risk of adverse pregnancy outcomes is increased. Clearly, as noted above in the discussion regarding amniotic fluid production and removal, polyhydramnios arises from either overproduction or under-removal or a combination of both.

Since measurements of both fetal urinary flow and swallowing are not adequately precise for clinical measurement, the typical clinical associations with excess amniotic fluid have been catalogued (see Table 49.4).[25,26]

Regarding the pathophysiological connection between polyhydramnios and its clinical associations, little is known with certainty. The link between

Table 49.4 Clinical associations with polyhydramnios

Cause	Hill, 1987 (n = 107)	Many, 1995 (n = 275)
Idiopathic	66%	69%
Diabetes mellitus	15%	18%
Congenital malformations	13%	15%
Rh incompatibility	1%	–
Multiple gestation	5%	–

Adapted from Hill, 1987[25]; Many, 1995.[26]

the increased incidence of polyhydramnios with maternal hyperglycemia in diabetes has been proposed to arise from diuresis in the fetus in response to hyperglycemia as it does in the mother. With associated anatomic abnormalities such as esophageal atresia, congenital diaphragmatic hernia and chest masses, fetal swallowing is impaired, resulting in polyhydramnios. Fetuses with central nervous system (CNS) anomalies such as anencephaly and holoprosencephaly may develop polyhydramnios from altered CNS function.[27]

Fetal conditions associated with fetal anemia, cardiac overload or congestive failure often develop polyhydramnios. Examples include the recipient twin in twin-twin transfusion syndrome, Rhesus isoimmunization, parvovirus infection and fetal-maternal hemorrhage.[28,29] Regardless of etiology, polyhydramnios should be taken as an ominous sign, with perinatal mortality increases over pregnancies with normal amniotic fluid of 2–5 fold.[3]

Diagnosis

Several criteria have been proposed as defining polyhydramnios which, by definition, is approximately 2–5% of the upper levels of sonographically measured AFI or MVP. As in oligohydramnios, the boundaries of normal and abnormal amniotic fluid vary with gestational age. In the third trimester, this would coincide with MVP values above 7 cm or AFI exceeding 21 cm (95th percentile, see Table 49.3). Others have advocated a more restrictive definition, such that only 1–2% of cases are defined. Using the MVP, polyhydramnios is present when the deepest amniotic fluid pocket is more than 8 cm, and with the AFI 24–30 cm (mild), 31–35 cm (moderate) and above 35 cm (severe). A commonly accepted cut-off for polyhydramnios is 24 cm (AFI) or 8 cm (MVP).

Evaluation
Sonography

Evaluate sonographically for fetal cardiac failure, anemia or anomalies possibly altering fetal swallowing:[30]

- Pericardial effusion, poor ventricular function, structural cardiac defect.
- Middle cerebral artery peak systolic velocity above 1.5 multiples of median for gestational age.
- CNS defect, e.g., Arnold-Chiari malformation, holoprosencephaly.
- Thoracic mass, e.g., diaphragmatic hernia, pulmonary sequestration, cystic adenomatoid malformation.
- Gastrointestinal tract obstruction, e.g., duodenal atresia, esophageal atresia.
- Sonographic markers of aneuploidy.

Laboratory screening

Undertake laboratory screening for:

• gestational diabetes
• Rh isoimmunization
• fetal infection (rubella, toxoplasmosis, parvovirus, CMV, syphilis)
• thalassemia especially alpha-thalassemia
• Kleihauer-Betke
• toxicology for substance abuse.

Amniocentesis

Consider amniocentesis for fetal karyotype.

A study of 672 pregnancies reported that the risk of aneuploidy was 10% when the fetus had sonographic anomalies and only 1% when no anomalies were found on sonogram.[31] Although the risk of aneuploidy is much lower when no anomalies are noted on sonogram, the risk of aneuploidy of 1% is still greater than the risk of fetal loss with an amniocentesis.

Complications

• Uterine distention can lead to a number of obstetrical complications including:
• Premature labor: In one study of 275 singleton pregnancies, premature delivery occurred in 19% of patients and the degree of polyhydramnios did not change this risk.[26]
• Preterm premature rupture of membranes.
• Malpresentation due to increased fetal mobility.
• Umbilical cord prolapse.
• Cesarean delivery.
• Placental abruption following PROM.
• Postpartum hemorrhage due to uterine overdistention.
• Maternal respiratory compromise due to mechanical pressure on the maternal diaphragm.
• Fetal mortality: In a study of over 40,000 singleton pregnancies, the risk of fetal mortality was increased as compared to patients with a normal AFI (49 per 1000 births vs 14 per 1000 births, $P < 0.001$). This finding remained significant when controlled for the presence of diabetes.[32]

Treatment options

It is not clear that any medical intervention improves the outcome of most cases of polyhydramnios. When a clear-cut etiology is evident, e.g., diabetes or isoimmunization, the underlying problem should be addressed. When polyhydramnios is caused by a congenital anomaly or is idiopathic, treatment is expectant and focused on closely monitoring the fetus and intervening for maternal complications. Importantly, a significant number of cases of mild polyhydramnios will resolve spontaneously.

Monitor for cervical length for preterm labor

Since polyhydramnios is associated with increased risk of premature PROM and preterm birth, sonographic monitoring of cervical length may provide advanced warning of impending labor. Cervical length should be assessed as dictated by clinical circumstances and gestational age, but typically a cervical length measurement every 2 weeks from 24 to 33 weeks may provide guidance regarding when to admit the patient for antenatal steroids. Finding a cervix less than 1.5 to 2.0 cm, especially with a positive cervical fetal fibronectin with gestational age less than 34 weeks should prompt evaluation for hospitalization and steroid treatment.[33]

Labor management

Delivery should occur at term or when fetal lung maturity is documented. While a vaginal delivery is usually optimal, care must be taken during labor to ensure that the presenting part remains vertex and the obstetrical team is ready to manage complications of sudden uterine decompression including abruption, change to a non-vertex fetal position, umbilical cord prolapse and postpartum hemorrhage.

Amnioreduction

Amnioreduction refers to reducing the amount of amniotic fluid through a large volume amniocentesis (100 mL to more than 1000 mL).[34] Typical indications include maternal respiratory compromise or severe abdominal pain/contractions. While there are no trials demonstrating efficacy, amnioreduction is a common therapy applied to stage 1 or stage 2 twin-twin transfusion syndrome. To give guidance on exactly how much fluid to remove, there is data that demonstrates a linear relationship between the AFI and the volume of amniotic fluid drained.[35]

Typically, an 18-gauge needle is inserted sterilely under ultrasonographic guidance into a free pocket of amniotic fluid. Tubing is either connected to wall suction or a three-way stopcock to permit removal with a large syringe. Fluid should be removed no faster than 1000 mL over 20 minutes and the procedure is terminated when the AFI returns to a normal range. One study of over 200 amnioreduction procedures including a large number of twin-twin transfusion syndrome cases with a median of 1500 mL of amniotic fluid removed during each procedure.[34] Complications of amnioreduction (approximately 3%) include chorioamnionitis, fetal bradycardia, placental abruption and preterm rupture of membranes.[36] The procedure is repeated if symptoms recur and gestational age is less than 33 weeks.

Indomethacin

Indomethacin, a prostaglandin synthetase inhibitor, decreases fetal urine output.[37] An important side effect of indomethacin is constriction of the fetal ductus arteriosus. Prior to 30 weeks, this effect is usually not significant. Treatment after 30 weeks should be considered with caution, and accompanied by daily sonographic assessment of fetal cardiac function. The starting dose is 25 mg orally three times daily, but may be increased to as much as 150 mg daily.[38] The AFI should be monitored daily and treatment stopped when the AFI returns to the upper normal range.

Biophysical monitoring of the fetus and amniotic fluid volume

Most cases of polyhydramnios resolve with advancing gestation. The frequency of monitoring of amniotic fluid volume should be determined by clinical circumstances and patient complaint. Usually every 3–4 weeks is adequate. However, because of the increased risk of fetal death with polyhydramnios, fetal biophysical status should be monitored carefully after the gestational age of viability. Typically, fetal movement counting is used nightly from 28 weeks[39] and twice-weekly modified biophysical profiles utilized from 32–34 weeks onward.[15]

Summary

Polyhydramnios occurs in 1–5% of pregnancies and is associated with significantly increased perinatal morbidity and mortality. A thorough laboratory and sonographic evaluation will aid in accurate recognition of the operative etiology and guide any subsequent therapy.

References

1 Chauhan SP, Sanderson M, Hendrix NW, Magann EF, Devoe LD. Perinatal outcome and amnionitc fluid index in the antepartum and intrapartum periods: a meta-analysis. *Am J Obstet Gynecol* 1999;181:1473–8.

2 Moore TR, Longo J, Leopold GR, Casola G, Gosink BB. The reliability and predictive value of an amniotic fluid scoring system in severe second-trimester oligohydramnios. *Obstet Gynecol* 1989;73(5 Pt 1):739–42.

3 Magann EF, Chauhan SP, Doherty DA, Lutgendorf MA, Magann MI, Morrison JC. Review of idiopathic hydramnios and pregnancy outcomes. *Obstet Gynecol Surv* 2007;62(12);795–802.

4 Brace RA, Wolf EJ. Normal amniotic fluid volume changes throughout pregnancy. *Am J Obstet Gynecol* 1989;161(2):382–8.

5 Brace RA. Physiology of amniotic fluid volume regulation. *Clin Obstet Gynecol* 1997; 40(2):280–9.

6 Moore TR, Cayle JE. The amniotic fluid index in normal human pregnancy. *Am J Obstet Gynecol* 1990;162:1168–73.

7 Phelan JP, Smith CV, Broussard P, Small M. Amniotic fluid volume assessment using the four-quadrant technique in the pregnancy between 36 and 42 weeks gestation. *J Reprod Med* 1987;32:601–4.

8 Magann EF, Doherty DA, Chauhan SP, Busch FW, Mecacci F, Morrison JC. How well do the amniotic fluid index and single deepest pocket indices (below the 3rd and 5th and above the 95th and 97th percentiles) predict oligohydramnios and hydramnios? *Am J Obstet Gynecol* 2004;190(1):164–9.

9 Nabhan AF, Abdelmoula YA. Amniotic fluid index versus single deepest vertical pocket as a screening test for preventing adverse pregnancy outcome. *Cochrane Database Syst Rev* 2008;(3): CD006593.

10 Magann EF, Sanderson M, Martin JN, Chauhan S. The amniotic fluid index, single deepest pocket, and two-diameter pocket in normal human pregnancy. *Am J Obstet Gynecol* 2000;182:1581–8.

11 Sarno AP Jr, Ahn MO, Brar HS, Phelan JP, Platt LD. Intrapartum Doppler velocimetry, amniotic fluid volume, and fetal heart rate as predictors of subsequent fetal distress. I. An initial report. *Am J Obstet Gynecol* 1989;161(6 Pt 1):1508–14.

12 Perlman M, Levin M. Fetal pulmonary hypoplasia, anuria, and oligohydramnios: clinicopathologic observations and review of the literature. *Am J Obstet Gynecol* 1974;118(8):1119–23.

13 Laudy JA, Wladimiroff JW. The fetal lung. II. Pulmonary hypoplasia. Ultrasound Obstet Gynecol 2000; 16:482–494.

14 Tanigaki S, Miyakoshi K, Tanaka M, *et al.* Pulmonary hypoplasia: prediction with use of ratio of MR imaging-measured fetal lung volume to US-estimated fetal body weight. *Radiology* 2004;232(3):767–72.

15 Magann EF, Doherty DA, Field K, Chauhan SP, Muffley PE, Morrison JC. Biophysical profile with amniotic fluid volume assessments. *Obstet Gynecol* 2004;104(1):5–10.

16 Pitt C, Sanchez-Ramos L, Kaunitz AM, Gaudier F. Prophylactic amnioinfusion for intrapartum oligohydramnios: a meta-analysis of randomized controlled trials. *Obstet Gynecol* 2000;96(5 Pt 2):861–6.

17 Regi A, Alexander N, Jose R, Lionel J, Varghese L, Peedicayil A. Amnioinfusion for relief of recurrent severe and moderate variable decelerations in labor. *J Reprod Med* 2009;54(5):295–302.

18 Chhabra S, Dargan R, Nasare M. Antepartum transabdominal amnioinfusion. *Int J Gynecol Obstet* 2007;97:95–9.

19 Darmstadt GL, Yakoob MY, Haws RA, *et al.* Reducing stillbirths: interventions during labour. *BMC Pregn Childbirth* 2009;9(Suppl 1):S6.

20 Oosterhof H, Haak MC, Aarnoudse JG. Acute maternal rehydration increases the urine production in the near-term human fetus. *Am J Obstet Gynecol* 2000;183:226–9.

21 Goodlin RC, Anderson JC, Gallagher TF. Relationship between amniotic fluid volume and maternal plasma volume expansion. *Am J Obstet Gynecol* 1983;146(5):505–11.

22 Hofmeyr GJ, Gülmezoglu AM. Maternal hydration for increasing amniotic fluid volume in oligohydramnios and normal amniotic fluid volume. *Cochrane Database Syst Rev* 2002;(1): CD000134.

23 Kilpatrick SJ, Safford KL. Maternal hydration increases amniotic fluid index in women with normal amniotic fluid. *Obstet Gynecol* 1993;81(1):49–52.

24 Doi S, Osada H, Seki K, Sekiya S. Effect of maternal hydration on oligohydramnios: a comparison of three volume expansion methods. *Obstet Gynecol* 1998;92(4 Pt 1):525–9.

25 Hill L, Breckle R, Thomas ML, Fires JK. Polyhydramnios:; ultrasonically detected prevalence and neonatal outcome. *Obstet Gynecol* 1987;69:21–25.

26 Many A, Hill LM, Lazebnik N, Martin JG. The association between polyhydramnios and preterm delivery. *Obstet Gynecol* 1995;86(3):389–91.

27 Panting-Kemp A, Nguyen T, Castro L. Substance abuse and polyhydramnios. *Am J Obstet Gynecol* 2002;187(3):602–5.

28 Krause S, Ebbesen F, Lange AP. Polyhydramnios with maternal lithium treatment. *Obstet Gynecol* 1990; 75:504.

29 Ang MS, Thorp JA, Parisi VM. Maternal lithium therapy and polyhydramnios. *Obstet Gynecol* 1990; 76:517.

30 Cicero S, Sacchini C, Rembouskos G, Nicolaides KH. Sonographic markers of fetal aneuploidy – a review. *Placenta* 2003;24 Suppl B:S88–98.

31 Dashe JS, McIntire DD, Ramus RM, Santos-Ramos R, Twickler DM. Hydramnios: anomaly prevalence and sonographic detection. *Obstet Gynecol* 2002;100(1):134–9.

32 Biggio JR, Wenstrom KD, Dubard MB, Cliver SP. Hydramnios prediction of adverse perinatal outcome. *Obstet Gynecol* 1999;94(5 Pt 1):773–7.

33 Tekesin I, Wallwiener D, Schmidt S. The value of quantitative ultrasound tissue characterization of the cervix and rapid fetal fibronectin in predicting preterm delivery. *J Perinat Med* 2005;33(5):383–91.

34 Elliott JP, Sawyer AT, Radin TG, Strong RE. Large-volume therapeutic amniocentesis in the treatment of hydramnios. *Obstet Gynecol* 1994;84(6):1025–7.

35 Denbow ML, Sepulveda W, Ridout D, Fisk NM. Relationship between change in amniotic fluid index and volume of fluid removed at amnioreduction. *Obstet Gynecol* 1997;90(4):529–32.

36 Leung WC, Jouannic JM, Hyett J, Rodeck C, Jauniaux E. Procedure-related complications of rapid amniodrainage in the treatment of polyhydramnios. *Ultrasound Obstet Gynecol* 2004;23(2):154–8.

37 Kramer WB, van den Veyver IB, Kirshon B. Treatment of polyhydramnios with indomethacin. *Clin Perinatol* 1994;21(3):615–30.

38 Cabrol D, Jannet D, Pannier E. Treatment of symptomatic polyhydramnios with indomethacin. *Eur J Obstet Gynecol Reprod Biol* 1996;66(1):11–15.

39 Moore TR, Piacquadio K. A prospective evaluation of fetal movement screening to reduce the incidence of antepartum fetal death. *Am J Obstet Gynecol* 1989;160:1075–80.

PROTOCOL 50

Preeclampsia

Baha M. Sibai

University of Cincinnati College of Medicine, Cincinnati, OH, USA

Overview

Hypertension complicates 7 to 10% of pregnancies, of which 70% are due to gestational hypertension–preeclampsia and 30% are due to chronic essential hypertension.

Risk factors include:

- nulliparity
- obesity
- multiple gestation
- family history of preeclampsia or eclampsia
- preexisting hypertension or renal disease
- previous preeclampsia or eclampsia
- diabetes mellitus
- nonimmune hydrops
- antiphospholipid antibody syndrome
- molar pregnancy.

Preeclampsia rarely develops before 20 weeks. In this early stage, rule out underlying renal disease or molar pregnancy.

Pathophysiology

Preeclampsia is a disorder of unknown etiology that is peculiar to human pregnancy. The pathophysiological abnormalities in preeclampsia include inadequate maternal vascular response to placentation, endothelial dysfunction, abnormal angiogenesis, and exaggerated inflammatory response with resultant generalized vasospasm, activation of platelets and abnormal hemostasis. These abnormalities result in pathophysiological vascular lesions in peripheral vessels and uteroplacental vascular beds, as well as in various organ systems, such as the kidneys, liver, lungs and brain.

Protocols for High-Risk Pregnancies, 5th edition. Edited by J.T. Queenan, J.C. Hobbins and C.Y. Spong. © 2010 Blackwell Publishing Ltd.

Consequently, these pregnancies, particularly those with severe preeclampsia, are associated with increased maternal and perinatal mortality and morbidity due to reduced uteroplacental blood flow, abruptio placentae and preterm delivery. Recent evidence indicates that preeclampsia is an endothelial disorder. Thus, in some patients the disease may manifest itself in the form of either a capillary leak, fetal growth restriction, or a spectrum of abnormal hemostasis with multiple organ dysfunction.

Diagnosis

Preeclampsia is now defined by the new onset of hypertension and proteinuria.

Gestational hypertension
- Systolic blood pressure ≥140 mmHg.
- Diastolic blood pressure ≥90 mmHg.
- The above pressures should be observed on at least two occasions 6 hours apart, no more than 7 days apart.
- Blood pressure readings can vary with the type of equipment used, cuff size, position of the arm, position of the patient, duration of rest period, obesity, smoking, anxiety, and the Korotkoff sound used to assess diastolic blood pressure. Only Korotkoff sound V should be used to establish diastolic BP.
- Severe hypertension: sustained elevations in systolic blood pressure to at least 160 mmHg and/or in diastolic blood pressure to at least 110 mmHg for at least 6 hours.

Proteinuria
- ≥0.3 g in a 24-hour urine collection or ≥0.1 g/L (≥2+ on the dipstick) in at least two random samples collected 6 hours or more apart, but no more than 7 days apart.
- Preeclampsia is characterized by intermittent vasospasm of the renal vessels, resulting in variable amounts of proteins in different spot urine samples.
- Protein excretion in the urine increases in normal pregnancy from approximately 5 mg/dL in the first and second trimesters to 15 mg/dL in the third trimester. These low levels are not detected by dipstick. The concentration of urinary protein is influenced by contamination with vaginal secretions, blood, bacteria, or amniotic fluid. It also varies with urine specific gravity and pH, exercise and posture.
- Proteinuria usually appears after hypertension in the course of the disease process.

Edema

- Excessive weight gain >4 lb/week (>1.8 kg/week) in the third trimester may be the first sign of the potential development of preeclampsia.
- 39% of eclamptic patients do not have edema.

Severe preeclampsia

Preeclampsia is labeled as severe in the presence of any of the following abnormalities.

- Systolic blood pressure ≥160 mmHg or diastolic blood pressure ≥110 mmHg on two occasions at least 6 hours apart with the patient at bed rest.
- Proteinuria of ≥5 g on 24-hour urine collection. Urine dipsticks are not accurate for this purpose.
- Oliguria (≤500 mL in 24 hours).
- Persistent cerebral or visual disturbances or cerebral edema.
- Persistent epigastric pain with nausea or vomiting, or both.
- Pulmonary edema.
- Thrombocytopenia.

Chronic hypertension with superimposed preeclampsia

- Chronic hypertension: persistent elevation of blood pressure to at least 140/90 mmHg on two occasions more than 24 hours apart before 20 weeks' gestation, or more than 42 days postpartum.
- Superimposed preeclampsia: the development of new-onset proteinuria.
- The development of new-onset proteinuria and/or development of thrombocytopenia or persistent cerebral symptoms.

Management

Delivery is the only available cure for preeclampsia. The ultimate goals of any management plan must be the safety of the mother first and then delivery of a live mature newborn who will not require intensive and prolonged neonatal care. The decision between immediate delivery and expectant management will depend on one or more of the following: maternal and fetal conditions at the time of evaluation, fetal gestational age, presence of labor, severity of the disease process, Bishop cervical score and maternal desire.

Mild hypertension–preeclampsia

Figure 50.1 provides a management algorithm for mild hypertension–preeclampsia.

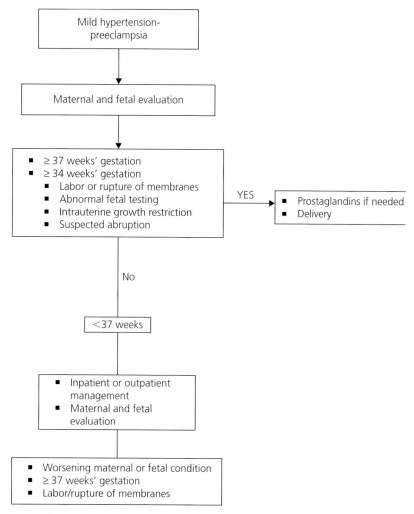

Figure 50.1 Recommended management of mild gestational hypertension or preeclampsia.

Beyond 37 weeks
- ≥37 weeks' gestation: induction. Induce also for any signs of maternal-fetal distress.
- Prostaglandins can be used for cervical ripening in those with Bishop score <6.

Less than 37 weeks
- In all patients the maternal and fetal conditions should be evaluated.
- Outpatient management is possible if the patient's systolic blood pressure is ≤150 mmHg and/or diastolic blood pressure is ≤100 mmHg,

with no significant proteinuria (<1 g/24 h), a platelet count $\geq 100,000/$ μL, normal liver enzymes and reassuring fetal testing. The patient should also have no subjective symptoms, and should be compliant and reliable.

- Whether the patient is in the hospital or being managed at home, the following should be observed:
  - Salt restriction, diuretics, antihypertensive drugs, and sedatives are not used.
  - Patient should have relative rest, daily dipstick measurement of protein, daily blood pressure monitoring, 1–2 times per week fetal testing, and laboratory evaluation of hematocrit and platelets, and liver function tests once or twice a week. Patient should be educated about preeclampsia warning signs, such as headache, visual disturbances, epigastric pain, nausea and vomiting. Patient should be instructed about daily kick counts and labor signs or vaginal bleeding.
- Fetal testing should consist of at least weekly non-stress testing (NST), and measurement of amniotic fluid volume as needed, in addition to assessment of fetal growth by ultrasonography every 3 weeks. Testing is considered nonreassuring if:
  - NST is nonreactive with abnormal fetal biophysical profile.
  - NST shows repetitive late deceleration, repetitive moderate to severe variable decelerations, or prolonged deceleration.
  - Oligohydramnios is present (AFI persistently ≤ 5.0 cm).
  - Estimated fetal weight is less than 10th percentile for gestational age.
- Prompt hospitalization is needed for disease progression: acute severe hypertension, development of significant proteinuria (2 g/24 h), outpatient management unsatisfactory for the specific patient, or abnormal fetal testing.

Severe preeclampsia

Figure 50.2 provides a management algorithm for severe preeclampsia.

- Beyond 34 weeks: induction and delivery. There is no need for assessment of fetal lung maturity.
- 33 to 34 weeks: steroids for fetal lung maturity. Delivery after 48 hours.
- 23 weeks 6 days to 32 weeks 6 days: expectant management and steroids.
- Less than 23 weeks: offer termination with prostaglandin E_2 (PGE_2) vaginal suppository, laminaria and oxytocin (Pitocin), or dilatation and evacuation. Overall perinatal survival without termination is 6.7%. If patient does not elect to terminate, manage expectantly, but counsel about maternal risks and poor perinatal outcome.

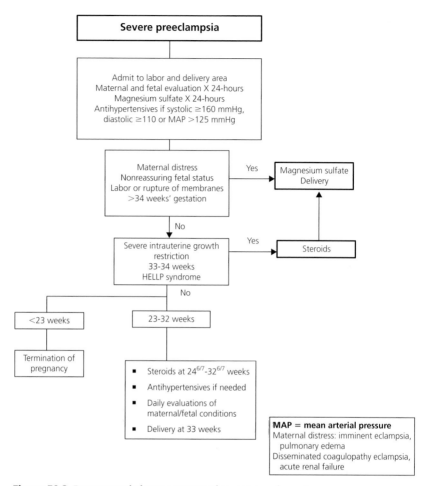

Figure 50.2 Recommended management of severe preeclampsia.

Conservative management of severe preeclampsia

In a tertiary care center:

- Initial intravenous magnesium sulfate for 24 hours.
- Antihypertensives: intravenous boluses, then shift to oral administration, nifedipine, labetalol.

  Hydralazine: 5 to 10 mg boluses every 20 to 30 minutes (maximum dose 20 mg).

  Labetalol: 20 to 40 mg boluses (maximum dose 220 mg). Then 200 mg orally every 8 hours (maximum 600 mg every 6 hours).

  Nifedipine: 10 to 20 mg orally every 30 minutes (maximum 50 mg). Then 10–20 mg every 4–6 hours (maximum 120 mg/day).

Aim: Diastolic blood pressure 90 to 100 mmHg and systolic blood pressure 140 to 150 mmHg. Avoid normal blood pressure because of the risk of decreased uteroplacental perfusion. Adequate therapeutic response is expected in 12 hours.

- Give steroids for immature lungs and attempt to delay delivery at least for steroid benefit (48 hours).
- Daily fetal-maternal testing.

The majority of patients with severe preeclampsia managed conservatively will require delivery within 2 weeks of admission. Indications for delivery of these patients include the following:

- Maternal indications: thrombocytopenia or HELLP (hemolysis, elevated liver enzymes, low platelets), disseminated intravascular coagulation (DIC), pulmonary edema, renal failure, eclampsia, uncontrolled severe hypertension, suspected abruptio placentae, labor or rupture of membranes, ascites; warning signs: persistent and severe headache, blurring of vision, epigastric pain.
- Fetal indications: Fetal distress irrespective of gestational age or lung maturity, persistent severe oligohydramnios, severe intrauterine growth restriction (IUGR; <5th percentile), or gestational age greater than 34 weeks achieved.

Hemolysis, elevated liver enzymes, low platelet count (HELLP)

- Hemolysis: abnormal peripheral blood smear; increased bilirubin ≥1.2 mg/dL; low haptoglobin levels.
- Elevated liver enzymes: increased lactic dehydrogenase greater than twice the upper limit of normal; increased SGOT >70 IU/L.
- Low platelets: <100 × 10^3/μL.
- Occurs in 10 to 12% of severe preeclamptic patients. More frequent in whites and multiparas.
- Complaints of nausea and vomiting (50%), malaise of a few days' duration (90%), epigastric or right upper quadrant pain (65%), or swelling. Others will have vague abdominal pain, flank or shoulder pain, jaundice, hematuria, gastrointestinal bleeding, or gum bleeding.
- Onset antepartum in 70% of the cases and postpartum in 30% of the cases.
- In the postpartum period, the time of onset of the clinical manifestations may range from a few hours to one week, with the majority developing within 48 hours.
- Hypertension may be absent in 20% and mild in 30% of the cases.
- Temporary management of HELLP for 48 hours is only possible in the absence of DIC, particularly for benefit of corticosteroid administration.

Intrapartum management of severe preeclampsia and HELLP

- The first priority is to assess and stabilize maternal condition and then to evaluate fetal well-being. Finally, a decision must be made as to whether immediate delivery is indicated (Table 50.1).

Table 50.1 Management outline of antepartum HELLP syndrome

---

1 Assess and stabilize maternal condition

   a Antiseizure prophylaxis with magnesium sulfate

   b Treatment of severe hypertension

   c Transfer to tertiary care center if appropriate

   d Computed tomography or ultrasound of the abdomen if subcapsular hematoma of the liver
     is suspected

2 Evaluate fetal well-being

   a If fetal lung maturity or >34 weeks' gestation → delivery

   b If immature fluid or ≤34 weeks' → steroids → delivery in 24–48 hours

Deliver if abnormal fetal assessment

Deliver if progressive deterioration in maternal condition

- Intravenous magnesium sulfate: 6 g loading dose over 20 minutes (6 g in 150 mL 5% dextrose in water) followed by the maintenance dose of 2 g/h during labor and for 12 to 24 hours postpartum (40 g in 1 L lactated Ringer's solution at 50 mL/h or 20 g in 1 L lactated Ringer's solution at 100 mL/h). This may also be offered to patients considered to have mild disease. Remember that the risk of eclamptic convulsion in those with severe disease is less than 2%. For mild preeclampsia, the risk is less than 0.5%.
- For HELLP patients, type and cross-match with 2 units of blood.
- Accurate measurement of fluid input and output: Foley catheter, restrict total intake to 100 mL/h to avoid pulmonary edema. If pulmonary edema is suspected, chest x-ray is done and diuretics can be given.
- Frequent monitoring of pulse, blood pressure and respiration.
- Monitor for signs of magnesium toxicity and have a magnesium level drawn if needed; be ready to counteract magnesium toxicity with 10 mL of 10% calcium gluconate intravenously, and intubation if the patient develops respiratory arrest. Be ready to deal with convulsions.
- Continuous fetal monitoring.
- Oxytocin induction and allow normal vaginal delivery for favorable cervix or gestational age of 30 weeks or beyond. If the cervix is unripe and gestational age is less than 30 weeks, consider elective cesarean delivery or cervical ripening with PGE_2.
- Anesthesia: intermittent small doses of meperidine IVP, 25 to 50 mg. Epidural anesthesia is preferred to general anesthesia in case of abdominal delivery if personnel skilled in obstetric anesthesia are available. Pudendal block and epidural are not advisable in HELLP patients as it might result in hematoma formation.
- If thrombocytopenia is present, it should be corrected before surgery: Transfuse with 10 units of platelets in all patients with a platelet count less than $40 \times 10^3/\mu L$.

- In HELLP patients to minimize the risk of hematoma formation: the bladder flap should be left open, a subfascial drain is used, and the wound is left open. The wounds can be successfully closed within 72 hours after drain removal.

Postpartum management
- Adequate observation of the mother in the recovery room for 12 to 24 hours under magnesium sulfate coverage. Remember that 25 to 30% of the eclampsia cases and 30% of the HELLP cases occur in the post-partum period.
- Most patients will show evidence of resolution of the disease process within 24 hours after delivery. Some, especially those with severe disease in the midtrimester, HELLP, or eclampsia, require close monitoring for 2 to 3 days.
- By the time of discharge, most patients will be normotensive. If hyper-tension persists, antihypertensive medications are prescribed for 1 week, after which the patient is re-evaluated.

Complications of preeclampsia and HELLP

Complications include abruptio placentae, pulmonary edema, acute renal failure, liver hematoma with possible rupture, postpartum hem-orrhage, wound or intraabdominal hematomas, DIC and multiorgan failure, including liver, kidneys and lungs (adult respiratory distress syndrome). Neurologic-like eclampsia, hypertensive encephalopathy, ischemia, infarcts, edema and hemorrhage can also occur, as can cardi-orespiratory arrest.

Follow-up and maternal counseling

Women who develop preeclampsia in their first pregnancy are at increased risk (20%) for development of preeclampsia in subsequent pregnancies. The risk of preeclampsia in the sister of a patient with preeclampsia is 14%.

With severe disease in a first pregnancy, the risk of recurrence is about 30%. With severe disease in the second trimester, the risk of recurrent preeclampsia is 50%. In 21% of the cases, the disease also occurs in the second trimester. HELLP recurs in about 5% of the cases.

There is increased risk of chronic hypertension and undiagnosed renal disease. This is especially true in patients with two episodes of severe preeclampsia in the second trimester. These patients should have adequate medical evaluation postpartum. There is also increased risk of intrauterine growth restriction in a subsequent pregnancy.

Suggested reading

Koopmans CM, Biglenga D, Groen H, *et al.*, for the HYPITAT study group. Induction of labour versus expectant monitoring for gestational hypertension or mild pre-eclampsia after 36 weeks' gestation (HYPITAT): a multicentre, open-label randomised controlled trial. *Lancet* 2009;374:979–88.

National High Blood Pressure Education Program Working Group. Report on high blood pressure in pregnancy. *Am J Obstet Gynecol* 2000;183:S1–22.

Sibai BM. Diagnosis and management of gestational hypertension and preeclampsia. *Obstet Gynecol* 2003;102:181–92.

Sibai BM. Hypertension. In: Gabbe SG, Niebyl JR, Simpson JL (eds) *Obstetrics: Normal and Problem Pregnancies*, 5th edn. New York: Churchill Livingstone, 2009; pp. 945–1004.

Sibai BM. Diagnosis, controversies and management of the syndrome of hemolysis, elevated liver enzymes, and low platelet count. *Obstet Gynecol* 2004;103:981–91.

Sibai BM. Magnesium sulphate prophylaxis in preeclampsia: lessons learned from recent trials. *Am J Obstet Gynecol* 2004;190:1520–6.

Sibai BM, Barton JR. Expectant management of severe preeclampsia remote from term: patient selection, treatment, and delivery indications. *Am J Obstet Gynecol* 2007;196:514.e1–514.e9.

PROTOCOL 51

Fetal Growth Restriction

Ray Bahado Singh

Department of Obstetrics and Gynecology, Wayne State University and Hutzel Women's Center, Detroit, MI, USA

Clinical significance

Fetal growth restriction (FGR) is defined in the United States as an estimated fetal weight obtained by ultrasound of <10th percentile for gestational age. Small for gestational age (SGA) refers to actual birth weight <10th percentile for gestation. The frequency of FGR is estimated to be between 4% and 8% of pregnancies in the United States. It is associated with increased perinatal mortality and morbidities, the rates of which increase dramatically with the decline in fetal weight percentiles. There is an eight-fold increase in perinatal mortality for weight <10th percentile, rising to an approximately twenty-fold increase for weight below the 3rd percentile.

Pathophysiology

The etiology of FGR is diverse and so are the pathogenic mechanisms. Broadly speaking the pathophysiological mechanisms fall into three categories: (1) decreased fetal growth potential due to intrinsic causes; (2) placental dysfunction and maternal vascular diseases and (3) other disorders limiting nutrient supply.

Placental dysfunction is the major cause of FGR. Abnormalities of the uteroplacental vasculature, arising frequently from maternal vascular disorders, constitute the most significant etiological group in FGR. Failure of dilation of spiral arteries in the uterine wall occurs along with reduced branching and invasion of the trophoblast carrying fetal vessels into which maternal nutrients are transported. Profound disturbance in nutrient

Protocols for High-Risk Pregnancies, 5th edition. Edited by J.T. Queenan, J.C. Hobbins and C.Y. Spong. © 2010 Blackwell Publishing Ltd.

transport function of the placenta has been documented in human FGR. These include reduced transport of glucose to the fetus, which leads to increase catabolism of fetal proteins and lipids, disturbances of amino acids and lipid transport and reduced clearance of metabolic end products such as lactic acid.

Diagnosis

Precise documentation of gestational dates is critical to diagnosis. This includes determination of date of last menstrual period, menstrual history, date of first positive pregnancy test and first perception of fetal movement. Accurate sonographic dating can be achieved with measurement of mean gestational sac diameter before the appearance of the embryo and thereafter crown−rump length measurement. The crown−rump length has a margin of error of ± 3−5 days. Between 14−20 weeks biometry dating has an accuracy of ± 7−10 days. The margin of error increases to 2.0 to 3.0 weeks between 20 and 26 weeks and thereafter the error is ± 3.0 to 4.5 weeks. Less commonly used measurements such as transcerebellar diameter and biorbital diameter are accurate methods of dating a pregnancy of 14−20 weeks and may be used particularly when menstrual dates are unavailable. Studies reveal large variations (27% to 86%) in the sensitivity of fundal height measurement in the detection of FGR, diminishing its value as a screening test. The diagnosis of FGR in the United States is based on sonographic estimated fetal weight (EFW) <10th percentile. Fetal weight formulas utilize measurements of BPD (biparietal diameter), HC (head circumference), AC (abdominal circumference) and FL (femur length). The larger the number of variables measured, the higher will be the accuracy of the formula. Generally a margin of error of ± 15% is achieved in estimation of fetal weight in 95% cases. The determination of growth rate requires serial measurements of the EFW.

The majority of fetuses with EFW <10th percentile, 40−75%, are constitutionally small and not at increased risk for perinatal morbidities. It is therefore important to distinguish the constitutionally small from the pathologically growth restricted fetus in order to avoid unwarranted testing and interventions. The sensitivity of EFW for the detection of FGR in high-risk women has a range of 33.3% to 89.2% with an associated specificity range of 53.7% to 90.9%. The sensitivity range for AC <10th percentile for comparable specificities is 72.9% to 94.5%, justifying the utilization of both the EFW and AC percentiles in the diagnosis of pathological FGR. A normal AC significantly reduces the likelihood of FGR.

Having confirmed small fetal size, a careful obstetric and medical history must be taken to identify common risk factors for FGR. The presence of an important risk factor significantly increases the odds of FGR.

The search for additional manifestations of growth dysfunction helps to objectively confirm the diagnosis. Doppler velocimetry of the umbilical artery and amniotic fluid assessment should be performed. Reduced amniotic fluid volume, when identified, strongly indicates the presence of FGR due to uteroplacental insufficiency. On the other hand, severe or early-onset FGR with normal amniotic fluid could suggest a congenital anomaly such triploidy or trisomy 18. Amniotic fluid index (AFI) assessment does not appear to be superior to a largest single pocket vertical measurement. Sonographic assessment of the placenta for the presence of abnormalities is required as is targeted anatomical survey of the fetus.

Karyotyping should be reserved for cases with findings of abnormalities on ultrasonography, e.g., severe early-onset IUGR, particularly in the presence of normal or increased amniotic fluid volume, or severe FGR with normal Doppler finding.

Fetal infection accounts for <5% of FGR. Toxoplasma, rubella, CMV and malaria have been significantly implicated in reduced fetal growth. Maternal TORCH tests are not routinely indicated in the evaluation of FGR. Data suggests that the yield is low and that such testing is not cost effective. Ultrasonographic findings suggestive of fetal infections as a cause of IUGR is an indication for TORCH testing and amniotic fluid microbiology.

Uterine artery Doppler measurement performed in the first and second trimester appears to be a poor screening test for FGR in the general population. Similarly, routine third trimester ultrasonographic screening did not result in improved outcome in FGR.

Treatment

The use of antenatal steroids is the only accepted therapy in FGR. Current guidelines require the use of antenatal steroids in pregnancies <34 weeks at risk for preterm delivery. FGR is no exception. Bed rest at home or in hospital is widely utilized; however, while the risks are well known — increased risk of venous thromboembolism and possible maternal bone and weight loss — there is no evidence of benefit. Other therapies such as maternal oxygen administration or the use of nitric oxide patch to induce vasodilation, aspirin use, dietary manipulation, calcium channel blockers and antioxidant therapy have not proven to be useful.

Complications

The complications of FGR are well documented and include perinatal asphyxia and death. Prematurity is a significant end result and complication of FGR. The rate of FGR increases with the severity of prematurity. Neonatal problems include respiratory distress syndrome, necrotizing enterocolitis, retinopathy of prematurity, intracranial hemorrhage and chronic lung disease. For the affected fetus, long-term effects extending into adulthood include obesity, hypertension, type 2 diabetes and hypercholesterolemia.

Surveillance

Once the diagnosis has been established or suspected, serial monitoring is of paramount importance. Umbilical artery Doppler velocimetry remains the most important modality for monitoring FGR pregnancies and is endorsed by the American College of Obstetricians and Gynecologists. Histological confirmation of decreased number of placental arteries with abnormal umbilical artery Doppler indices has been reported in several studies. Meta-analysis of randomized studies by the Cochrane library have confirmed benefits of fetal Doppler in high risk situations such as FGR. They include reduction of unnecessary hospitalizations and labor inductions and reduced perinatal mortality when compared to cases without surveillance. Other systematic reviews have confirmed a reduction of cesarean delivery. Thus, there exists level 1 evidence of improved outcome with the use of umbilical artery Doppler surveillance. No other parameter has achieved this level of confirmation. Other fetal Doppler modalities are being used with increasing frequency in specialist centers. In FGR, due to placental insufficiency, redistribution of blood flow from the trunk to the brain, heart and adrenals occurs with deterioration of fetal status and is a mechanism of preventing oxygenation of these vital organs. Doppler surveillance of the middle cerebral artery will detect these changes which manifest as increased end-diastolic velocity [reduced resistance index (RI), pulsatility index (PI) and ratio of peak systolic to diastolic blood flow velocity (S/D)] and increased peak systolic velocity. Proof of clinical benefit based on large randomized trials is currently lacking.

Impaired cardiac function leading to decreased myocardial contractility and compliance develops in the later stages of IUGR. The end result is reduced forward flow of blood from feeding veins entering the heart with associated venous hemodynamic changes. These may manifest on venous Doppler velocimetry as increased pulsatility with decreased forward velocity or even reversal of flow during the atrial contraction phase in the ductus venosus and inferior vena cava along with enhanced pulsatility of the umbilical vein waveforms in the seriously compromised fetus. There is an absence of optimally designed large-scale randomized studies of venous Doppler, with supporting evidence of its benefit limited to level 2 and 3.

Cardiotocography is the most widely used surveillance measure for monitoring FGR pregnancies. Regrettably, there is poor intra- and inter-observer agreement in interpretation of non-stress testing. While a tracing with good variability provides strong reassurance of good fetal oxygenation, abnormal tracings poorly correlate with fetal status and has a high false-positive rate. There is a lack of uniform evidence of the clinical benefits of this modality in FGR monitoring and evidence of its utility must be considered as level 2 to 3. Overall, non-stress testing must be considered a secondary test and should ideally not be used by itself for FGR monitoring. The biophysical profile is a dynamic test of fetal well-being that also suffers from important limitations. Randomized trials have not demonstrated the of the biophysical profile improves outcomes in high-risk pregnancies. Non-randomized studies indicate a correlation between a normal biophysical profile and good outcome, and an abnormal BPP score, 4–6, and increased perinatal death. The biophysical profile must also be considered a secondary test for FGR surveillance.

Maximum vertical pocket or AFI is used to assess amniotic fluid volume. Either an AFI ≤5 cm or <10th percentile for gestational age may be used to define oligohydramnios. Meta-analysis data confirm the association between oligohydramnios and low Apgar score in high-risk pregnancy. However, evidence based on randomized trials demonstrating improvement in pregnancy outcomes with amniotic fluid volume surveillance is currently lacking.

There is no consensus on the frequency of monitoring for FGR. In the absence of abnormal umbilical artery Doppler or low amniotic fluid volume, monitoring can be reduced to 2-weekly intervals and should arguably consist of umbilical artery Doppler, amniotic fluid volume assessment and non-stress testing (or possible biophysical profile). Serial EFW and AC measurements should arguably be performed at 3–4 weeks. With EFW <5th percentile or maternal disease, e.g., preeclampsia, the frequency of Doppler and biophysical measurements should be increased to weekly, even in the presence of nomal umbilical Doppler. Mild or moderate abnormalities of umbilical Doppler or reduced fluid volume requires twice-weekly biophysical monitoring with weekly Doppler measurements. All outpatient FGR cases should be instructed to perform daily fetal movement count. FGR cases with absent or reversed end-diastolic velocity in the umbilical artery, a persistent non-reactive or concerning non-stress test, biophysical profile ≤4 and moderate to severe oligohydramnios or abnormalities on biophysical testing should be hospitalized and evaluated for delivery or intensive fetal monitoring. The same applies for deterioration in maternal condition.

Management

The timing of delivery is perhaps the most challenging aspect of the management of FGR pregnancies. The most important considerations are gestational age and status of fetal testing. Generally, FGR pregnancies should be delivered at 37 weeks since the excellent neonatal outcome at this age does not justify the risk of continued intrauterine existence. FGR fetuses delivered <26 weeks with EFW <600 g reportedly have a low chance of survival, suggesting that conservative management be instituted at this stage. Antenatal steroids should be administered for preterm delivery between 24–34 weeks. Fetuses between 26–34 weeks with abnormalities in biophysical testing, prolonged non-reactive non-stress test, late decelerations, severe variable decelerations or biophysical profile score <4–6 should be delivered. Limited data indicates that between 25–30 weeks' gestation, prolonging intrauterine stay in FGR even by only a few days significantly decreases perinatal mortality. There is thus a great deal of interest in identifying the optimal time when the risk of stillbirth begins to exceed the benefits of intrauterine residence in the preterm fetus. Research by a number of groups suggests that there is a sequence of deterioration of Doppler and biophysical indices preceding the need for delivery or of fetal death in FGR. While there is some variation in the abnormal biophysical and Doppler findings, in general the earliest change appear to be an increase in the umbilical artery Doppler resistance which is often found at the time of diagnosis of FGR. Absent umbilical artery end-diastolic velocity develops in 50% of patients, approximately 7–9 days prior to delivery. The pulsatility index in the middle cerebral artery was found to be abnormal in 50% of patients approximately 4 days prior to delivery and reversal of diastolic velocities in the umbilical artery and ductus venosus develops in 50% of patients 1–2 days before the need for delivery. Reversal of flow in the ductus venosus and umbilical artery generally precedes non-reactive non-stress test, abnormal biophysical profile and the need for delivery by a few days. Taken together, this information gives a time line over which fetal deterioration and ultimately delivery is likely to occur. The current clinical standard is to await the development of abnormal non-stress test or biophysical profile before delivery of FGR fetuses <34 weeks' gestation. A large randomized study, the 'Growth Restriction Intervention Trial' (GRIT), compared the effect of early delivery against conservative management in FGR fetuses of 26–33 weeks, many with Doppler abnormalities, in which there was uncertainty regarding ideal timing of delivery. There was no significant difference in perinatal deaths and in serious long-term morbidity on 2-year follow-up of survivors. There appeared to be a trend toward more favorable neurological performance for Tae group managed in utero. Thus, premature delivery at this GA to improve neurological outcome appears not to be justified.

For fetuses between 34 and <37 weeks without Doppler or biophysical abnormalities, close surveillance and delivery at term appears appropriate. The development of Doppler abnormalities with or without equivocal biophysical testing would justify amniocentesis for lung maturity and pos-sible delivery. FGR do not preclude an attempt at vaginal delivery. Such attempts are particularly appropriate >34 weeks and in the presence of a favorable cervix. In the case of an unfavorable cervix, particularly <32 weeks, opting for an elective cesarean delivery rather than a pro-longed stressful induction might be the more prudent course.

Conclusion

FGR is a common problem and a major cause of stillbirth, prematurity and neonatal, pediatric and (based on more recent evidence) adult dis-eases. Obtaining the most precise dating in all pregnant women is critical to the detection and management of FGR. Sonographic diagnosis should be based on both EFW and AC percentiles. Umbilical artery Doppler is the only surveillance method proven to improve outcome. This may be supplemented with non-stress testing and fluid volume assessment. While timing of delivery in preterm gestation is currently based on the development of abnormalities of non-stress testing and biohysical profile, multi-vessel arterial and venous Doppler may be useful in providing a time course on the extent of cardiovascular and metabolic deterioration of the fetus.

Suggested reading

American College of Obstetricians and Gynecologists. Practice Bulletin #12, January 2000. *Intrauterine Growth Restriction. Clinical Management Guidelines for Obstetrician-Gynecologists.*

Barker, DJP. Adult consequences of fetal growth restriction. *Clin Obstet Gynecol* 2006;49:270–83.

Baschat AA. Fetal responses to placental insufficiency: an update. *Br J Obstet Gynaecol* 2004;111:1031–41.

Cosmi E, Ambrosini G, D'Antona D, Saccardi C, Mari G. Doppler, cardiotocography, and biophysical profile changes in growth-restricted fetuses. *Obstet Gynecol* 2005;106:1240–5.

Hui L, Challis D. Diagnosis and management of fetal growth restriction: the role of fetal therapy. *Best Pract Res Clin Obstet Gynaecol* 2008;22:139–58.

Mari G, Hanif F. Intrauterine growth restriction: how to manage and when to deliver. *Clin Obstet Gynecol* 2007;50:497–509.

Maulik, D. Management of fetal growth restriction: an evidence-based approach. *Clin Obstet Gynecol* 2006;49:320–34.

Neilson JP, Alfirevic Z. Doppler ultrasound for fetal assessment in high-risk pregnancies. *Cochrane Database Syst Rev* 2005. Cochrane Library.

Pattison N, McCowen L. Cardiotocography for antepartum fetal assessment. *Cochrane Database Syst Rev* 2003;(1). Cochrane Library.

Royal College of Obstetricians and Gynecologists. *The investigation and management of the small-for-gestational-age fetus.* Guideline No.31, November 2002.

Rh and Other Blood Group Alloimmunizations

Kenneth J. Moise Jr

Department of Obstetrics and Gynecology and Department of Surgery, Baylor College of Medicine, Houston, TX, USA

Overview

Once a significant cause of perinatal loss, alloimmunization to red cell antigens is infrequently encountered today in obstetrical practice. Sensitization to the RhD antigen remains the leading cause of hemolytic disease of the fetus/newborn (HDFN) accounting for over 50% of cases.[1] 2002 was the last year that the Centers for Disease Control reported the incidence of rhesus alloimmunization through birth certificate data. In that year, the incidence was 6.7/1000 live births.[2] In a report of 37 506 female patients at two New York blood centers, 1.1% of samples contained an antibody associated with HDFN. After anti-D, Kell antibodies were next most frequent (29%) followed by Duffy (7%), MNS (6%), Kidd and anti-U.[1] Despite the frequency of this disease, significant advances in diagnostic tools have occurred with the addition of genetic testing of the fetus and Doppler ultrasonography for the detection of fetal anemia.

Pathophysiology

The fetal-maternal interface was once thought to be an impervious barrier. However, more recent evidence suggests there is considerable trafficking of many types of cells between the fetus and its mother throughout gestation. In most cases, the antigenic load of incompatible antigen on the fetal erythrocytes and erythrocytic precursors is insufficient to stimulate the maternal immune system. However, in the case of a large antenatal feto-maternal hemorrhage, or a feto-maternal hemorrhage at delivery, B-lymphocyte clones that recognize the foreign red cell antigen are established. The initial

---

Protocols for High-Risk Pregnancies, 5th edition. Edited by J.T. Queenan, J.C. Hobbins and C.Y. Spong. © 2010 Blackwell Publishing Ltd.

maternal IgM antibody response is short-lived with a rapid change to IgG antibody.

Although the fetus of the sensitizing pregnancy often escapes the effects of the maternal antibody, subsequent fetuses are at risk for HDFN. Maternal IgG crosses the placenta and attaches to fetal erythrocytes that have expressed the paternal red cell antigen. These cells are then sequestered by macrophages in the fetal spleen where they undergo extravascular hemolysis producing fetal anemia. In cases of HDFN related to the Kell (anti-K1) antibody, in vitro and in vivo evidence suggest an additional mechanism for the fetal anemia – suppression of erythropoiesis.[3,4] Hydrops fetalis is the most significant manifestation of the fetal anemia although its exact pathophysiology remains unknown. An elevated central venous pressure has been reported in these fetuses and may cause a functional blockage of the lymphatic system at the level of the thoracic duct as it empties into the left brachiocephalic vein. Reports of poor absorption of red cells transfused into the peritoneal cavity in cases of hydrops support this theory.

Management of the first alloimmunized pregnancy

- Obtain an antibody screen on all pregnant women at their first prenatal visit. If the antibody screen returns positive, the antibody should be identified to see if it has been associated with HDFN (see Table 52.1). If this is the case, an antiglobulin titer should be undertaken.
- Obtain an early ultrasound examination for pregnancy dating.
- Determine the paternal antigen status.
  - If negative and paternity is assured, no further evaluation is necessary.
  - If positive, serologic testing can be used in consultation with a blood bank pathologist to determine the paternal zygosity (homozygous or heterozygous) for most red cell antigens. The one exception is the RhD antigen where the lack of a 'd' antigen is secondary to the non-expression of the RhD gene. In this situation, testing for paternal zygosity should be undertaken through DNA methods at a reference laboratory.
- Repeat titers every month until 24 weeks' gestation; then every 2 weeks for the remainder of the pregnancy. Perform titers with the older tube technology (gel methods have not been correlated with clinical outcome). Use an experienced blood bank; most commercial laboratories use enhancement techniques that will elevate titers.
- If the titer is 1:32 or greater (use a titer of 1:8 for the Kell antibody), there is a risk for fetal hydrops. Consult a maternal-fetal medicine specialist for further management.

Table 52.1 Non-RhD antibodies and associated hemolytic disease of the fetus or newborn

Antigen system	Specific antigen	Antigen system	Specific antigen	Antigen system	Specific antigen
Frequently associated with severe disease					
Kell	-K (K1)				
Rhesus	-c				
Infrequently associated with severe disease					
Colton	-Coa	MNS	-Mur	Scianna	-Sc2
	-Co3		-MV		-Rd
Diego	-ELO		-s	Other Ag's	-Bi
	-Dia		-sD		-Good
	-Dib		-S		-Heibel
	-Wra		-U		-HJK
	-Wrb		-Vw		-Hta
Duffy	-Fya	Rhesus	-Bea		-Jones
Kell	- Jsb		-C		-Joslin
	-k (K2)		-Ce		-Kg
	-Kpa		-Cw		-Kuhn
	- Kpb		-ce		-Lia
	-K11		-E		-MAM
	-K22		-Ew		-Niemetz
	-Ku		-Evans		-REIT
	- Ula		-G		-Reiter
Kidd	-Jka		-Goa		-Rd
MNS	-Ena		-Hr		-Sharp
	-Far		-Hro		-Vel
	-Hil		-JAL		-Zd
	-Hut		-Rh32		
	-M		-Rh42		
	-Mia		-Rh46		
	-Mta		-STEM		
	-MUT		-Tar		
Associated with mild disease					
Duffy	-Fyb	Kidd	-Jkb	Rhesus	-Riv
	-Fy3		-Jk3		-RH29
Gerbich	-Ge2	MNS	-Mit	Other	-Ata
	-Ge3	Rhesus	-CX		-JFV
	-Ge4		-Dw		-Jra
	-Lsa		-e		-Lan
Kell	- Jsa		-HOFM		
			-LOCR		

- In cases of a heterozygous partner, perform amniocentesis by 24 weeks' gestation to assess the fetal blood type through DNA analysis. Send maternal and paternal blood samples to the reference laboratory with the amniotic aliquot to minimize errors due to gene rearrangements in the parents. In the case of RhD, free fetal DNA in the maternal serum can now be used to test the antigen status of the fetus in a non-invasive fashion.
- The antigen-positive fetus can be monitored for the development of anemia by ultrasonography using the peak middle cerebral artery systolic velocity serially every 1–2 weeks.
  - A value of greater than 1.5 multiples of the median (MOM) for gestational age is highly suggestive for fetal anemia (see Fig. 52.1).[5] MCA's can be obtained as early as 18 weeks but are less useful after 35 weeks gestation.
  - Serial amniocenteses for ΔOD_{450} using the Queenan curve (see Fig. 52.2) is reserved for cases where access to a center experienced in MCA Doppler is not readily available. A transplacental approach should be avoided to decrease the chance for enhanced maternal sensitization.
- If the MCA Doppler is >1.5 MOM or the ΔOD_{450} value enters the *Rh positive (affected)* zone of the Queenan curve, perform cordocentesis with blood readied for intrauterine transfusion for a fetal hematocrit of <30%.
- Initiate antenatal testing with non-stress testing or biophysical profiles at 32 weeks' gestation.

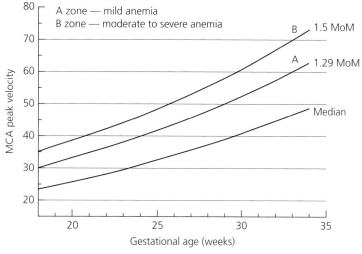

Figure 52.1 Middle cerebral artery peak systolic Doppler velocity. Reproduced with permission from: Moise KJ. Modern management of Rhesus alloimmunization in pregnancy. *Obstet Gynecol* 2002;100:600–11. Elsevier Science Company, Copyright © 2002.

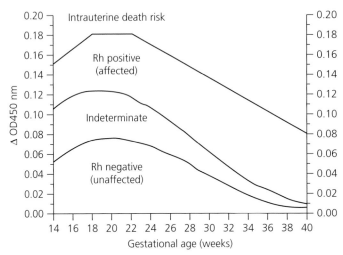

Figure 52.2 Queenan curve for ΔOD_{450} values (with permission) from: Queenan JT, Tomai TP, Ural SH, King JC. Deviation in amniotic fluid optical density at a wavelength of 450 nm in Rh-immunized pregnancies from 14 to 40 weeks' gestation: a proposal for clinical management. *Am J Obstet Gynecol* 1993;168:1370–6. Mosby, Inc., Copyright © 2001.

- After 35 weeks' gestation, there is minimal data on the sensitivity of the MCA Doppler to predict fetal anemia. False-negative values have been reported with the fetal heart rate accelerations that are more common at this gestation.[6] If values have remained normal up to this gestational age, an amniocentesis may be warranted to determine management for the remainder of the pregnancy. A test for fetal lung maturity and ΔOD_{450} value should be obtained.
  - If mature lungs are found and the ΔOD_{450} value has not reached the *Rh positive (affected)* zone of the Queenan curve or higher, induce by 37–38 weeks' gestation to allow for hepatic maturity in an effort to prevent hyperbilirubinemia.
  - If mature lungs are found and the ΔOD_{450} value has reached the *Rh positive (affected)* zone or *intrauterine transfusion* zone of the Queenan curve, delivery is indicated.
  - If immature lungs are found and the ΔOD_{450} value has reached the *Rh positive (affected)* zone, consider antenatal steroids and 7 days of maternal phenobarbital (30 mg oral dose TID); induce labor in 1 week. This will accelerate fetal hepatic maturity and allow for more efficient neonatal conjugation of bilirubin.[7] In these cases, a unit of packed red blood cells cross-matched to the pregnant patient should be prepared prior to the delivery so that it would be available in the event that the pediatrician must perform an emergency neonatal transfusion.

- If immature lungs are found and the ΔOD_{450} value is not in the *Rh positive (affected)* zone, repeat the amniocentesis for lung maturity in 10–14 days.

Management of a subsequent alloimmunized pregnancy

(Previously affected fetus that has undergone intrauterine transfusions or an infant that has undergone neonatal transfusions)
- Maternal titers are *not* helpful in predicting the onset of fetal anemia after the first affected gestation.
- In cases of a heterozygous paternal phenotype, perform amniocentesis at 15 weeks' gestation to determine the fetal red cell antigen status. In the case of RhD, free fetal DNA can be used to determine the fetal 'D' status. If an antigen-negative fetus is found and paternity is assured, no further testing is warranted.
- Begin serial MCA Doppler assessments at 18 weeks' gestation. Repeat at 1- to 2-week intervals.
- If a rising value for MCA Doppler >1.5 MOM, perform cordocentesis with blood readied for intrauterine transfusion for a fetal hematocrit of <30%.
- If the MCA Doppler remains normal, follow the same protocol for antenatal monitoring and delivery as previously noted for the management of the first sensitized pregnancy.

Treatment

Since it was first introduced in 1963,[8] the intrauterine transfusion (IUT) of donor red blood cells has clearly contributed to the survival of countless fetuses with severe HDFN worldwide. Today the direct intravascular transfusion (IVT) using the umbilical cord for access is the technique most widely used in the United States. Typically, a unit of donor red cells that has been recently donated and lacking the putative red cell antigen is used. The donor should be negative for antibody to cytomegalovirus. The unit is cross-matched to the pregnant patient and then packed to a final hematocrit of 75–85% to allow a minimal blood volume to be administered to the fetus during the IUT. The blood is then leukoreduced with a special filter and irradiated with 25 Gy to prevent graft-versus-host reaction.

The patient is usually admitted to the labor and delivery suite for an outpatient procedure. Conscious sedation is used in conjunction with local anesthetic. Prophylactic antibiotics are given but tocolytics are rarely required. Continuous ultrasonographic guidance is used to find the umbilical cord insertion. After the initial puncture of the umbilical vein, a sample of fetal blood is sent for hematocrit and other values. A small dose of a paralytic agent is administered to cause cessation of fetal movement. Donor red cells are then transfused based on the initial fetal hematocrit and formulas to calculate the fetoplacental blood volume using ultrasound-estimated fetal weight.[9] A final sample is obtained to measure the fetal hematocrit at the conclusion of the procedure. After the procedure, the patient undergoes continuous fetal monitoring until there is resumption of fetal movement. Ultrasonography is performed the following day to assess fetal viability.

IUTs are rarely successful prior to 18 weeks' gestation; excellent rates of neonatal survival in today's nurseries have led most centers to limit IUTs to gestational ages of less than 35 weeks. If the fetus is severely anemic and the gestational age is less than 24 weeks, the fetal hematocrit is only partially corrected with the first IVT.[10] A subsequent procedure is planned 48 hours later to correct the fetal hematocrit into the normal range. In other cases, the second procedure is usually planned 7–10 days after the first with an expected decrease in the fetal hematocrit of approximately 1%/day. Subsequent procedures are repeated at 2- to 3-week intervals based on fetal response.

After the last procedure, the patient is scheduled for induction of labor at 38–39 weeks' gestation to allow for fetal hepatic and pulmonary maturity. It is rare for these infants to require prolonged phototherapy or exchange transfusions. Breastfeeding is not contraindicated.

Outcome and follow-up

In experienced centers, the overall perinatal survival with IUTs is 85–90%.[11] Fetuses with hydrops have a markedly lower rate of survival, particularly if the hydrops does not resolve after two or three procedures. Suppression of fetal erythropoiesis results in prolonged bone marrow suppression after birth. These infants should be followed weekly with hematocrits and reticulocyte counts until there is evidence of reticulocytosis. Simple neonatal transfusions of red cells may be required in as many as 50% of cases, particularly if the neonate becomes symptomatic from its anemia.[12]

Neurodevelopmental follow-up of neonates transfused by IVT are limited in number. Most studies point to over a 90% chance of intact survival.[13] Hydrops fetalis does not seem to impact this outcome. Sensineural hearing loss may be slightly increased due to prolonged exposure of the fetus to high levels of bilirubin. A hearing screen should be performed during the early neonatal course and repeated by 2 years of age.

Prevention

Only RhD alloimmunization can be prevented through the use of a specific immune globulin (RhIG). Although this product is manufactured from human serum, clinical trials are under way with synthesized monoclonal antibodies. Prevention of alloimmunization to other red cell antigens is currently not possible as specific prophylactic immune globulins are not available. In some countries, such as Australia, Kell-negative female children and women of reproductive age are cross-matched to receive Kell-negative blood when they require a transfusion. This policy has not been adopted in the United States due to the low frequency of the Kell antigen in the general population.

Patients whose initial blood type at the first prenatal visit returns RhD negative, weak Rh positive (formerly called Du positive), have fewer RhD antigenic sites expressed on their red cells. For this reason they are not at risk for rhesus alloimmunization and therefore do not require RhIG. If an RhD-negative patient's initial antibody screen is negative, further diagnostic testing is unnecessary until 28 weeks' gestation. Unless the patient's partner is documented to be RhD negative, a 300 μg dose of RhIG should then be administered. A repeat antibody screen at 28 weeks is recommended by the American Association of Blood Banks (AABB), although the American College of Obstetricians and Gynecologists has left this to the discretion of the clinician.[14]

At the time of the delivery of an RhD-negative patient, cord blood should be tested for RhD typing. If the neonate is determined to be RhD positive, a second dose of 300 μg should be administered within 72 hours of delivery. Routine screening of all women for excessive feto-maternal bleeding at the time of delivery is now recommended by the AABB. Typically this involves a rosette test that is read qualitatively as positive or negative. If negative, one vial of RhIG (300 μg) is given as this will be sufficient to protect the patient from a 30 mL fetal bleed. If positive, the volume of the bleed is quantitated with a Kleihauer-Betke stain or fetal cell stain using flow cytometry. Blood bank consultation should then be undertaken to determine the number of doses of RhIG to administer. If RhIG is inadvertently omitted after delivery, some protection from sensitization has been shown with administration within 13 days. RhIG should not be withheld as late as 28 days after delivery if the need arises.[14]

Additional indications for RhIG are listed in Table 52.2. The use of RhIG for threatened abortion has not been well studied. If minimal vaginal bleeding is noted, it can probably be omitted; however if significant clinical bleeding is present, a dose should be administered. Although a 50 μg RhIG dose can be used up to 13 weeks' gestation; in practical terms most hospitals no longer stock this preparation and the cost is comparable

Table 52.2 Other indications for Rhesus immune globulin administration

---

- Spontaneous abortion
- Threatened abortion
- Elective abortion
- Ectopic pregnancy
- Hydatidiform mole
- Amniocentesis
- Chorionic villus biopsy
- Placenta previa with bleeding
- Suspected abruption
- Fetal death
- Blunt trauma to the abdomen (including motor vehicle accidents)
- External cephalic version

---

to the standard 300 μg dose. Repeat doses should be given at 12-week intervals if bleeding persists. A second indication for RhIg that is often overlooked is blunt trauma to the maternal abdomen, particularly at the time of a motor vehicle accident. Finally, if 300 μg of RhIG are given late in gestation for external cephalic version or third trimester amniocentesis for fetal lung maturity, a repeat dose is unnecessary if delivery occurs within 3 weeks as long as a feto-maternal hemorrhage in excess of 30 mL is not documented. The use of a repeat dose of RhIG after 40 weeks' gestation or its use after postpartum tubal ligation remains controversial.

Conclusion

The prevention and treatment of HDFN secondary to rhesus alloimmunization represents a true victory of modern perinatal care. Advances in DNA technology now allow for routine non-invasive RhD red cell typing of the fetus from maternal serum. In the near future, these same techniques may allow RhD-negative pregnant women who carry RhD-negative fetuses to forego antenatal rhesus immune globulin. Maternal immunomodulation will probably negate the need for intrauterine transfusion in the coming years.

References

1 Geifman-Holtzman O, Wojtowycz M, Kosmas E, Artal R. Female alloimmunization with antibodies known to cause hemolytic disease. *Obstet Gynecol* 1997;89:272.
2 Martin JA, Hamilton BE, Sutton PD, Ventura SJ, Menacker F, Munson ML. Births: final data for 2002. *Natl Vital Stat Rep* 2003;52:1.

3 Vaughan JI, Warwick R, Letsky E, Nicolini U, Rodeck CH, Fisk NM. Erythropoietic suppression in fetal anemia because of Kell alloimmunization. *Am J Obstet Gynecol* 1994;171:247.

4 Vaughan JI, Manning M, Warwick RM, Letsky EA, Murray NA, Roberts IA. Inhibition of erythroid progenitor cells by anti-Kell antibodies in fetal alloimmune anemia [see comments]. *N Engl J Med* 1998;338:798.

5 Mari G, for the Collaborative Group for Doppler Assessment of the Blood Velocity in Anemic Fetuses. Noninvasive diagnosis by Doppler ultrasonography of fetal anemia due to maternal red-cell alloimmunization. *N Engl J Med* 2000;342:9.

6 Swartz AE, Ruma MS, Kim E, Herring AN, Menard MK, Moise KJ. The effect of fetal heart rate on the peak systolic velocity of the middle cerebral artery. *Obstet Gynecol* 2009;113:1225.

7 Trevett T, Dorman K, Lamvu G, Moise KJ. Does antenatal maternal administration of phenobarbital prevent exchange transfusion in neonates with alloimmune hemolytic disease? *Am J Obstet Gynecol* 2003;189:S214.

8 Liley AW. Intrauterine transfusion of foetus in haemolytic disease. *Br Med J* 1963;2:1107.

9 Mandelbrot L, Daffos F, Forestier F, MacAleese J, Descombey D. Assessment of fetal blood volume for computer-assisted management of in utero transfusion. *Fetal Ther* 1988;3:60.

10 Radunovic N, Lockwood CJ, Alvarez M, Plecas D, Chitkara U, Berkowitz RL. The severely anemic and hydropic isoimmune fetus: changes in fetal hematocrit associated with intrauterine death. *Obstet Gynecol* 1992;79:390.

11 Schumacher B, Moise KJ, Jr. Fetal transfusion for red blood cell alloimmunization in pregnancy. *Obstet Gynecol* 1996;88:137.

12 Saade GR, Moise KJ, Belfort MA, Hesketh DE, Carpenter RJ. Fetal and neonatal hematologic parameters in red cell alloimmunization: predicting the need for late neonatal transfusions. *Fetal Diagn Ther* 1993;8:161.

13 Hudon L, Moise KJ, Jr., Hegemier SE, *et al.* Long-term neurodevelopmental outcome after intrauterine transfusion for the treatment of fetal hemolytic disease. *Am J Obstet Gynecol* 1998;179:858.

14 American College of Obstetricians and Gynecologists. *Prevention of RhD alloimmunization.* ACOG Practice Bulletin # 4, 1999.

Preterm Labor

Vincenzo Berghella

Department of Obstetrics and Gynecology, Division of Maternal-Fetal Medicine, Thomas Jefferson University, Philadelphia, PA, USA

Clinical significance

Preterm labor is responsible for approximately 50% of preterm births. Preterm birth is the foremost problem in obstetrics and accounts for most perinatal death. Preterm birth occurs in 12.7% (2007 data) of the over 4 million births in the United States. As such, there are over 500,000 preterm births in the United States each year. Over 75% of perinatal deaths related to preterm birth occur in babies born between 22 and 31 weeks. The rate of perinatal morbidity is also indirectly proportional to gestational age at birth (Table 53.1).

Pathophysiology

The pathophysiology of preterm labor is not well understood. At least four different mechanisms have been described: inflammation/infection, abruption (decidual bleeding), maternal and/or fetal stress, and excessive mechanical stretching of the uterus. Although arising from different pathways, and often more than just one, all spontaneous preterm births utilize a final common biochemical conduit that includes increased genital tract prostaglandin and protease production coupled with functional progesterone withdrawal related to progesterone receptor function. Disparities in preterm birth rates between racial groups may reflect both environmental stressors and differing genetic predispositions.

Diagnosis

Unfortunately there are many differing definitions of preterm labor. The classic definition involves 'uterine contractions ($\geq$6/60 min) and documented

Protocols for High-Risk Pregnancies, 5th edition. Edited by J.T. Queenan, J.C. Hobbins and C.Y. Spong. © 2010 Blackwell Publishing Ltd.

Table 53.1 Survival and major morbidities by gestational age at birth in 2008

GA (weeks)	Survival (%)	Chronic lung disease (%)	Severe IVH (%)	Necrotizing enterocolitis (%)	Severe ROP (%)
<22	3.3	33.3	33.3	33.3	66.7
22	6.0	77.8	52.0	11.1	57.9
23	34.3	79.2	33.8	15.9	46.9
24	59.2	74.7	29.5	12.4	34.7
25	75.3	65.9	20.1	11.6	26.2
26	80.0	51.7	17.2	10.2	14.2
27	89.4	35.9	9.7	6.8	7.0
28	91.2	25.8	6.3	7.2	3.0
29	94.3	16.2	4.3	4.9	1.0
30	96.8	11.0	1.9	3.4	0.7
31	96.7	7.3	1.9	2.4	0.6
32	97.5	4.1	1.3	1.7	0.2
33	98.1	3.1	1.4	1.0	0.9
34	98.4	4.4	1.5	0.9	0.0

GA, gestational age.
Chronic lung disease is defined as need for oxygen therapy at 36 weeks of postmenstrual age.
Severe IVH: grades III and IV.
Necrotizing enterocolitis includes medical and surgical.
Severe ROP (retinopathy of prematurity) is defined as >grade 2.
Data from (with permission): Vermont Oxford Network 2007 *Very Low Birth Weight Summary*. Horbar JD, Carpenter JH, Kenny M, Editors. Vermont Oxford Network, Burlington, VT. 2008. Courtesy of Kevin Dysart, MD.

cervical change by manual examination with intact membranes at 20–36 6/7weeks'. Most women with this diagnosis of preterm labor deliver at term (≥37weeks) even without intervention. Transvaginal ultrasound (TVU) cervical length (CL) and fetal fibronectin (FFN) are currently the two tests with the best data for good prediction of preterm birth in women with preterm labor. Therefore we like to add other criteria to this definition: 'in presence of TVU CL ≤20 mm, *or* TVU 20–30 mm and positive FFN'. The vast majority of these women would deliver preterm with this definition. Instead, women with preterm uterine contractions and manual cervical change but a TVU CL ≥30 mm have a <2% chance of delivering within 1 week and <10% chance of delivering <35 weeks.

Treatment

Preterm labor is better prevented than treated. The management of a woman with true preterm labor involves several approaches:
• Treating only the women with true preterm labor and a real risk of preterm birth. A randomized trial[1] has shown benefit (reduction in preterm

birth and quicker triage time) when women with threatened preterm labor are managed according to the algorithm shown in Fig. 53.1.
- Optimization of fetal status:
  - *Transfer*: Assess for transfer to appropriate level hospital, usually with level III nursery.
  - *Corticosteroids for fetal maturity*: A course of antenatal corticosteroids should be given to all women with true preterm labor, or at high risk for preterm birth within the next 7 days when between 23 and 34 weeks 6 days. All pregnant women between 24 and 34 weeks at high risk of preterm birth within 7 days should be offered treatment with a single course of antenatal corticosteroids (ACS). This single course of ACS consists of two doses of 12 mg betamethasone given intramuscularly 24 hours apart; or four doses of

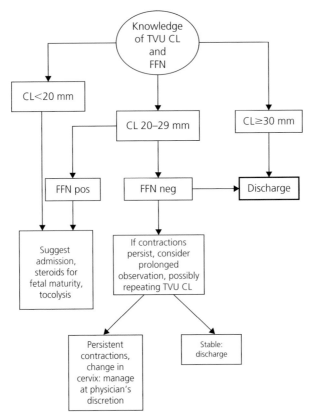

Figure 53.1 A proposed algorithm for combined cervical length (TVU CL) and fetal fibronectin (FFN) screening for women with symptoms of threatened preterm labor. TVU, transvaginal ultrasound; CL, cervical length; FFN, fetal fibronectin. Modified from Ness A, Visintine J, Ricci E, Berghella V. Does knowledge of cervical length and fetal fibronectin affect management of women with threatened preterm labor? A randomized trial. *Am J Obstet Gynecol* 2007;197(4):426.e1–7.

6 mg dexamethasone given intramuscularly 12 hours apart. A single course of ACS administered to women at increased risk of preterm birth between 24 and 34 weeks reduces morbidity (RDS, IVH, NEC, NICU admission, etc.) and mortality in infants. Regarding the effects of betamethasone compared with dexamethasone, a meta-analysis shows a lower incidence of IVH with betamethasone. The current benefit and risk data are insufficient to support routine use of repeat or rescue courses of ACS in clinical practice. When a course of ACS has been given before 28 weeks, one rescue course can be considered when >14 days after the first course, explaining risks and benefits.

- Tocolysis
  - The goal of tocolysis is to prevent imminent preterm birth, in order to have sufficient time to administer corticosteroids and, if necessary, allow for maternal in utero transfer to a hospital with appropriate neonatal care.
  - Given their safety profiles and effectiveness at delaying delivery for both 48 hours and 7 days, nifedipine (as usual first line) and indomethacin (for ≤48 hours) are the primary tocolyics we use clinically.
  - There is no evidence to support the use of maintenance tocolysis after successful arrest of preterm labor. There is not sufficient evidence to administer tocolysis once ACS have been administered.
- Magnesium for neuroprotection
  - Magnesium sulfate has been shown in five trials enrolling over 6000 women to significantly decrease cerebral palsy from 5.3% in placebo controls to 4.1%.[2] The American College of Obstetricians and Gynecologists and the Society for Maternal Fetal Medicine) have stated that "physicians electing to use magnesium sulfate for fetal neuroprotection should develop specific guidelines regarding inclusion criteria, treatment regimens, concurrent tocolysis, and monitoring in accordance with one of the larger trials."[3]
- Other interventions
  - There is insufficient data to recommend hydration, bed rest or decreased activity, progesterone or antibiotic therapy for prevention of preterm birth in women with preterm labor. Therefore these interventions should be avoided, or reserved for clinical trials.

Complications

Preterm birth is associated with severe complications for the neonate. These include both short- and long-term complications for the baby born too soon. Short-term, at times devastating, complications are listed in Table 53.1. Long-term complications include, among others, cerebral

palsy, cognitive defects (e.g. low IQ), school difficulties, behavioral problems and diminished long-term survival and reproduction.

Follow-up

An episode of preterm labor usually does not give rise to a preterm birth.
After administering ACS in the hospital, the woman can usually be discharged home. There are no interventions that are proven to prevent
preterm birth between discharge and eventual delivery. Bed rest, frequent
visits, and education on contractions have either been insufficiently studied or not proven beneficial so far. If the woman does have a preterm birth,
postpartum counseling regarding how to prevent a recurrent preterm birth is
extremely important.[4]

Table 53.2 Suggested prevention strategies to avoid preterm births

Preconception	Avoid extremes of age
	Aim for desirable inter-pregnancy interval (highest risk of PTB with interval <6 months)
	Avoid multiple gestations, with an emphasis on responsible ART
	Folate supplementation
	Vaccinations (especially varicella, rubella, hepatitis B)
	Balanced diet
	Exercise
	Avoid <120 lb maternal weight or BMI <19 kg/m^2
	Avoid illicit drug use and alcohol use
	Avoid sexually transmitted infections
	Optimize any medical disease (e.g., diabetes, hypertension, hypothyroidism, hyperthyroidism, asthma, lupus, HIV)
	Stop or substitute with safer medications any teratogenic drug
Prenatal care	Early ultrasound
	Screen for and treat asymptomatic bacteriuria
	Balanced diet
	Proper weight gain (at least 15 kg over 40 weeks for non-obese women)
	Avoid smoking, illicit drug use and alcohol
	Avoid prolonged standing >3h/day
	Avoid long work hours >39 h/week
	Avoid shift work
	Avoid vaginal douching
	Screen for domestic violence and provide resources
	Screen for and treat sexually transmitted infections

PTB, preterm birth; ART, assisted reproductive technologies; BMI, body mass index.

Prevention

Prevention is of most importance. Several preventive interventions have been shown to be successful in reducing the risk of preterm birth (Table 53.2). These should be widely implemented, both at the local level (doctor–patient), and at the national level (government incentives and policies to assure implementation).

Conclusions

The incidence of preterm birth has increased >30% in the last 20 years in the United States. This is mostly due to increases in use of assisted reproduction (and consequent multiple gestations), and indicated preterm birth. Among other causes, coding of births at 22–24 weeks as preterm instead of miscarriages has undoubtedly increased the incidence in the United States. Very recent data seems to show that the incidence of spontaneous preterm birth is starting to decrease in singleton gestations. Implementation of preventive strategies (as shown in Table 53.2) will help decrease this trend.

References

1 Ness A, Visintine J, Ricci E, Berghella V. Does knowledge of cervical length and fetal fibronectin affect management of women with threatened preterm labor? A randomized trial. *Am J Obstet Gynecol* 2007;197:426e1–426e7.
2 Doyle LW, Crowther CA, Middleton P, Marret S, Rouse D. Magnesium sulphate for women at risk of preterm birth for neuroprotection of the fetus. *Cochrane Database Syst Rev* 2009:CD004661.
3 American College of Obstetricians and Gynecologists. Magnesium Sulfate before anticipated preterm birth for neuroprotection. Committee Opinion No. 455. *Obstet Gynecol* 2010;115:669–71.
4 Spong CY. Prediction and prevention of recurrent spontaneous preterm birth. *Obstet Gynecol* 2007;110:405–15.

Premature Rupture of the Membranes

Brian Mercer

Case Western University and Department of Obstetrics and Maternal-Fetal Medicine, MetroHealth Medical Center, Cleveland, OH, USA

Overview

Premature rupture of the membranes (PROM) complicates approximately 10% of pregnancies, and 3% of pregnancies delivering before term. It is responsible for one-third of preterm deliveries, and is more common as a cause of preterm birth in populations of lower socioeconomic status.

Pathophysiology

Spontaneous membrane rupture occurs physiologically at term either before or after the onset of symptomatic contractions. This is believed to be related to progressive weakening of the membranes seen with advancing gestation, largely due to collagen remodeling and cellular apoptosis. When PROM occurs before term, the process of membrane weakening may be accelerated by a number of factors such as stretch, infection, inflammation and local hypoxia. Some clinical risk factors for preterm PROM are shown in Table 54.1.[1-3] In asymptomatic women, a short cervix on transvaginal ultrasound (relative risk 3.2) and a positive cervico-vaginal fetal fibronectin (fFN) screen (relative risk 2.5) are also associated with increased risks of preterm birth due to PROM.[3] However, routine screening with these modalities is not recommended as they fail to identify the majority of women delivering preterm due to PROM.

Protocols for High-Risk Pregnancies, 5th edition. Edited by J.T. Queenan, J.C. Hobbins and C.Y. Spong. © 2010 Blackwell Publishing Ltd.

Table 54.1 Clinical risk factors for preterm premature rupture of membranes.

Risk factor	Odds ratio
Previous preterm PROM	3.3–6.3
Previous preterm delivery	1.9–2.8
Cigarette smoking	2.1
Bleeding during pregnancy	
During first trimester	2.4
During second trimester	4.4
During third trimester	6.4
More than one trimester	7.4
Acute pulmonary disease	1.8
Bacterial vaginosis	1.5

Clinical implications

The hallmarks of PROM are brief latency from membrane rupture to delivery, increased risk of intrauterine and neonatal infection, and oligo-hydramnios.

At term, 95% of expectantly managed women will deliver within ~28 hours of membrane rupture, but when women with preterm PROM are managed conservatively to prolong gestation, approximately half will deliver within 1 week. With PROM near the limit of viability, approximately one in four women will remain undelivered at least 1 month after membrane rupture. Because the benefits of conservative management include time for acceleration of fetal maturity with antenatal corticosteroids (24–48 hours latency required) and reduction of gestational age dependent morbidity (extended latency $\geq$1 week required), serious consideration should be given to expeditious delivery if the fetus is considered to be at low risk for gestational age dependent morbidity near or at term, or if adequate time to accrue corticosteroid benefit and/or extended latency for fetal maturation are not anticipated.

Clinical chorioamnionitis is common after preterm PROM and increases with decreasing gestational age at membrane rupture. Clinical chorioamnionitis and endometritis complicate 13–60% and 2–13% of pregnancies, respectively, with PROM remote from term. Positive amniotic fluid cultures are obtained from amniocentesis specimens in 25 to 35% of women with preterm PROM.[4] Maternal sepsis is a rare but serious complication of conservatively managed PROM affecting ~1% women with PROM remote from term.

Fetal demise complicates approximately 1–2% of conservatively managed cases of preterm PROM. This risk increases in the face of chorioamnionitis, and when PROM occurs near the limit of potential viability. It is believed that in most cases demise results from umbilical cord compression, though loss due to fetal infection and placental abruption can occur. Cord prolapse is an uncommon complication of PROM.

Abruptio placentae complicates about 4 to 12% of patients with pre-term PROM. Placental bleeding may occur before or after the onset of membrane rupture. The benefits of conservative management should be reassessed if placental abruption is suspected. Attempts at extended latency should be reserved only for those who have minimal bleeding, no change in maternal cardiovascular status, and whose fetus is at high risk for death due to extreme prematurity with immediate delivery.

Diagnosis

Diagnosis of PROM can usually be made clinically based on a suggestive history combined with a sterile speculum examination. Demonstration of fluid passing per os is diagnostic of membrane rupture. Ancillary test-ing of vaginal fluid for an alkaline pH (>6.0–6.5) with nitrazine paper is supportive, but can be falsely positive (17%) due to the presence of blood, semen, alkaline antiseptics or bacterial vaginosis, and can be falsely negative (9%) with prolonged leakage. The presence of a ferning pattern on microscopic examination of dried vaginal secretions can also be con-firmatory and is less commonly falsely positive (6%) due to the presence of cervical mucus within the specimen (false-negative rate 13%). Repeat speculum examination after prolonged recumbency may be helpful if the diagnosis is suspected but initial examination is not confirmatory.

A number of biochemical markers have been found to be present in the vagina after PROM, and some of these are placental alpha microglobu-lin-1 (PAMG-1), insulin-like growth factor-binding protein-1 (IGFBP-1), fetal fibronectin, alpha-fetoprotein, diamino-oxydase, total T4 and free T4, prolactin, human chorionic gonadotropin and interleukin-6. Tests based on these markers are unnecessary when the diagnosis is evident clinically, and these have not generally been evaluated for their accuracy when the diagnosis of PROM is unclear. Though the concept of these ancillary tests is appealing, most are not available for clinical care and it is unclear that available tests are adequately helpful.[5,6] Ultrasonographic evidence of oligohydramnios is supportive of a clinical diagnosis but is not diagnostic as low amniotic fluid can occur for other reasons (e.g., fetal growth restric-tion, urinary tract anomalies), and the amniotic fluid volume may be within normal limits despite membrane rupture. The diagnosis can be con-firmed unequivocally through ultrasound-guided amnio-infusion of indigo carmine (1 mL in 9 mL of sterile normal saline) followed by observation for passage of blue dye per vaginum.

Evaluation

Initial evaluation of the woman presenting with preterm PROM includes:

1 Cervical cultures for *Neisseria gonorrheae* and *Chlamydia trachomatis*, ano-vaginal culture for group B streptococcus (GBS), and urinalysis with urine culture as appropriate.

2 If the diagnosis of PROM is suspected, digital cervical examinations should be avoided until the diagnosis of PROM has been excluded. Digital vaginal examinations after PROM have been shown to shorten the latency period from membrane rupture to delivery and increase the risk of chorioamnionitis, while adding little information regarding cervical dilatation and effacement over that obtained by visual examination.[7]

3 Initial maternal uterine activity and fetal heart rate monitoring should be performed to evaluate for evidence of labor, umbilical cord compression, and for fetal well-being if the limit of potential fetal viability has been reached. If conservative management is being considered, initial extended monitoring for ~6–12 hours followed by intermittent monitoring at least daily is appropriate. A non-reactive fetal heart rate can be a sign of intrauterine infection, particularly if testing had previously been reactive.

4 Clinical assessment for chorioamnionitis including assessment of maternal and fetal heart rates, maternal temperature, uterine tenderness, and vaginal discharge. The combination of fever (≥38.0°C or 100.4°F) with uterine tenderness and/or maternal or fetal tachycardia in the absence of an other evident source for infection is suggestive of chorioamnionitis and is an indication for delivery regardless of gestational age.

5 A maternal white blood cell count (WBC) above 16,000 is supportive of suspicious clinical findings or chorioamnionitis. There is significant variation in WBC count between patients and the WBC count is elevated in pregnancy and for 5–7 days after administration of antenatal corticosteroids. As such, this test should not be used in isolation. It is helpful to obtain a baseline WBC count, when conservative management is considered, for initial assessment and for subsequent comparison.

6 Perform ultrasonographic examination to determine fetal position and presentation, exclude fetal malformations associated with PROM (e.g., hydrops fetalis, intestinal obstruction, diaphragmatic hernia may cause uterine stretch due to polyhydramnios), estimate fetal weight, assess amniotic fluid volume and perform a biophysical profile should initial fetal heart rate testing be non-reactive.

7 Ultrasound-guided amniocentesis to evaluate for intraamniotic infection can be helpful if the diagnosis is suspected clinically, but the diagnosis is not clear. Care should be paid to avoid the umbilical cord, which can be mistaken for a small amniotic fluid pocket if there is severe oligo-hydramnios. Amniotic fluid can be sent for Gram's stain, white blood cell count ($\geq$30 cells/μL considered abnormal), glucose (<16–20 considered abnormal), and culture for aerobic and anaerobic bacteria.[8,9] *Mycoplasma* is a common microorganism identified from amniotic fluid after PROM but it is not visible on Gram's stain. *Mycoplasma* cultures are not available in all laboratories.

8 Women presenting with PROM at term generally do not require additional specific evaluations once the diagnosis is made, unless other complicating circumstances are present, or in the unlikely event that conservative management is being considered.

Management

Conditions that mandate delivery after preterm or term PROM include clinical chorioamnionitis, non-reassuring fetal testing, significant vaginal bleeding, advanced labor and concurrent pregnancy complications indicating delivery (e.g., severe preeclampsia). In the absence of amnionitis, placental abruption, fetal distress or advanced labor, conservative management of women with preterm PROM may be appropriate. A gestational age-based approach to conservative management should be considered. The patient should be appraised of available current data regarding neonatal morbidity and mortality according to gestational age at delivery,[4] in order to make appropriate decisions regarding the potential benefits of conservative management as opposed to expeditious delivery.

Term ($\geq$ 37 weeks)

While labor will spontaneously ensue within 12 hours in 50%, and by 24 hours in 70% of women with PROM at term, the risk of chorioamnionitis increases with the duration of membrane rupture (2% <12 hours, 6% 12–24 hours and 24% by 48 hours). Because of this, and because current data do not suggest an increased risk of infection or operative delivery with early induction, those with PROM at term are best served by labor induction/augmentation as needed, with cesarean delivery reserved for clinical indications. PROM is not a contraindication for pre-induction cervical priming with prostaglandin E_2 gel.[10] GBS prophylaxis should be administered to those with positive ano-vaginal cultures in the current pregnancy.[11] GBS prophylaxis should also be initiated for those without a recent negative culture (<6 weeks) who have membrane rupture

≥18 hours. Women with intrapartum fever should receive broad-spectrum antimicrobial therapy, including agents effective against Gram-positive and Gram-negative organisms, regardless of GBS culture status.

Preterm (34 weeks–36 weeks 6 days)

Because women with PROM near term (34–36 weeks) are at relatively low risk of serious acute morbidity which is not likely to be reduced with the relatively brief anticipated latency at this gestation, and because antenatal steroids are not generally recommended for fetal maturation at this gestation, these women are best treated by expeditious delivery as noted above for the term patient with PROM. Although there are risks of morbidity at this gestation, the risks of infection and umbilical cord compression outweigh the potential benefits of conservative management. As many of these women will not have had a recent ano-vaginal GBS culture and because of the increased risk of neonatal infection in low birth-weight infants, intrapartum GBS prophylaxis should be given in the absence of a recent (<6 weeks) negative ano-vaginal GBS culture.

Preterm (32 weeks–33 weeks 6 days)

In the absence of an indication for delivery, evaluate fetal lung maturity status on amniotic fluid collected from the vaginal pool or by amniocentesis [foam stability index ≥47 or phosphatidyl glycerol (PG) positive, or lecithin sphingomyelin (L/S) ratio ≥2/1 or FLM II ≥55 considered mature]. If there is blood- or meconium-stained amniotic fluid, vaginal pool specimens for L/S ratio or FLM may be falsely immature and should not be relied upon. However, delivery should be considered in these women because of the potential for fetal compromise.

If testing reveals a mature fetal pulmonary profile, expeditiously deliver according to the recommendations for PROM at 34–36 weeks.

If testing reveals an immature lung profile or if fluid cannot be obtained:

1 Induction of fetal pulmonary maturation with antenatal corticosteroids followed by delivery in 24–48 hours or at 34 weeks' gestation is recommended.

2 If conservative management is pursued, broad-spectrum antibiotic treatment should be administered to reduce maternal and neonatal infections, to prolong latency in order to enhance steroid induced and spontaneous maturation.

3 Once antenatal corticosteroid benefit has been achieved, the patient should be assessed regarding the potential for extended latency (≥1 week) before 34 weeks' gestation. If the patient is more than 330 weeks of gestation at this time, it is unlikely that further delay of delivery to 34 weeks will result in substantial spontaneous fetal maturation. Delivery is recommended before complications ensue.

4 During conservative management, maternal and fetal assessment, as delineated below for PROM at 23–31 weeks, should be initiated.

5 If antenatal corticosteroids and antibiotics are not given in this setting, consideration should be given to delivery before infection or other complications ensue.

Preterm (23 weeks–31 weeks 6 days)

Because the risks of neonatal morbidity and mortality due to prematurity is high with immediate delivery at 23–31 weeks' gestation, these women are generally best served by in-hospital conservative management to prolong pregnancy and reduce gestational age-dependent morbidity in the absence of evident infection, abruption, advanced labor or fetal compromise. Should the patient be initially admitted to a facility without resources for emergent care of the mother and a very premature newborn, she should be transferred to a facility capable of providing care for these patients if possible after initial assessment and before acute complications occur.

During conservative management, the following should be considered:

1 Initial extended continuous fetal and maternal monitoring (~6–12 hours) for contractions, non-reassuring fetal heart rate patterns, including umbilical cord compression.

2 At least daily clinical assessment for evidence of labor, chorioamnionitis, placental abruption. In addition, vital signs (temperature, pulse and blood pressure) should be documented at least each shift.

3 Antenatal corticosteroids for fetal maturation are recommended unless a full course has previously been given. Recent meta-analysis has suggested such treatment to be effective in reducing neonatal respiratory distress and intraventricular hemorrhage after PROM, without increasing the risk of neonatal infection.[12] Either betamethasone, 12 mg intramuscularly 24 hours apart × 2 doses, or dexamethasone, 6 mg intramuscularly 12 hours apart × 4 doses is appropriate.

4 Broad-spectrum antibiotic therapy should be administered during initial conservative management of preterm PROM to treat or prevent ascending subclinical decidual infection in order to prolong pregnancy, and to reduce neonatal infectious and gestational age-dependent morbidity. Intravenous therapy (48 hours) with ampicillin (2 g IV q 6 h) and erythromycin (250 mg IV q 6 h) followed by limited duration oral therapy (5 days) with amoxicillin (250 mg PO q 8 h) and enteric-coated erythromycin base (333 mg PO q 8 h) is recommended.[13] Shorter duration therapy has not been shown to offer similar neonatal benefits, and is not recommended. Although not specifically studied, recent shortages in antibiotic availability have led to the need for substitution of alternative antibiotic treatments. Oral ampicillin, erythromycin and azithromycin are likely appropriate substitutions for the above agents, as needed.

Although a large multicenter study has suggested that broad-spectrum antibiotic therapy might increase the risk of necrotizing enterocolitis,[14] this finding is at variance with those of the NICHD-MFMU trial finding a reduced stage 2–3 necrotizing enterocolitis with broad-spectrum antibiotic therapy in a higher risk population and this risk has not been found in a meta-analysis of studies regarding this issue.

Management of the known GBS carrier after the initial 7 days of antibiotic therapy has not been well defined. In the absence of any studies addressing this issue, options include:

i No further antepartum therapy, with intrapartum GBS prophylaxis of all known carriers.

ii Continued narrow-spectrum GBS prophylaxis of all known carriers from completion of the initial 7-day course through delivery.

iii Follow-up ano-vaginal culture after completion of the 7-day course, with continued narrow-spectrum therapy against GBS until delivery.

iv Follow-up ano-vaginal culture of those having extended latency after initial antibiotic treatment, with repeat treatment of women with subsequently positive cultures (as well as intrapartum prophylaxis for all known carriers).

5 At least daily non-stress fetal heart rate and contraction monitoring to observe for evidence of subclinical contractions, fetal heart rather decelerations due to umbilical cord compression, sustained tachycardia, or evidence of fetal compromise. A Biophysical profile score or 6/10 or greater may be helpful when the fetal heart rate pattern is not reactive. A fetal heart rate pattern that is reactive on initial testing but becomes non-reactive on follow-up tests, or a worsening biophysical profile score, should raise suspicion regarding the possibility of developing intrauterine infection or fetal compromise. Under such circumstances, prolonged monitoring and repeat biophysical testing should be considered.

6 White blood cell count monitoring can be helpful, but an elevated white blood cell count alone is not an indication for delivery. We perform an initial baseline white blood cell count for reference before administration of antenatal corticosteroids, and repeat testing if the initial result is elevated, or if equivocal clinical findings for intrauterine infection ensue. Repeat testing is not needed if the diagnosis of intrauterine infection is clear.

7 Treat specific cervico-vaginal pathogens and urinary tract infections.

8 Ultrasound should be performed every 3 to 4 weeks to assess fetal growth. It is not necessary to repeat amniotic fluid volume estimates frequently as persistent or worsening oligohydramnios is not an indication for delivery. Initial severe oligohydramnios has been associated with briefer latency to delivery, but this finding is an inaccurate predictor of latency or neonatal outcomes.

9 Data for efficacy of tocolysis of women with preterm PROM are not compelling. Treatment has been shown reduce the likelihood of delivery at 24–48 hours in some studies. However, such treatment has not been shown to improve neonatal outcomes. Tocolytic therapy should not be administered after preterm PROM if there is suspicion of intrauterine infection, fetal compromise or placental abruption. Amniocentesis to exclude concurrent intraamniotic infection may be helpful when tocolysis is being considered.

10 Because pregnancy and inactivity are risk factors for thromboembolic complications, preventative measures such as leg exercises and/or anti-embolic stockings and/or prophylactic doses of subcutaneous heparin may be of value in preventing this outcome during conservative management with bed rest.

11 The patient who remains stable without evidence of infection, abruption or fetal compromise should generally be delivered at 34 weeks' gestation because of the ongoing but low risk of fetal loss with conservative management and the high likelihood of survival without long-term sequelae with delivery at this gestational age. Assessment of fetal pulmonary maturity at 34 weeks, with continued conservative management of those with immature studies after further discussion of the risks and benefits of further conservative management, is acceptable.

12 Amnioinfusion has not been shown to be of benefit in preventing fetal compromise, or extending latency after preterm PROM. During labor, amnioinfusion is not recommended routinely, and should be reserved for the indication of ameliorating significant umbilical cord compression (variable heart rate decelerations) that is unresponsive to maternal repositioning.

Preterm (< 23 weeks)

When PROM occurs prior to the limit of viability, a 'best gestational age' determination should be made based on the earliest available ultrasonography and menstrual history. These patients should be counseled with a realistic appraisal of potential fetal and neonatal outcomes. Regarding maternal morbidity, conservative management of mid-trimester PROM is associated with a high risk of chorioamnionitis (39%), endometritis (14%), abruptio placentae (3%) and retained placenta with postpartum hemorrhage requiring curettage (12%). The risk of stillbirth during conservative management of mid-trimester PROM is approximately 15%, some of which is due to non-intervention for fetal distress when delivery occurs before the limit of viability. Most of these pregnancies will deliver before or near the limit of viability, where neonatal death is either assured or common. The risk of long-term sequelae will depend on the gestational age at delivery. Persistent oligohydramnios is a poor prognostic indicator after PROM before 20 weeks, placing the fetus at high risk of lethal pulmonary hypoplasia regardless of extended latency.

Management options for women with PROM before 23 weeks include:

1 Labor induction with the following according to individual clinical circumstances
   i high-dose intravenous oxytocin
   ii intravaginal prostaglandin E_2
   iii oral or intravaginal prostaglandin E_1 (misoprostol).

2 Dilatation and evacuation. Intracervical laminaria placement prior to labor induction or dilatation and evacuation may be helpful.

3 Conservative management. Should conservative management be pursued, the following should be considered:
   i The patient should be monitored initially for the development of infection, labor or placental abruption. Strict pelvic rest and modified bed rest with bathroom privileges should be encouraged to enhance the potential for membrane resealing, and to reduce the potential for ascending infection. Given the absence of data regarding the superiority of either, initial inpatient or outpatient monitoring may be appropriate according to individual clinical circumstances.
   ii Serial ultrasound is recommended to evaluate or fetal pulmonary growth and for persistent oligohydramnios. Fetal pulmonary growth can be estimated by ultrasound measurement of the thoracic/abdominal circumference ratio or chest circumference. A low thoracic/abdominal circumference ratio in the setting of persistent oligohydramnios is highly predictive of lethal pulmonary hypoplasia after PROM.[15] When identified before the limit of viability, this finding may help the patient regarding the decision between continued conservative management and delivery.
   iii Women with PROM before 23 weeks gestation have been included in some studies of antibiotic therapy after PROM. Treatment as described above for women at 23–31 weeks is appropriate. However, this population has not been studied separately, and it is not known if treatment is beneficial.
   iv Once the patient with pre-viable premature rupture of the membranes reaches the limit of viability, many physicians will admit the patient to hospital for ongoing bed rest. The purpose of admission at this time is to allow for early diagnosis and intervention for infection, abruption, labor and non-reassuring fetal heart rate patterns (see conservative management of PROM at 23 weeks–31 weeks 6 days above). Because these women remain at high risk for early delivery, administration of antenatal corticosteroids for fetal maturation may be appropriate at this time. It is unlikely that delayed administration of broad-spectrum antibiotics for pregnancy prolongation will assist this population.

v Novel treatments for membrane sealing after pre-viable PROM, including serial amnioinfusion, membrane plugging with Gelfoam or fibrin-platelet-cryoprecipitate plugs, and indwelling transcervical infusion catheter have been studied. Further research regarding the maternal and fetal risks and benefits of these interventions is needed before membrane sealing is incorporated in clinical practice.

Special circumstances

Cerclage

When the cerclage is removed on admission for preterm PROM, the risk of adverse perinatal outcomes is not higher than for those women with preterm PROM no cerclage. Studies comparing cerclage retention or removal after preterm PROM have suggested trends towards increased maternal infection with retained cerclage; however, no individual study has reached statistical significance. Alternatively, no study has found a significant reduction in the infant morbidity with cerclage retention subsequent to preterm PROM, and one study found increased neonatal death due to infection with cerclage retention. As such, cerclage should generally be removed when PROM occurs. Should the cerclage be retained during attempts to enhance fetal maturation with antenatal corticosteroids, concurrent antibiotic administration should be considered to reduce the risk of infection and the stitch should be removed after antenatal steroid benefit has been achieved (24–48 hours).

Herpes simplex virus

A history of herpes simplex virus infection is not a contraindication for expectant management of PROM remote from term. If herpetic lesions are present at the onset of labor, a cesarean section is indicated. Alternatively, with PROM at 30 weeks or thereafter, the presence of primary or secondary herpetic lesions should lead to consideration of expeditious cesarean delivery.

Human immunodeficiency virus

Intrapartum vertical transmission of HIV increases with increasing duration of membrane rupture. Given the poor prognosis of perinatally acquired HIV infection, expeditious abdominal delivery after PROM at any gestational age after the limit of fetal viability is recommended. Vaginal delivery may be appropriate for women with HIV, if the viral titer is low (see Protocol 38). If conservative management of the patient with PROM at or before the limit of viability is undertaken, multi-agent antiretroviral therapy with serial monitoring of maternal viral load and CD4 counts should be initiated.

Resealing of the membranes

A small number of women will experience cessation of leakage with resealing of the membranes. Under this circumstance, we continue monitoring in hospital for approximately 1 week after cessation of leakage and normalization of the amniotic fluid index to encourage healing of the membrane rupture site. These women are subsequently discharged to modified bed rest and pelvic rest, with frequent re-evaluation.

Prevention of recurrent preterm PROM

Women with a history of preterm birth, especially that due to preterm PROM, are at increased risk for recurrent preterm birth due to PROM. Women with a prior preterm birth due to PROM have a 3.3-fold higher risk of recurrence, and a 13.5-fold higher risk of preterm PROM before 28 weeks' gestation. In addition to general guidance regarding adequate nutrition, smoking cessation, avoidance of heavy lifting and prolonged standing without breaks, weekly intramuscular injections with 17-hydroxyprogesterone caproate (250 mg) has been shown to reduce the risk of a recurrence.[16] Daily vaginal progesterone suppositories (100 mg) have also been shown to prevent preterm birth in high-risk women, but progesterone vaginal gel (90 mg) has not. Though vitamin C deficiency could potentially result in preterm PROM, vitamin C supplementation is not helpful and may be harmful.[17,18]

References

1 Naeye RL. Factors that predispose to premature rupture of the fetal membranes. *Obstet Gynecol* 1992;60:93.

2 Harger JH, Hsing AW, Tuomala RE, *et al*. Risk factors for preterm premature rupture of fetal membranes: a multicenter case-control study. *Am J Obstet Gynecol* 1990;163:130.

3 Mercer BM, Goldenberg RL, Meis PJ, Moawad AH, Shellhaas C, Das A, Menard MK, Caritis SN, Thurnau GR, Dombrowski MP, Miodovnik M, Roberts JM, McNellis D, and the NICHD-MFMU Network. The preterm prediction study: Prediction of preterm premature rupture of the membranes using clinical findings and ancillary testing. *Am J Obstet Gynecol* 2000;183:738–45.

4 Mercer BM. Preterm premature rupture of the membranes. *Obstet Gynecol* 2003;101(1):178–93.

5 Chen FC, Dudenhausen JW. Comparison of two rapid strip tests based on IGFBP-1 and PAMG-1 for the detection of amniotic fluid. *Am J Perinatol* 2008;25:243–6.

6 Lee SM, Lee J, Seong HS, Lee SE, Park JS, Romero R, Yoon BH. The clinical significance of a positive Amnisure test in women with term labor with intact membranes. *J Matern Fetal Neonat Med* 2009;22:305–10.

7 Alexander JM, Mercer BM, Miodovnik M, *et al.* The impact of digital cervical examination on expectantly managed preterm rupture of membranes. *Am J Obstet Gynecol* 2000;183:1003–7.

8 Romero R, Yoon BH, Mazor M, *et al*. A comparative study of the diagnostic performance of amniotic fluid glucose, white blood cell count, interleukin-6, and Gram stain in the detection of microbial invasion in patients with preterm premature rupture of membranes. *Am J Obstet Gynecol* 1993;169:839–51.

9 Belady PH, Farhouh LJ, Gibbs RS. Intra-amniotic infection and premature rupture of the membranes. *Clin Perinatol* 1997;24:43–57.

10 Hannah ME, Ohlsson A, Farine D, *et al*. Induction of labor compared with expectant management for prelabor rupture of the membranes at term. TERMPROM Study Group. *N Engl J Med* 1996;334:1005–10.

11 American College of Obstetricians and Gynecologists. ACOG Committee Opinion #279, December 2002. Prevention of early-onset group B streptococcal disease in newborns. *Obstet Gynecol* 2002;100:1405–12.

12 Harding JE, Pang J, Knight DB, Liggins GC. Do antenatal corticosteroids help in the setting of preterm rupture of membranes? *Am J Obstet Gynecol* 2001;184:131–9.

13 Mercer B, Miodovnik M, Thurnau G, Goldenberg R, Das A, Merenstein G, Ramsey R, Rabello Y, Thom E, Roberts J, McNellis D, and the NICHD-MFMU Network. Antibiotic therapy for reduction of infant morbidity after preterm premature rupture of the membranes: a randomized controlled trial. *JAMA* 1997;278:989–95.

14 Kenyon SL, Taylor DJ, Tarnow-Mordi W; Oracle Collaborative Group. Broad spectrum antibiotics for preterm, prelabor rupture of fetal membranes: the ORACLE I randomized trial. *Lancet* 2001;357:979–88.

15 D'Alton M, Mercer B, Riddick E, Dudley D. Serial thoracic versus abdominal circumference ratios for the prediction of pulmonary hypoplasia in premature rupture of the membranes remote from term. *Am J Obstet Gynecol* 1992;166:658–63.

16 Meis PJ, Klebanoff M, Thom E, Dombrowski MP, Sibai B, Moawad AH, Spong CY, Hauth JC, Miodovnik M, Varner MW, Leveno KJ, Caritis SN, Iams JD, Wapner RJ, Conway D, O'Sullivan MJ, Carpenter M, Mercer B, Ramin SM, Thorp JM, Peaceman AM, Gabbe S; National Institute of Child Health and Human Development Maternal-Fetal Medicine Units Network. Prevention of recurrent preterm delivery by 17 alpha-hydroxyprogesterone caproate. *N Engl J Med* 2003;348:2379–85.

17 Casanueva E, Ripoll C, Tolentino M, Morales RM, Pfeffer F, Vilchis P, Vadillo-Ortega F. Vitamin C supplementation to prevent premature rupture of the chorioamniotic membranes: a randomized trial. *Am J Clin Nutr* 2005;81:859–63.

18 Spinnato JA 2nd, Freire S, Pinto e Silva JL, *et al*. Antioxidant supplementation and premature rupture of the membranes: a planned secondary analysis. *Am J Obstet Gynecol* 2008;199:433.e1–8.

PROTOCOL 55

Prevention of Cerebral Palsy

Dwight Rouse

Maternal-Fetal Medicine Division, Women & Infants Hospital of Rhode Island; Department of Obstetrics and Gynecology, Warren Alpert School of Medicine at Brown University, Providence, RI, USA

Clinical significance

Cerebral palsy is a related group of disorders characterized by abnormal control of movement or posture that arise due to non-progressive damage or dysfunction of the developing fetal or infant brain. The result of this abnormal control is limitation of activity. Cerebral palsy is a leading cause of chronic childhood disability; it has been estimated that over 200,000 American children between the ages of 3 and 13 suffer from this disorder. Preterm birth is a major risk factor for cerebral palsy – infants born at the extreme of viability face up to a 50-fold increased risk of cerebral palsy compared to those born at term. In fact, half of all cerebral palsy is associated with prematurity.

Pathophysiology

The pathophysiology of cerebral palsy is generally poorly understood. Factors associated with cerebral palsy include genetic disorders, thrombophilias and maternal infection or fever in the antepartum period. Intrapartum asphyxiating events give rise to a minority of cerebral palsy cases. The preterm fetal brain is especially vulnerable to the damaging effects of cytokines and excitatory amino acids that characterize the inflammatory milieu of early spontaneous preterm birth. Approximately half of cerebral palsy cases in preterm infants are presaged by severe neonatal cranial ultrasound abnormalities, e.g., cystic periventricular leukomalacia or grade III or IV intraventricular hemorrhage.

Protocols for High-Risk Pregnancies, 5th edition. Edited by J.T. Queenan, J.C. Hobbins and C.Y. Spong. © 2010 Blackwell Publishing Ltd.

Diagnosis

In its more severe forms, a diagnosis of cerebral palsy can be made in the first year of life. Milder forms of what appears to be cerebral palsy may not persist, and thus a definitive diagnosis should be delayed until the age of at least 2 if the condition is mild.

Cerebral palsy should be diagnosed on the basis of the following three factors by a clinician trained and experienced in the diagnosis: (1) minimum 30% delay in gross motor development milestones; (2) abnormalities in muscle tone such as scissoring, 4+ or absent deep tendon reflexes, or movement abnormality such as posturing or gait asymmetry; and (3) persistence of primitive, or absence of protective, reflexes. Findings in at least two of these three categories must be present. When cerebral palsy is diagnosed, the Gross Motor Function Classification Scale can be used to assess its severity.[1]

Prevention

That magnesium sulfate ($MgSO_4$) administered to mothers delivering prematurely could prevent cerebral palsy in their offspring was first suggested by a case–control study performed by Drs Karin Nelson and Judy Grether.[2] In their study, children with cerebral palsy were much less likely to have been exposed to $MgSO_4$ than controls (odds ratio 0.14, 95% confidence interval [CI] 0.05–0.51). This protective association persisted after controlling for confounders, and has biological plausibility, because magnesium has the potential to reduce vascular instability, forestall hypoxic damage and mitigate cytokine or excitatory amino acid damage.[3]

Since the report of Nelson and Grether, three large, randomized placebo-controlled trials of antenatal $MgSO_4$ for fetal neuroprotection have been conducted and reported. Alone and in combination, the results of these trials support the use of $MgSO_4$ to lower the risk of cerebral palsy among the survivors of early preterm birth.

The first of these trials was by Crowther and colleagues who studied 1062 women expected to deliver before 30 weeks' gestation.[4] In this trial, $MgSO_4$ was administered as a 4 g intravenous bolus followed by a constant intravenous infusion of 1 g/h for up to 24 hours. The combined outcome of stillbirth or death before age 2 was less frequent among the offspring of women randomized to $MgSO_4$ than among those randomized to placebo, 13.8% vs 17.1% (relative risk [RR] 0.83, 95% CI 0.64–1.09). Substantial gross motor dysfunction (equivalent to moderate or severe cerebral palsy in the NINDS/NICHD MFMU trial discussed below[1]) was significantly less frequent among surviving children in the $MgSO_4$ group, 3.4% vs 6.6% (RR 0.51, 95% CI 0.29–0.91).

The second major trial to be reported was the NINDS/NICHD MFMU Network trial that enrolled 2241 women deemed to be at imminent risk of delivery between 24 and 31 weeks' gestation.[1] In this trial, $MgSO_4$ was administered as a 6 g loading dose followed by a constant infusion of 2 g/h for up to 12 hours. The primary study outcome was the composite of fetal/infant death or moderate or severe cerebral palsy (inability to walk unaided by the age of 2). Although $MgSO_4$ had no significant effect on this primary combined outcome, 11.3% in the $MgSO_4$ group vs 11.7% in the placebo group (RR 0.97, 95% CI 0.77–1.2), it significantly reduced the risk of the pre-specified secondary outcome of moderate or severe cerebral palsy among surviving children, 1.9% vs 3.5% (RR 0.55; 95% CI 0.32–0.95). In an unadjusted analysis, $MgSO_4$ was associated with a slight but non-significant increase in the risk of fetal or infant death, 9.5% vs 8.5% (RR 1.1, 95% CI 0.85–1.5). However, after the exclusion of infants with major congenital malformations discovered after birth, the apparent increased risk for death was for all purposes eliminated, 8.3% vs 8.1% (RR 1.0, 95% CI 0.77–1.4). However, the decreased risk for cerebral palsy persisted virtually unchanged, 1.8% vs 3.2% (RR 0.56, 95% CI 0.32–0.99). Among the offspring of women randomized prior to 28 weeks, $MgSO_4$ was associated with a larger absolute risk reduction, 2.7% vs 6.1% (RR 0.45, 95% CI 0.23–0.87).

The most recently reported major trial was conducted by Marret *et al.* who studied 573 mothers.[5] In their trial, randomization was to either $MgSO_4$ administered as a 4 gm bolus immediately prior to delivery or to placebo. The women randomized to $MgSO_4$ were less likely to die, 9.7% vs 11.3% (RR 0.85, 95% CI 0.55–1.3), and also less likely to be suffer from cerebral palsy, 7.0% vs 10.2% (RR 0.69, 95% CI 0.41–1.2).

These three trials and two more have recently been incorporated into a Cochrane Systematic Review.[6] The two additional trials include a small study of 150 women that was conducted as a feasibility trial and reported in a research letter and another study whose primary intent was to test the maternal anticonvulsant effectiveness of $MgSO_4$. Overall in these five trials, 6145 children were enrolled as fetuses and their outcomes included in the systematic review. $MgSO_4$ was associated with a significant reduction in cerebral palsy (RR 0.68, 95% CI 0.54–0.87) without an effect on fetal or infant mortality (RR 1.04, 95% CI 0.92–1.17). In four trials (4446 children) neuroprotection was the specific outcome. In these trials, not only was $MgSO_4$ associated with a reduction in cerebral palsy, but also with a reduction in the combined outcome of cerebral palsy or fetal/infant death (RR 0.85, 95% CI 0.74–0.98).[6]

As detailed above, the protocols for $MgSO_4$ administration varied among the three neuroprotective trials. The protocol utilized in the NINDS/NICHD MFMU Network trial[1] was a 6 g loading dose given over 20–30 minutes, followed by a constant infusion of 2 g/h for up to 12 hours (Table 55.1). If after 12 hours delivery did not seem imminent, the infusion was

Table 55.1 Protocol: magnesium sulfate (MgSO₄) for the prevention of cerebral palsy*

Eligible candidates

Gestational age: 24–31 weeks' gestation

At risk of immediate delivery

   Preterm premature rupture of membranes

   Advanced preterm labor (cervix ≥4 cm)

   Indicated (severe fetal growth restriction)

Magnesium administration

Initial therapy

6 g intravenous load over 20–30 minutes

2 g/h constant infusion until delivery

If delivery not imminent, infusion discontinued

Retreatment

When delivery again threatens prior to 34 weeks

If <6 hours from discontinuation, no MgSO₄ bolus

Monitor

Deep tendon reflexes

Urine output

Serum Mg⁺⁺ concentrations (e.g., renal dysfunction)

---

*Rouse DJ, Hirtz DG, Thom E, Varner MW, Spong CY, Mercer BM, *et al.* A randomized, controlled trial of magnesium sulfate for the prevention of cerebral palsy. *N Engl J Med* 2008;359:895–905.

discontinued, with the intent of restarting it when delivery again threatened before 34 weeks' gestation. The bolus was re-given if 6 hours had elapsed since the constant infusion was stopped. Eligible candidates included those with preterm premature rupture of membranes (who often receive the full 12 hours of infusion, after which the magnesium is turned off and restarted when labor threatens), those in advanced (≥4 cm) preterm labor with intact membranes, and those whose delivery was planned within 24 hours for fetal indications (e.g., severe fetal growth restriction).

The number needed to treat with MgSO₄ to prevent cerebral palsy is in line with the current use of MgSO₄ for the prevention of eclamptic convulsions: treating 63 women threatening to deliver prior to 32 weeks will prevent one case of moderate or severe cerebral palsy. In contrast, approximately 100 women with preeclampsia need to be treated to prevent one eclamptic convulsion.[7] If treatment were limited to 28 weeks or below, the NINDS/NICHD MFMU Network trial suggests that treating only 29 women would prevent one case of moderate or severe cerebral palsy.

Complications

Although MgSO₄ has a high margin of safety, and was associated with no life-threatening events in the over 3000 maternal exposures in the

Cochrane review, it should be utilized only with close monitoring of maternal reflexes (neuromuscular depression occurs at Mg^{++} concentrations of 10 mEq/L and above) and urine output (Mg^{++} is renally excreted). The administration of $MgSO_4$ in the face of renal dysfunction requires especial vigilance. Suspicion of significant hypermagnesiumenia should be evaluated by measurement of serum Mg^{++} concentration and in many cases by discontinuation of the $MgSO_4$ infusion. Frank respiratory depression (and the even rarer cardiopulmonary arrest) is treated by administration of 1 g of intravenous calcium gluconate, discontinuation of the $MgSO_4$ infusion, and ventilatory support as necessary.[8]

Conclusion

Recently published research demonstrates that $MgSO_4$ offers a rare opportunity to improve the neurodevelopmental prognosis of fetuses destined to deliver at early gestational ages. In the United States, 2% of women deliver prior to 32 weeks' gestation, approximately 75% of them spontaneously. If the mothers of all of these infants received $MgSO_4$ for fetal neuroprotection, and it were as effective as in the NINDS/NICHD MFMU Network trial, then over 1000 children a year in the United States alone could be spared from handicapping cerebral palsy.

References

1 Rouse DJ, Hirtz DG, Thom E, *et al.* A randomized, controlled trial of magnesium sulfate for the prevention of cerebral palsy. *N Engl J Med* 2008;359:895–905.
2 Nelson KB, Grether JK. Can magnesium sulfate reduce the risk of cerebral palsy in very low birthweight infants? *Pediatrics* 1995;95:263–9.
3 Hirtz DG, Nelson KN. Magnesium sulfate and cerebral palsy in premature infants. *Curr Opin Pediatr* 1998;10:131–7.
4 Crowther CA, Hiller JE, Doyle LW, Haslam RR. Effect of magnesium sulfate given for neuroprotection before preterm birth birth: a randomized controlled trial. *JAMA* 2003;290:2669–76.
5 Marret S, Maroeau L, Follet-Bouhamed C, *et al.* Effect of magnesium sulphate on mortality and neurologic morbidity of the very preterm newborn with two-year neurological outcome: results of the prospective PREAMAG trial. *Gynecologie Obstetrique & Fertilite* 2008;36:278–88.
6 Doyle LW, Crowther CA, Middleton P, Marret S, Rouse D. Magnesium sulphate for women at risk of preterm birth for neuroprotection of the fetus. *Cochrane Database Syst Rev* 2009;(1): CD004661. DOI: 10.1002/14651858.CD004661.pub3.
7 Lucas MJ, Leveno KJ, Cunningham FG. A comparison of magnesium sulfate with phenytoin for the prevention of eclampsia. *N Engl J Med* 1995;333:201–5.
8 Cunningham FG, Leveno KJ, Bloom SL, Hauth JC. *Williams Obstetrics*, 22nd edn. New York: McGraw-Hill Medical Publishing, 2005; p. 789.

Cooling for Hypoxic Ischemic Encephalopathy

Rosemary D. Higgins

Center for Developmental Biology and Perinatal Medicine, Eunice Kennedy Shriver National Institute of Child Health and Human Development, National Institutes of Health, Bethesda, MD, USA

Clinical significance

Hypoxic ischemic encephalopathy (HIE) is a serious neurological condition affecting 1–2 per 1000 infants in the United States. Though relatively uncommon, the chances for serious sequelae are high as a result of hypoxia, ischemia, or a combination of the two. Short-term complications include serious morbidity including encephalopathy, cardiovascular compromise, respiratory failure and renal impairment/failure. Mortality remains high from HIE. Short- and long-term neurodevelopment can be compromised in a significant proportion of survivors.

Pathophysiology

HIE can result whenever there is compromised blood flow (ischemia) or compromised oxygen delivery (hypoxia) or a combination of both to the brain. Without appropriate blood flow and adequate oxygenation, the brain is at high risk for reverting from aerobic to anaerobic metabolism. Anaerobic glycolysis results and causes depletion of high-energy phosphate, increases in lactic acid, calcium, free radical production, and deterioration of cellular function. If the hypoxia, and ischemia are severe and/or prolonged, cell death or apoptosis can result. Cellular injury and death can be acute and chronic.

A large number of animal studies[1–5] have shown the effects of hypoxia, ischemia and the combination of hypoxia and ischemia. Animal studies investigating the impact of cooling following hypoxic-ischemic injury showed significant promise and formed the basis of translational research to large-scale clinical studies. Animal studies can be controlled precisely

---

Protocols for High-Risk Pregnancies, 5th edition. Edited by J.T. Queenan, J.C. Hobbins and C.Y. Spong. © 2010 Blackwell Publishing Ltd.

to know the timing, duration and severity of hypoxia and ischemia. The clinical situation may not be as clear as laboratory investigations.

HIE in infants usually results following a catastrophic event which can include prolapsed cord, uterine rupture, placenta previa, placental abruption and other causes of interrupted fetal or uterine blood flow. There is an acute injury involving lack of oxygen and nutrients resulting in energy failure, followed by reperfusion of the affected area(s) of the brain. The reperfusion phase involves edema of the brain or specific areas of the brain and potential apoptosis.

Diagnosis

HIE in recently reported clinical trials selected patients that were strictly defined. In the major randomized clinical trials,[6,7] infants eligible for study needed to meet criteria for moderate to severe encephalopathy. These consist of:

1 Evidence of peripartum or intrapartum acute events such as cord prolapse, uterine rupture, placental abruption or other catastrophic event leading to fetal hypoxia, ischemia or both.
2 The infants generally had Apgar scores of ≤5 at 10 minutes of age, mechanical ventilation or continued need for resuscitation at 10 minutes of age, and a cord pH or initial pH of <7.0–7.15 (or base deficit at least 12 mmol/L).
3 Evidence of encephalopathy as defined by Sarnat staging of stage 2 or higher.

The American Academy of Pediatrics' Committee on Fetus and Newborn and the American College of Obstetricians and Gynecologists' Committee on Practice have defined criteria for acute intrapartum hypoxia sufficient to cause cerebral palsy as the following:[8]

1 Metabolic acidosis in the fetal umbilical cord blood obtained at delivery (pH <7 and base deficit ≥12 mmol/L).
2 Early onset of moderate to severe neonatal encephalopathy in infants born at 34 or more weeks' gestation.
3 Cerebral palsy of the spastic quadriplegic or dyskinetic type.
4 Exclusion of other identifiable etiologies, such as trauma, coagulation disorders, infectious conditions or genetic causes.

Treatment

Until very recently, treatment consisted of supportive therapies for infants with HIE. Head cooling and whole body cooling have been shown to improve the outcome from moderate to severe HIE in two large controlled trials.[6,7] Infants were randomized by 6 hours in the interventional cooling trials performed thus far.

In the CoolCap study,[6] infants received head cooling by a cooling cap device (Olympic Medical Cool Care System) with maintained rectal temperature of 34–35°C for a total of 72 hours. The control group received standard care via a radiant warmer with skin temperature adjusted to maintain rectal temperature 36.8–37.2°C.

In the NICHD Whole Body Cooling Trial,[7] infants randomized to cooling were placed on a pre-cooled infant cooling blanket (Blanketrol II, Cincinnati SubZero) which was servo-controlled to an esophageal temperature of 33–34°C for 72 hours. The control group received standard care.

Both trials[6,7] showed improvement in outcome with cooling therapy. Additional smaller trials and pilot studies[9–11] have been performed and a Cochrane meta-analysis[12] has concluded that there is benefit of therapeutic hypothermia for term infants with HIE and that cooling decreases death without increasing major disability in survivors. Additional trials including the TOBY[13] and ICE[14] trials are awaiting peer review publication.

The Committee on Fetus and Newborn[15] has published that cooling, if offered, should be performed using published protocols. Longer-term outcomes are not available at this time, but are under way.[16,17]

Complications

Several studies have been published reporting complications or safety outcomes. Eicher et al.[18] reported higher rates of bradycardia and lower heart rate measurements, longer use of vasopressors, higher prothrombin times, lower platelet levels and higher rates of seizures in the cooled infants. Cooled infants have lower heart rates.[7] Mild hypothermia did not affect arterial blood pressure or initial treatment with inotropic agents or volume administration in the CoolCap Study, though infants in the cooled arm of the trial had slower withdrawal of these therapies.[19] Inotropic support, blood transfusion, platelet transfusion, volume expansion, use of nitric oxide, use of extracorporeal membrane oxygenation (ECMO), and non-central nervous system organ dysfunction were similar between the cooled and control groups in the NICHD Whole Body Cooling Trial.[20]

Lower encephalopathy grade, lower birth weight, greater amplitude-integrated electroencephalographic (aEEG) amplitude, and absence of seizures were associated with better outcomes in the CoolCap Study.[21] Elevated temperatures have been reported to be associated with adverse outcomes in both the CoolCap[21] and NICHD Whole Body Cooling[22] trials.

Follow-up

The trials conducted thus far have evaluated infants at 18–22 months and have shown a reduction in death without an increase in neurodevelopmental impairment in infants receiving hypothermia therapy.[6,7] Follow-up consisted of Bayley Scales of infant development II (BSID II), assessment of cerebral palsy, hearing impairment/deafness assessment, and blindness. Based on AAP[15] recommendations, follow-up should be undertaken if infants receive cooling therapy. Longer-term follow-up is under way.[16,17]

Knowledge gaps

Significant knowledge gaps remain in the area of cooling for HIE.[23] The longer-term impact (i.e., school-age follow-up) of hypothermia for HIE remains unknown; COOLCAP and NICHD trial participants are being followed through school age.[16,17] More information for evidence-based guidelines for care of infants with HIE will be available when results from the TOBY Trial and ICE Trial are published. Depth, duration and rewarming strategies need further study. Time to cooling is being investigated currently in an NICHD whole-body cooling trial enrolling patients 6–24 hours of age.[24] Head and whole body cooling comparisons have not been performed in a randomized controlled trial.

Conclusion

Based on the available data and large knowledge gaps, hypothermia appears to be a potentially promising therapy for HIE. Long-term efficacy and safety are yet to be established. Clinicians choosing to offer this treatment should therefore understand all of the limitations of the available evidence, keep up-to-date on evidence on this topic as it evolves, counsel parents and family about the limitations of the current evidence, and adhere to AAP recommendations.[15]

Note: Subsequent to writing this protocol, the TOBY trial has been published (N Engl J Med. 2009 Oct 1;361(14):1349–58) and concluded that induction of moderate hypothermia for 72 hours in infants who had perinatal asphyxia did not significantly reduce the combined rate of death or severe disability but resulted in improved neurologic outcomes in survivors. A meta analysis (BMJ. 2010 Feb 9;340:c363. doi: 10.1136/bmj.c363) incorporating the TOBY Trial results concludes that infants with hypoxic-ischaemic encephalopathy, moderate hypothermia is associated with a consistent reduction in death and neurological impairment at 18 months.

References

1 Laptook AR, Corbett RJ. Sterett R, Burns DK, Tollefsbol G, Garcia D. Modest hypothermia provides partial neuroprotection for ischemic neonatal brain. *Pediatr Res* 1994;35:436–42.

2 Thoresen M, Penrice J, Lorek A, *et al.* Mild hypothermia after severe transient hypoxia-ischemia ameliorates delayed cerebral energy failure in the newborn piglet. *Pediatr Res* 1995;37:667–70.

3 Edwards AD, Yue X, Squier MV, *et al.* Specific inhibition of apoptosis after cerebral hypoxia-ischaemia by moderate post-insult hypothermia. *Biochem Biophys Res Commun* 1995;217:1193–9.

4 Gunn AJ, Gunn TR, de Haan HH, Williams CE, Gluckman PD. Dramatic neuronal rescue with prolonged selective head cooling after ischemia in fetal lambs. *J Clin Invest* 1997;99:248–56.

5 Gunn AJ, Gunn TR, Gunning MI, Williams CE, Gluckman PD. Neuroprotection with prolonged head cooling before post ischemic seizures in fetal sheep. *Pediatrics* 1998;102:1098–106.

6 Gluckman PD, Wyatt JS, Azzopardi D, *et al.* Selective head cooling with mild systemic hypothermia after neonatal encephalopathy: multicenter randomized trial. *Lancet* 2005;365:663–70.

7 Shankaran S, Laptook AR, Ehrenkranz R, Tyson J, McDonald S, Donovan E, Fanaroff AA, Poole WK, Wright LL, Higgins RD, Finer NN, Carlo WA, Duara S, Oh W, Cotten CM, Stevenson DK, Stoll BJ, Lemons JA, Guillet R, Jobe AH; National Institute of Child Health and Human Development Neonatal Research Network. Whole-body hypothermia for neonates with hypoxic-ischemic encephalopathy. *N Engl J Med* 2005;353(15):1574–84.

8 American College of Obstetrics and Gynecology. Committee Opinion #348. Umbilical Cord Blood Gas and Acid-Base Analysis. *Obstet Gynecol* 2006;108:1319–22.

9 Eicher DJ, Wagner CL, Katikaneni LP, *et al.* Moderate hypothermia in neonatal encephalopathy: efficacy outcomes. *Pediatr Neurol* 2005;32:11–17.

10 Lin ZL, Yu HM, Lin J, Chen SQ, Liang ZQ, Zhang ZY. Mild hypothermia via selective head cooling as neuroprotective therapy in term neonates with perinatal asphyxia: an experience from a single neonatal intensive care unit. *J Perinatol* 2006;26(3):180–4.

11 Gunn AJ, Gluckman PD, Gunn TR. Selective head cooling in newborns infants after perinatal asphyxia: a safety study. *Pediatrics* 1998;102:885–92.

12 Jacobs S, Hunt R, Tarnow-Mordi W, Inder T, Davis P. Cooling for newborns with hypoxic ischaemic encephalopathy. *Cochrane Database Syst Rev* 2007;(4):CD003311.

13 Azzopardi D, Brocklehurst P, Halliday H, Levene M, Thoresen M, Whitelaw A; TOBY Study Group. The TOBY Study. Whole body hypothermia for the treatment of perinatal asphyxial encephalopathy: a randomised controlled trial. *BMC Pediatr* 2008;8:17.

14 Jacobs SE, Stewart M, Inder TE, Doyle L, Morley C. Feasibility of a pragmatic randomised controlled trial of whole body cooling for term newborns with hypoxic-ischaemic encephalopathy. *Hot Topics in Neonatology.* Washington, DC; 2002.

15 Blackmon LR, Stark AR; American Academy of Pediatrics Committee on Fetus and Newborn. Hypothermia: a neuroprotective therapy for neonatal hypoxic-ischemic encephalopathy. *Pediatrics* 2006;117(3):942.

16 http://clinicaltrials.gov/ct2/show/NCT00581581?term=coolcap&rank=1

17 http://clinicaltrials.gov/ct2/show/NCT00005772?term=cooling+and+infant&rank=2

18 Eicher DJ, Wagner CL, Katikaneni LP, *et al.* Moderate hypothermia in neonatal encephalopathy: safety outcomes. *Pediatr Neurol* 2005;32:18–24.

19 Battin MR, Thoresen M, Robinson E, Polin RA, Edwards AD, Gunn AJ; Cool Cap Trial Group. Does head cooling with mild systemic hypothermia affect requirement for blood pressure support? *Pediatrics* 2009;123(3):1031–6.

20 Shankaran S, Pappas A, Laptook AR, McDonald SA, Ehrenkranz RA, Tyson JE, Walsh M, Goldberg RN, Higgins RD, Das A; NICHD Neonatal Research Network. Outcomes of safety and effectiveness in a multicenter randomized, controlled trial of whole-body hypothermia for neonatal hypoxic-ischemic encephalopathy. *Pediatrics* 2008;122(4):e791–8.

21 Wyatt JS, Gluckman PD, Liu PY, Azzopardi D, Ballard R, Edwards AD, Ferriero DM, Polin RA, Robertson CM, Thoresen M, Whitelaw A, Gunn AJ; CoolCap Study Group. Determinants of outcomes after head cooling for neonatal encephalopathy. *Pediatrics* 2007;119(5):912–21.

22 Laptook A, Tyson J, Shankaran S, McDonald S, Ehrenkranz R, Fanaroff A, Donovan E, Goldberg R, O'Shea TM, Higgins RD, Poole WK; National Institute of Child Health and Human Development Neonatal Research Network. Elevated temperature after hypoxic-ischemic encephalopathy: risk factor for adverse outcomes. *Pediatrics* 2008;122(3):491–9.

23 Higgins RD, Raju TNK, Perlman J, Azzopardi DV, Blackmon LR, Clark RH, Edwards AD, Ferriero DM, Gluckman PD, Gunn AJ, Jacobs SE, Eicher DJ, Jobe AH, Laptook AR, LeBlanc MH, Palmer C, Shankaran S, Soll RF, Stark AR, Thoresen M, Wyatt J for the NICHD Hypothermia Workshop Speakers and Discussants. Hypothermia and perinatal asphyxia: executive summary of the National Institute of Child Health and Human Development workshop. *J Pediatr* 2006;148:170–5.

24 http://clinicaltrials.gov/ct2/show/NCT00614744?term=infant+and+encephalopathy&rank=1

PROTOCOL 57

Amnionitis

George A. Macones[1] and Sindhu K. Srinivas[2]

Department of Obstetrics & Gynecology, Washington University School of Medicine,
St Louis, MO, USA

Overview

Amnionitis (chorioamnionitis, intraamniotic infection) is common, occurring
in 1–5% of term deliveries and up to 25% of preterm deliveries. Amnionitis
may be a causative factor in preterm births due to preterm labor or preterm
premature rupture of membranes (PPROM).

Depending on the type and severity of the infection as well as the
gestational age at which it occurs, amnionitis may lead to a variety of
outcomes including spontaneous abortion, stillbirth, prematurity (and
the various complications that might result from prematurity), neonatal
sepsis, infectious maternal morbidity and even sepsis and shock.

Pathophysiology

It is believed that amnionitis results from an ascending infection from
the lower genital tract into the amniotic cavity, although hematogenous
and transplacental etiologies have also been proposed. In the early stages
of an ascending bacterial invasion of the choriodecidual interface, there
may be no maternal symptomatology (subclinical intrauterine infection).
However, as the infection ascends and continues, clinical manifestations
may become apparent.

Amnionitis is a polymicrobial infection and most commonly involves
bacteria that are part of the normal vaginal flora. These bacteria include:
Bacteroides (25%), *Gardnerella* (25%), *streptococcus* species (25%), *E. coli* and
other Gram-negative rods (20%) and mycoplasmas.

In term patients amnionitis seems to occur more as a consequence of
multiple risk factors such as prolonged rupture of membranes or multiple
vaginal examinations. However, in preterm patients it is believed that
amnionitis might incite preterm labor or PPROM. There are multiple

Protocols for High-Risk Pregnancies, 5th edition. Edited by J.T. Queenan, J.C. Hobbins and
C.Y. Spong. © 2010 Blackwell Publishing Ltd.

hypotheses regarding how amnionitis may trigger PPROM or premature labor. One theory is that the infection may trigger prostaglandin synthesis and release from amniotic membranes, which may lead to preterm labor or PPROM. A second hypothesis is that the there is bacterial lipopolysaccharide (endotoxin) release causing release of cytokines (Il-1, Il-6, tumor necrosis factor, etc.) which then increase the production of collagenases and matrix metalloproteinases (which can lead to membrane weakening and PPROM).

Risk factors

Many factors have been associated with amnionitis. Established risk factors include long labor, nulliparity, low socioeconomic status, multiple vaginal examinations, internal fetal monitoring, length of internal monitoring and maternal bacterial vaginosis infection as well as other lower genital tract infections such as *Chlamydia trachomatis*, *Neisseria gonorrheae*, and *Ureoplasma urealyticum*. Other associated risk factors are cigarette smoking and history of prior preterm delivery or PPROM.

Clinical presentation

There are two main categories of patients in which amnionitis should be suspected.

1 Term pregnancies, in which there are clinical symptoms suggestive of infection. In this scenario, amnionitis is defined as: maternal fever (>100.4°F or 38°C) and one of the following additional findings:
   • maternal tachycardia (>100 beats/minute)
   • fetal tachycardia (>160 beats/minute)
   • uterine tenderness
   • leukocytosis (>18,000 white blood cell count)
   • foul-smelling vaginal discharge.

Other conditions in the differential diagnosis include pyelonephritis or urinary tract infection, appendicitis, viral illnesses and respiratory infections.

2 Patients presenting with preterm labor or PPROM.

Some patients who present with preterm labor or PPROM may also have clinical symptoms that strongly suggest amnionitis (same criteria as above). In subjects with preterm labor or PPROM who do not exhibit any of these classic signs or symptoms, physicians must still be concerned about a subclinical intrauterine infection. For women in preterm labor, amnionitis is common in those who are failing first-line tocolytic therapy.

Diagnosis and management

1 In patients at term, amnionitis is primarily a clinical diagnosis: maternal fever with one of the following additional signs: maternal tachycardia, fetal tachycardia, uterine tenderness, leukocytosis, or foul-smelling vaginal discharge.
  • Delivery is indicated when the diagnosis of amnionitis is made at term in order to minimize infectious morbidity to both the mother and fetus.
  • If fetal heart monitoring is reassuring, labor should be induced and an attempt should be made at a vaginal delivery.
  • If a non-reassuring fetal heart rate pattern is detected, a cesarean delivery should be performed (note that indications for cesarean delivery are standard obstetrical indications. Amnionitis in itself is not an indication for cesarean delivery).
  • Once the diagnosis of amnionitis is made, broad-spectrum antibiotics should be started immediately (i.e., ampicillin 2 g IV q 6 hours and gentamicin 1.5 mg/kg q 8 hours, or other broad-spectrum regimens).
2 Patients who present with PPROM or preterm labor should be considered at high risk for having amnionitis. Overall, the management of patients with PPROM or preterm labor depends on gestational age at presentation and the presence or absence of clinical symptoms.
  (a) *Preterm labor/PPROM with symptoms of amnionitis*
    • Once diagnosis is made, delivery is indicated regardless of gestational age.
    • Broad-spectrum antibiotics should be utilized.
    • Vaginal delivery is preferred, with cesarean reserved for standard obstetrical indications.
  (b) *Preterm labor/PPROM without clinical symptoms*
    • This group is at risk of having amnionitis.
    • Monitor closely for maternal symptoms (fever, uterine tenderness) or fetal symptoms (tachycardia, non-reactive non-stress test) of infection.
    • Consider amniocentesis for diagnosis if vague/unclear clinical symptoms.
    • If an amniocentesis is needed, send the transabdominally obtained fluid for culture (aerobic, anaerobic) and for the following tests: Gram stain, glucose concentration and white blood cell count (WBC). In some institutions, IL-6 and leukocyte esterase may also be obtained. The gold standard for diagnosis is a positive amniotic fluid culture. Delivery should be strongly considered if bacteria are seen on Gram stain or if the amniotic fluid culture is positive. If any of the other parameters listed in Table 57.1 are abnormal,

Table 57.1 Abnormal results in diagnosing amnionitis

Amniotic fluid glucose <15 mg/dL
Amniotic fluid WBC >30 cells/µL
Amniotic fluid Il-6 ≥7.9 ng/mL
Amniotic fluid leukocyte esterase ≥1; positive reaction
Amniotic fluid Gram stain any organism on an oil immersion field
Amniotic fluid any positive growth of an aerobic or anaerobic microorganism

the entire clinical picture should be taken into account and delivery should not be pursued based on a single abnormal value.
- If amnionitis is diagnosed via amniocentesis results or based on high level of clinical suspicion, broad-spectrum antibiotics should be initiated and a move toward delivery should be undertaken.

3 Patients who present with fever without a clear source. These cases can be challenging to manage. Take care to entertain a wide differential diagnosis of which amnionitis should be considered. Other diagnoses include pyelonephritis, appendicitis, gastroenteritis, etc. The other clinical manifestations will help to distinguish between these diagnoses. If the diagnosis is uncertain, an amniocentesis may be appropriate to rule out amnionitis since the presence of an intrauterine infection would warrant delivery.

Table 57.1 contains laboratory values used in diagnosing amnionitis.

Treatment

Once the diagnosis of amnionitis is made either clinically or by amniocentesis, preparations for delivery should be undertaken. Additionally, given that amnionitis is polymicrobial in nature, broad-spectrum antibiotics should be initiated. The most common recommended regimen is ampicillin 2 g every 6 hours and gentamicin 1.5 mg/kg every 8 hours although other regimens that offer similar coverage may be utilized. If the patient undergoes a cesarean delivery, clindamycin may be added. Further, antibiotics should be used after cesarean delivery until the patient has been afebrile for 24–48 hours.

Complications

In patients with amnionitis, an increased cesarean delivery rate (30–40%) is seen, mostly secondary to arrest disorders. Patients with amnionitis are also at increased risk of postpartum hemorrhage, endometritis and post cesarean delivery wound infection.

Prevention

Several risk factors have been identified for amnionitis and care should be taken to avoid these when possible. These include extended duration of labor, prolonged rupture of membranes (>18 hours), multiple vaginal examinations and internal monitoring. Other risk factors associated with amnionitis that are not preventable include young maternal age, low socioeconomic status and nulliparity.

Additionally, some infection control measures have been evaluated such as chlorhexidine vaginal washes, and have been found to be ineffective in preventing amnionitis. Antepartum treatment of bacterial vaginosis has also not been shown to prevent amnionitis. The effective preventive strategies that have been proven to decrease the incidence of amnionitis are: active labor management, induction of labor after PROM at term and the use of antibiotics in selected patients.

Conclusion

The diagnosis of amnionitis is typically clinical and based upon the presence of maternal fever (>100.4°F or 38°C) and one of the following additional criteria: maternal tachycardia (>100 beats/minute), fetal tachycardia (>160 beats/minute), uterine tenderness, leukocytosis (>18,000 white blood cell count) or foul-smelling vaginal discharge.

Amniocentesis for amniotic fluid culture is the best diagnostic test for subclincial amnionitis or in uncertain clinical presentations.

Maternal complications include bacteremia, labor abnormalities (mainly arrest disorders) and hemorrhage. In addition, cesarean delivery in the presence of amnionitis increases risk of hemorrhage and wound infection.

Amnionitis has been linked to long-term neurodevelopmental delay and cerebral palsy in children. Continuous intrapartum fetal monitoring is recommended for cases of amnionitis in order to observe evidence of fetal compromise.

Immediate delivery has not been shown to improve outcome in cases of amnionitis where there is reassuring intrapartum testing and antibiotic administration. However, the true cure for amnionitis is delivery, so induction should be expeditious and cesarean delivery should be performed for standard obstetric indications. Amnionitis in itself is not an indication for cesarean delivery.

Amnionitis is polymicrobial in nature. Broad-spectrum antibiotics should be initiated once the diagnosis is made to minimize maternal and neonatal morbidity. Antibiotics are recommended postpartum after a cesarean delivery until the patient has been afebrile for 24 hours.

Suggested reading

Creasy RK, Resnick R, Iams JD (eds) *Creasy & Resnik's Maternal-Fetal Medicine: Principles and Practice*, 6th edn. Philadelphia: Saunders Elsevier, 2009.

Gibbs RS, Duff P. Progress in pathogenesis and management of clinical intra-amniotic infection. *Am J Obstet Gynecol* 1991;164:1317.

Newton ER. Preterm labor, preterm premature rupture of membreanes, and chorioamnionitis. *Clin Perinatol* 2005;32:571–600.

Romero R, Espinoza J, Goncalves LF, Kusanovic JP, Friel L, Hassan S. The role of inflammation and infection in preterm birth. *Semin Reprod Med* 2007;25:21–39.

Romero R, Sirtori M, Oyarzun, E, *et al.* Infection and Labor V. Prevalence, microbiology and clinical significance of intra-amniotic infection in women with preterm labor and intact membranes. *Am J Obstet Gynecol* 1989;161:817.

Yoon, BH, Romero, R, Moon JB, *et al.* Clinical significance of intra-amniotic inflammation in patients with preterm labor and intact membranes. *Am J Obstet Gynecol* 2001;185:1130–6.

Third Trimester Bleeding

Yinka Oyelese

UMDNJ-Robert Wood Johnson Medical School, Jersey Shore University Medical Center, Neptune, NJ, USA

Bleeding complicates approximately 3% of pregnancies in the third trimester. Bleeding can be a cause of major perinatal and maternal morbidity and mortality. Bleeding in the third trimester always warrants prompt and thorough evaluation.

Pathophysiology

Bleeding in the third trimester is most frequently due to placental separation. In the case of placenta previa, the placenta is abnormally implanted into the lower uterine segment, and separates when the cervix starts to dilate. When labor starts, bleeding is inevitable. A normally located placenta may separate prior to labor or delivery of the baby, a condition known as placental abruption. Bleeding may also result from the rupture of a fetal vessel. This typically occurs when there is a vasa previa, which refers to fetal vessels running freely in the membranes over the cervix, unsupported by placental tissue or umbilical cord. Other causes of third trimester bleeding include preterm labor, infections of the lower genital tract, trauma, foreign bodies and neoplasms. Very rarely, the urinary tract or lower gastrointestinal tract may be the source of bleeding, and may be confused with vaginal bleeding. In about one-half of cases, no cause is found. However, when bleeding is heavy, it is generally the result of placenta previa or placental abruption.

Placenta previa refers to a placenta that is abnormally located in the lower uterine segment, either overlying or in close proximity to the internal os. It complicates approximately 1 in 250 pregnancies. When labor starts, and the cervix dilates, placental separation occurs, resulting in heavy bleeding. Consequently, these patients usually require cesarean delivery.

Protocols for High-Risk Pregnancies, 5th edition. Edited by J.T. Queenan, J.C. Hobbins and C.Y. Spong. © 2010 Blackwell Publishing Ltd.

Placenta previa typically presents with painless hemorrhage in the early third trimester (as compared to the usually painful bleeding of placental abruption). This bleeding probably results from placental separation that occurs with development of the lower uterine segment. However, it is now common, using ultrasonography, to diagnose placenta previa in asymptomatic patients in the second trimester. It has been observed that over 90% of cases of placenta previa diagnosed by sonography in the second trimester will resolve prior to term. As the lower uterine segment develops with advancing gestation, the placenta appears to move away from the cervix.

The main risk factor for placenta previa is prior cesarean delivery. Other risk factors include any surgery that disrupts the endometrial lining, such as myomectomy or curettage of the uterine cavity. Smoking, multiparity, multifetal pregnancies, maternal age and cocaine use have also been shown to be associated with increased risk of placenta previa. Patients who have a placenta previa and a prior cesarean are at increased risk of placenta accreta, a condition in which the placenta abnormally adheres to the myometrium or actually invades it. Consequently, it is not possible to separate the placenta at delivery, and these women typically suffer massive postpartum hemorrhage. The risk of placenta accreta increases with the number of prior cesareans. The risk may be as high as 67% with three prior cesareans.

Placental abruption refers to placental separation before the birth of the baby. Abruption may be revealed, when blood escapes through the cervix into the vagina, or concealed, with blood accumulating behind the placenta, with no obvious vaginal bleeding. The consequences of abruption depend on the degree of placental separation, and the gestational age at which it occurs. The vast majority of abruptions involve only small degrees of placental separation and have few clinical consequences. However, abruption, even in minor cases, carries an increased risk of preterm labor and birth, preterm premature rupture of the membranes, intrauterine growth restriction, perinatal death and other adverse perinatal outcomes. When over 50% of the placenta separates, fetal death often results. Placental abruption may result from acute events such as direct or indirect abdominal trauma and cocaine use. It may also be associated with longstanding pathological processes such as hypertension, intrauterine growth restriction and placental dysfunction. Risk factors for abruption include smoking, trauma, hypertension and preeclampsia, cocaine use, intrauterine infection, oligohydramnios and preterm premature rupture of the membranes. The rapid uterine decompression that occurs when the membranes rupture in patients with polyhydramnios may also lead to abruption. Patients with abruption may present in shock that is out of proportion to the apparent blood loss, especially when the abruption is concealed. Similarly, concealed abruption may be associated with disseminated intravascular coagulopathy, especially when fetal death occurs. There is consumption of coagulation factors and fibrinogen, with resultant failure of coagulation.

Vasa previa is a condition in which the umbilical cord inserts into the membranes rather than into the placenta. Fetal vessels run over the cervix and under the presenting part. These vessels are unsupported by umbilical cord or placental tissue and can rupture when the membranes rupture, resulting in fetal hemorrhage and often exsanguination and death. Unfortunately, fetal death is not uncommon due to the condition not being recognized before the membranes rupture. Risk factors include a second trimester low-lying placenta, multifetal gestations, pregnancies with bilobed placentas and those resulting from in vitro fertilization. Vasa previa can be diagnosed prenatally with ultrasonography and color Doppler. A high index of suspicion is crucial to making the diagnosis. Prenatal diagnosis and cesarean delivery prior to rupture of the membranes are essential to achieving good perinatal outcomes. In the absence of prenatal diagnosis, perinatal mortality exceeds 50%.

Diagnosis

The diagnosis of placental abruption is a clinical one, and is based on a high index of suspicion, as well as recognition of the symptoms and signs associated with abruption. The diagnosis of placenta previa is made using imaging, typically sonography. Perhaps the most important differentiating diagnostic features between placenta previa and abruption are the presence or absence of pain, and the presence or absence of a placenta previa on ultrasonographic examination. The bleeding associated with placenta previa is generally painless, while that of abruption is typically associated with pain. However, there are exceptions to this rule. Placenta previa may be associated with painful contractions in cases where there is preterm labor. Conversely, abruption may be painless. In fact, when abruption occurs with a posterior placenta, backache may be the only symptom. A carefully taken history is essential. The patient may previously have had ultrasonography that revealed a placenta previa. History of recent intercourse, trauma, drug use or hypertension may aid in the diagnosis. If the mother is stable, a sonogram should be performed to determine the placental location; a placenta that is not located in the lower uterine segment suggests that placental abruption is responsible for the bleeding. Digital examination is contraindicated in cases of vaginal bleeding in which the placental location has not been established. A digital examination in the presence of placenta previa may result in torrential hemorrhage. In cases in which the lower uterine segment and the lower placental edge cannot be adequately visualized by transabdominal sonography, transvaginal sonography should be performed. Transvaginal sonography is more accurate for diagnosing placenta previa than transabdominal sonography, and is safe, not associated with increased bleeding, and is well tolerated. In patients with placenta previa and prior cesareans, a high index of suspicion for placenta accreta is essential. Perhaps the most reliable sonographic sign of placenta accreta is the presence of large vascular lacunae in the placenta in the lower uterine segment, giving a 'moth-eaten' appearance. Sonography is of limited utility in the diagnosis of placental abruption. In cases of acute revealed abruption, blood frequently does not accumulate behind the placenta. Thus the absence of any sonographic findings does not rule out placental abruption. Findings of retroplacental hematoma, free clot floating in the amniotic cavity, a thickened heterogenous placenta, or a subchorionic hematoma all have a good positive predictive value for abruption.

If possible, sonographic examination of the region over the cervix with color Doppler should be performed in order to rule out a vasa previa. Fetal vessels will have the appearance of linear echolucent structures on gray-scale sonography. Pulsed Doppler may reveal a fetal vessel waveform. The uterus is generally soft and non-tender to palpation in cases of placenta previa. In abruption, there is often some uterine tenderness. Frequently contractions may be palpated, while in large abruptions, the uterus may feel hard to palpation. When placenta previa has been ruled out, a speculum examination should be performed. This may reveal other causes of bleeding such as vaginal candidiasis, cervical ectropion, lacerations of the vagina or cervix (that may occasionally follow intercourse), foreign bodies, polyps, or more rarely, neoplasms of the lower genital tract. Fetal heart rate monitoring in abruption may reveal variable or late decelerations, bradycardia, reduced variability, or a sinusoidal pattern. There are often low-amplitude, high-frequency uterine contractions. These heart rate patterns may also occur with vasa previa. Tests for fetal blood in the vaginal blood such as the Apt test were previously used to rule out a ruptured vasa previa, but are generally no longer in wide use.

Management

The management of women who present with third trimester bleeding depends on the gestational age, the degree of bleeding and the stability of the mother and fetus. In all cases, the first step is evaluation and stabilization of the mother and fetus. However, in cases where bleeding is heavy enough to lead to maternal or fetal compromise, expeditious delivery, usually by cesarean, with simultaneous maternal resuscitation is warranted. Similarly, a suspicion of a ruptured vasa previa should lead to immediate cesarean delivery. Intravenous access with wide-bore catheters should be established. Blood should be taken for complete blood count, type and screen. In cases of abruption, coagulation studies should be performed. Blood may be taken in a tube without anticoagulant and inverted every few minutes. Failure to clot within 10 minutes suggests coagulopathy. In cases of placenta previa, when there is coagulaopathy, or when blood loss is in excess of 500 mL, blood should be cross-matched. Coagulopathy should be corrected. Blood should be replaced promptly and adequately initially with crystalloid and subsequently with blood as required.

The fetus should be monitored continuously until it is clear that fetal status is both stable and reassuring. Steroids should be given to promote fetal lung maturation in gestations less than 34 weeks. Rh immune globulin should be administered to women who are Rh negative. Generally, any significant bleeding after 37 weeks warrants delivery. Delivery should be by the safest route for mother and fetus. In cases of placenta previa where the placental edge covers or lies within 2 cm of the internal os, delivery should be by cesarean. When the placental edge is more than 2 cm from the internal os, vaginal birth is safe as long as there are no other contraindications. Women with placenta previa who have active bleeding after 34 weeks should be delivered promptly by cesarean. In those cases where there is no bleeding, an amniocentesis at 36 to 37 weeks followed by elective cesarean delivery is recommended. This will allow the patient to be delivered in a controlled situation, rather than as an emergency if severe bleeding were to occur.

When placenta previa presents with bleeding in the third trimester prior to 34 weeks, the patient should be admitted for at least 48 hours. If bleeding continues, the patient should remain in hospital. However, if she has not bled for 48 hours, consideration may be given to management as an outpatient provided the patient is reliable, and has good and quick access to the hospital. Women who have low-lying placentas who have a vaginal delivery are still at risk of postpartum hemorrhage since the lower uterine segment is non-contractile. In cases of minor abruption at term where the fetus and mother are stable, the mother may be allowed to labor as long as both mother and fetus are monitored very carefully, and emergent cesarean can be performed quickly. In cases of fetal compromise, cesarean is the safest option for the fetus. When fetal death has occurred, the patient is often in advanced labor, and if labor progresses rapidly, and the mother is stable, a vaginal delivery is desirable. Coagulopathy is a particular problem in these cases, and the patient should be carefully monitored for evidence of impaired clotting, and clotting factors should be replaced aggressively.

In cases of abruption prior to 34 weeks, if the mother and fetus are both stable, conservative management in hospital may help achieve an increased gestational age at delivery. However, these pregnancies should be monitored very closely, since there is a significant risk of sudden worsening abruption with fetal death. Only in cases in which the fetus and mother have been shown to be stable on prolonged monitoring, and in which there is no bleeding, should outpatient management be considered. Tocoloytics may be used with extreme caution in women with abruption who are stable and contracting. The importance of close monitoring in these cases cannot be overemphasized.

Vasa previa carries a risk of rupture of the membranes with rupture of the vessels. Therefore, these cases should be delivered by elective cesarean at 35–36 weeks, or earlier should bleeding, labor or rupture of the membranes occur. Patients known to have a vasa previa should be admitted to hospital at 32 weeks to provide rapid access to the operating room should the membranes rupture. Steroids should be administered to promote fetal lung maturation. It is important to deliver these pregnancies in centers with adequate neonatal care.

The risk of placenta accreta is high in women who have both a placenta previa and a prior cesarean delivery and increases with the number of prior cesareans. There is evidence that outcomes with placenta accreta are optimized when the condition is diagnosed prenatally, and delivery occurs in a scheduled manner, and delivery management is by a multidisciplinary approach, involving specialties such as anesthesiology, neonatology, blood bank, urology, maternal fetal medicine, interventional radiology and gynecologic oncology.

Complications

Perhaps the most important complication of third trimester bleeding is hypovolemic shock, which may be severe and life threatening. There may be severe morbidity or even death of the fetus or the mother. Disseminated intravascular coagulopathy may occur in abruption, and sometimes with placenta previa when there has been massive blood loss with volume replacement deficient in coagulation factors. Hypovolemia may result in renal failure. Abruption may also be associated with acute renal cortical necrosis. Sheehan syndrome or postpartum pituitary infarction is rarely seen in the Western world, but may result from severe hemorrhage. Finally, the patient is at risk from anesthetic and surgical complications.

Conclusion

Bleeding in the third trimester is often a serious complication of pregnancy that carries a significant risk of perinatal death and severe maternal morbidity. It should always be treated seriously and with a high index of suspicion. Careful evaluation should be performed; ultrasonography is an important tool to assist in the diagnosis. Accurate diagnosis and appropriate treatment will optimize outcomes for mother and fetus in most cases.

Suggested reading

Bhide A, Thalinganathan B. Recent advances in the management of placenta previa. *Curr Opin Obstet Gynecol* 2004;16:447–51.

Comstock CH. Antenatal diagnosis of placenta accreta. *Ultrasound Obstet Gynecol* 2005; 26:89–96.

Oyelese Y, Ananth CV. Placental abruption. *Obstet Gynecol* 2006;108(4):1005–16.

Oyelese Y, Smulian JC. Placenta previa, placenta accreta, and vasa previa. *Obstet Gynecol* 2006;107(4):927–41.

PROTOCOL 59

Amniotic Fluid Embolus

Robert Resnik
Department of Reproductive Medicine, UCSD School of Medicine, Solana Beach, CA, USA

Since the entity was first described by Meyer,[1] amniotic fluid embolism has come to be recognized as a dramatic and dire event, responsible for more than 10% of maternal mortalities in the United States. The clinical presentation is that of a term or near-term patient, more frequently multiparous, in whom the sudden onset of agitation, dyspnea, anxiety and respiratory arrest develops during labor, delivery or in the first few hours postpartum. Early publications suggested a mortality rate of 50% or higher, but more recent studies report lower death rates, ranging from 21% to 30%.[2–4] This is likely due to more rapid recognition and aggressive cardiopulmonary support. Predisposing factors include maternal age >35, placenta previa and cesarean delivery.[2] Among those who survive the acute event, left ventricular failure may develop in a clinical picture consistent with adult respiratory distress syndrome as well as disseminated intravascular coagulation.

Pathophysiology and diagnosis

The pathophysiology of amniotic fluid embolism (AFE) has not been entirely clarified. However, combining data from animal models[5,6] and humans,[7,8] an understanding of the disease mechanism can be pieced together. Rapid infusion of amniotic fluid with particulate matter into the maternal circulation leads initially to an immediate and sharp increase in mean pulmonary artery pressure, pulmonary vascular resistance and resultant systemic hypoxia due to disordered ventilation-perfusion. This is followed by a second phase of left ventricular failure. Data obtained from patients with AFE, monitored with pulmonary artery catheters, reveal a severe reduction in left ventricular systolic work index and secondary increase in pulmonary wedge and diastolic pressures.[8] Information

---

Protocols for High-Risk Pregnancies, 5th edition. Edited by J.T. Queenan, J.C. Hobbins and C.Y. Spong. © 2010 Blackwell Publishing Ltd.

collected from the National Amniotic Fluid Embolism Registry suggests that the syndrome is similar to anaphylaxis and septic shock, conditions also triggered by foreign toxins which enter the intravascular space.[9]

Amniotic fluid rich in tissue factor triggers the intrinsic clotting system, with rapid defibrination and hemorrhage, thus aggravating an already complex cardiovascular picture. The differential diagnosis includes acute pulmonary edema, pulmonary emboli from the peripheral venous circulation, and cardiac arrhythmias. During resuscitative efforts, it is advisable to obtain blood from the pulmonary artery via central lines to look for fetal squame cells (Attwood stain) and mucin (Giemsa stain).[9] This observation will confirm the diagnosis in those patients who survive.

Management

Given this clinical picture, the following represents an appropriate management format:

1 Institute endotracheal intubation, with maintenance of oxygen flow rates dictated by monitoring arterial blood gases.
2 Cardiac resuscitative measures may be needed. Crystalloids should be administered to maintain intravascular volume and cardiac output. Inotropic agents may be required to treat hypotension and heart failure. The appropriate use of these agents necessitates continuous intensive care cardiopulmonary monitoring. Use of a triple-lumen pulmonary catheter is required.
3 Careful attention should be paid to blood loss following delivery and measurement of clotting factors. Blood should be obtained for measurement of clotting factors, partial thromboplastin time, platelets, fibrin split products and fibrinogen. In addition, while awaiting these results, one should observe the time required for blood to form a solid clot in a red-top tube (normal, less than 8 min). In the presence of disseminated intravascular clotting, component therapy should be initiated with fresh frozen plasma or platelets, or both. (Fresh frozen plasma contains approximately 1g fibrinogen/unit; each unit of platelets raises the platelet count by approximately 8000/μL.). The use of recombinant factor VIIa may be considered, although extensive experience is lacking.

Patients who survive the cardiopulmonary event may have a 2- to 5-day course of mild to substantial respiratory insufficiency, probably due to adult respiratory distress syndrome, and complicated by pulmonary edema secondary to diminished left ventricular function.

References

1 Meyer JR. Embolia pulmonar amnio-casiosa. *Brazil Med* 1926;2:301.
2 Abenhaim HA, Azoulay L, Kraner MS, *et al.* Incidence and risk factors of amniotic fluid embolisms: a population-based study on 3 million births in the United States. *Am J Obstet Gynecol* 2008;199:49.e1–49.e8.
3 Gilbert WM, Danielsen B. Amniotic fluid embolism: decreased mortality in a population-based study. *Obstet Gynecol* 1999;93:973.
4 Tuffnell DJ. United Kingdom amniotic fluid embolism register. *Br J Obstet Gynecol* 2005;112:1625.
5 Reis RL, Pierce WS, Eehrendt DM. Hemodynamic effects of amniotic fluid embolism. *Surg Gynecol Obstet* 1965;129:45.
6 Attwood HD, Downing SE. Experimental amniotic fluid and meconium embolism. *Surg Gynecol Obstet* 1965;120:255.
7 Clark SL, Montz FJ, Phelan JP. Hemodynamic alterations associated with amniotic fluid embolism: a reappraisal. *Am J Obstet Gynecol* 1985;151:617.
8 Clark SL, Cotton DB, Gonik B, Greenspoon J, Phelan JP. Central hemodynamic alterations in amniotic fluid embolism. *Am J Obstet Gynecol* 1988;158:1124.
9 Clark SL, Hankins GDV, Dudley DA, *et al.* Amniotic fluid embolism: analysis of a national registry. *Am J Obstet Gynecol* 1995;172:1158.
10 Resnik R, Swartz WH, Plumer MH, et al. Amniotic fluid embolism with survival. Obstet Gynecol 1976;47:295.

PART 6

Labor and Delivery

PROTOCOL 60

Maternal Transport

Jean Rex[1] and Jerome Yankowitz[2]

[1] Department of Pediatrics, Washington University School of Medicine, St Louis, MO, USA
[2] Division of Maternal-Fetal Medicine, University of Iowa College of Medicine, Iowa City, IA, USA

Overview

One of the scientific triumphs of the twentieth century was the dramatic reduction in mortality rates for many segments of the population. One area of medicine, in particular, that has enjoyed a sharp decline in mortality in the past century is maternal and neonatal care. Much of this success is attributable to the development of perinatal centers, which began in Scandinavia and the Netherlands in the late 1940s. Urban hospitals in the United States were quick to emulate these centers. Mortality committees were also developed to devise strategies for improving outcomes in the perinatal period. Perinatal centers generally provide subspecialist care for high-risk obstetric patients, as well as the latest technology and expertise in neonatal intensive care. As technology has progressed, a greater variety of diseases have been successfully managed, with improvements in outcomes for younger and smaller infants, as well as pregnant women with coexisting medical problems. During the 1970s and 1980s, in an effort to extend the benefits of these perinatal centers to residents of rural areas, many states devised regionalized systems of perinatal care in which physicians working in community hospitals provide the bulk of perinatal care, but work in close conjunction with the tertiary care subspecialists.

An essential component of regionalized perinatal care is maternal transport. Before regionalization, many high-risk infants were transferred to tertiary perinatal centers after birth in order to receive intensive treatment. With the advent of regionalization, these neonatal transport programs were often strengthened, but were also joined by the option of maternal transport, allowing the mother to go to the tertiary center before delivery, either because of a concomitant maternal medical problem or if there might be reason to believe the neonate at risk for complications. In this way, the neonate may begin receiving intensive care immediately after birth with the ultimate goal of improved neonatal outcomes. This

Protocols for High-Risk Pregnancies, 5th edition. Edited by J.T. Queenan, J.C. Hobbins and C.Y. Spong. © 2010 Blackwell Publishing Ltd.

protocol will outline indications commonly used for maternal transport, as well as guidelines regarding the details of maternal transport. The protocol will discuss conflicting results in the medical literature concerning the appropriate level of specialization at the delivering medical centers.

Indications for maternal transport

Many studies have reported the common reasons for maternal transport. Maternal factors are responsible for the majority of maternal transports. Most of these transfers, however, are initiated with the health of the fetus in mind. A review by Giles revealed that over 40% of maternal transports occur because of more than one indication. In another review, Knox and Schnitker noted that many maternal transports are dependent on the possibility of a premature delivery. In the United Kingdom, it was shown that 52% of transfers were related to preterm labor with and without ruptured membranes and an additional 20% were related to preterm ruptured membranes without labor.

Premature rupture of the membranes was cited by many studies as a common indication for maternal transport. Giles noted that since the late 1970s there has been increased encouragement to attempt to prevent delivery en route by transporting pregnant women before active labor begins. Therefore, there appears to be a low threshold for transporting women who have experienced PROM, but are not yet in active labor.

Several authors also cited preterm labor as an indication for maternal transport. Several studies that have shown increased benefit for neonates of certain gestational ages or birthweights to be delivered at tertiary care centers support preterm labor as an indicator for transport.

The recommendations for which infants should be transported have changed greatly within the past two decades. A 1987 study by Paneth et al. recommended that infants <37 weeks or <2250 g be delivered in a facility with neonatal intensive care. In 1993 Strobino et al. found that those infants <32 weeks would likely benefit from maternal transfer, a recommendation echoed by Walsh-Sukys and Fanaroff in 1997, who also added the indication to transfer infants <1500 g. Most recently in 2003 Lee et al. provided evidence that for pregnancies prior to 29 weeks' gestation, newborns benefit from delivery at a tertiary care center. The neonates may not receive benefit from tertiary care, in the absence of other risk factors after this gestational age. For women in advanced preterm labor, Elliott et al. cautioned that other risk factors must be taken into account when deciding to transfer a pregnant woman, including the distance between hospitals, the expected time needed for transport, the personnel available to serve on the transport team, the facilities available at the referring hospital, and the speed of progression of labor.

In the history of perinatal care, there has been a steady progression from establishment of NICUs in the 1960s and 1970s, to regionalization of neonatal intensive care in the mid-1970s. The initial expectation was that hospitals with no or intermediate NICUs were to refer infants that weighed 2000 g or less to a regional NICU. Since then there has been marked change in the provision of care with diffusion of neonatal expertise into the community. Is there any evidence available today as to what appropriate care should be? Cifuentes *et al.* evaluated mortality of infants weighing less than 2000 g at those hospitals with no NICUs, intermediate NICUs, low-volume community NICUs and high-volume (census >15) NICUs to regional NICUs as the reference. Only the high volume community NICUs could approach the lower level of mortality of the regional NICUs. Bartels *et al.* had analogous findings for very low birthweight infants (VLBW, those weighing less than 1500 g). They found that in Germany, the mortality rate in small NICUs (<36 VLBW infants/year) was increased significantly compared to large NICUs for deliveries <29 weeks. California, like many parts of the United States, went through a marked expansion in non-tertiary care NICUs. Gould *et al.* found that while the regional and the community NICUs with California Children's Services (CCS) Program NICU designation had comparable outcomes, primary care hospitals, intermediate NICUs and non-CCS designated NICUs had worse outcomes for neonates below 1000 g. It has been shown that the rate of severe intraventricular hemorrhage is greater for infants born at level I hospitals and transported to a tertiary care hospital than similar inborn infants at that tertiary care center. Some of the better outcomes might be explained by a higher level of maternal corticosteroid administration at tertiary care centers.

Modanlou *et al.* generalized the indications for maternal transport with the statement that pregnant women are often referred antenatally to tertiary centers for chronic problems, while maternal transport often occurs for acute conditions that threaten the life of the fetus. Other acute conditions often responsible for maternal transport include antenatal bleeding, preeclampsia/eclampsia, chorioamnionitis, placental abruption and abnormal/transverse lie. Chronic conditions, however, may become indications for maternal transport if they have gone undiagnosed due to lack of prenatal care or if the severity increases suddenly. Examples of such circumstances include pregnancy-induced hypertension/chronic hypertension, multiple gestation, maternal diabetes and Rh sensitization. Other indications for transport cited less frequently include intrauterine death, fetal anomalies, need for cesarean section, maternal cardiac disease, sickle cell crisis, obstructed labor, incompetent cervix, post-dates pregnancy, and placenta previa. Table 60.1 provides a summary of commonly cited indications and contraindications for maternal transport. Ultimately the decision to transfer a pregnant patient must be made by physicians at both the referring

Table 60.1 Indications and contraindications for maternal transport

Maternal indications	Fetal indications	Contraindications
Premature rupture of membranes	Low gestational age	Maternal/fetal cardiovascular instability
Preterm labor	Cervical incompetence	
Preeclampsia/eclampsia/ hypertension	Anomalies requiring surgery	Advanced cervical dilation (>3 cm) not arrested by tocolytics
Multiple gestation	Rh sensitization/ hemolytic disorder	Preterm contractions without other risk factor
Antenatal bleeding	Need for ventilation	
Serious infection	Fetal arrhythmia or bradycardia	Delivery en route highly likely
Poorly controlled diabetes		
Renal disease/decreased function	Unexplained intrauterine death	
Drug overdose	Non-reassuring fetal testing	
	Intrauterine growth restriction	
Trauma	Breech/transverse lie	
Acute abdominal emergencies	Severe oligohydramnios	
Collagen vascular disease (lupus)	Need for cesarean section	
Hepatic disease		
Cardiac disease		
Thyroid storm, thyrotoxicosis		
Malignancy		
Sickle cell crisis		

and receiving hospitals, with full knowledge of the referring hospital's capabilities and with the primary goal of maintaining maternal safety. Referring physicians should responsibly and ethically assess their hospital's capability to care for neonates, particularly those delivered at less than 28–30 weeks gestation.

Guidelines for maternal transport

The American Academy of Pediatrics and the American College of Obstetricians and Gynecologists have published guidelines for use when transporting patients, including information regarding personnel, equipment, transport procedures, and outreach education. Additionally, other authors have presented suggestions that may be useful in designing protocols for maternal transport, such as standardized equipment kits, personnel qualifications and guidelines for treatment of common maternal conditions during transport.

Transport options are not, of course, limited to maternal transport alone, and it should not be assumed that every maternal-fetal pair that encounters a problem during late pregnancy should be transported to a tertiary center. Unless there is a substantial risk to the mother or infant, it may be ideal for the woman to receive treatment at the local hospital, by her local physician. This option allows for treatment by a familiar physician in a location close to home and to the support of family, as well as sparing the financial costs of transport and high intensity care. In some cases a telephone consult with a specialist physician may be all that is needed. In other cases it may be convenient for the specialist physician to travel to the local center to provide care. Maternal transport may be considered if there is an identified maternal or fetal risk for which the referring hospital is unequipped to treat, the maternal-fetal pair can be stabilized for transport, and both referring and receiving physicians agree that tertiary care is needed. Finally, neonatal, rather than maternal, transport may be necessary in cases of unexpected morbidities, advanced labor with delivery likely before transport can be completed, or any other reason that maternal transport is thought to be ill-advised.

The transport team should be composed of specially trained personnel who are familiar with a variety of emergency conditions that may occur in obstetric and neonatal patients. Each regional system should be directed by a tertiary care physician with training in high-risk obstetrics or neonatology. This consultant must be familiar with the latest technology in the field, as well as with the capabilities of the community hospitals in the region. The personnel who accompany the patient during maternal transport may include a wide variety of specialists, including physicians, neonatal or labor and delivery nurses, respiratory therapists, anesthesiologists and emergency medical technicians. It may be optimal for a team to be dispensed from the tertiary center in order to best deal with complications that occur en route; however, teams are often composed of personnel from the referring hospital. Indeed, it may provide relief to the patient to have her own physician or local nurses with her during transport. In any case, the members of the transport team must be individualized for each particular transport; for example, in the case of congestive heart failure a respiratory therapist may be essential. When transporting more stable patients, however, emergency medical technicians can often provide safe transport in the absence of specialized personnel. The responsibility for the patient generally falls upon the referring hospital until arrival at the tertiary center, including during any time spent planning the transport. If, however, the specialty center sends its own transport team, the responsibility may shift to the receiving facility at the time transport begins.

The equipment needed for maternal transport should be considered carefully for each case, keeping in mind the maternal and fetal risk factors, distance to be traveled, type of transport vehicle, and resources available locally. An advantage of maternal over neonatal transport is the reduced need for extra equipment for neonatal transport. The AAP and ACOG guidelines broadly suggest for all transports the following: equipment for monitoring physiologic functions, temperature, and pulse oximetry, resuscitation and support equipment, portable medical gas tanks if ventilators are needed, and electrical equipment compatible with sources in the transport vehicle. Each piece of equipment should be tested regularly in the harshest conditions to be expected in the region. Other authors describe individual components of maternal transport kits that may be considered, such as standard medications, intravenous solutions, and supplies needed for delivery.

The choice of transport vehicle often depends on the distance of the transport. Ambulance is likely the most effective for short-distance travel up to about 50 to 60 miles, except in urban areas with heavy traffic. Helicopter may be the most appropriate option for the 60 to 100 mile range, while aircraft should be considered for longer distances. When using air transportation the pilot becomes an essential team member in the decision to transport. It must be remembered that the pilot has the final decision on whether an air transport will take place as he or she is responsible for the safety of not only the patient but also the entire crew and transport team.

The maternal transport itself should begin with a coordinated decision between referring and receiving hospitals on the utility of the transfer. The receiving physician should provide recommendations before the transport is initiated on such issues as use of tocolytics, antibiotics, steroids and any other medication needed. Before transport can begin, necessary personnel, equipment and medical records must be assembled for transport, as well as consent obtained from the patient. Table 60.2 provides an overview of the essential steps that must be considered for maternal transport to occur. During transport it is important to observe the patient continuously, as well as monitor vital signs, oximetry, ventilatory pressures, cervical status, uterine contractions and fetal heart rates as appropriate. The transport team should also be prepared to handle an imminent delivery or perform procedures such as chest tube placement and intubation if the patient's clinical condition changes during transport. Another priority of the team is to provide supportive care for the patient in order to decrease her anxiety. Constant communication

Table 60.2 Steps in maternal transport

1	Notify perinatologist
2	Notify labor and delivery personnel
3	Notify neonatal intensive care unit personnel
4	Notify neonatologist
5	Notify relevant subspecialists
6	Notify admitting office personnel
7	Transfer patient's records

with the receiving hospital is important in case the patient's condition changes en route.

A final responsibility of the regional center staff is to provide outreach education to the community hospitals in the region, as well as to the public. A study by Gibson *et al.* suggests the utility of establishing protocols by the regional center for maternal transport in the region in order to standardize procedures, enhance communication and hopefully improve outcomes. Regional centers should also collect data on transport outcomes and community hospital capabilities, educate staff at referring centers on new technologies and treatments in high-risk obstetric and neonatal care, and inform the public about services provided and the structure of the regional network.

Based all the data and guidelines, the American College of Obstetricians and Gynecologists suggests that maternal transport to a tertiary care center before delivery be considered for pregnancies at the threshold of viability less than 750 to 1000 g and/or less than 26 weeks.

Conclusion

The development of maternal transport systems has been a relatively recent advance in the field of perinatology, but has proved beneficial for a variety of maternal and fetal acute and chronic conditions in providing improved access to specialty care. In making the decision to transport a pregnant woman to a tertiary center, one must take into account several factors including the patient's condition, the presumed risks to the neonate and the capabilities of the referring hospital. Of course, any decision for transport must be made jointly by the referring and receiving physicians. The development of protocols for maternal transport situations may help improve communication, as well as standardize the necessary procedures involved in order to maximize patient outcomes. It must be kept in mind, however, that each transport must be planned according to the needs of the individual patient.

References and suggested reading

American Academy of Pediatrics/American College of Obstetricians and Gynecologists. Interhospital care of the perinatal patient. In: *Guidelines for Perinatal Care*, 6th edn. AAP and ACOG; 2007.

American College of Obstetricians and Gynecologists. *Perinatal care at the threshold of viability.* Practice Bulletin # 38, September 2002.

Bartels DB, Wypij D, Wenzlaff P, Dammann O, Poets CF. Hospital volume and neonatal mortality among very low birth weight infants. *Pediatrics* 2006;117:2206–14.

Boehm FH, Haire MF. One-way maternal transport: an evolving concept. *Am J Obstet Gynecol* 1979;134:484–9.

Brown FB. The management of high-risk obstetric transfer patients. *Obstet Gynecol* 1978;51:674–6.

Chien LY, Ohlsson A, Seshia MM, Boulton J, Sankaran K, Lee SK, Canadian Neonatal Network. Variations in antenatal corticosteroid therapy: a persistent problem despite 30 years of evidence. *Obstet Gynecol* 2002;99:401–8.

Cifuentes J, Bronstein J, Phibbs CS, Phibbs RH, Schmitt SK, Carlo WA. Mortality in low birth weight infants according to level of neonatal care at hospital of birth. *Pediatrics* 2002;109:745–51.

Delaney-Black V, Lubchenco LO, Butterfield J, Goldson E, Koops BL, Lazotte DC. Outcome of very-low-birth-weight infants: are populations of neonates inherently different after antenatal versus neonatal referral?. *Am J Obstet Gynecol* 1989;160:545–52.

Elliott JP, Sipp TL, Balazs KT. Maternal transport of patients with advanced cervical dilatation – to fly or not to fly? *Obstet Gynecol* 1992;79:380–2.

Fenton AC, Ainsworth SB, Sturgiss SN. Population-based outcomes after acute antenatal transfer. *Paediatr Perinat Epidemiol* 2002;16:278–85.

Gibson ME, Bailey CF, Ferguson JE. Transporting the incubator: effects upon a region of the adoption of guidelines for high-risk maternal transport. *J Perinatol* 2001;21:300–6.

Giles HR. Maternal transport. *Clin Obstet Gynaecol* 1979;6:203–13.

Gould JB, Marks AR, Chavez G. Expansion of community-based perinatal care in California. *J Perinatol* 2002;22:630–40.

Knox GE, Schnitker KA. In-utero transport. *Clin Obstet Gynaecol* 1984;27:11–16.

Lee SK, McMillan DD, Ohlsson A, Boulton J, Lee DSC, Ting S, Liston R. The benefit of preterm birth at tertiary care centers is related to gestational age. *Am J Obstet Gynecol* 2003;188:617–22.

Miller TC, Densberger M, Krogman J. Maternal transport and the perinatal denominator. *Am J Obstet Gynecol* 1983;147:19–24.

Modanlou HD, Dorchester W, Freeman RK, Rommal C. Perinatal transport to a regional perinatal center in a metropolitan area: maternal versus neonatal transport. *Am J Obstet Gynecol* 1980;138:1157–64.

Paneth N, Kiely JL, Wallenstein S, Susser M. The choice of place of delivery: effect of hospital level on mortality in all singleton births in New York City. *Am J Dis Child* 1987;141:60–64.

Powell SL, Holt VL, Hickok DE, Easterling T, Connell FA. Recent changes in delivery site of low-birth-weight infants in Washington: impact on birth weight-specific mortality. *Am J Obstet Gynecol* 1995;173:1585–92.

Souma ML. Maternal transport: behind the drama. *Am J Obstet Gynecol* 1979;134:904–9.

Strobino DM, Frank R, Oberdorf MA, Shachtman R, Kim YJ, Callan N, Nagey D. Development of an index of maternal transport. *Med Decis Making* 1993;13:64–73.

Towers CV, Bonebrake R, Padilla G, Rumney P. The effect of transport on the rate of severe intraventricular hemorrhage in very low birth weight infants. *Obstet Gynecol* 2000;95:291–5.

Walsh-Sukys MC, Fanaroff AA. Perinatal Services and Resources. In: *Neonatal-Perinatal Medicine: Diseases of the Fetus and Infant*, 6th edn. St Louis, MO: Mosby, 1997.

Wilson AK, Martel M-J, and the Clinical Practice Obstetrics Committee. Maternal transport policy. *J Obstet Gynaecol Can* 2005;27:956–8.

Intrapartum Fetal Heart Rate Monitoring

Roger K. Freeman
University of California Irvine, Long Beach, CA, USA

Rationale

Intrapartum fetal heart rate monitoring was developed in the mid-1960s after patterns of heart rate change in relation to uterine contractions had been described by Hon, Caldero-Barcia and Hammacher. At the time of development of fetal heart rate monitoring it was believed that most cases of congenital neurological abnormalities were due to fetal hypoxia proximate to birth. When the method was first developed, there were numerous non-randomized studies comparing electronically monitored patients to either historical controls or low-risk patients who were monitored by auscultation which was not rigorous. It was clear early on that the intrapartum fetal death rate was significantly less in electronically monitored patients than in the non-randomized controls, even if the controls were low risk and the electronically monitored patients were high risk.

In the mid-1970s Haverkamp[1] did the first prospectively randomized controlled study where the study group was openly electronically monitored and the control group had the electronic fetal monitor covered up so the caregivers could not use the information in patient management. The control group was monitored by auscultation with a rigorous protocol of listening every 15 minutes in the first stage of labor and every 5 minutes in the second stage by a dedicated one-on-one nurse assigned to each patient. The results of this study and of several more randomized prospective trials revealed no benefit to electronic fetal heart rate monitoring during the intrapartum period when compared to intensive auscultation.[2] Several of the studies also found higher cesarean delivery rates in the electronically monitored group. The only statistically significant benefit was shown in the large Dublin trial where the electronically monitored patients had neonates

---

Protocols for High-Risk Pregnancies, 5th edition. Edited by J.T. Queenan, J.C. Hobbins and C.Y. Spong. © 2010 Blackwell Publishing Ltd.

with fewer seizures but on follow-up the incidence of cerebral palsy was not different between the electronically monitored patients and those with intensive auscultation.[3]

Today as we look back it has been pointed out that, even with the introduction of electronic fetal monitoring in the majority of laboring patients, there has been no reduction in the incidence of cerebral palsy.[4] This finding has indicated to some that the technique has no benefit. However, if we accept the reduction in term intrapartum deaths in electronically monitored patients compared to those with non-intensive auscultation from the original non-randomized trials,[5] and also compare the marked increase in perinatal survival over the past 30 years, we must conclude that some fetuses that used to die intrapartum now survive damaged and some that used to survive damaged now survive intact. Thus electronic intrapartum fetal monitoring probably has been valuable. Nevertheless, it is clear that the vast majority of non-reassuring patterns do not result in neurological damage and to the epidemiologist this high false-positive rate makes the technique invalid.[6] However, if the technique were perfect, intervention based on the fetal monitor pattern would prevent all cases of cerebral palsy due to intrapartum hypoxia and there would be zero correlation with neurological outcome, rendering the technique not predictive of future outcome, which is the standard used by epidemiologists.

Pattern interpretation

Baseline fetal heart rate characteristics[7] include rate with tachycardia defined as >160 bpm (beats per minute) and bradycardia defined as <10 bpm. Variability is classified as absent, minimal (1 to 5 bpm), moderate (5–25 bpm) and increased (>25 bpm).

There are five periodic fetal heart rate patterns[7] that have been described.

1 Fetal heart rate acceleration with an amplitude of 15 bpm and a duration of 15 seconds from onset to offset is seen in most patients beyond 32 weeks' gestation and signifies good fetal oxygenation and an umbilical arterial pH of ≥7.20. If accelerations are not present spontaneously, one can evoke fetal heart rate accelerations with fetal scalp stimulation after membrane rupture or with vibroacoustic stimulation before membrane rupture. This technique can be useful when following a problematic fetal heart rate pattern where spontaneous or evoked accelerations may allow one to avoid intervention.[8]

2 Early deceleration is a uniform pattern with slow onset and offset that is a mirror image of the contraction. This is believed to be due to fetal

head compression and is mediated as a vagal reflex. It is not associated with fetal hypoxia or acid–base change and requires no intervention.

3 Variable deceleration is a pattern characterized by rapid onset and rapid offset and usually has an amplitude of 30 to 40 bpm or more. It is believed to be due to umbilical cord compression giving rise to a vagal response. Unless the deceleration is prolonged beyond 40 to 60 seconds on a repetitive basis, is associated with a rising baseline rate or decreased fetal heart rate variability, or the return to baseline is prolonged, it is considered reassuring and does not require intervention. However, if cord compression is sufficient to produce more than transient fetal hypoxia, the findings of tachycardia, decreased variability and/or slow return to baseline indicate that hypoxia may be more than transient and intervention may be indicated.

4 Late deceleration is characterized as a uniform decrease in fetal heart rate beginning after the peak of a contraction of normal duration and with a return to baseline after the contraction is over. The onset and offset are gradual. It is believed to be due to decreased oxygen transfer across the placenta, which may be due to decreased uteroplacental blood flow or maternal hypoxemia. Initially late deceleration is usually associated with average fetal heart rate variability and is believed to be due to a vagal reflex but, as hypoxia increases and the fetus develops metabolic acidosis, the variability decreases and at this point the mechanism for the late deceleration is believed to be due to myocardial depression.

5 The last periodic change that is described is prolonged deceleration which usually lasts more than 2 minutes and by definition <10 minutes. Its onset may be similar to a late deceleration or a variable deceleration. This pattern is usually seen with a sentinel event such as a prolapsed cord, ruptured uterus or sudden complete abruption.

The National Institute of Child Health and Human Development (NICHD) conducted workshops in 1997[9] and 2008[10] designed to address issues of definitions and recommendations for future research in electronic fetal monitoring. In the 2008 conference the terms reassuring and non-reassuring fetal heart rate tracings were abandoned due to the lack of precision and agreement attributed to these terms. At this meeting fetal heart rate patterns were subdivided into three categories with category I indicating good oxygenation and no need for intervention. Category III indicated patterns consistent with ongoing hypoxic damage and or death. While there was good agreement among the participants on these two categories, category II includes all patterns between categories I and III and it remains unclear what the significance of category II patterns are and management recommendations were sought from the American College of Obstetricians and Gynecologists and future research findings.

Within category II it appears that, if moderate variability is preserved, significant ongoing hypoxia is unlikely but further research is necessary for specific management recommendations.

Finally, inter- and intraobserver variation in fetal heart rate pattern interpretation is significant[11,12] and it is hoped that the new three-category classification will improve this problem.

Fetal inflammatory response to maternal chorioamnionitis

Recently reports have indicated that fetal inflammatory response to maternal infection may result in the elaboration of proinflammatory cytokines that may be responsible for damage in the periventricular areas of the premature fetal brain resulting in spastic diplegia. In term infants this fetal inflammatory response may result in damage to the same cortical and subcortical watershed areas of the motor cortex that are affected by prolonged intermittent hypoxia resulting in spastic quadriplegia. Fetal heart rate patterns have not been described in these situations but in this author's anecdotal experience there are commonly findings of tachycardia with decreased variability, usually in association with maternal fever, and inconsistent deceleration patterns may be present. While antibiotics are advisable when maternal chorioamnionitis is suspected, there have been no strategies that have proven effective in preventing neurological damage due to the fetal inflammatory response.[13,14]

Medical-legal implications

While there may be disagreement on the overall value of intrapartum fetal heart rate monitoring, in the courtroom, the fetal monitor strip is usually the main focus when a lawsuit alleges negligence in cases of cerebral palsy believed to be due to intrapartum fetal asphyxia. Thus there are important considerations for the obstetrician when there is concern at the time of birth about the neonatal condition. The determination of a cord arterial pH of greater than 7.0 and a Base deficit >12.0 mm/liter indicates that fetal hypoxia proximate to birth cannot be implicated as a cause of later neurological damage. The presence of chorioamnionitis and funisitis may indicate that the cause of later neurological damage could be due to a fetal inflammatory response to maternal infection. Thus when delivery of a depressed infant occurs or when fetal heart rate patterns have been of concern it is often helpful to get fetal cord arterial blood gases and to save the placenta in order to later determine the likely cause of any neurological developmental problems.

References

1 Haverkamp AD, Thompson HE, McFee JG, *et al.* The evaluation of continuous fetal heart rate monitoring in high risk pregnancy. *Am J Obstet Gynecol* 1976;125:310.

2 Freeman RK. Intrapartum fetal monitoring – a disappointing story. *N Eng J Med* 1990;322:624–6.

3 Grant A, O'Brien N, Joy MT, Hennessy E, MacDonald D. Cerebral palsy among children born during the Dublin randomized trial of intrapartum monitoring. *Lancet* 1989;2:1233–6.

4 Stanley FJ, Watson L. The cerebral palsies in western Australia: trends 1968–1981. *Am J Obstet Gynecol* 1988;158:89.

5 *Antenatal Diagnosis. Report of a Consensus Development Conference.* NIH Publication #79-1973. Bethesda, MD: April 1979.

6 Nelson KB, Dambrosia DM, Ting TY, Grether JK. Uncertain value of electronic fetal monitoring in predicting cerebral palsy. *N Eng J Med* 1996;334:613–18.

7 Freeman RK, Garite TJ, Nageotte MP. *Fetal Heart Rate Monitoring,* 3rd edn. Philadelphia, PA: Lippincott Williams & Wilkins, 2003.

8 Clark SL, Gimovsky ML, Miller FC. Fetal heart rate response to scalp blood sampling. *Am J Obstet Gynecol* 1982;44:706.

9 National Institute of Child Health and Human Development. Electronic fetal heart rate monitoring: research guidelines for interpretation. *Am J Obstet Gynecol* 1997; 177:1385–90.

10 Macones G, Hankins G, Spong C, Hauth J, & Moore T. The 2008 National Institute of Child Health and Human Development Report on Electronic Fetal Monitoring. *Obstet Gynecol* 2008;112:661–6.

11 Beaulieu M, Fabia J, Leduc B, *et al.* The reproducibility of intrapartum cardiotocogram interpretation. *Can Med Assoc J* 1982;127:214–16.

12 Chauhan S, Klauser C, Woodring T, *et al.* Intrapartum nonreassuring fetal heart rate tracing and prediction of adverse outcomes: interobserver variability. *Am J Obstet Gynecol* 2008;199:623e1–623e5.

13 Royal College of Obstetricians and Gynecologists. *Intrauterine infection and perinatal brain injury.* Scientific Advisory Committee Opinion Paper #3. November 2002.

14 American College of Obstetricians and Gynecologists and American Academy of Pediatrics. *Neonatal encephalopathy and cerebral palsy: defining the pathogenesis and pathophysiology.* January 2003.

PROTOCOL 62

Abnormal Labor

Alan Peaceman

Division of Maternal-Fetal Medicine, Northwestern University Feinberg School of Medicine, Chicago, IL, USA

Dystocia, from the Greek, meaning difficult or abnormal labor, is the term given to laboring patients whose progress in labor stalls prior to delivery. Some practitioners use this term for all patients having cesarean delivery for inadequate progress in labor. Dystocia is the leading indication listed for cesarean in nulliparous patients, and accounts for approximately one-third of all cesareans performed. Conversely, dystocia is very uncommon among multiparous patients, occurring in <2% of women with prior vaginal deliveries. The frequency of cesarean for dystocia has risen dramatically over the past three decades, occurring in less than 2% of labors in 1970 and between 8% and 10% of labors currently. This increased frequency is a major reason for the rise in the primary cesarean delivery rate in this country, which has also fueled the rise in repeat cesareans being performed. The diagnosis of dystocia can be described by a number of other terms, including failed induction of labor, active phase arrest of dilatation, and second stage arrest of descent, but these terms related more to the timing of the diagnosis rather than the cause. Rates of dystocia vary markedly among practitioners, hospitals, states, regions of the country, and among countries, which likely is more a result of differences in labor management strategies rather than differences in patient characteristics. Success in decreasing the incidence of dystocia among nulliparous patients would have a major impact on the overall rate of cesarean birth.

Definition

Part of the reason for variation in rates of cesarean delivery for dystocia is because a strict definition of dystocia is not established. No discrete end-point exists in the latent phase to describe the length of time when

---

Protocols for High-Risk Pregnancies, 5th edition. Edited by J.T. Queenan, J.C. Hobbins and C.Y. Spong. © 2010 Blackwell Publishing Ltd.

vaginal delivery is no long accomplishable, and agreement does not exist regarding the length of time for active phase arrest before intervention is appropriate. For nulliparous patients, Friedman described the upper limit of normal for the length of the latent phase as 20 hours, and the lower limit of normal for rate of cervical dilatation in the active phase as 1.2 cm/h. These numbers were derived from the analysis of 500 patients more than 50 years ago, with a cesarean delivery rate of 1.8% and a forceps rate of 51%. Further, management of labor, including use of oxytocin and regional anesthesia, is much different today.

A number of investigators have questioned the applicability of Friedman's findings in today's labor units. In 2002, Zhang *et al.* found a markedly different labor curve, with labors being much slower today. They found that rates of dilatation less than 1 cm/h were not uncommon among women delivering vaginally, and many patients without any dilatation noted for 2 or more hours still delivered vaginally. The recommendation that 2 hours of arrest in the active phase may be sufficient for a diagnosis of dystocia has also been challenged. Among nulliparous women with active phase arrest for 2 hours, Rouse *et al.* found that 74% of patients still delivered vaginally if oxytocin was continued for at least another 2 hours. In our labor unit, we found that nulliparous women had an average rate of dilatation in the active phase of 1.7 cm/h, with the lower 5th percentile being 0.7 cm/h. Further, 39% of patients delivering vaginally had a rate of dilatation less than the 1.2 cm/h, the lower limit of normal described by Friedman.

Causes of dystocia

The main causes of dystocia are listed in Table 62.1. Inefficient uterine action is the most common cause, and it is comprised of a number of clinical situations. Induction of labor has been associated with a two-fold increase in the rate of cesarean delivery, and some increased risk persists even after the patient reaches 4 cm of dilatation. This risk is even higher among patients starting induction with an unfavorable cervix, and cervical ripening does not necessarily lower this risk. For patients undergoing induction of labor and those who present in spontaneous labor, some cases of dystocia could be avoided with increased or longer uterine stimulation with oxytocin. While most patients who deliver vaginally have at least 200 Montevideo units as measured by intrauterine pressure catheter, individual patients may progress with more stimulation. In other situations, more frequent or more intense contractions cannot be attained, often due to intrauterine infection or fetal intolerance to labor as perceived by interpretation of the fetal heart rate monitor, and dystocia is the result.

Table 62.1 Causes of dystocia

Inefficient uterine action
    Induction
    Inadequate stimulation of contractions
    Failure of uterine response to stimulation
Malposition
    Occiput posterior
    Asynclitism
    Inadequate cephalic flexion
Cephalo-pelvic disproportion

Malposition of the cephalic presentation is also a significant factor that can lead to dystocia, especially in the second stage. Arrest of descent occurs less frequently if the largest diameter of the fetal head is aligned with the largest diameter of the maternal pelvis. This is not necessarily a recurring issue in future pregnancies, and may explain why many patients with arrest of descent can have a subsequent successful trial of labor with a similar-sized fetus. Some studies have associated an increased frequency of malposition with epidural anesthesia, but more recent studies with more dilute concentrations of local anesthetic, with or without narcotic, have challenged this association.

Cephalo-pelvic disproportion (CPD) is a commonly used reason given for dystocia. Risk factors include both large fetal size and small maternal pelvic size. However, there are no established criteria for this diagnosis, and it is often made based on the lack of progress in the presence of regular uterine contractions without regard to position of the occiput. X-ray pelvimetry has not been found to be helpful in clarifying the diagnosis. In the absence of a contracted pelvis, such as seen with android pelvic architecture or pelvic deformity, the diagnosis of CPD is uncertain, and dystocia could be more a function of fetal position or uterine action.

Complications associated with dystocia can occur and should be anticipated. Prolonged labors have higher rates of intrauterine infection, and are associated with an increased risk of uterine atony after delivery. On rare occasions, obstructed labor can lead to a constriction ring in the uterus, or rupture of the uterus. Compression of the sigmoid colon during prolonged obstructed labor is still a cause of rectovaginal fistula formation in underdeveloped regions of the world. Of more relevance to developed nations, the rising rate of cesarean delivery for a diagnosis of dystocia has led to an increased number of pregnancies occurring among patients with a prior abdominal delivery. This increase in turn has led to more complications seen with vaginal birth after cesarean, as well as major hemorrhage associated with placenta accreta.

Management

Principles for labor management in an effort to reduce or manage dystocia include:

1 Induction increases the risk of dystocia over spontaneous labor. Elective induction should be undertaken with caution in the nulliparous patient, especially with an unfavorable cervix.

2 Interventions to stimulate contractions with prolonged latent labor are often unsuccessful. When a patient in the latent phase has amniotomy and labor stimulation, the labor frequently is similar to induced labor. Another option is maternal sedation if she is exhausted.

3 Amniotomy can stimulate contractions, and should be performed prior to a diagnosis of dystocia.

4 Uterine rupture is a rare event in nulliparous labor. Most mothers and fetuses tolerate labor stimulation with oxytocin without complication.

Dosing of oxytocin remains a controversial issue, with the optimal rate of infusion not determined. Most obstetric units utilize a low dose protocol, often starting at 1 mU/min, and increasing by increments of 1–2 mU/min until a target contraction frequency is reached. A contraction frequency of more than 5 in 10 minutes is termed tachysystole, and the oxytocin infusion rate should be decrease if this persists. Nonetheless, a number of randomized trials have suggested a benefit to labor augmentation with a higher rate of oxytocin infusion, with lower rates of cesareans and shorter labors. Not all studies, however, have shown this benefit, and some have seen an increase in the incidence of tachysystole, although without a demonstrated adverse impact on the newborns. The 'active management of labor' has been utilized successfully at some institutions, but is reserved for nulliparous patients at term, in spontaneous labor with cephalic presentation. As initially described, it involves utilizing higher rates of oxytocin infusion, but also focusing more on the quality of the contractions rather than frequency for the diagnosis of labor, and companionship during labor. Regardless of the method of labor management that is chosen, a protocol that lowers the rate of cesarean for dystocia without an increase in adverse neonatal outcomes is desirable.

Suggested reading

Friedman EA. Primigravid labor: a graphicostatistical analysis. *Obstet Gynecol* 1955;6:567–87.

Lopez-Zeno JA, Peaceman AM, Adashek JA, Socol ML. A controlled trial of a program for the active management of labor. *N Engl J Med* 1992;326:450–4.

Rouse DJ, Owen J, Hauth JC. Active-phase labor arrest: oxytocin augmentation for at least 4 hours. *Obstet Gynecol* 1999;93:323–8.

Zhang J, Troendle JF, Yancey MK. Reassessing the labor curve in nulliparous women. *Am J Obstet Gynecol* 2002;187:824–8.

PROTOCOL 63

Breech Delivery

Martin L. Gimovsky

Department of Obstetrics and Gynecology, Mount Sinai School of Medicine, New York and
Department of Obstetrics and Gynecology, Newark Beth Israel Medical Center, Newark, NJ, USA

Overview

The management of labor and delivery for the fetus presenting breech has long been recognized as a complex clinical challenge. Breech presentation complicates approximately 3 to 4% of labor and deliveries at term and is even more frequent earlier in gestation.

Perinatal morbidity and mortality are significantly increased in infants born from breech presentation. The adverse outcome is primarily attributable to: increased rates of congenital anomalies, frequency of premature birth, and labor and delivery-related asphyxia and trauma. Frequently these three major contributors are interrelated. In addition the subset of problems associated with breech presentation is fundamentally different from the risks seen with breech labor and delivery.

Diagnosis

Early diagnosis of breech presentation increases the options available for management. Since breech presentation has a tendency to recur, the past obstetrical history is a logical starting point to make the diagnosis. Women with multiple leiomyomata, previous uterine surgery and grand multiparity are more likely to have breech-presenting fetuses, especially in the third trimester. During prenatal care, assessment of fetal lie should be performed routinely after 36 weeks. Clinical suspicion and Leopold maneuvers, liberally supplemented with ultrasonography, are commonly used in making the diagnosis antepartum. When a fetus is confirmed to be in breech presentation after 36 weeks of gestation, we recommend the following approach.

Protocols for High-Risk Pregnancies, 5th edition. Edited by J.T. Queenan, J.C. Hobbins and C.Y. Spong. © 2010 Blackwell Publishing Ltd.

Management

A Discussion with the patient and her family about the inherent problems seen in association with breech labor and delivery.

B Although an 18–20 week level II ultrasound will exclude most anomalies, bedside scan at the time of presentation to labor and delivery is warranted to estimate fetal weight, the attitude of the fetal cervical spine and placental location. A biophysical profile and careful determination of the amniotic fluid index should also be obtained. This same evaluation should be performed regardless of whether the patient is for a trial of labor or a cesarean section (C/S).

C With appropriate consent, we offer our patients a trial of external cephalic version (ECV) when a breech fetus is diagnosed after 36 weeks. A beta-mimetic agent is used routinely. A prior C/S is not considered a contraindication to an attempt at version. Whether ECV is successful or not, we perform fetal surveillance twice a week post-ECV until delivery.

D If version is unsuccessful, contraindicated, or not acceptable to the patient, discuss with the patient a potential trial of labor by protocol, or by scheduled cesarean section. The vast majority of patients and physicians will opt for C/S, particularly if the diagnosis of breech presentation is made before the onset of labor. ACOG Committee Opinion # 265 cites the Term Breech Trial (Hannah et al., 2000) in support of this common practice. Controversy exists regarding the management of a patient presenting in advanced labor with breech presentation. Additionally, when a second twin presents as breech, one option includes vaginal delivery by breech extraction or by assisted breech delivery.

E A selective trial of labor may be chosen on a case-by-case basis provided:

1 The estimated gestational age of the fetus is 37 to 42 weeks

2 The fetus is estimated to weigh 2000 to 3500 g at the onset of labor

3 The fetus is in the frank or complete breech presentation

4 Computed tomographic (CT) pelvimetry and/or bedside ultrasonography confirms that the fetal head is not hyperextended and that the arms are flexed upon the fetal chest, in addition to excluding women with a borderline or small pelvis. If CT is performed, the following criteria are useful in excluding a borderline bony pelvis: (a) anteroposterior (AP) diameter at the pelvic inlet is >11 cm; (b) transverse diameter at the pelvic inlet is >12 cm; (c) interspinous diameter at the midpelvis is >10 cm.

F During the trial of labor

1 Continuous electronic fetal heart rate monitoring is employed, supplemented by acoustic stimulation or tactile stimulation as indicated to assess fetal acid–base balance when necessary.

2 The Friedman curve is carefully followed with hourly evaluation of the progress of labor. Greater than 1.2 cm/h in the nullipara, and greater than 1.5 cm/h in the multipara, are guidelines for the minimal acceptable rates of progression in active labor. Oxytocin is utilized as indicated by uterine activity. Failure to progress, or any borderline situation, calls for prompt cesarean section.

G The second stage of labor is managed in the delivery room or in the operating room as a 'double setup'. Support from anesthesia, pediatrics and the operating room staff assists a delivery team of two gowned and gloved obstetricians.

H The delivery itself is treated with watchful waiting. The less force employed by the accoucheur, and the greater the reliance on force from the patient, the more likely the fetal body will maintain flexion in the delivery process. This will minimize the risk of traumatic birth. Continuous fetal monitoring in the delivery room, as well as the availability of a portable ultrasound machine, is advisable.

I The fetus is encouraged to deliver with the back anterior insofar as possible. A Mauriceau maneuver or one of its variants allows for easy delivery of the aftercoming head. If necessary, forceps are easily applied to the fetal head as a pelvic application. An episiotomy is made after the buttocks have crowned. A cord sample for acid–base analysis is obtained and analyzed as indicated by the need for neonatal resuscitation.

J At C/S delivery, the same fundamental principles apply. Upon entering the abdominal cavity, the fetus is palpated and the degree of uterine rotation determined. At term delivery, a transverse uterine incision usually suffices. In opening the uterus, great care should be taken to avoid fetal laceration. Our approach is to employ Allis clamps to elevate the myometrium away from the fetus. A simple snap is then used to rupture the membranes. The fetal buttocks are positioned at the incision. The primary operator calls for direct fundal pressure to assist with the delivery of the body. When the fetal scapula is reached, the shoulders are delivered by rotation and the arms swept downward if necessary. The aftercoming head is also delivered by direct fundal pressure to maintain cranial flexion.

K At preterm delivery the choice of transverse or vertical uterine incisions is determined by individual circumstances upon entry to the abdominal cavity. A vertical or 'classical' incision is will facilitate delivery if premature rupture of membranes has occurred, the fetus is less than 30 weeks, or has an estimated fetal weight of less than 1000 g. Intravenous nitroglycerin may be given for brief and dramatic uterine relaxation. As with vaginal delivery, undue haste is avoided.

Conclusion

Regardless of the mode of delivery, the breech fetus challenges the clinician to balance the risks of operative delivery (C/S) to the mother with the risks of vaginal delivery to the fetus. In either situation, injury to mother or child is infrequent. However, it should be noted that a breech infant may also sustain injury at C/S delivery. Additionally, the mother may also suffer serious morbidity whether a C/S or a trial of labor is chosen. A balanced approach to delivery, beginning with early recognition during the antepartum period, should include consideration of external cephalic version followed by C/S for the majority of patients. The protocol recommended above offers an alternative approach to minimize the risks to both mother and fetus when a selective trial of labor is chosen.

Suggested reading

American College of Obstetricians and Gynecologists. *Mode of term singleton breech delivery.* ACOG Committee Opinion #265. Washington, DC: ACOG, 2001.

Alarab M, Regan C, O'Connell M, Keane D, O'Herlihy C, Foley M. Singleton vaginal delivery at term: still a safe option. *Obstet Gynecol* 2004;103:407–12.

Albertson S, Rasmussen S, Reigstad H. Evaluation of a protocol for selecting fetuses in breech presentations for vaginal delivery or cesarean section. *Am J Obstet Gynecol* 1997;177:586–92.

Deering S, Brown J, Hodor J, Satin A. Simulation training and resident performance of singleton breech delivery. *Obstet Gynecol* 2006;107:86–90.

Gimovsky M, Wallace R, Schifrin B, Paul R. Randomized management of the non frank breech presentation at term: a preliminary report. *Am J Obstet Gynecol* 1983;146:34–40.

Gimovsky ML, Rosa E, Bronshtein E. Update in breech management. *Contemp ObGyn* September 2007;52(9):66–73.

Gimovsky M. Breech presentation. In: O'Grady J, Gimovsky M, Bayer-Zwirello L, Giordano K (eds) *Operative Obstetrics,* 2nd edn. New York: Cambridge University Press, 2008.

Glezerman M. Five years to the term breech trial: the rise and fall of a randomized controlled trial. *Am J Obstet Gynecol* 2006;194:20–5.

Hannah M, Hannath W, Hewson S, Hodnett E, Saigai S, Willan A. Planned cesarean section versus planned vaginal birth for breech presentation at term: a randomized multicentre trial. *Lancet* 2000;356:1375–83.

Queenan J. Teaching infrequently used skills: vaginal breech delivery. *Obstet Gynecol* 2004;103:405–6.

Smith J, Hernandez D Wax J. Fetal laceration injury at cesarean section. *Obstet Gynecol* 1997;90:344–6.

Whyte H, Hannah M, Saigal S. Outcomes of children at 2 years of age in the term breech trial. *Am J Obstet Gynecol* 2003;189(Suppl):S57.

PROTOCOL 64

Vaginal Birth After Cesarean

James R. Scott

Department of Obstetrics and Gynecology, University of Utah Medical Center, Salt Lake City, UT, USA

The cesarean delivery rate in the United States has dramatically risen from 5% in 1970 to 32.8% today. Many believe the current cesarean rate and rising rates in other countries are too high, and VBAC (vaginal birth after cesarean) has long been promoted as one way to lower them. Despite >1000 citations in the literature and the current emphasis on evidence-based medicine, there has never been a randomized trial to prove definitively that maternal and neonatal outcomes are better with either a trial of labor after cesarean or repeat cesarean delivery. Contemporary issues that affect VBAC rates include the right for women to have a cesarean with no medical indication ('on request'), the possibility of future pelvic support disorders after vaginal delivery, and medical legal risks should uterine rupture occur. Consequently, deciding between trial of labor and repeat cesarean is a challenge for both physicians and patients. The purpose of this protocol is to outline a careful and safe approach to VBAC.

Pre-labor counseling

The decision for a trial of labor (TOL) after a previous cesarean involves balancing risks vs benefits (Fig. 64.1). Trial of labor in a carefully selected patient with a low transverse cesarean scar is usually desirable, but physicians and patients need to know about potential adverse outcomes. Most studies on VBAC have been conducted in university or tertiary-level centers under ideal conditions with 24-hour staff coverage and in-house anesthesia. Yet many women in the United States are delivered in smaller community hospitals where obstetricians and anesthesiologists may not be available in-house on nights and weekends. Although patients were carefully selected in initial studies, the list of obstetric conditions reportedly

Protocols for High-Risk Pregnancies, 5th edition. Edited by J.T. Queenan, J.C. Hobbins and C.Y. Spong. © 2010 Blackwell Publishing Ltd.

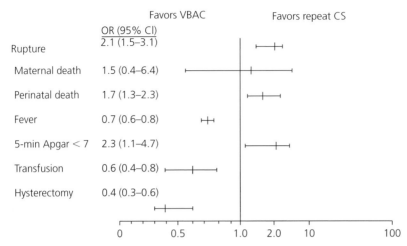

Figure 64.1 Odds ratio graph comparing morbidity of trial of labor with elective repeat cesarean delivery. Reproduced with permission. American College of Obstetricians and Gynecologists. *Vaginal Birth After Previous Cesarean Delivery.* Practice Bulletin # 54, July 2004. Washington, DC: ACOG.

appropriate for VBAC rapidly expanded. Usually derived from small series, they included unknown uterine scar, twins, post-term pregnancy and suspected macrosomia. Understanding limitations of this literature and preparation for the possibility of an emergency cesarean is important when attempting VBAC in these situations. Common sense should prevail.

It is reasonable to encourage appropriately selected women to undertake trial of labor in a safe setting, but potential complications should be discussed. Thorough, impartial, and fact-based counseling beginning early in pregnancy provides the best preparation for trial of labor. Medical records should be obtained to review the circumstances surrounding the indication for the previous cesarean(s) and to confirm the type of uterine incision.

Vaginal delivery is associated with fewer complications, is less expensive, has a faster recovery, and for many women there is an important satisfaction factor. Published series indicate that about 60–80% of trial of labor after a previous cesarean result in successful vaginal births. However, these rates often represent a selected population. Patients inappropriate for trial of labor usually have been excluded, so the exact percentage of women with a previous cesarean who undergo trial of labor is not known. A woman who has delivered vaginally at least once before or after her previous cesarean is more likely to have a successful trial of labor than the woman who has not yet delivered vaginally. The chance of success for those with a previous diagnosis of dystocia is consistently lower (40–70%) than for those with non-recurring indications. Clinical judgment is also important since no scoring system is totally reliable in predicting a successful trial of labor. For example, successful VBAC is more likely for a woman whose indication for the first cesarean was breech presentation than it is for a woman <5 ft. tall whose first 4300 g infant was delivered by cesarean because of a deep transverse arrest.

Conversely, repeat cesarean may be more practical and safe in certain settings. It can be scheduled, is predictable, avoids a failed trial of labor with its frustration and morbidity, and essentially eliminates uterine rupture with its potential catastrophic outcome and litigation. However, elective cesarean carries with it a likelihood of more cesareans with their future risks. Placenta previa and accreta have become significant problems associated with multiple cesareans. Taken together, previa and accreta occur in <5% of women with no prior cesarean, but the prevalence progressively increases with each cesarean and is as high as 67% with four or more previous cesareans. Severe bleeding associated with these conditions now accounts for over half of peripartum hysterectomies. These are difficult cases, often requiring extensive preoperative preparation, and associated with extensive surgery, bladder and ureter injury, excessive blood loss, and even maternal death.

Criteria most predictive of a safe and successful trial of labor

1 One (or two) prior low segment transverse cesareans.
2 Clinically adequate pelvis and normal fetal size.
3 No other uterine scars, anomalies or previous rupture.
4 Patient enthusiasm and consent.
5 Spontaneous labor.
6 Physician available capable of monitoring labor, the fetus, and performing a cesarean.
7 Anesthesia, blood bank and personnel available, and simulation training for emergency cesarean.

Potential contraindications

1 Prior classical or T-shaped incision or previous uterine surgery.
2 Contracted pelvis and/or macrosomia.
3 Medical or obstetric condition precluding vaginal delivery.
4 Patient refusal.
5 Unripe cervix, induction and augmentation.
6 Inability to perform emergency cesarean because of unavailable obstetrician, anesthesia, staff or inadequate facility.

The final decision for trial of labor vs repeat cesarean should be made by the patient and her physician after careful consideration and discussion (Fig. 64.2). A plan of management should then be outlined and documented

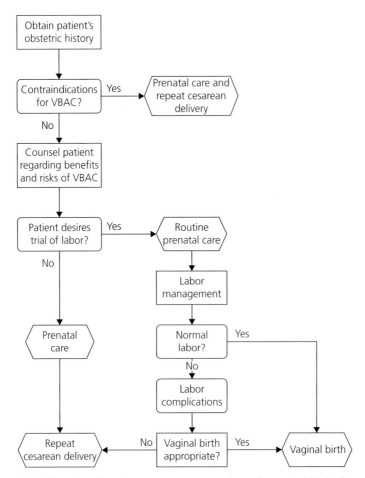

Figure 64.2 Flow sheet showing one management scheme for vaginal birth after cesarean. Reproduced with permission from Porter TF, Scott JR. Cesarean delivery. In: Scott JR, Gibbs RS, Karlan BY, Haney AF (eds) *Obstetrics and Gynecolog,*. 9th edn. Philadelphia: Lippincott Williams & Wilkins, 2003: pp. 449–60.

in the prenatal record. Once the decision for trial of labor is made, the patient deserves support and encouragement. This does not mean that the plan cannot be altered if the situation changes.

Management of labor and delivery

Each hospital should develop a protocol for management of VBAC patients. Epidural anesthesia is not contraindicated. In fact, adequate pain relief may allow more women to choose trial of labor. The safety of induction of labor with prostaglandin gel and augmentation with oxytocin remains controversial, and misoprostol is contraindicated. Once labor has begun, the patient should be promptly evaluated and monitored; continuous electronic monitoring is usually preferable. It is important for personnel to be familiar with the potential complications of VBAC and to watch closely for fetal heart tone abnormalities and inadequate progress of labor. These women are at high risk for labor problems in view of the 20% to 40% rate of unsuccessful trial of labor. Timely diagnosis and prompt management of labor abnormalities are essential in any woman with a uterine scar to avoid the added risk of obstructed labor. Prospective simulation training that allows for a prompt and organized response to any maternal or fetal emergency is highly desirable.

There is nothing particularly unique about delivery of the infant after trial of labor. The necessity for routine exploration of the uterus after successful VBAC is controversial. If there is excessive vaginal bleeding or signs of hypovolemia, immediate assessment of the scar and entire genital tract is necessary. There is an increased incidence of infection and morbidity in patients who require cesarean because of a failed trial of labor.

Uterine rupture

Rupture of the uterine scar is the most serious complication of VBAC, and it can be life threatening for both mother and baby. During labor, the rupture usually involves the previous scar and lower uterine segment, but it may be stellate and extend intraperitoneally or retroperitoneally. Associated factors include excessive amounts of oxytocin, dysfunctional labor, more than one cesarean delivery, multiparity and even a previous non-pregnant uterine perforation. However, in most cases the reason for rupture is unclear, and adverse outcomes can occur even in appropriate VBAC candidates. The rate of rupture is related to the type and location of the previous incision. The risk of uterine rupture with a classical or T incision is 4–9%, with a low transverse incision it is 0.5–1.5%, and the risk with a low vertical incision is estimated to be between 1 and 4%.

Diagnosis

Uterine rupture is sometimes difficult to diagnose, and close surveillance is necessary. Signs and symptoms may progress gradually or rapidly. The most common presenting signs are fetal heart rate abnormalities. A fetal heart rate pattern with subtle variable decelerations may rapidly evolve into late decelerations, bradycardia and undetectable fetal heart tones. Uterine or abdominal pain most commonly occurs in the area of the previous incision but may range from mild to 'tearing' in nature. Uterine contractions often diminish in intensity and frequency. Vaginal or intraabdominal bleeding produces anxiety, restlessness, weakness, dizziness, gross hematuria, shoulder pain and shock. This clinical picture has sometimes been mistaken for abruption. Loss of station of the presenting part on vaginal examination is diagnostic.

Treatment

Any of these findings in a patient undergoing trial of labor warrant immediate exploratory laparotomy. The condition of the infant is dependent on the severity of the rupture and relationship to the placenta and umbilical cord. The outcome is not always favorable even when delivery occurs within 30 minutes. The combined rate of fetal death and severe long-term neurological impairment when rupture occurs is as high as 20–25%. Repair of the uterus is possible in the majority of patients. In others, hemorrhage from extension of the rupture into the broad ligament or extensive damage to the uterus requires hysterectomy.

Summary

VBAC was enthusiastically supported by many groups during the past three decades. With more experience, it has become apparent that there are rare but significant risks to the mother and infant. Poor perinatal outcome associated with uterine rupture is now a common cause of litigation. Most problems occur when the patient is not under direct observation or the diagnosis of uterine rupture is delayed. The latest Practice Bulletin from the American College of Obstetricians and Gynecologists recommends that a physician capable of performing a cesarean should be 'immediately available'. Although outcomes from trial of labor and elective repeat cesarean are relatively equivalent, one may be better than the other for an individual case. With careful selection and close attention during labor, the majority of women can successfully deliver vaginally. In situations where attempted VBAC is not safe or the patient does not want it, elective cesarean is a reasonable alternative.

Suggested reading

American College of Obstetricians and Gynecologists. *Vaginal Birth After Previous Cesarean Delivery.* Practice Bulletin # 54, July 2004. Washington, DC: ACOG.

Cahill AG, Macones GA. Vaginal birth after cesarean delivery: evidence-based practice. *Clin Obstet Gynecol* 2007;50(2):518–25.

Dodd JM, Crowther CA, Huertas E, Guise J-M, Horey D. Planned elective repeat caesarean section versus planned vaginal birth for women with a previous caesarean birth.

Cochrane Database Syst Rev 2004;(4): CD004224. DOI: 10.1002/14651858.CD004224. pub2.

Landon MB, Hauth JC, Leveno KJ, *et al.* Maternal and perinatal outcomes associated with a trial of labor after prior cesarean delivery. *N Engl J Med* 2004;351:2581–9.

Landon MB. Vaginal birth after cesarean delivery. *Clin Perinatol* 2008;35:491–504.

Lavin JR Jr, Dipasquale L, Crane S, Stewart J Jr. A state-wide assessment of the obstetric, anesthesia, and operative team personnel who are available to manage the labors and deliveries and to treat the complications of women who attempt vaginal birth after cesarean delivery. *Am J Obstet Gynecol* 2002;187:611–14.

National Institutes of Health Consensus Development Conference Statement Vaginal Birth After Cesarean: New Insights, March 8–10, 2010. *Obstet Gynecol* 2010:115(6): (in press).

Porter TF, Scott JR. Cesarean delivery. In: Scott JR, Gibbs RS, Karlan BY, Haney AF (eds) *Obstetrics and Gynecology*, 9th edn. Philadelphia, PA: Lippincott Williams & Wilkins, 2003: pp. 449–60.

Scott JR. Avoiding labor problems during VBAC. *Clin Obstet Gynecol* 1997;40:533–41.

Scott JR, Porter TF. Cesarean Delivery. In Gibbs RS, Karlan BY, Haney AF, Nygaard I (eds) *Obstetrics and Gynecology*, 10th ed. Philadelphia, PA: Lippincott Williams & Wilkins, 2008: pp. 491–503.

Scott JR. Solving the Vaginal Birth After Cesarean (VBAC) Dilemma. *Obstet Gynecol* 2010:115(6): (in press).

Silver RM, Landon MB, Rouse DJ, *et al.* Maternal morbidity associated with multiple repeat cesarean deliveries. *Obstet Gynecol* 2006;107:1226–32.

Srinivas SK, Stamillo DM, Stevens EJ, *et al.* Predicting failure of a vaginal birth attempt after cesarean delivery. *Obstet Gynecol* 2007;109:800–5.

PROTOCOL 65

Placenta Accreta

Robert M. Silver

Department of Obstetrics & Gynecology, Division of Maternal-Fetal Medicine, University of Utah Health Sciences Center, Salt Lake City, UT, USA

Overview and clinical significance

Placenta accreta occurs when the placenta becomes abnormally adherent to the myometrium rather than the uterine decidua. After delivery, the placenta does not easily separate from the uterus, leading to potentially life-threatening hemorrhage. If the placenta actually invades the myometrium it is termed placenta increta. If it invades through the uterine serosa or into organs adjacent to the uterus it is termed placenta percreta. In many circumstances and during this Protocol, the term placenta accreta is used to describe accretas, percretas and incretas interchangeably as a single disease spectrum.

Placenta accreta is associated with considerable maternal morbidity including large volume blood transfusion, need for hysterectomy, intensive care unit (ICU) admission, infection, and prolonged hospitalization. Hemorrhage may be fatal and can lead to disseminated intravascular coagulation (DIC) and multi-organ failure. Fetal risks are similar to those for placenta previa and mostly consist of the complications of preterm birth.

Rates of placenta accreta are dramatically increasing, primarily due to the increase in the rate of cesarean delivery (see 'pathophysiology and risk factors'). The incidence has increased from a reported 1 in 30,000 in the 1960s to 1 in 533 in 2002. Every practitioner of obstetrics should be familiar with the risk factors, diagnosis and management of this increasingly common and life-threatening condition.

Pathophysiology and risk factors

The pathophysiology of placenta accreta remains somewhat uncertain. Under normal circumstances, trophoblast invades into the decidua, behaving somewhat like a cancer. Once the cytotrophoblast cells reach a certain level, termed

Protocols for High-Risk Pregnancies, 5th edition. Edited by J.T. Queenan, J.C. Hobbins and C.Y. Spong. © 2010 Blackwell Publishing Ltd.

Nitabuch's layer (or spongiosus layer of the decidua), they stop invading and differentiate. After cesarean delivery there may be a failure to reconstitute the endometrium or decidua basalis. Thus, if the placenta implants over the uterine scar from a prior cesarean, cytotrophoblast does not receive the normal 'stop' signal and keeps invading to an abnormal degree. Histology reveals trophoblast invading into myometrium without intervening decidua.

Relative hypoxia in the cesarean scar also may play a role in the development of accreta. Hypoxia stimulates cytotrophoblast invasion; these cells differentiate once they reach the spiral arterioles and increased oxygen tension. However, the cesarean scar is relatively avascular, acellular and hypoxic, promoting further invasion. In fact, the relative hypoxia of the scar may actually preferentially allow for the development of the early embryo, perhaps explaining why previas and accretas are more common in women with multiple cesareans.

Regardless of the pathophysiology, it is clear that the overwhelming risk factor for placenta accreta is *multiple prior cesarean* deliveries. The vast majority of women with accreta have had at least one prior cesarean delivery and the risk increases with the number of cesarean deliveries. Women having their fourth or fifth cesarean have over a 2% chance of accreta and the risk increases to almost 7% in those having their sixth or greater cesarean. The combination of placenta previa and prior cesarean dramatically increases the risk since the placenta overlies the uterine scar. A recent large cohort study estimates the risk of accreta in women with previa to be 3%, 11%, 40%, 61% and 67% for first, second, third, fourth and fifth or more cesarean deliveries, respectively. Indeed, women with two or more prior cesareans and a placenta previa are at extreme risk for placenta accreta. Since the rate of cesarean deliveries continues to escalate, the rate of placenta accreta will increase as well.

Prior uterine surgery such as uterine curettage, myomectomy, or hysteroscopic surgery is another risk factor for placenta accreta. Patients who develop Asherman syndrome after uterine curettage (or for any reason) are at especially high risk for accreta. Other risk factors include prior endometrial ablation, uterine artery or fibroid embolization, prior accreta and pelvic irradiation. In short, anything that might affect the normal architecture of the endometerial cavity increases the odds of accreta. Demographic risk factors include advanced maternal age and increasing parity. Also, placenta previa alone, even without prior cesarean, is a risk factor for accreta.

Diagnosis

The gold standard for the diagnosis of placenta accreta is histological examination of the placenta and uterus. Of course, this is only possible when a hysterectomy is performed. Although it is controversial, a clinical diagnosis of accreta may be made in cases of abnormally adherent placenta if a hysterectomy is not performed.

In order to optimize outcomes, it is highly desirable to diagnose placenta accreta prior to delivery. The best-studied modality for antenatal diagnosis is ultrasonography. The sensitivity of ultrasonography for the diagnosis of accreta has been reported to be 80–90% and the specificity for excluding the condition is 98%. It is important to note that almost all published studies have been conducted in women wherein there was a high index of suspicion (and major risk factors) for accreta. Thus, ultrasound may be less accurate for the identification of accreta in low-risk populations. Also, reported studies have been conducted in tertiary care centers with expertise in obstetric sonogram. Results may not be widely reproducible.

The single most helpful finding on sonogram is to determine whether or not there is a placenta previa (Protocol 58). If there is no previa, the risk for accreta is substantially less. In cases of normal placentation, there is a very uniform, homogenous appearance to the placenta and the bladder wall. In addition, there is a distinct echolucent zone (termed the myometrial zone) between the placenta and the bladder wall. In cases of accreta, there is a loss or disruption in the continuity of the echolucent myometrial zone. Also, there may be a disruption in the continuity of the bladder wall and sometimes the placenta will actually protrude into the bladder. The placenta may have irregularly shaped vascular spaces, termed lacunae, giving the placenta a 'Swiss cheese' appearance. Finally, there may be increased vascularity in the placenta–bladder interface or turbulence within the lacunae that can be demonstrated with Doppler velocimetry.

Magnetic resonance imaging (MRI) also has been used for the antenatal diagnosis of accreta. In centers with an interest and expertise, MRI has been reported to have a sensitivity of over 90% and a specificity of 99% for the diagnosis of accreta. Also, MRI may delineate the extent of placental invasion into adjacent organs more clearly than ultrasonograph. However, performance has been substantially worse in centers without such expertise. At present, it is probably best to consider MRI as an adjunctive tool for the diagnosis of accreta unless there is expertise in your center.

Several maternal blood tests have the potential to diagnose accreta. For the most part these are markers of placental damage or abnormal placental development. Examples include elevated levels of alpha-fetoprotein, free fetal DNA, placental mRNA, beta-human chorionic gonadotropin and creatinine kinase. Although of interest, none of these tests are recommended for clinical use at present.

Complications

The primary risk of placenta accreta is hemorrhage and associated complications such as DIC and multi-organ failure. In one recent series of 76 cases, blood transfusion was required in over 80% and transfusion of ≥ 4 units of packed red blood cells in over 40% of cases. Twenty-eight percent had DIC. Another series reported an average blood loss of 3000 mL and an average transfusion of 10 units of packed red blood cells.

The most common surgical complication is cystotomy. True rates are hard to ascertain since many reports include cases of intentional cystotomy. Ureteral injury has been reported in 10–15% of cases. Less common injuries occur to bowel, large vessels and pelvic nerves. Other relatively frequent morbidities include wound, abdominal and vaginal cuff infections and the need for a second operation (most often to control bleeding or treat infection).

Between one-quarter to one-half of patients require admission to the ICU. Rates of associated complications such as pyelonephritis, pneumonia and thromboembolism are increased. Maternal deaths may occur and have been reported in up to 7% of cases. Outcomes are influenced by the severity of the case (e.g., percreta) and the expertise of the center caring for the patient. There assuredly is under-reporting of this complication from centers seeing a low volume of the condition. Vesicovaginal fistula is an important late complication of cesarean hysterectomy for accreta.

Finally, perinatal morbidity is increased. This is primarily due to prematurity. However, maternal hemorrhage may lead to compromised fetal oxygenation/perfusion and associated complications. One series reported a perinatal death rate of 9%.

Management

The most important consideration for the management of accreta is prenatal diagnosis. This allows for the most advantageous obstetric management and a potential reduction in morbidity. In turn, antenatal diagnosis requires a high index of suspicion based on risk factors. This is especially true for women with multiple prior cesareans, placenta previa and Asherman syndrome.

There are no randomized clinical trials delineating the optimal obstetric management of accreta. The following recommendations are based on retrospective studies and expert opinion. Ideally, delivery should be accomplished in a hospital with a state-of-the-art blood bank, anesthesiologists experienced in critically ill patients and surgeons with experience in treating accreta and the ability to perform retroperitoneal dissection and bladder, ureteral and bowel surgery. In some cases, hemorrhage is life threatening in spite of the most optimal planning, surgeons and facilities. Placenta accretas are among the most difficult obstetric conditions to treat and require the utmost respect and preparation.

Antepartum obstetric care (suspected accreta)

1 Obstetric sonogram to assess the probability of accreta.
2 Consideration of MRI to assess the probability of accreta.
3 Pelvic rest.
4 Consideration of bed rest and/or hospitalization in cases of antepartum bleeding.
5 Administration of corticosteroids to enhance fetal pulmonary maturity in cases of antepartum bleeding at the time of hospital admission.
6 If there is no antepartum bleeding, empiric administration of corticosteroids to enhance fetal pulmonary maturity at 34 weeks' gestation.
7 Consultation with the patient and her family to discuss delivery options, risks of the disease, potential complications, and impact of treatment on fertility.
8 Consultation with a multidisciplinary team to plan the delivery (see below).
9 The optimal timing of delivery is uncertain. Ideally, it should be accomplished in a scheduled and controlled fashion. The risk of maternal hemorrhage must be weighed against the fetal risk of prematurity. In cases without antepartum bleeding, delivery at 34–36 weeks' gestation is advised. It is not necessary to assess fetal pulmonary maturity with amniocentesis.
10 In cases with episodic bleeding, delivery between 32–34 weeks' gestation is advised, depending upon the severity of bleeding.
11 Heavy bleeding may require earlier delivery.

Surgical (suspected accreta)

1 Care should be provided with a multidisciplinary team. This should include surgeons with experience in accreta, critical care specialists, anesthesiologists and blood bank specialists. Gynecological oncologists are ideal because of their experience with bladder and ureteral surgery in addition to difficult pelvic surgery. Interventional radiologists and vascular surgeons should be available.
2 If all of the requirements under (1) are not available, consider transfer to a center with appropriate expertise.
3 If possible, the case should be performed in the 'main' operating room rather than in the labor and delivery unit. In most centers the staff in the 'main' operating room is considerably more experienced with the care of critically ill patients than labor and delivery personnel.

4 Adequate blood products should be available. Ideally, this should include 20 units of packed red blood cells and fresh frozen plasma and 12 units of platelets. Additional blood products should be available in reserve. Recombinant activated factor VII also should be available.

5 A vertical skin incision should be made, regardless of prior abdominal or pelvic scars.

6 General anesthesia should be used.

7 The patient should be kept warm and a (relatively) normal pH maintained.

8 Strong consideration should be given to preoperative placement of ureteral stents. Our group has found this to be extremely helpful with minimal risk.

9 Consideration should be given to using an autologous blood salvage device. Although there are theoretical risks of contamination with amniotic fluid, blood obtained with a cell saver at time of cesarean delivery appears to be safe for maternal transfusion.

10 Consideration should be given to preoperative placement of either regular or balloon catheters in the uterine arteries. These can be infused with material for embolization or the balloons inflated after the delivery of the fetus. In turn, this may decrease blood loss at the time of hysterectomy or allow for the avoidance of hysterectomy (see below). Alternatively, catheters can be placed and only used if needed. This practice is controversial and serious adverse events with balloon placement have been reported.

11 Ideally, in cases of strongly suspected accreta, planned cesarean hysterectomy should be accomplished. A classical hysterotomy that does not compromise the placenta should be used to deliver the infant. *No attempt should be made to remove the placenta.* Placental removal has the potential to dramatically increase the risk of life-threatening hemorrhage. The hysterotomy should be quickly sutured to achieve some measure of hemostasis, followed by hysterectomy. If the case is difficult to accomplish or if the patient is unstable, consideration should be given to supracervical hysterectomy.

12 Umbrella packs or other 'tamponade' devices should be available.

13 Consideration may be given to hypogastric artery ligation. Our group has not found this to be helpful.

14 Consideration may be given to leaving the placenta in situ, closing the hysterotomy, and planning a 'delayed' hysterectomy in 6 weeks. In theory, this may allow some of the enhanced vascularity associated with pregnancy to 'regress', facilitating the hysterectomy. This approach has been advocated in women with percretas to avoid bladder resection. Our group has not found this to be helpful.

Surgical (unsuspected accreta)

1 Once an accreta is recognized, help should be summoned. This should include surgeons with experience in accreta, critical care specialists, anesthesiologists and blood bank specialists. Gynecological oncologists are ideal because of their experience with bladder and ureteral surgery in addition to difficult pelvic surgery. Interventional radiologists and vascular surgeons should be considered.

2 If the surgeon or medical center is not capable of caring for the patient, consideration should be given to performing a stabilizing procedure and transferring the patient to an appropriate center for definitive therapy. This may require packing the abdomen to control bleeding, transfusion, and medical stabilization of the patient. This is not always possible.

3 If labor and delivery personnel are uncomfortable with the case, personnel from the 'main' operating room should be recruited. Instruments and equipment may need to be obtained from the 'main' operating room as well.

4 The blood bank should be alerted to the need for adequate blood products. Many hospitals have a massive transfusion protocol. If so, this should be activated. Recombinant activated factor VII also should be available.

5 If a Pfannenstiel incision is used, a Mallard or Cherney incision can be used to allow better pelvic access.

6 The patient should be kept warm and a (relatively) normal pH maintained.

7 Consideration should be given to converting to general anesthesia.

8 Consideration should be given to using an autologous blood salvage device. Although there are theoretical risks of contamination with amniotic fluid, blood obtained with a cell saver at time of cesarean delivery appears to be safe for maternal transfusion.

9 The hysterotomy should be quickly sutured to achieve some measure of hemostasis, followed by hysterectomy. If the case is difficult to accomplish or if the patient is unstable, consideration should be given to supracervical hysterectomy.

10 Umbrella packs or other 'tamponade' devices should be available.

11 Consideration may be given to hypogastric artery ligation. Our group has not found this to be helpful.

12 Consideration may be given to leaving the placenta in situ, closing the hysterotomy, and planning a 'delayed' hysterectomy in 6 weeks. In theory, this may allow some of the enhanced vascularity associated with pregnancy to 'regress', facilitating the hysterectomy. This approach has been advocated in women with percretas to avoid bladder resection. Our group has not found this to be helpful.

Conservative management

There is an obvious and understandable desire on the part of some families with placenta accreta to preserve fertility. Numerous strategies have been employed in an attempt to avoid hysterectomy in cases of accreta and several successful cases have been reported. These include leaving the placenta in situ after delivery, surgical uterine devascularization, embolization of the uterine vessels, uterine compression sutures, oversewing of the placental vascular bed and the use of methotrexate to inhibit trophoblast growth and hasten postpartum involution of the placenta. However, our experience with attempted conservative management has been poor. In many cases, attempted conservative management delays but does not prevent hysterectomy. However, the delay may result in increased morbidity. For example, cases wherein the placenta is left in situ have led to severe infection and uncontrolled hemorrhage. Also, it is likely that complications of attempts at conservative management are under-reported in published literature. Finally, the risk of obstetric complications including recurrent accreta in subsequent pregnancies is uncertain. Women desiring preservation of fertility should be closely monitored and extensively counseled regarding the risks. Cases that may be relatively amenable to attempts at conservative management include posterior placenta previa/accreta, fundal accreta, and cases when the diagnosis of accreta is uncertain.

Prevention

The best strategy to avoid placenta accreta is to avoid multiple cesarean deliveries. In turn, the best strategy to avoid multiple cesarean deliveries is to avoid primary cesarean delivery. Also, vaginal birth after cesarean delivery should be available for appropriate candidates.

It is possible that alterations in the surgical technique for cesarean delivery may reduce the risk of accreta in subsequent pregnancies. For example, a two-layer versus one-layer closure of the hysterotomy may facilitate reconstitution of the decidua basalis. A variety of other surgical techniques and/or the use of topical agents may promote revascularization of the cesarean scar. As the cesarean rate continues to rise, this should be an active area of investigation.

Follow-up

The patient should be offered a postpartum visit at 1–2 weeks to assess surgical complications and emotional well-being and to offer support. Patients often go through a difficult time trying to recover from a major surgery and illness while trying to care for their infant. Also, there is often a period of anger and mourning for their lost fertility and their inability to choose when this would occur. Counseling may be helpful and should be offered. Another visit should be scheduled at 6 weeks postpartum. Women who did not have a hysterectomy should be advised that the risk in subsequent pregnancies is uncertain. Close monitoring and careful preparation for possible recurrent accreta seems prudent in subsequent pregnancies.

Conclusion

Placenta accreta is an increasingly common cause of major maternal morbidity and mortality. The most important risk factor is multiple prior cesarean deliveries. Patients with identified risk factors should be evaluated with obstetric sonogram by a specialist familiar with the condition. In cases of suspected accreta, care should be delivered by a multidisciplinary team in a large center with a state-of-the-art blood bank. Planned cesarean hysterectomy should be scheduled under optimal circumstances prior to the onset of hemorrhage.

Suggested reading

Bauer ST, Bonanno C. Abnormal placentation. *Semin Perinatol* 2009;33:88–96.

Comstock CH. Antenatal diagnosis of placenta accreta: a review. *Ultrasound Obstet Gynecol* 2005;26:89–96.

Eller AG, Porter TF, Soisson P, Silver RM. Optimal management strategies for placenta accreta. *Br J Obstet Gynaecol* 2009;116:648–54.

Flood KM, Said S, Geary M, Robson M, Fitzpatrick C, Malone FD. Changing trends in peripartum hysterectomy over the past 4 decades. *Am J Obstet Gynecol* 2009;200:632. e1–632.e6.

Oyelese Y, Smulian JC. Placenta previa, placenta accreta, and vasa previa. *Obstet Gynecol* 2006;107:927–41.

Rosen T. Placenta accreta and cesarean scar pregnancy: overlooked costs of the rising cesarean section rate. *Clin Perinatol* 2008;35:519–29.

Silver RM, Landon MB, Rouse DJ, Leveno KJ, Spong CY, Thim EA, *et al.* Maternal morbidity associated with multiple repeat cesarean deliveries. *Obstet Gynecol* 2006; 107:1226–32.

Timmermans S, van Hof AC, Duvekot JJ. Conservative management of abnormal invasive placentation. *Obstet Gynecol Surv* 2007;62:529–39.

PROTOCOL 66

Shoulder Dystocia

Robert Gherman

Division of Maternal Fetal Medicine, Prince George's Hospital Center, Cheverly, MD, USA

Overview

All healthcare providers attending vaginal deliveries must be prepared to handle this unpredictable obstetric emergency. Knowledge of the maneuvers employed for the alleviation of shoulder dystocia is relevant not only for obstetric residents and attending house staff, but also for family practitioners, nurses and nurse midwives. The reported incidence varies in the literature, ranging from 0.2% to 3.0%.

Pathophysiology and diagnosis

In a normal delivery after expulsion of the fetal head, external rotation occurs, returning the head to a right angle position in relation to the shoulder girdle. The fetal shoulder during descent is in an oblique pelvic diameter. After expulsion and restitution the anterior fetal shoulder should emerge from the oblique axis under the pubic ramus.

Shoulder dystocia represents the failure of delivery of the fetal shoulder(s), whether it be the anterior, posterior or both. Shoulder dystocia results from a size discrepancy between the fetal shoulders and the pelvic inlet. A persistent anterior-posterior location of the fetal shoulders at the pelvic brim may occur with a large fetal chest relative to the biparietal diameter (e.g., an infant of a diabetic mother) or when truncal rotation does not occur (e.g., precipitous labor). Shoulder dystocia typically occurs when the descent of the anterior shoulder is obstructed by the pubic symphysis. It can also result from impaction of the posterior shoulder on the maternal sacral promontory.

The retraction of the fetal head against the maternal perineum accompanied by difficulty in accomplishing external rotation has been called

Protocols for High-Risk Pregnancies, 5th edition. Edited by J.T. Queenan, J.C. Hobbins and C.Y. Spong. © 2010 Blackwell Publishing Ltd.

Table 66.1 Risk (%) for shoulder dystocia based on fetal weight, diabetic status and method of delivery

Fetal weight (kg)	Non-diabetic	Diabetic: spontaneous delivery	Diabetic: assisted delivery
4–4.25	5	8	12
4.26–4.5	9	12	17
4.51–4.75	14	20	27
4.76–5	21	24	35

the 'turtle sign'.' Most authors have defined shoulder dystocia to include those deliveries requiring maneuvers in addition to gentle downward traction on the fetal head to effect delivery. Several studies have proposed defining shoulder dystocia as a prolonged head-to-body delivery interval (60 seconds) and/or the use of ancillary obstetric maneuvers.

The risk of shoulder dystocia increases significantly as birth weight increases; it must be remembered, however, that approximately 50% to 60% of shoulder dystocias occur in infants weighing less than 4000 g. Even if the birth weight of the infant is over 4000 g, shoulder dystocia will only complicate 3.3% of the deliveries.

No single associated condition or combination of antenatal factors, however, allows for clinically useful positive predictive values for shoulder dystocia. Risks for shoulder dystocia based on known (but not estimated) fetal weight are listed in Table 66.1.

Management

There are no randomized clinical trials to guide physicians in the order of maneuvers that are to be performed. A single randomized trial assessing prophylactic usage of the McRoberts maneuver showed no difference in head-to-body delivery times. The best evidence available shows fetal injury to be associated with all described maneuvers to relieve shoulder dystocia.

The length of delay that results in permanent brain injury will depend on the condition of the fetus at the time that the shoulder dystocia is diagnosed. It may be as short as 4 to 5 minutes, or as long as 15 to 20 minutes. Most, if not all, of the commonly encountered shoulder dystocia episodes can be relieved within several minutes.

1 The patient should stop pushing after the shoulder dystocia is initially recognized.
2 Maternal expulsive efforts will need to be restarted after the fetal shoulders have been converted to the oblique diameter, in order to complete the delivery.

3 Additional assistance may be obtained by summoning other obstetricians, an anesthetist or anesthesiologist, additional nursing support, or a pediatrician.

4 Ask someone to note the time.

5 The McRoberts maneuver is typically used as the first technique for shoulder dystocia alleviation. This can be done by having the patient grasp her posterior thighs and flexing the legs against her abdomen or by having birth attendants (or family members) flex the patient's legs in a similar position. McRoberts' position causes cephalic rotation of the pubic symphyisis and flattening of the sacrum. Care should be taken to avoid prolonged or overly aggressive application of McRoberts.

6 Suprapubic pressure, commonly administered by nursing personnel, is typically used immediately prior to or in direct conjunction with the McRoberts maneuver. This pressure is usually directed posteriorly, but other described techniques have included lateral application from either side of the maternal abdomen or alternating between sides using a rocking pressure.

7 If these techniques fail to accomplish delivery, attempt to deliver the posterior arm. Posterior arm extraction replaces the bisacromial diameter with the axilloacromial diameter, thereby reducing the obstructing diameter in the pelvis. Pressure should be applied at the antecubital fossa in order to flex the fetal forearm. The arm is subsequently swept out over the infant's chest and delivered over the perineum. Rotation of the fetal trunk to bring the posterior arm anteriorly is sometimes required. Grasping and pulling directly on the fetal arm, as well as application of pressure onto the mid-humeral shaft, should be avoided as bone fracture may occur.

8 If after delivery of the posterior fetal arm, delivery of the baby cannot be accomplished, perform rotation of the posterior shoulder 180° to the anterior position while simultaneously rotating the anterior shoulder 180° to the posterior position. If the fetus is facing the mother's right side, rotation should be attempted in a counterclockwise direction as a first step.

9 Some physicians are more comfortable attempting fetal rotational maneuvers before attempting to deliver the posterior arm. In the Woods corkscrew maneuver, the practitioner attempts to abduct the posterior shoulder by exerting pressure onto its anterior surface. In the Rubin (reverse Woods) maneuver, pressure is applied to the posterior surface of the most accessible part of the fetal shoulder (either the anterior or posterior shoulder). If the anterior shoulder is tightly wedged underneath the symphysis pubis, it may be necessary to push the fetus slightly upwards in order to facilitate the rotation.

10 Shoulder dystocia is considered to be a 'bony dystocia' and therefore episiotomy alone will not release the impacted shoulder. The need for cutting a generous episiotomy or proctoepisiotomy must be based on clinical circumstances, such as a narrow vaginal fourchette in a nulliparous patient.

11 Attendants should refrain from applying fundal pressure as a maneuver for the alleviation of shoulder dystocia. Pushing on the fundus serves only to further impact the anterior shoulder behind the symphysis pubis. Fundal pressure can be employed to assist with delivery of the fetal body, but only if the shoulder dystocia has already been alleviated.

12 Attempts at traction on the fetal head should be in keeping with the long axis of fetal spine. The provider should not attempt to rotate the fetal head.

Extraordinary maneuvers

If neither rotational maneuvers nor extraction of the posterior arm is possible, bilateral shoulder dystocia or posterior arm shoulder dystocia may be present. In this case the anterior arm is lodged behind the symphysis pubis and/or the posterior shoulder is lodged high in the pelvis at or near the sacral promontory. Under these circumstances, consideration should be given to 'heroic' maneuvers.

Gaskin maneuver

The mother's position is rotated 180° from the supine position to one in which the mother is positioned on her hands and knees, with the maternal back pointing toward the ceiling. This change in maternal position is thought to allow for a change in fetal position within the maternal pelvis. An attempt is now made to deliver the posterior shoulder by downward (toward the floor) traction followed by delivery of the anterior fetal shoulder by gentle upward traction.

Cephalic replacement (Zavanelli maneuver)

The fetal head is rotated back to a pre-restitution occiput anterior position and then gently flexed. Constant firm pressure is used to push the fetal head back into the vagina and cesarean delivery is subsequently performed. Halothane or other general anesthetics, in conjunction with tocolytic agents, may be administered. Oral or intravenous nitroglycerin may be used as well.

Abdominal rescue

A low transverse uterine incision can be performed, the anterior shoulder manually rotated into the oblique diameter by the surgeon doing the uterine incision, and vaginal delivery accomplished. This requires at least two skilled delivery attendants and should rarely be used.

Symphysiotomy
This should be performed only as a last-ditch effort to deliver a neurologically intact fetus. It is uncommonly used in the United States.

Documentation

Documentation of delivery maneuvers and the sequence of these maneuvers is an essential part of patient care and risk management. The use of a pre-printed form listing important elements is suggested for use in cases of shoulder dystocia, regardless of apparent fetal injury at the time of delivery.

Suggested documentation for shoulder dystocia
- When and how shoulder dystocia was diagnosed.
- Position and rotation of infant's head.
- Which shoulder was anterior.
- Presence of episiotomy, if performed.
- Estimate of head-to-body time interval.
- Estimation of force of traction applied.
- Order, duration and results of maneuvers employed.
- Additional medical personnel present for assistance.
- Birth weight.
- 1-minute and 5-minute Apgar scores.
- Venous and/or arterial umbilical cord blood gas evaluation.
- Inform patient that shoulder dystocia has occurred.

Suggested reading

American College of Obstetricians and Gynecologists. *Shoulder Dystocia*. Practice Bulletin #40. Washington, DC: ACOG, 2002.

Crofts JF, Fox R, Ellis D, Winter C, Hinshaw K, Draycott TJ. Observations from 450 shoulder dystocia simulations: lessons for skills training. *Obstet Gynecol* 2008;112:906–12.

Gherman RB, Chauhan S, Ouzounian JG, Lerner H, Gonik B, Goodwin TM. Shoulder dystocia: the unpreventable obstetric emergency with empiric management guidelines. *Am J Obstet Gynecol* 2006;195:657–72.

Gherman RB, Ousounian JG, Goodwin TM. Obstetric maneuvers for shoulder dystocia and associated fetal morbidity. *Am J Obstet Gynecol* 1998;1126–30.

Hope P, Breslin S, Lamont L, *et al*. Fatal shoulder dystocia: a review of 56 cases reported to the Confidential Enquiry into Stillbirths and Deaths in Infancy. *Br J Obstet Gynaecol* 1998;105:1256–61.

MacKenzie IZ, Shah M, Lean K, Dutton S, Newdick H, Tucker DE. Management of shoulder dystocia: trends in incidence and maternal and neonatal morbidity. *Obstet Gynecol* 2007;110:1059–68.

Nesbitt TS, Gilbert WM, Herrchen B. Shoulder dystocia and associated risk factors with macrosomic infants born in California. *Am J Obstet Gynecol* 1998;179:476–80.

Ouzounian JG, Gherman RB. Shoulder dystocia: Are historic risk factors reliable predictors? *Am J Obstet Gynecol* 2005;192:1933–38.

Poggi SH, Spong CY, Allen RH. Prioritizing posterior arm delivery during severe shoulder dystocia. *Obstet Gynecol* 2003;101:1068–72.

Spong CY, Beall M, Rodrigues D, *et al.* An objective definition of shoulder dystocia: prolonged head-to-body delivery intervals and/or the use of ancillary obstetric maneuvers. *Obstet Gynecol* 1995;86:433–6.

PROTOCOL 67

Twins, Triplets and Beyond

Mary E. D'Alton and Karin M. Fuchs

Department of Obstetrics and Gynecology, Columbia University College of Physicians and Surgeons, New York Presbyterian Hospital, New York, NY, USA

Clinical significance

Compared to singletons, multifetal pregnancies face a higher risk of both maternal and fetal complications. Women carrying multiples are at risk of a number of pregnancy complications in both the antepartum and postpartum period. Although multiple gestations represent only a fraction of all pregnancies in the United States, they account for a disproportionate amount of infant deaths. The increased risk of perinatal morbidity and mortality results largely from preterm delivery, intrauterine growth restriction (IUGR) and congenital anomalies. Given these maternal and fetal risks, patients carrying multiples require close monitoring and frequent follow-up throughout pregnancy as well as careful planning of delivery.

Pathophysiology

Multiple gestations result either from the fertilization of multiple ova or from the division of a single fertilized ovum into more than one fetus. The terms 'monozygotic' and 'dizygotic' refer to the number of ova responsible for the multiple gestations. A monozygotic pregnancy results from a single fertilized ovum that splits into two distinct fetuses. By definition, monozygotic pregnancies are genetically identical. In contrast, dizygotic pregnancies originate from the fertilization of two separate ova and are therefore genetically dissimilar.

The frequency of monozygotic twins is constant worldwide at 4 per 1000 births. In contrast, the frequency of dizygotic twins varies by maternal age, parity, family history, maternal weight, nutritional state,

Protocols for High-Risk Pregnancies, 5th edition. Edited by J.T. Queenan, J.C. Hobbins and C.Y. Spong. © 2010 Blackwell Publishing Ltd.

race and the use of infertility drugs. In the United States, two-thirds of twins are dizygotic and one-third are monozygotic.

The frequency of dizygotic twinning is increased with increasing serum concentrations of follicle-stimulating hormone (FSH) and luteinizing hormone (LH). As a result of these higher gonadotropin levels, multiple ovulations can occur in a single menstrual cycle, increasing the likelihood of dizygotic twinning. Gonadotropin levels fluctuate depending on maternal age, weight, nutrition, parity and heredity. For these reasons, both infertility treatments and advanced maternal age are associated with increased frequency of dizygotic twinning.

Placentation

Although multiple gestations can be classified as monozygotic or dizygotic, it is clinically important to determine the placentation and amnionicity of multiple pregnancies. Dizygotic pregnancies are by definition dichorionic diamniotic. Chorionicity of monozygotic gestations is determined by the time at which division of the fertilized ovum occurs and can be dichorionic-diamniotic, monochorionic-diamniotic or monochorionic-monoamniotic.

In the United States, 20% of twin pregnancies are monochorionic and approximately 80% are dichorionic. Determination of chorionicity in multiple gestations is essential for proper management of the pregnancy. Approximately 20% of monochorionic diamniotic twin gestations are complicated by twin-twin transfusion syndrome, whereas monochorionic monoamniotic gestations are at risk of conjoining or cord entanglement.

Diagnosis

Delayed diagnosis of multiple gestation can result in an increased risk of complications. Therefore, early diagnosis is essential.
1 *Clinical examination.* Multifetal gestations should be suspected if the uterine size is greater than expected or if multiple fetal heart tones are detected.
2 *Maternal serum alpha-fetoprotein.* Multiple gestation should be excluded if a elevated level of maternal serum alpha-fetoprotein is noted on second trimester serum screening.
3 *Ultrasonography.* Ultrasonography can be used to diagnosis multiple gestations in the first trimester as well as later in gestation. In the first trimester, visualization of two distinct gestational sacs suggests a dichorionic twin gestation. Visualization of a single gestational sac with two fetal poles and two yolk sacs suggests a monochorionic diamniotic twin gestation. Visualization of a single gestational sac with two fetal poles but one yolk sac suggests a monochorionic monoamniotic twin pregnancy.

Later in gestation, ultrasonography can be used to determine the number of fetuses, the number of placentas, and fetal sex, and to assess the presence and thickness of a dividing membrane.

Determining chorionicity

1 *Placental number.* If two placental disks are seen, the pregnancy is dichorionic.
2 *Fetal sex.* If the fetuses are opposite sex, the pregnancy is dichorionic.
3 *Dividing membrane.* If the membrane is thick (>2 mm) or has three to four visible layers, consider dichorionic diamniotic. Visualization of a triangular projection of placenta between the layers of the dividing membrane (known as the twin peak or lambda sign) is also useful in diagnosis of dichorionicity, but its absence is not as reliable to predict monochorionicity. If membrane is thin, consider monochorionic diamniotic. Consider a monochorionic monoamniotic gestation if no membrane is seen.
4 *Postpartum.* Confirm chorionicity by examining the placenta after delivery, including gross and histological examination.

Among same-sex dichorionic gestations, genetic studies are required to definitively determine zygosity.

Treatment

Antepartum treatment
Early ultrasonography
Ultrasonography should be performed early in gestation to confirm pregnancy dating and to assess chorionicity. If a fetal size discrepancy is noted, use biometry of the larger fetus for dating purposes.

Medications and nutritional requirements
Women carrying multiples should be counseled regarding the additional caloric and nutritional requirements. The American College of Obstetricians and Gynecologists recommends daily intake of 300 kcal more than with a singleton gestation, and a total weight gain of 35–45 pounds for women with a normal pre-pregnancy BMI. Daily folic acid (1 mg) and elemental iron (60 mg) is recommended in addition to a daily prenatal vitamin.

Prenatal diagnosis
• *Aneuploidy screening.* In dizygotic twin pregnancies, each fetus has its own independent risk of aneuploidy and, therefore, the chance of at least one abnormal fetus is increased. Both first and second trimester serum markers are approximately twice as high in twin pregnancies as in singleton

pregnancies. Interpretation of abnormal serum screening results is difficult because it is not possible to determine which of the fetuses is responsible for the abnormal analyte concentration. Nuchal translucency measurement, which assesses each fetus independently, is a reasonable alternative to serum testing for aneuploidy screening in multiple gestations.

- *Maternal serum alpha-fetoprotein screening to determine neural tube defect (NTD) risk.* Maternal serum alpha-fetoprotein levels are approximately double in twins compared to singletons. A level greater than 4.0 MoM in twins is associated with an increased risk of neural tube and ventral wall defect and should be addressed with a detailed sonographic survey of these structures. Amniocentesis is offered if an open defect is suspected or ultrasound examination is inadequate.

- *Prenatal diagnosis.* All women, regardless of age, should be counseled about the option for either screening or diagnostic testing for fetal aneuploidy. Amniocentesis may be performed on one sac only if monozygosity is certain. Otherwise, amniocentesis for karyotype should be done on all sacs. Genetic amniocentesis in multiples is usually diagnosed using an ultrasound-guided multiple-needle approach. Indigo carmine dye may be used to confirm proper needle placement. Although pregnancy loss rates after genetic amniocentesis in twins has been considered similar to singletons, recent literature suggests an increased risk of loss after amniocentesis of twin gestations. Chorionic villus sampling offers the advantage of earlier diagnosis, and can be performed between 10 and 13 weeks with a loss rate similar to amniocentesis.

- *Congenital anomalies.* Careful sonographic assessment of fetal anatomy is indicated in multifetal pregnancies because both monozygotic and dizygotic pregnancies are at increased risk for many structural anomalies. Anomalies unique to multiple gestations include acardia and conjoined twins. If one fetus in a multiple gestation has a major malformation, selective termination of the affected fetus may be offered.

Preterm birth prevention
Preterm birth occurs in more than 40% of twin and 75% of triplet gestations.

Ultrasound surveillance of cervical length and fetal fibronectin testing can identify those multiple gestations at increased risk of preterm delivery. A transvaginal measurement of cervical length of <2.5 cm at 24 weeks is associated with an increased risk of preterm delivery before 32 weeks (odds ratio, 6.9). Similarly, a positive FFN at 28 weeks is associated with an increased risk of preterm delivery before 32 weeks (odds ratio, 9.4).

There is no evidence that prophylactic cervical cerclage, bed rest, outpatient uterine monitoring, or long-term use of prophylactic tocolytic agents are effective in preventing preterm labor or prolonging pregnancy in multiple gestations. Similarly, prophylactic progesterone has not been shown to decrease the rate of preterm birth among twin gestations.

Patient education regarding the early signs of preterm labor in multiple gestations is important. Cervical length should be measured every 2 weeks from 16 to 24 weeks in multiple gestations thought to be at highest risk for preterm delivery. Tocolysis should be reserved for women with documented preterm labor, and may be administered to delay delivery and allow administration of antenatal steroids. Antenatal steroids should be administered if preterm delivery is expected within 7 days and the gestational age is between 24 and 34 weeks.

Diabetes screening
A 1-hour glucose challenge test is recommended at 24 to 28 weeks to screen for gestational diabetes. If positive, a 3-hour glucose tolerance test should be performed to establish diagnosis of gestational diabetes.

Fetal growth assessment
Serial ultrasonography is the most accurate method to assess fetal growth in multiple gestations. Serial ultrasonographic examinations should be performed every 3–4 weeks beginning at approximately 20 weeks' gestation. Singleton growth charts may be used. Discordance should be expressed as a percentage of the larger fetal weight.

Antepartum testing
Routine antepartum testing of multiple gestations has not been shown to have benefit. Surveillance with non-stress testing or biophysical profile is, however, recommended for multiple gestations complicated by discordant growth (>20%), intrauterine growth restriction, oligohydramnios, twin-twin transfusion or specific maternal medical conditions. Doppler velocimetry may also be used to evaluate fetal well-being in multiple gestations complicated by significant growth restriction or discordance.

Delivery
Timing of delivery
Perinatal mortality among dichorionic twin pregnancies nadirs at approximately 38 weeks, and at approximately 35 weeks for triplet gestations. Elective delivery of dichorionic twins by 39 weeks and of uncomplicated triplet gestations by 36 weeks is therefore warranted. There is increasing evidence that, even in the setting of intensive fetal surveillance, there is a significant risk of fetal death at each gestational age in monochorionic twin gestations. Accordingly, it may be reasonable to offer elective delivery of uncomplicated monochorionic twins by 34 to35 weeks' gestation after a detailed discussion of the associated risks and benefits.

Table 67.1 Frequency of presentation

Vertex/vertex	40%
Vertex/breech	26%
Breech/vertex	10%
Breech/breech	10%
Vertex/transverse	8%
Miscellaneous	6%

Source: MacLennan AH. Multiple gestation: clinical characteristics and management. In: Creasy RK, Resnik R (eds) *Maternal-Fetal Medicine: Principles and Practice.* Philadelphia, PA: WB Saunders, 1994; pp. 589–601.

Mode of delivery

Several factors must be evaluated to determine the route of delivery for a patient with multiple gestations including gestational age, estimated fetal weight (EFW), fetal presentation and availability of an obstetric provider skilled in assisted breech deliveries and total breech extractions (Table 67.1).

- *Vertex/vertex.* It is reasonable to plan for vaginal delivery for all estimated fetal weights.
- *Vertex/non-vertex.* Route of delivery should be determined by estimated fetal weights and provider experience. In our practice, trial of labor with possible external cephalic version or breech extraction is offered if the EFW of both fetuses is greater than 1500 g and there is less than 20% discordance. If the EFW of either fetus is <1500 g or if there is more than 20% discordance (with B > A), external cephalic version can be attempted of the second twin, but – if version is unsuccessful – cesarean delivery is performed.
- *Non-vertex/vertex or non-vertex/non-vertex.* Cesarean delivery is indicated for all fetal weights section if the presenting twin is non-vertex.
- *Triplets and beyond.* Cesarean delivery is indicated for all fetal weights.

Other considerations

- Continuous electronic fetal monitoring should be used throughout labor.
- The use of prostaglandins for induction and oxytocin for induction or augmentation of labor is acceptable in twin gestations.
- If a trial of labor is elected, epidural anesthesia should be recommended to allow a full range of obstetric interventions to be performed if needed.

- If vaginal delivery is attempted, an operating room should be available at all times, given the potential need for emergent cesarean delivery of one or both twins.
- If vaginal delivery is attempted, ultrasonography should be available to evaluate position of twin B after delivery of twin A.
- Twin gestation is not a contraindication to VBAC (vaginal birth after cesarean delivery).

Complications

Maternal and fetal complications of multifetal pregnancies are listed in Tables 67.2 and 67.3.

Table 67.2 Maternal complications in multifetal pregnancies

Hyperemesis
Urinary tract infection
Anemia
Cholestasis
Gestational diabetes
Preeclampsia
HELLP syndrome
Acute fatty liver of pregnancy
Placental abruption
Placenta previa
Vasa previa
Preterm labor
Preterm premature rupture of membranes
Cesarean delivery
Postpartum hemorrhage

Table 67.3 Fetal complications in multifetal pregnancies

Vanishing twin
Congenital anomalies
Intrauterine growth restriction
Discordant growth
Umbilical cord entanglement (monoamniotic gestations)
Twin transfusion syndrome (monochorionic gestations)
Prematurity
Perinatal mortality
Locking twins (non-vertex/vertex presentation)

Specific complications

Monoamniotic pregnancies

Monoamniotic gestations are associated with increased perinatal mortality secondary to cord entanglement. Consider administering steroids and delivery by cesarean delivery at 34 weeks' gestation. Deliver before 34 weeks if any evidence of intrauterine growth restriction or significant discordance accompanied by abnormal non-stress test, biophysical profile, or Doppler studies.

Twin-twin transfusion

Occurs only in monochorionic pregnancies as a result of arteriovenous communications. Ultrasound diagnosis requires presence of a single placenta, gender concordance, amniotic fluid discordance (polyhydramniotic recipient/oligohydramniotic donor); may be accompanied by abnormal umbilical artery Dopplers and hydrops or cardiac dysfunction. Perinatal mortality up to 70%. Treatment includes selective laser photocoagulation of communicating vessels, septostomy, or serial amnioreduction. Intensive fetal surveillance should be performed when viability is reached.

Single fetal demise

Incidence of fetal death of one twin after 20 weeks ranges from 2.6% to 6.8% and may be as high as 17% in triplets and higher-order multiples. The concept of an increased risk of clinically significant maternal coagulopathy after demise of one fetus of a multiple gestation has been refuted and generally is not accepted. Obtain baseline platelet count, prothrombin time, partial thromboplastin time and fibrinogen level and, if normal, no further surveillance is necessary. The main risk to the surviving fetus is prematurity. Due to vascular anastomoses of monochorionic pregnancies, hemodynamic changes associated with the demise of one fetus renders an approximately 20% risk of multicystic encephalomalacia in the viable twin. Delivery after single fetal demise does not improve outcome. Continue antenatal surveillance including non-stress testing and serial ultrasonographic examination for assessment of fetal growth and cervical length. MRI of fetal brain approximately 2 weeks after single fetal demise may help to determine the presence of cerebral injury in the surviving twin.

Prevention

Over the last several decades, the twin birth rate in the United States has increased every year, to a rate of over 30 per 1000 total births. The number of triplet, quadruplet and higher-order multiple births increased over 400% before peaking in recent years. The two major factors accounting for these increases are the widespread availability of assisted reproductive technologies and increasing maternal age at childbirth.

Multifetal pregnancy reduction

The goal of multifetal pregnancy reduction is to reduce the number of live fetuses present in the uterus and thereby decrease the risk of preterm delivery in multiple gestations. The procedure is usually performed transabdominally by injecting potassium chloride into the fetal thorax. Multifetal pregnancy reduction is usually performed between 9 weeks and 13 weeks of gestation. Although the benefit of the procedure for triplet gestation remains controversial, the majority of multifetal pregnancy reduction procedures are performed to reduce triplets to twins. A large series of 1000 cases demonstrated that the pregnancy loss rate before 24 weeks remained constant at about 5.4% in the hands of an experienced operator with the starting number of fetuses ranging from 2 to 5. Those pregnancies finishing with two or three fetuses delivered at similar gestational ages as non-reduced twins and triplets.

Selective termination

The management options available in the event of discovering an abnormality of one fetus is often an important consideration in the decision-making process involved in formulating a screening and/or diagnostic strategy. These options are expectant management (do nothing), termination of the pregnancy (both abnormal and normal fetuses), or selective termination of the abnormal fetus or fetuses. Among dichorionic gestations, selective termination is usually performed by transabdominal fetal intracardiac injection of potassium chloride. Among monochorionic gestations, selective termination can be performed using radiofrequency ablation of the cord of the anomalous twin or using other methods of cord ligation. Results of a large series of 200 cases demonstrated an overall pregnancy loss rate of 4%. Factors affecting pregnancy loss included a greater number of starting fetuses and reduction of more than one fetus.

Conclusion

Twin gestations and higher-order multifetal pregnancies comprise a significant proportion of births in the United States. Given the risk of both maternal and fetal complications, close surveillance of maternal and fetal status throughout gestation is warranted. Early confirmation of pregnancy dating and sonographic diagnosis of chorionicity are important to assess risk of specific complications. Timing of delivery should be determined based on chorionicity, and mode of delivery should be determined by gestational age, fetal weight, intertwin discordance and fetal presentation.

Suggested reading

American College of Obstetricians and Gynecologists. *Multiple Gestation: Complicated Twin, Triplet, and High-Order Multifetal Pregnancy*. Practice Bulletin # 56. Washington, DC: ACOG, 2004.

American College of Obstetricians and Gynecologists. *Screening for Fetal Chromosomal Abnormalities*. Practice Bulletin # 77. Washington, DC: ACOG, 2007.

Blickstein I, Keith LG. Outcome of triplets and high-order multiple pregnancies. *Curr Opin Obstet Gynecol* 2003;15:113.

Cahill AG, Macones GA, Stamilio DM, *et al.* Pregnancy loss rate after mid-trimester amniocentesis in twin pregnancies. *Am J Obstet Gynecol* 2009;200:257.

D'Alton ME, Dudley DK. The ultrasonographic prediction of chorionicity in twin gestation. *Am J Obstet Gynecol* 1989;160:557.

Goldenberg RL, Iams JD, Miodovnik M, National Institute of Child Health and Human Development Maternal-Fetal Medicine Units Network. The preterm prediction study: Risk factors in twin gestations. *Am J Obstet Gynecol* 1996;175:1047.

Kahn B, Lumey H, Zybert PA, *et al.* Prospective risk of fetal death in singleton, twin, and triplet gestations: implications for practice. *Obstet Gynecol* 2003;102;685.

Lee YM, Cleary-Goldman J, Thaker HM, *et al.* Antenatal sonographic prediction of twin chorionicity. *Am J Obstet Gynecol* 2006;195:863.

Malone FD, D'Alton ME. Multiple pregnancy: clinical characteristics and management. In: Creasy RK (ed.) *Maternal Fetal Medicine*, 6th edn. Philadelphia, PA: Saunders Elsevier, 2009.

Martin JA, Hamilton BE, Sutton PD, *et al.* Births: Final Data for 2004. *Natl Vital Stat Rep* 2006;55(1):80.

Petersen IR, Nyholm J. Multiple pregnancies with single intrauterine demise. *Acta Obstet Gynecol Scand* 1999;78:202.

Senat MV, Deprest J, Boulvain M, Paupe A, Winer N. Ville Y. Endoscopic laser surgery versus serial amnioreduction for severe twin-to-twin transfusion syndrome. *N Engl J Med* 2004;351:136.

Sperling L, Tabor A. Twin pregnancy: the role of ultrasound in management. *Acta Obstet Gynecol Scand* 2001;80:287.

Stone J, Eddleman K, Lynch L, Berkowitz RL. A single center experience with 1000 consecutive cases of multifetal pregnancy reduction. *Am J Obstet Gynecol* 2002;187:1163.

Winn HN, Cimino J, Powers J, *et al.* Intrapartum management of nonvertex second-born twins: a critical analysis. *Am J Obstet Gynecol* 2001;185:1204.

PROTOCOL 68

Postpartum Hemorrhage

Gary S. Eglinton

Department of Obstetrics and Gynecology, New York Hospital Queens, Flushing, New York;
Department of Obstetrics and Gynecology, Weill Medical College of Cornell University, New York,
NY, USA

Clinical significance

Worldwide, obstetrical hemorrhage has been identified as the single most important cause of maternal death, associated with half of all maternal deaths in developing countries. In countries with greater resources, more women survive obstetrical hemorrhage, but it still accounts for a large percentage of maternal deaths. A recent review in the United Kingdom found the majority of deaths from hemorrhage were associated with substandard care.

Most obstetrical hemorrhage is associated with the intrapartum or immediate postpartum period. Primary postpartum hemorrhage occurs within the first 24 postpartum hours. It results from bleeding from the placental site, lacerations or damage to the genital tract or nearby tissues or both. Survival of the mother depends upon immediate expert care and availability of blood products. The penalty for not having blood products available is severe. Jehovah's Witnesses who declined blood products suffered a 44-fold higher risk of maternal death associated with obstetrical hemorrhage.

Risks for and causes of immediate postpartum hemorrhage are listed in Table 68.1.

Pathophysiology

Cardiac output is the volume of blood pumped per minute. It is the product of heart rate and stroke volume. Stroke volume depends upon preload, myocardial contractility and afterload. Preload is the volume of venous blood filling the heart before each heart beat. It is determined by

---

Table 68.1 Predisposing factors and causes of immediate postpartum hemorrhage

---

Bleeding from placental implantation site

  Hypotonic myometrium – uterine atony
    Some general anesthetics – halogenated hydrocarbons
    Poorly perfused myometrium – hypotension
      Hemorrhage
      Conduction analgesia
    Overdistended uterus – large fetus, twins, hydramnios
    Following prolonged labor
    Following very rapid labor
    Following oxytocin-induced or augmented labor
    High parity
    Uterine atony in previous pregnancy
    Chorioamnionitis
  Retained placental tissue
    Avulsed cotyledon, succenturiate lobe
    Abnormally adherent – accreta, increta, percreta
Trauma to the genital tract

  Large episiotomy, including extensions
  Lacerations of perineum, vagina, or cervix
  Ruptured uterus
Coagulation defects

  Intensify all of the above

Source: *Williams Obstetrics*, 22nd edn. Cunningham FG, Leveno KJ, Bloom SL, Hauth JC, Gilstrap III LC, Wenstrom KD (eds). New York: McGraw Hill, 2005; Table 35-5, p. 824.

the difference between mean venous systemic pressure and right atrial pressure. Preload determines the degree of myocardial stretch, which determines contractility. Afterload is the pressure the heart must overcome to force blood through the arterial system.

The human can survive the loss of 80% of the liver and adrenals, 75% of the kidneys, 75% of the red blood cell mass, and loss of more than one lung. Acute loss of 35% of *blood volume* can be fatal. The cardiovascular system operates with a small blood volume and a steep Starling curve (volume-dependent ventricle).

The venous system is a reservoir or capacitance system that stores the volume necessary for cardiac output. It has two components. The first component is the volume that would remain if the venous pressure dropped to zero. Most of this volume is preserved during hemorrhage, but it does not contribute to preload. Some of it is lost into the second component. The second component is the above-zero-pressure volume. This component contributes to cardiac output and is lost during hemorrhage.

A useful definition of shock is inadequate organ perfusion and tissue oxygenation. With loss of venous volume come early compensatory changes including endogenous catecholamines creating progressive vasoconstriction and increasing peripheral vascular resistance and increasing heart rate and diastolic pressure. Increasing heart rate and diminution of pulse pressure are two early warning signs of shock. Rising diastolic pressure does little to increase organ perfusion.

As perfusion deteriorates, many vasoactive substances, including histamine, bradykinin, beta-endorphins, prostanoids and other cytokines, create many effects on micro-circulation and membrane permeability. Additional salt water is lost from the intravascular space into the interstitium and into dysfunctional cells with disturbed membrane function. At the cellular level, hypoperfusion leads to intracellular aberrations resulting in anaerobic metabolism and elaboration of lactic acid. Metabolic acidosis ensues, usually with lactic acid partially trapped in the periphery because of profound peripheral vasoconstriction. If the process is not reversed through improved perfusion, further tissue swelling and cellular death result.

Administration of isotonic crystalloid in sufficiently large quantities facilitates improved perfusion. Adequate oxygenation, ventilation and fluid resuscitation are the three stanchions upon which successful resuscitation depends. Resuscitation may be accompanied by increasing interstitial edema, in part cased by reperfusion injury owing to leaky capillary membranes. This further increases the requirement for volume infusion to complete resuscitation.

The initial treatment of shock is aimed at restoring cellular and organ perfusion with adequately oxygenated blood volume. Control of bleeding and restoration of blood volume are the goals. Return of pre-hemorrhage vital signs and adequate urine output are the markers of success. Advanced trauma life support (ATLS) discourages administration of vasopressors in management of hemorrhagic shock. In this circumstance, vasopressors worsen perfusion. As resuscitation continues, packed red blood cells and additional blood products might be necessary. Blood products should be employed in response to specific laboratory abnormalities.

Diagnosis

The definition of postpartum hemorrhage varies and is never precise. Traditional definitions of 500 mL after vaginal delivery and 1000 mL after cesarean delivery clearly are misleading. A fall of hematocrit of 10% is a late finding and is not useful acutely. Blood loss commonly is underestimated by as much as 100%. Training can improve the estimation of blood volume loss. Protecting the gravida are the blood volume expansion of normal pregnancy and compensatory mechanisms which might delay disturbances of maternal vital signs until after acute loss of as much as 25% of her blood volume. Leveno has provided a method to estimate non-pregnant and pregnant blood

Table 68.2 Calculation of maternal total blood volume (TBV)

Non-pregnant TBV

$$\frac{[\text{Maternal height (inches)} \times 50] + [\text{Maternal weight (pounds)} \times 25]}{2} = \text{TBV (mL)}$$

Pregnant TBV

Add 50% to non-pregnant TBV but remember normal pregnancy blood volume *increase* varies between 30% and 60% of non-pregnant TBV and increases with gestational age

Pregnancy TBV increase is less in severe preeclampsia or eclampsia and more with multiple fetuses

Pregnant TBV in serious hemorrhage

Assume acute return to non-pregnant TBV because normal pregnancy hypervolemia has been acutely lost

From Leveno and colleagues, 2003. Williams Obstetrics, 22nd edition, Cunningham FG, Leveno KJ, Bloom SL, Hauth JC, Gilstrap III LC, Wenstrom KD, eds. McGraw Hill, New York, 2005, Table 35-6, p. 825.

volume (see Table 68.2). Severe hypertension and preeclampsia can interfere with the blood volume expansion of normal pregnancy, rendering patients with these conditions at greater risk from severe hemorrhage. In the acute phase of large volume blood loss, hematocrit does not change and cannot be used as an indicator of the volume of blood lost. There are methods available to estimate blood volume and to estimate the amount of hemorrhage encountered by the patient. Careful observation of vital signs, including urine output, with comparison to pre-delivery values is crucial. It is likely that far more patients in obstetrics suffer significant hemorrhage than are diagnosed. Acute loss of blood volume greater than equivalent to a class I hemorrhage (see Table 68.3) is an emergency that requires the attention of the attending physician responsible for the patient. Classifying the patient in the correct class I through class IV hemorrhage category requires attention to the most disordered symptom or sign the patient expresses. It is dangerous to await more signs or symptoms to be certain the blood loss is important. Any disturbance of blood pressure or heart rate in the victim of blood loss requires attention and intervention before the patient deteriorates further. Physician delay causes patient harm.

Treatment

With recognition of excessive obstetrical bleeding, many interventions should occur nearly simultaneously. Before delivery the patient should have had a 16-gauge peripheral intravenous catheter inserted. While performing uterine massage, the delivery attendant must call for assistance and direct the placement of a second large bore peripheral intravenous

Table 68.3 Estimated fluid and blood losses[1] based on patient's initial presentation

	Class I	Class II	Class III	Class IV
Blood loss (mL)	Up to 750	750–1500	1500–2000	>2000
Blood loss (% blood volume)	Up to 15%	15%–30%	30%–40%	>40%
Pulse rate	<100	100–120	120–140	>140
Blood pressure	Normal	Normal	Decreased	Decreased
Pulse pressure (mmHg)	Normal or increased	Decreased	Decreased	Decreased
Respiratory rate	14–20	20–30	30–40	>35
Urine output (mL/h)	>30	20–30	5–15	Negligible
CNS/mental status	Slightly anxious	Mildly anxious	Anxious, confused	Confused, lethargic
Fluid replacement (3:1 rule)[2]	Crystalloid	Crystalloid	Crystalloid and blood	Crystalloid and blood

[1]For a 70 kg man.

[2]The 3-for-1 rule, which derives from the empiric observation that most patients in hemorrhagic shock require as much as 300 mL of electrolyte solution for each 100 mL of blood loss. Applied blindly, these guidelines can result in excessive or inadequate fluid administration. For example, a patient with a crush injury to the extremity may have hypotension out of proportion to his or her blood loss and require fluids in excess of the 3:1 guidelines. In contrast, a patient whose ongoing blood loss is being replaced by blood transfusion requires less than 3:1. The use of bolus therapy with careful monitoring of the patient's response can moderate these extremes.

Source: *Advanced Trauma Life Support for Doctors Student Course Manual*, 8th edn. American College of Surgeons Committee on Trauma, Chicago, 2008; Table 3-1, p. 61.

catheter. Initial fluid resuscitation requires 1 to 2 L of warmed Ringer's lactate solution as quickly as possible. Aggressive uterine massage and compression is not a gentle art (see Fig. 68.1).

Atony is responsible for 80% of immediate postpartum hemorrhage. Aggressive uterine massage and compression will almost always terminate or significantly slow excessive postpartum uterine bleeding. Dilute intravenous oxytocin solution should already be infusing or intramuscular uterotonic should have already been administered before the atony is discovered. If oxytocin administration was not started before the emergency it should be administered now. Oxytocin should not be administered as an intravenous bolus because dangerous side effects may occur. If atony is not responsive to massage/compression and oxytocin infusion, administration of alternative uterotonics might be helpful. Table 68.4 lists alternative uterotonics.

If the uterus seems adequately contracted and bleeding continues, immediate careful inspection of the vagina, cervix and uterus for lacerations is mandatory. This requires adequate analgesia/anesthesia, retraction and

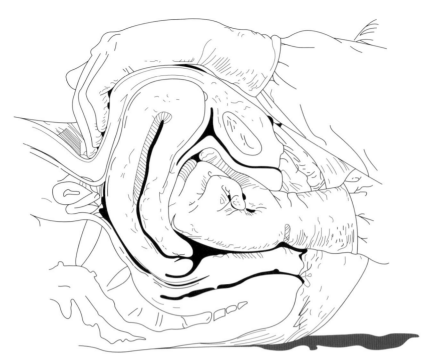

Figure 68.1 Postpartum hemorrhage. Bimanual compression of the uterus and massage with the abdominal hand usually effectively controls hemorrhage from uterine atony. Source: Cunningham FG, Leveno KJ, Bloom SL, Hauth JC, Gilstrap III LC, Wenstrom KD (eds) *Williams Obstetrics*, 22nd edn. New York: McGraw Hill, 2005; Figure 35-16, p. 827.

Table 68.4 Uterotonic agents

Uterotonic agent	Dose	Uses	Comments
Oxytocin continuous IV infusion	10 to 160 IU per liter	Administer after delivery of the placenta. Higher dose may be required with cesarean	Most common uterotonic regimen used in the US
Oxytocin IM	5 IU or 10 IU IM	Administer after delivery of anterior shoulder, after delivery of baby or after delivery of placenta	Administration before placental delivery might be associated with entrapment of placenta
15-methyl prostaglandin $F_{2\alpha}$ (Carboprost tromethamine, Hemabate)	250 μg (0.25 mg) IM	Repeat as necessary every 15 to 90 minutes to a maximum of 8 doses	20% of patients with diarrhea, hypertension, emesis, fever, flushing and/or tachycardia. Avoid with asthma, hypertension and hypotension

(*Continued*)

Table 68.4 (Continued)

Uterotonic agent	Dose	Uses	Comments
Dinoprostone (Prostin E$_2$)	20 mg suppository (rectal or vaginal)	Repeat as necessary every 2 hours	Avoid with hypotension. Fever is common. Stored frozen. Must thaw before use
Misoprostol (Cytotec)	600 to 1000 μg per rectum	Not effective for prophylaxis. May be used for patients who fail to respond to other agents	Possible prostaglandin side effects similar to above
Methylergonovine-Methylergometrine (Methergine)	0.2 mg 1 mL ampoule IM	May be repeated every 2 to 4 hours. May be administered IV, but not intraarterial. IM is safer. May be combined with oxytocin	More nausea, emesis and hypertension than with oxytocin. Avoid with hypertension
Ergonovine-Ergometrine	500 μg 1 mL ampoule IM; 200–500 μg IV	IM administration preferred. Administer IV only for emergencies	More nausea, emesis and hypertension than with oxytocin alone. Avoid with hypertension. May give rise to widespread and dangerous vasoconstriction and rarely acute pulmonary edema
Combined 0.5 mg ergometrine + 5 IU oxytocin (Syntometrine)	1 mL ampoule IM	Slightly more effective than IM oxytocin alone	More nausea, emesis and hypertension than with oxytocin alone. Avoid with hypertension. May give rise to widespread and dangerous vasoconstriction and rarely acute pulmonary edema

IU, international units

Administration of any uterotonic before delivery of the entire fetus and/or placenta could lead to undesired results including difficulty with delivery/extraction.

assistance. Lacerations are the second most common cause for immediate postpartum hemorrhage.

Retained placental or membrane fragments may interfere with the ability of uterine contractions to establish and maintain hemostasis. Blunt curettage with a sponge or gauze-wrapped finger or a large blunt curette may immediately improve hemostasis. Placental site bleeding may continue. If the uterus is open, oversewing and suture ligation may improve hemostasis.

If the patient will receive definitive care without transfer to another institution, initiation and maintenance of aggressive volume replacement with Ringer's lactate solution at three times the volume of estimated blood loss is mandatory. The victim of hemorrhagic shock is short of intravascular salt water because of hemorrhage and because of leakage out of the vascular space. There is no evidence from randomized trials that volume expansion with colloid solutions is superior to crystalloid, and there are credible data suggesting crystalloid is superior to albumin. Colloid does not replace the large volume of lost salt water. Colloid does increase cardiac output more than crystalloid, but survival is not improved with colloid and might be diminished with colloid. If the patient must be transferred to a higher level of care for management of postpartum hemorrhage, some level of continued permissive hypotension might be better than aggressive fluid resuscitation before transfer.

If blood loss exceeds the expected volume expansion of normal pregnancy, packed red blood cell transfusion probably is necessary to maintain required oxygen transport capability. If the patient is severely preeclamptic or hypertensive she might not have experienced the normal blood volume expansion of pregnancy. She will be more susceptible to hypovolemic shock and may require earlier packed red blood cell transfusion. In a young healthy patient with cessation of active bleeding, and anticipation of no additional bleeding or surgery, 7 g of hemoglobin is adequate and does not require transfusion of red cells. If the patient continues to bleed actively and/or probably will require surgical exploration, 9 to 10 g of hemoglobin probably is a better target. It is not necessary to treat to a higher level, and treating to a higher level might increase mortality. Other blood products should be administered based upon laboratory abnormalities. It seldom is necessary to employ other blood products until after infusion of 5 to 10 units of packed red blood cells. Fresh frozen plasma should not be infused solely to expand intravascular volume.

If aggressive uterine massage and compression and application of uterotonic medications and endovaginal exploration and repair of obstetrical lacerations leave the patient still bleeding excessively, internal uterine compression or interventional radiology embolization of arteries supplying bleeding vessels might terminate hemorrhage. Internal compression is applied by insertion of the Bakri balloon or similar substitute with pressure applied predominantly to the lower uterine segment, but depending upon the size of the uterine cavity, internal pressure throughout the uterine cavity might be possible. If all of these actions fail to control hemorrhage, and/or continued occult hemorrhage is suspected, surgical exploration is mandatory. Delaying necessary interventions threatens loss of life and/or function. Early and rapid decisions are necessary. Unnecessary delay results in continued deterioration of the patient, which delays recovery and prejudices the possibility of recovery without patient injury and deficit.

After the initial phase of resuscitation, the patient's response to resuscitation informs further management (see Table 68.5). The most common causes of failure of resuscitation of the hemorrhagic shock victim are inadequate resuscitation and occult continuing hemorrhage. If volume loss is large enough to result in transfusion, it is wise to perform blood gas analysis. It is likely that crystalloid resuscitation has been inadequate. Markers include elevated base deficit and/or lactate. Discovery of metabolic acidosis usually should prompt more aggressive oxygenation, probably through intubation and mechanical ventilation, and increasing crystalloid and packed cells infusion. In general, administration of bicarbonate is not appropriate.

Surgical exploration beyond visual inspection and palpation per vaginum requires laparotomy or extension of the surgical management beyond the standard cesarean procedure. Surgical control of obstetrical hemorrhage requires careful exploration of the abdomen and surgical sites to confirm or establish hemostasis. Uterine atony is most common and requires a systematic approach. If surgical exploration is necessary, massage, compression and uterotonics probably have failed. If superficial intraabdominal bleeding is discovered, achieving hemostasis may require revision of suture lines and additional hemostatic sutures.

Additional control of hemorrhage may be possible by attempting to reduce blood flow to the uterus. Internal iliac (hypogastric) artery ligation

Table 68.5 Responses to initial fluid resuscitation[1]

	Rapid response	Transient response	No response
Vital signs	Return to normal	Transient improvement, then recurrence of decreased BP and increased HR	Remain abnormal
Estimated blood loss	Minimal (10%–20%)	Moderate and ongoing (20%–40%)	Severe (> 40%)
Need for more crystalloid	Low	High	High
Need for blood	Low	Moderate to high	Immediate
Blood preparation	Type and cross-match	Type-specific	Emergency blood release
Need for operative intervention	Possibly	Likely	Highly likely
Early presence of surgeon	Yes	Yes	Yes

[1]2000 mL Ringer's lactate solution in adults, 20 mL/kg Ringer's lactate bolus in children.
Source: *Advanced Trauma Life Support for Doctors Student Course Manual*, 8th edn. American College of Surgeons Committee on Trauma, Chicago, 2008; Table 3-2, p. 65.

is traditional but is difficult and probably dangerous for surgeons who have not practiced it. The success rate is less than 50%, so it has faded from favor. Uterine artery ligation in multiple locations along the uterine border and infundibulopelvic artery ligation are far simpler to perform. AbdRabbo described an orderly modification of uterine artery ligation and coined the phrase 'stepwise uterine devascularization'. This technique has been very successful, has been followed by normal menstrual function and pregnancies, and has been adopted internationally. The suture should be number 1 chromic catgut.

If the source of bleeding seems to be from the placental site, especially in the lower uterine segment, bleeding may continue despite apparently adequate uterine tone. If oversewing bleeding points in the placental site and other techniques described above fail to establish hemostasis, the Bakri balloon may be inserted before closure and inflated after closure of the uterus. The balloon should be seated firmly against the lower uterine segment, and inflated as illustrated in the manufacturer's instructions.

If atony persists, such that the endometrial space is very large, the uterine incision and atonic expanded intrauterine space should be closed using a compression suture as described by B-Lynch or one of the simpler compression techniques offered by Cho or Hayman. Ochoa has reported pyometra as a complication of compression suturing. Compression sutures were described without use of the Bakri balloon. Combining compression sutures with the balloon has been reported. With or without the balloon the suture material probably should be number 1 chromic catgut. If the surgeon chooses to combine the compression sutures and the balloon, sutures must be placed carefully so as not to perforate the balloon, not to prevent removal of the balloon, the balloon should be inserted before the compression sutures are tied down, and the balloon should be inflated carefully, acknowledging the diminished volume and distorted anatomy of the cavity after suturing.

If these measures have not stopped the bleeding an interventional radiology embolization may avoid hysterectomy. If all other available interventions have been attempted, hysterectomy is the remaining inter-vention. Try not to perform hysterectomy on a patient who still requires life-saving resuscitation. If possible, it is better to resort to hysterectomy before the patient deteriorates to this level. If necessary, apply clamps, sponges and pressure to slow the bleeding and allow the resuscitation to catch up (resuscitative surgery) and stabilize the patient before proceed-ing with definitive surgery. In some circumstances it might be preferable to move the patient from the operating room into the recovery area to continue intensive care and resuscitation with the abdomen open with clamps, sponges and pressure applied as necessary with a plan to return to the operating room when the patient is a better candidate for surgery.

Keep the patient warm, hydrated, oxygenated and prevent or reverse metabolic acidosis associated with cold and intense peripheral vasoconstriction and inadequate volume expansion.

Complications

The most common causes of failure of resuscitation of the hemorrhagic hypovolemic shock victim are inadequate resuscitation and occult continuing hemorrhage. Resuscitate and stop the bleeding.

Follow-up

Observe for inadequate resuscitation and continued or recurrent concealed hemorrhage.

Prevention

Outside of the United States, an intramuscular injection of oxytocin, ergot alkaloid or combined medication (Syntometrine) may be administered with delivery of the fetal shoulder or immediately after delivery of the fetus before delivery of the placenta. There is some risk that injection of an uterotonic before delivery of the entire baby and/or placenta could lead to entrapment and difficulty in completing the delivery, especially with an undiagnosed twin. In the United States, dilute oxytocin infusion begins after placental delivery. Comparison of oxytocin and Syntometrine for prevention of third stage atony found oxytocin safer. In the United States, administration of oxytocin most commonly occurs immediately after expulsion of the placenta. A randomized trial demonstrated no advantage to administration of dilute oxytocin infusion before delivery of the placenta and there might be disadvantages. Regardless of timing, 10 to 40 units of oxytocin per liter of normal saline or Ringer's lactate after vaginal delivery is the appropriate prophylactic intervention. The infusion rate should be approximately 10 mL per minute until it is clear that uterine tone is maintained. Then the infusion rate may be diminished to 1 to 2 mL per minute until the patient is ready for transfer to the postpartum area. Munn *et al.* demonstrated that prophylactic administration after cesarean of 80 units per 500 mL over 30 minutes reduced the frequency of uterine atony compared to 10 units in 500 mL. Oxytocin should not be administered as an intravenous bolus.

At term, 600 mL per minute is the estimated blood flow through the intervillous space. Failure of normal control mechanisms to prevent this volume of blood from escaping into the uterus after delivery requires rapid response and expert management. Creation of an obstetrical rapid response team with team members responding to special telecommunications devices and beepers can shorten response time for calls for help. Simulation of responses to emergencies through monitored drills with educational debriefing can improve responses to emergencies. Development of multi-disciplinary teams facilitates response.

In all cases of prior cesarean and in all cases of placenta previa, it is important to search for ultrasonographic findings suggestive of placenta accreta, increta or percreta. Sensitivity and specificity are not high for accreta, but are better for increta and percreta. In some institutions magnetic resonance imaging might be useful to attempt to identify accreta. Identification or suspicion of abnormal placental attachment permits planning to attempt to limit the risk of significant hemorrhage and morbidity. If the threshold permitting donation is adjusted down to hemoglobin of 10, autologous blood donation can bank several units of the patient's blood in the weeks before delivery. Amniocentesis for fetal lung maturity at 36 weeks' gestation permits scheduling the delivery early in the morning with all of the hospital's resources and consultants ready. It is easier to schedule the cell saver than to call for this support after the patient is in shock. Scheduling these cases in the main operating room instead of in the labor and delivery suite avoids tying up labor and delivery resources for long cases and provides expertise and equipment found more readily in the main operating room, where hysterectomies and response to major trauma and hemorrhage are more common.

Conclusion

Preparation for obstetrical hemorrhage improves outcomes. Multidisciplinary team approaches to critical emergencies improve outcomes. Resuscitation of hemorrhagic hypovolemic shock patients following current guidelines improves outcomes. There are some proponents for permissive hypotension in the resuscitation of victims of hypovolemia. But that concept is not incorporated in current ATLS teaching.

Suggested reading

AbdRabbo SA. Stepwise uterine devascularization: a novel technique for management of uncontrollable postpartum hemorrhage with preservation of the uterus. *Am J Obstet Gynecol* 1994;171:694–700.

Advanced Trauma Life Support for Doctors Student Course Manual, 7th edn. American College of Surgeons Committee on Trauma, Chicago, 2004, Protocol 3, Shock, pp. 69–102.

American College of Obstetricians and Gynecologists. Postpartum hemorrhage. ACOG Practice Bulletin #76. *Obstet Gynecol* 2006;108:1039–47.

Bakri YN, Amri A, Abdul Jabbar F. Tamponade-balloon for obstetrical bleeding. *Int J Gynecol Obstet* 2001;74:139–2.

B-Lynch CB, Coker A, Lawal AH, Abu J, Cowen MJ. The B-Lynch surgical technique for the control of massive postpartum haemorrhage: an alternative to hysterectomy? Five cases reported. *Br J Obstet Gynaecol* 1997;104:372–5.

Cho JH, Jun HS, Lee CNL. Hemostatic suturing technique for uterine bleeding during cesarean delivery. *Obstet Gynecol* 2000;96:129–31.

de Groot ANJA, van Dongen PWJ, Vree TB, Hekster YA, van Roosmalen J. Ergot alkaloids: current status and review of clinical pharmacology and therapeutic use compared with other oxytocics in obstetrics and gynaecology. *Drugs* 1998; 56: 523–35.

Dildy GA 3rd, Paine AR, George NC, Velasco C. Estimating blood loss: can teaching significantly improve visual estimation? *Obstet Gynecol* 2004;104:601–6.

Gutierrez G, Reines HD, Wulf-Gutierrez ME. Clinical review: hemorrhagic shock. *Crit Care* 2004;8:373–81.

Hayman RG, Arulkumaran S, Steer PJ: Uterine compression sutures: surgical management of postpartum hemorrhage. *Obstet Gynecol* 2002;99:502–6.

Munn MB, Owen J, Vincent R, Wakefield M, Chestnut DH, Hauth JC. Comparison of two oxytocin regimens to prevent uterine atony at cesarean delivery: a randomized controlled trial. *Obstet Gynecol* 2001;98:386–90.

Ochoa M, Allaire AD, Stitely ML. Pyometria after hemostatic square suture technique. *Obstet Gynecol* 2002;99:506–9.

Skupski DW, Lowenwirt IP, Weinbaum FI, Brodsky D, Danek M, Eglinton GS. Improving hospital systems for the care of women with major obstetric hemorrhage. *Obstet Gynecol* 2006;107:977–83.

Williams Obstetrics, 22nd edn. Cunningham FG, Leveno KJ, Bloom SL, Hauth JC, Gilstrap III LC, Wenstrom KD, eds. McGraw Hill, New York, 2005, Protocol 17, Normal labor and delivery, pp. 409–41 and Protocol 35, Obstetrical hemorrhage, pp. 809–54.

PROTOCOL 69

Vaginal and Vulvar Hematoma

Robert Resnik

Department of Reproductive Medicine, UCSD School of Medicine, Solana Beach, CA, USA

The formation of a pelvic hematoma in the puerperium is a rare but potentially life-threatening complication. The reported incidence ranges from as low as 1 in 300 to 1 in 10,000 deliveries, but if one considers only those cases that require surgical intervention, a more realistic frequency is approximately 1 in 1000 births. Early reports suggested a maternal mortality of up of 21% for vulvovaginal hematomas, although early recognition and prompt management consisting of blood transfusion, aggressive surgical intervention, and antibiotics will, in almost all cases, eliminate the risk of mortality and significant morbidity.[1]

Pathophysiology and diagnosis

Puerperal hematomas usually result from birth trauma or improper hemostasis at the time of episiotomy or vaginal laceration repair, although they may also occur following an uncomplicated spontaneous vaginal delivery. Associated factors include primiparity, operative delivery, large fetal weight, prolonged second stage of labor and vulvar varicosities. In most cases, the patient will present with exquisite perineal pain shortly following delivery, and examination in many cases will reveal an obvious vulvar hematoma. However, a paravaginal hematoma may also develop that is not obvious externally, and can only be diagnosed by vaginal examination. In this instance, it is common to have the hematoma mass occlude the vaginal canal and dissect into the ischiorectal fossa.

These hematomas can be classified into four groups, depending on their location.[2]

1 *Vulvar*: The bleeding is limited to the vulvar tissues, superficial to fascial planes.

2 *Vulvovaginal*: The hematoma is evident on the vulva, but extends into the paravaginal tissues.

Protocols for High-Risk Pregnancies, 5th edition. Edited by J.T. Queenan, J.C. Hobbins and C.Y. Spong. © 2010 Blackwell Publishing Ltd.

3 *Vaginal*: The hematoma is confined to the paravaginal tissues, and is not evident on external examination.

4 *Supravaginal or subperitoneal*: The hematoma may dissect retroperitoneally forming a mass palpable above Poupart's ligament, or may develop within the broad ligament. Intraligamentous hematomas will present with abdominal pain, hypotension, and tachycardia consistent with blood loss, and upward and lateral deviation of the uterus in the abdomen to the side opposite the hematoma.

Although perineal or rectal pain, or both, is the most common symptom, patients may present with continued vaginal bleeding, hypotension, or urinary retention.

Management

1 If the hematoma is relatively small, not enlarging and painless, expectant management is warranted.[3]

2 In the presence of an expanding and/or painful hematoma, more aggressive treatment is necessary. Blood should be made available for transfusion, inasmuch as the blood loss is usually well in excess of what is visible at the time of examination, and due to the anticipated blood loss during surgical evacuation. An initial hematocrit, as well as serial blood count monitoring, is indicated for 12 to 24 hours following resolution of bleeding. Under adequate anesthesia and in an operating setting, the hematoma should be opened, the clot evacuated, and any apparent bleeding sites ligated. The space should be closed with deep mattress sutures, a drain placed, and the vaginal mucosa and/or vulvar skin reapproximated without tension. In the presence of a paravaginal hematoma, the vagina should be packed tightly and a Foley catheter left in place.

3 If bleeding continues, or if there is reformation of the hematoma following surgical intervention, the next most effective step in management is that of angiographic embolization.[4–6] This requires passage of a catheter from the femoral artery, retrograde into the internal iliac artery to identify the area of contrast extravasation, followed by embolization with small gel foam particles. This will, in almost all cases, stop the bleeding rapidly, and allow for occlusion only of the bleeding vessel. Hypogastric artery ligation is frequently ineffective for stopping pelvic hemorrhage,[7] disrupts blood supply to a larger area than is necessary, and precludes subsequent pelvic catheterization for embolization.

4 Management of a hematoma within the broad ligament is dependent on its size and progression. A very large hematoma should be evacuated surgically with ligation of bleeding sites. If bleeding reoccurs, pelvic arteriography and embolization are again helpful for definitive therapy.

5 Patients should be treated with broad-spectrum antibiotics.

References

1 Sotto LSJ, Collins RJ. Perigenital hematomas. *Obstet Gynecol* 1958;12:259.

2 Pedowitz P, Pozner S, Adler N. Puerperal hematomas. *Am J Obstet Gynecol* 1961; 81:350.

3 Probst AM, Thorp JM. Traumatic vulvar hematoma: conservative versus surgical management. *South Med J* 1998;91:144.

4 Chin HG, Scott DR, Resnik R, *et al.* Angiographic embolization of intractable puerperal hematomas. *Am J Obstet Gynecol* 1989;160:434.

5 Gilbert WM, Moore TR, Resnik R, *et al.* Angiographic embolization in the manage-ment of hemorrhagic complications of pregnancy. *Am J Obstet Gynecol* 1992;166:493.

6 Clark SL, Phelan JP, Yeh SY, *et al.* Hypogastric artery ligation for obstetric hemor-rhage. *Obstet Gynecol* 1985;66:353.

7 Fargeaudo Y, Soyer P, Morel O, *et al.* Severe primary postpartum hemorrhage due to genital tract laceration after operative vaginal delivery: successful treatment with transcatheter arterial embolization. *Eur Radiol* 2009; May 5 (Epub).

PART 7
Clinical Reference Tables

APPENDIX A

Commonly Used Ultrasound Measurements

Antonino F. Barbera

Department of Obstetrics and Gynecology, Denver Health Medical Center, University of Colorado Denver School of Medicine, Denver, CO, USA

Protocols for High-Risk Pregnancies, 5th edition. Edited by J.T. Queenan, J.C. Hobbins and C.Y. Spong. © 2010 Blackwell Publishing Ltd.

Table A-1 Predicted menstrual age (MA) in weeks from crown–rump length (CRL) measurements (cm)*

CRL	MA	CRL	MA	CRL	MA	CRL	MA	CRL	MA	CRL	MA
0.2	5.7	2.2	8.9	4.2	11.1	6.2	12.6	8.2	14.2	10.2	16.1
0.3	5.9	2.3	9.0	4.3	11.2	6.3	12.7	8.3	14.2	10.3	16.2
0.4	6.1	2.4	9.1	4.4	11.2	6.4	12.8	8.4	14.3	10.4	16.3
0.5	6.2	2.5	9.2	4.5	11.3	6.5	12.8	8.5	14.4	10.5	16.4
0.6	6.4	2.6	9.4	4.6	11.4	6.6	12.9	8.6	14.5	10.6	16.5
0.7	6.6	2.7	9.5	4.7	11.5	6.7	13.0	8.7	14.6	10.7	16.6
0.8	6.7	2.8	9.6	4.8	11.6	6.8	13.1	8.8	14.7	10.8	16.7
0.9	6.9	2.9	9.7	4.9	11.7	6.9	13.1	8.9	14.8	10.9	16.8
1.0	7.2	3.0	9.9	5.0	11.7	7.0	13.2	9.0	14.9	11.0	16.9
1.1	7.2	3.1	10.0	5.1	11.8	7.1	13.3	9.1	15.0	11.1	17.0
1.2	7.4	3.2	10.1	5.2	11.9	7.2	13.4	9.2	15.1	11.2	17.1
1.3	7.5	3.3	10.2	5.3	12.0	7.3	13.4	9.3	15.2	11.3	17.2
1.4	7.7	3.4	10.3	5.4	12.0	7.4	13.5	9.4	15.3	11.4	17.3
1.5	7.9	3.5	10.4	5.5	12.1	7.5	13.6	9.5	15.3	11.5	17.4
1.6	8.0	3.6	10.5	5.6	12.2	7.6	13.7	9.6	15.4	11.6	17.5
1.7	8.1	3.7	10.6	5.7	12.3	7.7	13.8	9.7	15.5	11.7	17.6
1.8	8.3	3.8	10.7	5.8	12.3	7.8	13.8	9.8	15.6	11.8	17.7
1.9	8.4	3.9	10.8	5.9	12.4	7.9	13.9	9.9	15.7	11.9	17.8
2.0	8.6	4.0	10.9	6.0	12.5	8.0	14.0	10.0	15.9	12.0	17.9
2.1	8.7	4.1	11.0	6.1	12.6	8.1	14.1	10.1	16.0	12.1	18.0

*The 95% confidence interval is ±8% of the predicted age.
Source: Hadlock FP, Shah YP, Kanon DJ, Lindsey JV. Fetal crown–rump length: reevaluation of relation to menstrual age (5–18 weeks) with high-resolution real-time US. *Radiology* 1992;182:501–5.

Table A-2 Gestational sac measurement

Mean predicted gestational sac (cm)	Mean predicted gestational age (wk)	Gestational sac (cm)	Gestational age (wk)
1.0	5.0	3.6	8.8
1.1	5.2	3.7	8.9
1.2	5.3	3.8	9.0
1.3	5.5	3.9	9.2
1.4	5.6	4.0	9.3
1.5	5.8	4.1	9.5
1.6	5.9	4.2	9.6
1.7	6.0	4.3	9.7
1.8	6.2	4.4	9.9
1.9	6.3	4.5	10.0
2.0	6.5	4.6	10.2
2.1	6.6	4.7	10.3
2.2	6.8	4.8	10.5
2.3	6.9	4.9	10.6
2.4	7.0	5.0	10.7
2.5	7.2	5.1	10.9
2.6	7.3	5.2	11.0
2.7	7.5	5.3	11.2
2.8	7.6	5.4	11.3
2.9	7.8	5.5	11.5
3.0	7.9	5.6	11.6
3.1	8.0	5.7	11.7
3.2	8.2	5.8	11.9
3.3	8.3	5.9	12.0
3.4	8.5	6.0	12.2
3.5	8.6	–	–

Source: Hellman LM, Kobayashi M, Fillisti L, *et al*. Growth and development of the human fetus prior to the twentieth week of gestation. *Am J Obstet Gynecol* 1969;103:789.

Table A-3 Sac size versus hCG levels for normal pregnancies ($n = 56$)

Mean sac diameter (mm)	HCG level (mIU/mL) Predicted*	95% Confidence limits Lower	Upper
5	1,932	1,026	3,636
6	2,165	1,226	4,256
7	2,704	1,465	4,990
8	3,199	1,749	5,852
9	3,785	2,085	6,870
10	4,478	2,483	8,075
11	5,297	2,952	9,508
12	6,267	3,502	11,218
13	7,415	4,145	13,266
14	8,773	4,894	15,726
15	10,379	5,766	18,682
16	12,270	6,776	22,235
17	14,528	7,964	26,501
18	17,188	9,343	31,621
19	20,337	10,951	37,761
20	24,060	12,820	45,130
21	28,464	15,020	53,970
22	33,675	17,560	64,570
23	39,843	20,573	77,164

*$\log (HCG) = 2.92 + 0.073 (MSD)$, $R^2 = 0.93$, $P < 0.001$.
Source: Nyberg, DA, Filly, RA, Duane Filho, DL, *et al.* Abnormal pregnancy: early diagnosis by US and serum chorionic gonadotropin levels. *Radiology* 1986;158:393–6.

Table A-4 Reference values for length of nasal bone

Gestational age (wk)	Length of nasal bone (mm) −2 SD	Mean	+2 SD
14	3.3	4.2	5.0
16	3.1	5.2	7.3
18	5.0	6.3	7.6
20	5.7	7.6	9.5
22	6.0	8.2	10.4
24	6.8	9.4	12.0
26	7.2	9.7	12.3
28	7.8	10.7	13.6
30	8.3	11.3	14.4
32	8.0	11.6	15.2
34	7.5	12.3	17.0

Reproduced with permission from Guis F, Ville V, Vincent V, Doumerc S, Pons JC, *et al.* Ultrasound evaluation of the length of the fetal nasal bones throughout gestation. *Ultrasound Obstet Gynecol* 1995;5:304–7.

Table A-5 Biparietal diameter (BPD) and gestational age

BPD (cm)	Menstrual age (wk)	BPD (cm)	Menstrual age (wk)	BPD (cm)	Menstrual age (wk)	BPD (cm)	Menstrual age (wk)
2.0	12.2	4.0	18.0	6.0	24.6	8.0	32.5
2.1	12.5	4.1	18.3	6.1	25.0	8.1	32.9
2.2	12.8	4.2	18.6	6.2	25.3	8.2	33.3
2.3	13.1	4.3	18.9	6.3	25.7	8.3	33.8
2.4	13.3	4.4	19.2	6.4	26.1	8.4	34.2
2.5	13.6	4.5	19.5	6.5	26.4	8.5	34.7
2.6	13.9	4.6	19.9	6.6	26.8	8.6	35.1
2.7	14.2	4.7	20.2	6.7	27.2	8.7	35.6
2.8	12.5	4.8	20.5	6.8	27.6	8.8	36.1
2.9	14.7	4.9	20.8	6.9	28.0	8.9	36.5
3.0	15.0	5.0	21.2	7.0	28.3	9.0	37.0
3.1	15.3	5.1	21.5	7.1	28.7	9.1	37.5
3.2	15.6	5.2	21.8	7.2	29.1	9.2	38.0
3.3	15.9	5.3	22.2	7.3	29.5	9.3	38.5
3.4	16.2	5.4	22.5	7.4	29.9	9.4	38.9
3.5	16.5	5.5	22.8	7.5	30.4	9.5	39.4
3.6	16.8	5.6	23.2	7.6	30.8	9.6	39.9
3.7	17.1	5.7	23.5	7.7	31.2	9.7	40.5
3.8	17.4	5.8	23.9	7.8	21.6	9.8	41.0
3.9	17.7	5.9	24.2	7.9	32.0	9.9	41.5
–	–	–	–	–	–	10.0	42.0

Reproduced by permission from FP Hadlock, RL Deter, RB Harrist. Fetal biparietal diameter. *J Ultrasound Med* 1982;1:97.

Table A-6 Percentile values head circumference

Menstrual age (weeks)	Head circumference (cm) percentiles 3rd	10th	50th	90th	97th
14.0	8.8	9.1	9.7	10.3	10.6
15.0	10.0	10.4	11.0	11.6	12.0
16.0	11.3	11.7	12.4	13.1	13.5
17.0	12.6	13.0	13.8	14.6	15.0
18.0	13.7	14.2	15.1	16.0	16.5
19.0	14.9	15.5	16.4	17.4	17.9
20.0	16.1	16.7	17.7	18.7	19.3
21.0	17.2	17.8	18.9	20.0	20.6
22.0	18.3	18.9	20.1	21.3	21.9
23.0	19.4	20.1	21.3	22.5	23.2
24.0	20.4	21.1	22.4	23.7	24.3
25.0	21.4	22.2	23.5	24.9	25.6
26.0	22.4	23.2	24.6	26.0	26.8
27.0	23.3	24.1	25.6	27.0	27.9
28.0	24.2	25.1	26.6	28.1	29.0
29.0	25.0	25.9	27.5	29.1	30.0
30.0	25.8	26.8	28.4	30.0	31.0
31.0	26.7	27.6	29.3	31.0	31.9
32.0	27.4	28.4	30.1	31.8	32.8
33.0	28.0	29.0	30.8	32.6	33.6
34.0	28.7	29.7	31.5	33.3	34.3
35.0	29.3	30.4	32.2	34.1	35.1
36.0	29.9	30.9	32.8	34.7	35.8
37.0	30.3	31.4	33.3	35.2	36.3
38.0	30.8	31.9	34.2	36.2	36.8
39.0	31.1	32.2	34.2	36.2	37.3
40.0	31.5	32.6	34.6	36.6	37.7

Adapted from Hadlock FP, Deter RL, Harrist RB, Park SK. Estimating fetal age: computer-assisted analysis of multiple fetal growth parameters. *Radiology* 1984;152:497–501.

Table A-7 Reference values for abdominal circumference

Menstrual age (wk)	Abdominal circumference (cm) percentiles				
	3rd	10th	50th	90th	97th
14.0	6.4	6.7	7.3	7.9	8.3
15.0	7.5	7.9	8.6	9.3	9.7
16.0	8.6	9.1	9.9	10.7	11.2
17.0	9.2	10.3	11.2	12.1	12.7
18.0	10.9	11.5	12.5	13.5	14.1
19.0	11.9	12.6	13.7	14.8	15.5
20.0	13.1	13.8	15.0	16.3	17.0
21.0	14.1	14.9	16.2	17.6	18.3
22.0	15.1	16.0	17.4	18.8	19.7
23.0	16.1	17.0	18.5	20.0	20.9
24.0	17.1	18.1	19.7	21.3	22.3
25.0	18.1	19.1	20.8	22.5	23.5
26.0	19.1	20.1	21.9	23.7	24.8
27.0	20.0	21.1	23.0	24.9	26.0
28.0	20.9	22.0	24.0	26.0	27.1
29.0	21.8	23.0	25.1	27.2	28.4
30.0	22.7	23.9	26.1	28.3	29.5
31.0	23.6	24.9	27.1	29.4	30.6
32.0	24.5	25.8	28.1	30.4	31.8
33.0	25.3	26.7	29.1	31.5	32.9
34.0	26.1	27.5	30.0	32.5	33.9
35.0	26.9	28.3	30.9	33.5	34.9
36.0	27.7	29.2	31.8	34.4	35.9
37.0	28.5	30.0	32.7	35.4	37.0
38.0	29.2	30.8	33.6	36.4	38.0
39.0	29.9	31.6	34.4	37.3	38.9
40.0	30.7	32.4	35.3	38.2	39.9

Adapted from Hadlock FP, Deter RL, Harrist RB, Park SK. Estimating fetal age: computer-assisted analysis of multiple fetal growth parameters. *Radiology* 1984;152:497–501.

Table A-8 Reference values for femur length

Menstrual age (wk)	Femur length (cm) percentiles				
	3rd	10th	50th	90th	97th
14.0	1.2	1.3	1.4	1.5	1.6
15.0	1.5	1.6	1.7	1.9	1.9
16.0	1.7	1.8	2.0	2.2	2.3
17.0	2.1	2.2	2.4	2.6	2.7
18.0	2.3	2.5	2.7	2.9	3.1
19.0	2.6	2.7	3.0	3.3	3.4
20.0	2.8	3.0	3.3	3.6	3.8
21.0	3.0	3.2	3.5	3.8	4.0
22.0	3.3	3.5	3.8	4.1	4.3
23.0	3.5	3.7	4.1	4.5	4.7
24.0	3.8	4.0	4.4	4.8	5.0
25.0	4.0	4.2	4.6	5.0	5.2
26.0	4.2	4.5	4.9	5.3	5.6
27.0	4.4	4.6	5.1	5.6	5.8
28.0	4.6	4.9	5.4	5.9	6.2
29.0	4.8	5.1	5.6	6.1	6.4
30.0	5.0	5.3	5.8	6.3	6.6
31.0	5.2	5.5	6.0	6.5	6.8
32.0	5.3	5.6	6.2	6.8	7.1
33.0	5.5	5.8	6.4	7.0	7.3
34.0	5.7	6.0	6.6	7.2	7.5
35.0	5.9	6.2	6.8	7.4	7.8
36.0	6.0	6.4	7.0	7.6	8.0
37.0	6.2	6.6	7.2	7.9	8.2
38.0	6.4	6.7	7.4	8.1	8.4
39.0	6.5	6.8	7.5	8.2	8.6
40.0	6.6	7.0	7.7	8.4	8.8

Adapted from Hadlock FP, Deter RL, Harrist RB, Park SK. Estimating fetal age: computer-assisted analysis of multiple fetal growth parameters. *Radiology* 1984;152:497–501.

Table A-9 Length of fetal long bones (mm)

Week no.	Humerus percentile			Ulna percentile			Radius percentile			Femur percentile			Tibia percentile			Fibula percentile		
	5	50	95	5	50	95	5	50	95	5	50	95	5	50	95	5	50	95
11	–	6	–	–	5	–	–	5	–	–	6	–	–	4	–	–	2	–
12	3	9	10	–	8	–	–	7	–	–	9	–	–	7	–	–	5	–
13	5	13	20	3	11	18	–	10	–	6	12	19	4	10	17	–	8	–
14	5	16	20	4	13	17	8	13	12	5	15	19	2	13	19	6	11	10
15	11	18	26	10	16	22	12	15	19	11	19	26	5	16	27	10	14	18
16	12	21	25	8	19	24	9	18	21	13	22	24	7	19	25	6	17	22
17	19	24	29	11	21	32	11	20	29	20	25	29	15	22	29	7	19	31
18	18	27	30	13	24	30	14	22	26	19	28	31	14	24	29	10	22	28
19	22	29	36	20	26	32	20	24	29	23	31	38	19	27	35	18	24	30
20	23	32	36	21	29	32	21	27	28	22	33	39	19	29	35	18	27	30
21	28	34	40	25	31	36	25	29	32	27	36	45	24	32	39	24	29	34
22	28	36	40	24	33	37	24	31	34	29	39	44	25	34	39	21	31	37
23	32	38	45	27	35	43	26	32	39	35	41	48	30	36	43	23	33	44
24	31	41	46	29	37	41	27	34	38	34	44	49	28	39	45	26	35	41
25	35	43	51	34	39	44	31	36	40	38	46	54	31	41	50	33	37	42
26	36	45	49	34	41	44	30	37	41	39	49	53	33	43	49	32	39	43

(*Continued*)

Table A-9 (Continued)

Week no	Humerus percentile			Ulna percentile			Radius percentile			Femur percentile			Tibia percentile			Fibula percentile		
	5	50	95	5	50	95	5	50	95	5	50	95	5	50	95	5	50	95
27	42	46	51	37	43	48	33	39	45	45	51	57	39	45	51	35	41	47
28	41	48	52	37	44	48	33	40	45	45	53	57	38	47	52	36	43	47
29	44	50	56	40	46	51	36	42	47	49	56	62	40	49	57	40	45	50
30	44	52	56	38	47	54	34	43	49	49	58	62	41	51	56	38	47	52
31	47	53	59	39	49	59	34	44	53	53	60	67	46	52	58	40	48	57
32	47	55	59	40	50	58	37	45	51	53	62	67	46	54	59	40	50	56
33	50	56	62	43	52	60	41	46	51	56	64	71	49	56	62	43	51	59
34	50	57	62	44	53	59	39	47	53	57	65	70	47	57	64	46	52	56
35	52	58	65	47	54	61	38	48	57	61	67	73	48	59	69	51	54	57
36	53	60	63	47	55	61	41	48	54	61	69	74	49	60	68	51	55	56
37	57	61	64	49	56	62	45	49	53	64	71	77	52	61	71	55	56	58
38	55	61	66	48	57	63	45	49	53	62	72	79	54	62	69	54	57	59
39	56	62	69	49	57	66	46	50	54	64	74	83	58	64	69	55	58	62
40	56	63	69	50	58	65	46	50	54	66	75	81	58	65	69	54	59	62

Source: Jeanty P. Fetal Limb biometry (letter). *Radiology* 1983;147:602.

Table A-10 Fetal weight percentiles by gestational age

Gestational age (wk)	Fetal weight percentiles (g)				
	3rd	10th	50th	90th	97th
10	26	29	35	41	44
11	34	37	45	53	56
12	43	48	58	68	73
13	54	61	73	85	92
14	69	77	93	109	117
15	87	97	117	137	147
16	109	121	146	171	183
17	135	150	181	212	227
18	166	185	223	261	280
19	204	227	273	319	342
20	247	275	331	387	415
21	298	331	399	467	500
22	357	397	478	559	599
23	424	472	568	664	712
24	500	556	670	784	840
25	586	652	785	918	984
26	681	758	913	1,068	1,145
27	787	876	1,055	1,234	1,323
28	903	1,005	1,210	1,415	1,517
29	1,029	1,145	1,379	1,613	1,729
30	1,163	1,294	1,559	1,824	1,955
31	1,306	1,454	1,751	2,048	2,196
32	1,457	1,621	1,953	2,285	2,449
33	1,613	1,795	2,162	2,529	2,711
34	1,773	1,973	2,377	2,781	2,981
35	1,936	2,154	2,595	3,036	3,254
36	2,098	2,335	2,813	3,291	3,528
37	2,259	2,514	3,028	3,542	3,797
38	2,414	2,687	3,236	3,785	4,058
39	2,563	2,852	3,435	4,018	4,307
40	2,700	3,004	3,619	4,234	4,538
41	2.825	3,144	3,787	4,430	4,749
42	2.935	3,266	3,934	4,602	4,933

Ln. natural log; MA, menstrual age; wt, weight.

Note: Ln (wt) = 0.578 + 0.332 MA − 0.00354 × MA2; standard deviation = 12.7% of predicted weight.

Reproduced with permission from Hadlock FP, Harrist RB. Marinez-Poyer J. In utero analysis of fetal growth: a sonographic weight standard. *Radiology* 1991;181:129–33 (extrapolated to 42 weeks from 40 weeks).

Table A-11 Estimated fetal weights

Biparietal diameters	Abdominal circumferences																									
	15.5	16.0	16.5	17.0	17.5	18.0	18.5	19.0	19.5	20.0	20.5	21.0	21.5	22.0	22.5	23.0	23.5	24.0	24.5	25.0	25.5	26.0	26.5	27.0	27.5	28.0
3.1	224	234	244	255	267	279	291	304	318	332	346	362	378	395	412	431	450	470	491	513	536	559	584	610	638	666
3.2	231	241	251	263	274	286	299	312	326	340	355	371	388	405	423	441	461	481	502	525	548	572	597	624	651	680
3.3	237	248	259	270	282	294	307	321	335	349	365	381	397	415	433	452	472	493	514	537	560	585	611	638	666	695
3.4	244	255	266	278	290	302	316	329	344	359	374	391	408	425	444	463	483	504	526	549	573	598	624	652	680	710
3.5	251	262	274	285	298	311	324	338	353	368	384	401	418	436	455	475	495	517	539	562	587	612	638	666	695	725
3.6	259	270	281	294	306	319	333	347	362	378	394	411	429	447	466	486	507	529	552	575	600	626	653	681	710	740
3.7	266	278	290	302	315	328	342	357	372	388	404	422	440	458	478	498	519	542	565	589	614	640	667	696	725	756
3.8	274	286	298	310	324	337	352	366	382	398	415	432	451	470	490	510	532	554	578	602	628	654	682	711	741	772
3.9	282	294	306	319	333	347	361	376	392	409	426	444	462	482	502	523	545	568	592	616	642	669	697	727	757	789
4.0	290	303	315	328	342	356	371	386	403	419	437	455	474	494	514	536	558	581	606	631	657	684	713	743	773	806
4.1	299	311	324	338	352	366	381	397	413	430	448	467	486	506	527	549	572	595	620	645	672	700	729	759	790	828
4.2	308	320	333	347	361	376	392	408	424	442	460	479	498	519	540	562	585	609	634	660	688	716	743	776	807	841
4.3	317	330	343	357	371	387	402	419	436	453	472	491	511	532	554	576	600	624	649	676	703	732	762	793	825	859
4.4	326	339	353	367	382	397	413	430	447	465	484	504	524	545	567	590	614	639	665	692	719	749	779	810	843	877
4.5	335	349	363	377	393	408	425	442	459	478	497	517	538	559	581	605	629	654	680	708	736	765	796	828	861	896
4.6	345	359	373	388	404	420	436	454	472	490	510	530	551	573	596	620	644	670	696	724	753	783	814	846	880	915
4.7	355	369	384	399	415	431	448	466	484	503	523	544	565	588	611	635	660	686	713	741	770	801	832	865	899	934
4.8	366	380	395	410	426	443	460	478	497	517	537	558	580	602	626	650	676	702	730	758	788	819	851	884	919	954
4.9	376	391	406	422	438	455	473	491	510	530	551	572	594	617	641	666	692	719	747	776	806	837	870	903	938	975
5.0	387	402	418	434	451	468	486	505	524	544	565	587	610	633	657	683	709	736	765	794	824	856	889	923	959	996
5.1	399	414	430	446	463	481	499	518	538	559	580	602	625	649	674	699	726	754	783	812	843	876	909	944	980	1,017
5.2	410	426	442	459	476	494	513	532	552	573	595	618	641	665	690	717	744	772	801	831	863	895	929	964	1,001	1,039
5.3	422	438	455	472	489	508	527	547	567	589	611	634	657	682	708	734	762	790	820	851	883	916	950	986	1,023	1,061
5.4	435	451	468	485	503	522	541	561	582	604	627	650	674	699	725	752	780	809	839	870	903	936	971	1,007	1,045	1,084
5.5	447	464	481	499	517	536	556	577	598	620	643	667	691	717	743	771	799	828	859	891	924	958	993	1,030	1,068	1,107

Biparietal diameters																									
5.6	461	477	495	513	532	551	571	592	614	636	660	684	709	735	762	789	818	848	879	911	945	979	1,015	1,052	1,091	1,131
5.7	474	491	509	527	547	566	587	608	630	653	677	701	727	753	780	809	838	869	900	933	966	1,001	1,038	1,075	1,114	1,155
5.8	488	505	524	542	562	582	603	625	647	670	695	719	745	772	800	829	858	889	921	954	989	1,024	1,061	1,099	1,139	1,180
5.9	502	520	539	558	578	598	619	642	664	688	713	738	764	792	820	849	879	911	943	977	1,011	1,047	1,085	1,123	1,163	1,205
6.0	517	535	554	573	594	615	636	659	682	706	731	757	784	811	840	870	900	932	965	999	1,035	1,071	1,109	1,148	1,189	1,231
6.1	532	550	570	590	610	632	654	677	700	725	750	777	804	832	861	891	922	955	988	1,023	1,058	1,095	1,134	1,173	1,214	1,257
6.2	547	566	586	606	627	649	672	695	719	744	770	797	824	853	882	913	945	977	1,011	1,046	1,083	1,120	1,159	1,199	1,241	1,284
6.3	563	583	603	624	645	667	690	714	738	764	790	817	845	874	904	935	967	1,001	1,035	1,071	1,107	1,145	1,185	1,226	1,268	1,311
6.4	580	600	620	641	663	686	709	733	758	784	811	838	867	896	927	958	991	1,025	1,059	1,096	1,133	1,171	1,211	1,253	1,295	1,339
6.5	597	617	638	659	682	705	728	753	778	805	832	860	889	919	950	982	1,015	1,049	1,084	1,121	1,159	1,198	1,238	1,280	1,323	1,368

Biparietal diameters	Abdominal circumferences																							
	28.5	29.0	29.5	30.0	30.5	31.0	31.5	32.0	32.5	33.0	33.5	34.0	34.5	35.0	35.5	36.0	36.5	37.0	37.5	38.0	38.5	39.0	39.5	40.0
3.1	696	726	759	793	828	865	903	943	985	1,029	1,075	1,123	1,173	1,225	1,279	1,336	1,396	1,458	1,523	1,591	1,661	1,735	1,812	1,893
3.2	710	742	774	809	844	882	921	961	1,004	1,048	1,094	1,143	1,193	1,246	1,301	1,358	1,418	1,481	1,546	1,615	1,686	1,761	1,838	1,920
3.3	725	757	790	825	861	899	938	979	1,022	1,067	1,114	1,163	1,214	1,267	1,323	1,381	1,441	1,504	1,570	1,639	1,711	1,786	1,865	1,946
3.4	740	773	806	841	878	916	956	998	1,041	1,087	1,134	1,183	1,235	1,289	1,345	1,403	1,464	1,528	1,595	1,664	1,737	1,812	1,891	1,973
3.5	756	789	823	858	896	934	975	1,017	1,061	1,107	1,154	1,204	1,256	1,311	1,367	1,426	1,488	1,552	1,619	1,689	1,762	1,839	1,918	2,001
3.6	772	805	840	876	913	953	993	1,036	1,080	1,127	1,175	1,226	1,278	1,333	1,390	1,450	1,512	1,577	1,645	1,715	1,789	1,865	1,945	2,029
3.7	788	822	857	893	931	971	1,012	1,056	1,101	1,147	1,196	1,247	1,300	1,356	1,413	1,474	1,536	1,602	1,670	1,741	1,815	1,893	1,973	2,057
3.8	805	839	874	911	950	990	1,032	1,076	1,121	1,168	1,218	1,269	1,323	1,379	1,437	1,498	1,561	1,627	1,696	1,768	1,842	1,920	2,001	2,086
3.9	822	856	892	930	969	1,009	1,052	1,096	1,142	1,190	1,240	1,292	1,346	1,402	1,461	1,523	1,586	1,653	1,722	1,794	1,870	1,948	2,030	2,115
4.0	839	874	911	949	988	1,029	1,072	1,117	1,163	1,212	1,262	1,315	1,369	1,426	1,486	1,548	1,612	1,679	1,749	1,822	1,898	1,977	2,059	2,145
4.1	857	892	929	968	1,008	1,049	1,093	1,138	1,185	1,234	1,285	1,338	1,393	1,451	1,511	1,573	1,638	1,706	1,776	1,849	1,926	2,005	2,088	2,174
4.2	875	911	948	987	1,028	1,070	1,114	1,159	1,207	1,256	1,308	1,361	1,417	1,475	1,536	1,599	1,664	1,733	1,804	1,878	1,954	2,035	2,118	2,205
4.3	893	930	968	1,007	1,048	1,091	1,135	1,181	1,229	1,279	1,331	1,385	1,442	1,500	1,562	1,625	1,691	1,760	1,832	1,906	1,984	2,064	2,148	2,236
4.4	912	949	987	1,027	1,069	1,112	1,157	1,204	1,252	1,303	1,355	1,410	1,467	1,526	1,588	1,652	1,718	1,788	1,860	1,935	2,013	2,094	2,179	2,267
4.5	932	969	1,008	1,048	1,090	1,134	1,179	1,226	1,275	1,326	1,380	1,435	1,492	1,552	1,614	1,679	1,746	1,816	1,889	1,964	2,043	2,125	2,210	2,298
4.6	951	989	1,028	1,069	1,112	1,156	1,202	1,249	1,299	1,351	1,404	1,460	1,518	1,579	1,641	1,706	1,774	1,845	1,918	1,994	2,073	2,156	2,241	2,330

(Continued)

Table A-11 (Continued)

Abdominal circumferences

Biparietal diameters	28.5	29.0	29.5	30.0	30.5	31.0	31.5	32.0	32.5	33.0	33.5	34.0	34.5	35.0	35.5	36.0	36.5	37.0	37.5	38.0	38.5	39.0	39.5	40.0
4.7	971	1,010	1,049	1,091	1,134	1,178*	1,225	1,273	1,323	1,375	1,430	1,486	1,545	1,605	1,669	1,734	1,803	1,874	1,948	2,024	2,104	2,187	2,273	2,363
4.8	992	1,031	1,071	1,113	1,156	1,201	1,248	1,297	1,348	1,401	1,455	1,512	1,571	1,633	1,697	1,763	1,832	1,904	1,978	2,055	2,136	2,219	2,306	2,396
4.9	1,013	1,052	1,093	1,135	1,179	1,225	1,272	1,322	1,373	1,426	1,482	1,539	1,599	1,661	1,725	1,792	1,861	1,934	2,009	2,086	2,167	2,251	2,339	2,429
5.0	1,034	1,074	1,115	1,158	1,203	1,249	1,297	1,347	1,399	1,452	1,508	1,566	1,626	1,689	1,754	1,821	1,891	1,964	2,040	2,118	2,200	2,284	2,372	2,463
5.1	1,056	1,096	1,138	1,181	1,226	1,273	1,322	1,372	1,425	1,479	1,535	1,594	1,655	1,718	1,783	1,851	1,922	1,995	2,071	2,150	2,232	2,317	2,406	2,498
5.2	1,078	1,119	1,161	1,205	1,251	1,298	1,347	1,398	1,451	1,506	1,563	1,622	1,683	1,747	1,813	1,882	1,953	2,027	2,103	2,183	2,266	2,351	2,440	2,532
5.3	1,101	1,142	1,185	1,229	1,276	1,323	1,373	1,425	1,478	1,533	1,591	1,651	1,713	1,777	1,843	1,913	1,984	2,059	2,136	2,216	2,299	2,386	2,475	2,568
5.4	1,124	1,166	1,209	1,254	1,301	1,349	1,399	1,452	1,506	1,562	1,620	1,680	1,742	1,807	1,874	1,944	2,016	2,091	2,169	2,250	2,333	2,420	2,510	2,604
5.5	1,148	1,190	1,234	1,279	1,327	1,376	1,426	1,479	1,534	1,590	1,649	1,710	1,773	1,838	1,906	1,976	2,049	2,124	2,203	2,284	2,368	2,456	2,546	2,640
5.6	1,172	1,215	1,259	1,305	1,353	1,402	1,454	1,507	1,562	1,619	1,678	1,740	1,803	1,869	1,938	2,008	2,082	2,158	2,237	2,319	2,403	2,491	2,582	2,677
5.7	1,197	1,240	1,285	1,332	1,380	1,430	1,482	1,535	1,591	1,649	1,709	1,770	1,835	1,901	1,970	2,041	2,115	2,192	2,272	2,354	2,439	2,528	2,619	2,714
5.8	1,222	1,266	1,311	1,358	1,407	1,458	1,510	1,564	1,621	1,679	1,739	1,802	1,866	1,934	2,003	2,075	2,150	2,227	2,307	2,390	2,475	2,564	2,657	2,752
5.9	1,248	1,292	1,338	1,386	1,435	1,486	1,539	1,594	1,651	1,710	1,770	1,834	1,899	1,966	2,037	2,109	2,184	2,262	2,342	2,426	2,512	2,602	2,694	2,790
6.0	1,274	1,319	1,366	1,414	1,464	1,515	1,569	1,624	1,682	1,741	1,802	1,866	1,932	2,000	2,071	2,144	2,219	2,298	2,379	2,463	2,550	2,640	2,733	2,829
6.1	1,301	1,346	1,393	1,442	1,493	1,545	1,599	1,655	1,713	1,773	1,835	1,899	1,965	2,034	2,105	2,179	2,255	2,334	2,416	2,500	2,588	2,678	2,772	2,869
6.2	1,328	1,374	1,422	1,471	1,522	1,575	1,630	1,686	1,745	1,805	1,868	1,932	1,999	2,069	2,140	2,215	2,291	2,371	2,453	2,538	2,626	2,717	2,811	2,909
6.3	1,356	1,403	1,451	1,501	1,552	1,606	1,661	1,718	1,777	1,838	1,901	1,967	2,034	2,104	2,176	2,251	2,328	2,408	2,491	2,577	2,665	2,757	2,851	2,949
6.4	1,385	1,432	1,481	1,531	1,583	1,637	1,693	1,751	1,810	1,872	1,935	2,001	2,069	2,140	2,213	2,288	2,366	2,446	2,530	2,616	2,705	2,797	2,892	2,991

Abdominal circumferences

Biparietal diameters	15.5	16.0	16.5	17.0	17.5	18.0	18.5	19.0	19.5	20.0	20.5	21.0	21.5	22.0	22.5	23.0	23.5	24.0	24.5	25.0	25.5	26.0	26.5	27.0	27.5	28.0
6.6	614	635	656	678	701	724	748	773	799	826	853	882	911	942	973	1,006	1,039	1,074	1,110	1,147	1,185	1,225	1,266	1,308	1,352	1,397
6.7	632	653	675	697	720	744	769	794	820	848	876	905	935	965	997	1,030	1,065	1,100	1,136	1,174	1,213	1,253	1,294	1,337	1,381	1,427
6.8	651	672	694	717	740	765	790	816	842	870	898	928	958	990	1,022	1,056	1,090	1,126	1,163	1,201	1,241	1,281	1,323	1,367	1,411	1,458
6.9	670	691	714	737	761	786	811	838	865	893	922	952	983	1,015	1,048	1,082	1,117	1,153	1,190	1,229	1,269	1,310	1,353	1,397	1,442	1,489
7.0	689	711	734	758	782	807	833	860	888	916	946	976	1,008	1,040	1,074	1,108	1,144	1,181	1,219	1,258	1,298	1,340	1,383	1,427	1,473	1,521
7.1	709	732	755	779	804	830	856	883	912	941	971	1,002	1,033	1,066	1,100	1,135	1,171	1,209	1,247	1,287	1,328	1,370	1,414	1,459	1,505	1,553

(Continued)

7.2	730	763	777	801	827	853	880	907	936	965	996	1,027	1,060	1,093	1,128	1,163	1,200	1,238	1,277	1,317	1,358	1,401	1,445	1,491	1,538	1,586
7.3	751	775	799	824	850	876	904	932	961	991	1,022	1,054	1,087	1,121	1,156	1,192	1,229	1,267	1,307	1,348	1,390	1,433	1,478	1,524	1,571	1,620
7.4	773	797	822	847	874	901	928	957	987	1,017	1,049	1,081	1,114	1,149	1,184	1,221	1,259	1,297	1,338	1,379	1,421	1,465	1,511	1,557	1,605	1,655
7.5	796	820	845	871	898	925	954	983	1,013	1,044	1,076	1,109	1,143	1,178	1,214	1,251	1,289	1,328	1,369	1,411	1,454	1,499	1,544	1,592	1,640	1,690
7.6	819	844	870	896	923	951	980	1,009	1,040	1,072	1,104	1,137	1,172	1,207	1,244	1,281	1,320	1,360	1,401	1,444	1,487	1,533	1,579	1,627	1,676	1,727
7.7	843	868	894	921	949	977	1,007	1,037	1,068	1,100	1,133	1,167	1,202	1,238	1,275	1,313	1,352	1,393	1,434	1,477	1,522	1,567	1,614	1,663	1,712	1,764
7.8	868	894	920	947	975	1,004	1,034	1,065	1,096	1,129	1,162	1,197	1,232	1,269	1,306	1,345	1,385	1,426	1,468	1,512	1,557	1,603	1,650	1,699	1,749	1,801
7.9	893	919	946	974	1,003	1,032	1,062	1,094	1,126	1,159	1,193	1,228	1,264	1,301	1,339	1,378	1,418	1,460	1,503	1,547	1,592	1,639	1,687	1,737	1,787	1,840
8.0	919	946	973	1,002	1,031	1,061	1,091	1,123	1,156	1,189	1,224	1,259	1,296	1,333	1,372	1,412	1,453	1,495	1,538	1,583	1,629	1,676	1,725	1,775	1,826	1,879
8.1	946	973	1,001	1,030	1,060	1,090	1,121	1,153	1,187	1,221	1,256	1,292	1,329	1,367	1,406	1,446	1,488	1,531	1,575	1,620	1,666	1,714	1,763	1,814	1,866	1,919
8.2	974	1,001	1,030	1,059	1,089	1,120	1,152	1,185	1,218	1,253	1,288	1,325	1,363	1,401	1,441	1,482	1,524	1,567	1,612	1,657	1,704	1,753	1,803	1,854	1,906	1,960
8.3	1,002	1,030	1,059	1,089	1,120	1,151	1,183	1,217	1,251	1,286	1,322	1,359	1,397	1,436	1,477	1,518	1,561	1,605	1,650	1,696	1,744	1,793	1,843	1,895	1,948	2,002
8.4	1,032	1,060	1,090	1,120	1,151	1,183	1,216	1,249	1,284	1,320	1,356	1,394	1,433	1,473	1,513	1,555	1,599	1,643	1,689	1,735	1,784	1,833	1,884	1,936	1,990	2,045
8.5	1,062	1,091	1,121	1,151	1,183	1,216	1,249	1,283	1,318	1,355	1,392	1,430	1,469	1,510	1,551	1,594	1,637	1,682	1,728	1,776	1,825	1,875	1,926	1,979	2,033	2,089
8.6	1,093	1,122	1,153	1,184	1,216	1,249	1,283	1,318	1,354	1,390	1,428	1,467	1,507	1,548	1,589	1,633	1,677	1,722	1,769	1,817	1,866	1,917	1,969	2,022	2,077	2,134
8.7	1,125	1,155	1,186	1,218	1,250	1,284	1,318	1,353	1,390	1,427	1,465	1,505	1,545	1,586	1,629	1,673	1,717	1,764	1,811	1,859	1,909	1,960	2,013	2,067	2,122	2,179
8.8	1,157	1,188	1,220	1,252	1,285	1,319	1,354	1,390	1,427	1,465	1,504	1,543	1,584	1,626	1,669	1,714	1,759	1,806	1,854	1,903	1,953	2,005	2,058	2,113	2,169	2,226
8.9	1,191	1,222	1,254	1,287	1,321	1,356	1,391	1,428	1,465	1,503	1,543	1,583	1,625	1,667	1,711	1,756	1,802	1,849	1,897	1,947	1,998	2,050	2,104	2,159	2,216	2,274
9.0	1,226	1,258	1,290	1,324	1,358	1,393	1,429	1,456	1,504	1,543	1,583	1,624	1,666	1,709	1,753	1,799	1,845	1,893	1,942	1,992	2,044	2,097	2,151	2,207	2,264	2,322
9.1	1,262	1,294	1,327	1,361	1,396	1,432	1,468	1,506	1,544	1,584	1,624	1,666	1,708	1,752	1,797	1,843	1,890	1,938	1,988	2,039	2,091	2,144	2,199	2,255	2,313	2,372
9.2	1,299	1,332	1,365	1,400	1,435	1,471	1,508	1,546	1,586	1,626	1,667	1,709	1,752	1,796	1,841	1,888	1,936	1,984	2,035	2,086	2,139	2,193	2,248	2,305	2,363	2,423
9.3	1,337	1,370	1,404	1,439	1,475	1,512	1,550	1,588	1,628	1,668	1,710	1,753	1,796	1,841	1,887	1,934	1,982	2,032	2,083	2,135	2,188	2,242	2,298	2,356	2,414	2,475
9.4	1,376	1,410	1,444	1,480	1,516	1,554	1,592	1,631	1,671	1,712	1,755	1,798	1,842	1,887	1,934	1,982	2,030	2,080	2,132	2,184	2,238	2,293	2,350	2,407	2,467	2,527
9.5	1,416	1,450	1,486	1,522	1,559	1,597	1,635	1,675	1,716	1,758	1,800	1,844	1,889	1,935	1,982	2,030	2,080	2,130	2,182	2,235	2,289	2,345	2,402	2,460	2,520	2,582
9.6	1,457	1,492	1,528	1,565	1,602	1,641	1,680	1,720	1,762	1,804	1,847	1,892	1,937	1,984	2,031	2,080	2,130	2,181	2,233	2,287	2,342	2,398	2,456	2,515	2,575	2,637
9.7	1,500	1,535	1,572	1,609	1,647	1,686	1,726	1,767	1,809	1,852	1,895	1,940	1,986	2,033	2,082	2,131	2,181	2,233	2,286	2,340	2,395	2,452	2,510	2,570	2,631	2,693
9.8	1,544	1,580	1,617	1,654	1,693	1,733	1,773	1,815	1,857	1,900	1,945	1,990	2,037	2,085	2,133	2,183	2,234	2,286	2,340	2,395	2,451	2,508	2,567	2,627	2,688	2,751
9.9	1,589	1,625	1,663	1,701	1,740	1,781	1,822	1,864	1,907	1,951	1,996	2,042	2,089	2,137	2,186	2,237	2,288	2,341	2,395	2,450	2,507	2,565	2,624	2,684	2,746	2,810
10.0	1,635	1,672	1,710	1,749	1,789	1,830	1,871	1,914	1,958	2,002	2,048	2,094	2,142	2,191	2,241	2,292	2,344	2,397	2,452	2,507	2,564	2,623	2,682	2,743	2,806	2,870

Table A-11 (Continued)

Biparietal diameters	Abdominal circumferences																							
	28.5	29.0	29.5	30.0	30.5	31.0	31.5	32.0	32.5	33.0	33.5	34.0	34.5	35.0	35.5	36.0	36.5	37.0	37.5	38.0	38.5	39.0	39.5	40.0
6.6	1,444	1,492	1,542	1,594	1,647	1,702	1,759	1,817	1,878	1,941	2,006	2,073	2,142	2,213	2,287	2,364	2,443	2,524	2,609	2,696	2,786	2,879	2,975	3,075
6.7	1,474	1,523	1,574	1,626	1,679	1,735	1,792	1,852	1,913	1,976	2,042	2,109	2,179	2,251	2,326	2,403	2,482	2,564	2,649	2,737	2,827	2,921	3,018	3,117
6.8	1,505	1,555	1,606	1,658	1,713	1,769	1,827	1,887	1,949	2,012	2,078	2,147	2,217	2,290	2,365	2,442	2,522	2,605	2,690	2,778	2,869	2,964	3,061	3,161
6.9	1,537	1,587	1,639	1,692	1,747	1,803	1,862	1,922	1,985	2,049	2,116	2,184	2,255	2,329	2,404	2,482	2,563	2,646	2,732	2,821	2,912	3,007	3,104	3,205
7.0	1,570	1,620	1,672	1,726	1,781	1,839	1,898	1,959	2,022	2,087	2,154	2,223	2,295	2,368	2,444	2,523	2,604	2,688	2,774	2,863	2,955	3,050	3,149	3,250
7.1	1,603	1,654	1,706	1,761	1,817	1,875	1,934	1,996	2,059	2,125	2,193	2,262	2,334	2,409	2,485	2,564	2,646	2,730	2,817	2,907	2,999	3,095	3,193	3,295
7.2	1,636	1,688	1,741	1,796	1,853	1,911	1,971	2,034	2,098	2,164	2,232	2,302	2,375	2,450	2,527	2,607	2,689	2,773	2,861	2,951	3,044	3,140	3,239	3,341
7.3	1,671	1,723	1,777	1,832	1,890	1,948	2,009	2,072	2,137	2,203	2,272	2,343	2,416	2,491	2,569	2,649	2,732	2,817	2,905	2,996	3,089	3,186	3,285	3,388
7.4	1,706	1,759	1,813	1,869	1,927	1,987	2,048	2,111	2,176	2,244	2,313	2,384	2,458	2,534	2,612	2,693	2,776	2,862	2,950	3,041	3,135	3,232	3,332	3,435
7.5	1,742	1,795	1,850	1,907	1,965	2,025	2,087	2,151	2,217	2,285	2,354	2,426	2,501	2,577	2,656	2,737	2,821	2,907	2,996	3,088	3,182	3,279	3,380	3,483
7.6	1,779	1,833	1,888	1,945	2,004	2,065	2,127	2,192	2,258	2,326	2,397	2,469	2,544	2,621	2,700	2,782	2,866	2,953	3,042	3,134	3,229	3,327	3,428	3,531
7.7	1,816	1,871	1,927	1,985	2,044	2,105	2,168	2,233	2,300	2,369	2,440	2,513	2,588	2,666	2,746	2,828	2,912	3,000	3,090	3,182	3,277	3,376	3,477	3,581
7.8	1,855	1,910	1,966	2,025	2,085	2,146	2,210	2,275	2,343	2,412	2,484	2,557	2,633	2,711	2,792	2,874	2,959	3,047	3,137	3,230	3,326	3,425	3,526	3,631
7.9	1,894	1,949	2,006	2,065	2,126	2,188	2,252	2,318	2,386	2,456	2,528	2,603	2,679	2,757	2,838	2,921	3,007	3,095	3,186	3,279	3,376	3,475	3,576	3,681
8.0	1,934	1,990	2,048	2,107	2,168	2,231	2,296	2,362	2,431	2,501	2,574	2,649	2,725	2,804	2,886	2,969	3,056	3,144	3,235	3,329	3,426	3,525	3,627	3,733
8.1	1,975	2,031	2,089	2,149	2,211	2,275	2,340	2,407	2,476	2,547	2,620	2,695	2,773	2,852	2,934	3,018	3,105	3,194	3,286	3,380	3,477	3,577	3,679	3,785
8.2	2,016	2,073	2,132	2,193	2,255	2,319	2,385	2,453	2,522	2,594	2,667	2,743	2,821	2,901	2,983	3,068	3,155	3,244	3,336	3,431	3,529	3,629	3,732	3,838
8.3	2,059	2,116	2,176	2,237	2,300	2,364	2,431	2,499	2,569	2,641	2,715	2,791	2,870	2,950	3,033	3,118	3,206	3,296	3,388	3,483	3,581	3,682	3,785	3,891
8.4	2,102	2,160	2,220	2,282	2,345	2,410	2,477	2,546	2,617	2,689	2,764	2,841	2,920	3,001	3,084	3,169	3,257	3,348	3,441	3,536	3,634	3,735	3,839	3,945
8.5	2,146	2,205	2,266	2,328	2,392	2,457	2,525	2,594	2,665	2,739	2,814	2,891	2,970	3,052	3,135	3,221	3,310	3,401	3,494	3,590	3,688	3,790	3,894	4,000
8.6	2,192	2,251	2,312	2,375	2,439	2,505	2,573	2,643	2,715	2,789	2,864	2,942	3,022	3,104	3,188	3,274	3,363	3,454	3,548	3,644	3,743	3,845	3,949	4,056
8.7	2,238	2,298	2,359	2,423	2,488	2,554	2,623	2,693	2,765	2,840	2,916	2,994	3,074	3,157	3,241	3,328	3,417	3,509	3,603	3,700	3,799	3,901	4,005	4,113

8.8	2,285	2,346	2,408	2,472	2,537	2,604	2,673	2,744	2,817	2,892	2,968	3,047	3,128	3,210	3,295	3,383	3,472	3,565	3,659	3,756	3,855	3,958	4,063	4,170
8.9	2,333	2,394	2,457	2,521	2,587	2,655	2,725	2,796	2,869	2,944	3,021	3,101	3,182	3,265	3,351	3,438	3,528	3,621	3,716	3,813	3,913	4,015	4,120	4,228
9.0	2,382	2,444	2,507	2,572	2,639	2,707	2,777	2,849	2,923	2,998	3,076	3,155	3,237	3,321	3,407	3,495	3,585	3,678	3,773	3,871	3,971	4,074	4,179	4,287
9.1	2,433	2,495	2,559	2,624	2,691	2,760	2,830	2,903	2,977	3,053	3,131	3,211	3,293	3,377	3,464	3,552	3,643	3,736	3,832	3,930	4,030	4,133	4,239	4,347
9.2	2,484	2,547	2,611	2,677	2,744	2,814	2,885	2,958	3,032	3,109	3,187	3,268	3,350	3,435	3,522	3,611	3,702	3,795	3,891	3,989	4,090	4,193	4,299	4,408
9.3	2,536	2,599	2,664	2,731	2,799	2,869	2,940	3,014	3,089	3,166	3,245	3,326	3,409	3,494	3,581	3,670	3,761	3,855	3,951	4,050	4,151	4,254	4,361	4,469
9.4	2,590	2,653	2,719	2,786	2,854	2,925	2,997	3,070	3,146	3,224	3,303	3,384	3,468	3,553	3,641	3,738	3,822	3,916	4,013	4,111	4,213	4,316	4,423	4,532
9.5	2,644	2,709	2,774	2,842	2,911	2,982	3,054	3,129	3,205	3,283	3,362	3,444	3,528	3,614	3,701	3,791	3,884	3,978	4,075	4,174	4,275	4,379	4,486	4,595
9.6	2,700	2,765	2,831	2,899	2,969	3,040	3,113	3,188	3,264	3,343	3,423	3,505	3,589	3,675	3,763	3,854	3,946	4,041	4,138	4,237	4,339	4,443	4,550	4,659
9.7	2,757	2,822	2,889	2,958	3,028	3,099	3,173	3,248	3,325	3,404	3,484	3,567	3,651	3,738	3,826	3,917	4,010	4,105	4,202	4,302	4,404	4,508	4,615	4,724
9.8	2,815	2,881	2,948	3,017	3,088	3,160	3,234	3,309	3,387	3,466	3,547	3,630	3,715	3,802	3,890	3,981	4,074	4,170	4,267	4,367	4,469	4,573	4,680	4,790
9.9	2,874	2,941	3,009	3,078	3,149	3,222	3,296	3,372	3,450	3,529	3,611	3,694	3,779	3,866	3,956	4,047	4,140	4,236	4,333	4,433	4,536	4,640	4,747	4,857
10.0	2,935	3,002	3,070	3,140	3,211	3,285	3,359	3,436	3,514	3,594	3,676	3,759	3,845	3,932	4,022	4,113	4,207	4,303	4,400	4,501	4,603	4,708	4,815	4,924

Log (birth weight) = 1.7492 + 0.166(BPD) + 0.046(AC) − 2.646 (AC + BPD)/1,000.

SD = ±106.0 g/kg of birth weight.

From Shepard MJ, Richards VA, Berkowitz RL, et al. An evaluation of two equations for predicting fetal weight by ultrasound. *Am J Obstet Gynecol* 1982;142:47–55, with permission.

Table A-12 Amniotic fluid index values in normal pregnancy

Gestational age (wk)	Amniotic fluid index percentile values (mm)				
	3rd	5th	50th	95th	97th
16	73	79	121	185	201
17	77	83	127	194	211
18	80	87	133	202	220
19	83	90	137	207	225
20	86	93	141	212	230
21	88	95	143	214	233
22	89	97	145	216	235
23	90	98	146	218	237
24	90	98	147	219	238
25	89	97	147	221	240
26	89	97	147	223	242
27	85	95	146	226	245
28	86	94	146	228	249
29	84	92	145	231	254
30	82	90	145	234	258
31	79	88	144	238	263
32	77	86	144	242	269
33	74	83	143	245	274
34	72	81	142	248	278
35	70	79	140	249	279
36	68	77	138	249	279
37	66	75	135	244	275
38	65	73	132	239	269
39	64	72	127	226	255
40	63	71	123	214	240
41	63	70	116	194	216
42	63	69	110	175	192

Source: Adapted from Moore TR, Coyle JE. The amniotic fluid index in normal human pregnancy. *Am J Obstet Gynecol* 1990;162:1168.

Table A-13 A nomogram of the transverse cerebellar diameter (TCD) (mm)

Gestational age (wk)	Percentile		
	10th	50th	90th
15	13	14	16
16	14	16	17
17	16	17	18
18	17	18	19
19	18	19	20
20	19	20	21
21	20	21	23
22	22	23	24
23	23	24	26
24	23	26	28
25	25	27	30
26	26	28	32
27	27	30	33
28	28	31	35
29	29	33	38
30	31	35	40
31	33	38	42
32	34	39	43
33	35	40	44
34	38	41	44
35	41	42	45
36	42	43	45
37	43	45	48
38	45	48	50
39	48	52	55
40	52	55	58

Source: Goldstein I, Reece EA, Pilu G, *et al*. Cerebellar measurements with ultrasonography in the evaluation of fetal growth and development. *Am J Obstet Gynecol*. 1987;156:1065–9, with permission.

Table A-14 Reference values for umbilical artery Doppler resistive index and systolic/diastolic ratio

Percentiles	5th		50th		95th	
GA (wk)	RI	S/D ratio	RI	S/D ratio	RI	S/D ratio
16	0.70	3.39	0.80	5.12	0.90	10.50
17	0.69	3.27	0.79	4.86	0.89	9.46
18	0.68	3.16	0.78	4.63	0.88	8.61
19	0.67	3.06	0.77	4.41	0.87	7.90
20	0.66	2.97	0.76	4.22	0.86	7.30
21	0.65	2.88	0.75	4.04	0.85	6.78
22	0.64	2.79	0.74	3.88	0.84	6.33
23	0.63	2.71	0.73	3.73	0.83	5.94
24	0.62	2.64	0.72	3.59	0.82	5.59
25	0.61	2.57	0.71	3.46	0.81	5.28
26	0.60	2.50	0.70	3.34	0.80	5.01
27	0.59	2.44	0.69	3.22	0.79	4.76
28	0.58	2.38	0.68	3.12	0.78	4.53
29	0.57	2.32	0.67	3.02	0.77	4.33
30	0.56	2.26	0.66	2.93	0.76	4.14
31	0.55	2.21	0.65	2.84	0.75	3.97
32	0.54	2.16	0.64	2.76	0.74	3.81
33	0.53	2.11	0.63	2.68	0.73	3.66
34	0.52	2.07	0.62	2.61	0.72	3.53
35	0.51	2.03	0.61	2.54	0.71	3.40
36	0.50	1.98	0.60	2.47	0.70	3.29
37	0.49	1.94	0.59	2.41	0.69	3.18
38	0.47	1.90	0.57	2.35	0.67	3.08
39	0.46	1.87	0.56	2.30	0.66	2.98
40	0.45	1.83	0.55	2.24	0.65	2.89
41	0.44	1.80	0.54	2.19	0.64	2.81
42	0.43	1.76	0.53	2.14	0.63	2.73

GA, gestational age; RI, resistive index; S/D ratio, systolic/diastolic ratio.

Note: $RI = 0.97199 - 0.01045 \times GA$ (SD = 0.06078); systolic/diastolic ratio = $11(1 - RI)$.

Data from Kofinas AD, Espeland MA, Penry M, Swain M, Hatjis CG. Uteroplacental Doppler flow velocity waveform indices in normal pregnancy: a statistical exercise and the development of appropriate reference values. *Am J Perinatol* 1992;9:94–101.

Table A-15 Fetal thoracic circumference measurements (cm)

Gestational age (wk)	Predictive percentile								
	#	2.5	5	10	25	50	75	90	95	97.5
16	6	5.9	6.4	7.0	8.0	9.1	10.3	11.3	11.9	12.4
17	22	6.8	7.3	7.9	8.9	10.0	11.2	12.2	12.8	13.3
18	31	7.7	8.2	8.8	9.8	11.0	12.1	13.1	13.7	14.2
19	21	8.6	91	9.7	10.7	11.9	13.0	14.0	14.6	15.1
20	20	9.5	10.0	10.3	11.7	12.9	13.9	15.0	15.5	16.0
21	30	10.4	11.0	11.3	12.6	13.7	14.8	15.8	16.4	16.9
22	18	11.3	11.9	12.5	13.5	14.6	15.7	16.7	17.3	17.8
23	21	12.2	12.8	13.4	14.4	15.5	16.6	17.6	18.2	18.8
24	27	13.2	13.7	14.3	15.3	16.4	17.5	18.5	19.1	19.7
25	20	14.1	14.6	15.2	16.2	17.3	18.4	19.4	20.0	20.6
26	25	15.0	15.5	16.1	17.1	18.2	19.3	20.3	21.0	21.5
27	24	15.9	16.4	17.0	18.0	19.1	20.2	21.3	21.9	22.4
28	24	16.8	17.3	17.9	18.9	20.0	21.2	22.2	22.8	23.3
29	24	17.7	18.2	18.8	19.8	21.0	22.1	23.1	23.7	24.2
30	27	18.6	19.1	19.7	20.7	21.9	23.0	24.0	24.6	25.1
31	24	19.5	20.0	20.6	21.6	22.8	23.9	24.9	25.5	26.0
32	28	20.4	20.9	21.5	22.6	23.7	24.8	25.8	26.4	26.9
33	27	21.3	21.8	22.5	23.5	24.6	25.7	26.7	27.3	27.8
34	25	22.3	22.8	23.4	24.4	25.5	26.6	27.6	28.2	28.7
35	20	23.1	23.7	24.3	25.3	26.4	27.5	28.5	29.1	29.6
36	23	24.0	24.6	25.2	26.2	27.3	28.4	29.4	30.0	30.6
37	22	24.9	25.5	26.1	27.1	28.2	29.3	30.3	30.9	31.5
38	21	25.9	26.4	27.0	28.0	29.1	30.2	31.2	31.9	32.4
39	7	26.8	27.3	27.9	28.9	30.0	31.1	32.2	32.8	33.3
40	6	27.7	28.2	28.8	29.8	30.9	32.1	33.1	33.7	34.2

GA, gestational age; #, number.

Data from Chitkara U, Rosenberg J, Chervenak F, *et al.* Prenatal sonographic assessment of fetal thorax: normal values. *Am J Obstet Gynecol* 1987:156:1069–74.

Table A-16 Expected peak velocity (cm/sec) of systolic blood flow in the middle cerebral artery as a function of gestational age

Gestational age (wk)	Multiple of the median			
	1.00	1.29	1.50	1.55
18	23.2	29.9	34.8	36.0
20	25.5	32.8	38.2	39.5
22	27.9	36.0	41.9	43.3
24	30.7	39.5	46.0	47.5
26	33.6	43.3	50.4	52.1
28	36.9	47.6	55.4	57.2
30	40.5	52.2	60.7	62.8
32	44.4	57.3	66.6	68.9
34	48.7	62.9	73.1	75.6
36	53.5	69.0	80.2	82.9
38	58.7	75.7	88.0	91.0
40	64.4	83.0	96.6	99.8

GA, gestational age.
Data from Mari G. Noninvasive diagnosis by Doppler ultrasonography of fetal anemia due to maternal red-cell alloimmunization. *N Engl J Med* 2000;342:9–14.

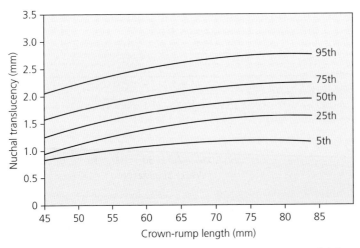

Figure A-1 Reference range of fetal nuchal translucency and chromosomal defects. Source: Nuchal translucency and chromosomal defects. In: KH Nicolaides, NJ Sebire, RJM Snijders (eds) The 11–14 week scan: the diagnosis of fetal abnormalities. New York: Parthenon Publishing, 1999.

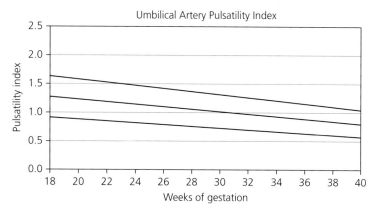

Figure A-2 Umbilical artery pulsatility index throughout gestation. Source: Ferrazzi E, Gementi P, Bellotti M, Rodolfi, M, Della Peruta S, Barbera A, Pardi G. Dopper velocimetry: critical analysis of umbilical, cerebral and aortic reference values. *Eur J Obstet Gynaecol* 1990;38:189–96.

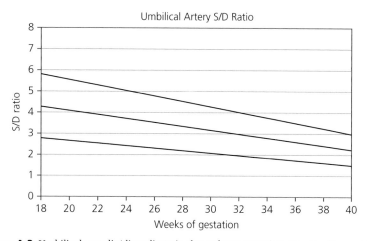

Figure A-3 Umbilical systolic/diastolic ratio throughout gestation. Source: Ferrazzi E, Gementi P, Bellotti M, Rodolfi, M, Della Peruta S, Barbera A, Pardi G. Dopper velocimetry: critical analysis of umbilical, cerebral and aortic reference values. *Eur J Obstet Gynaecol* 1990;38:189–96.

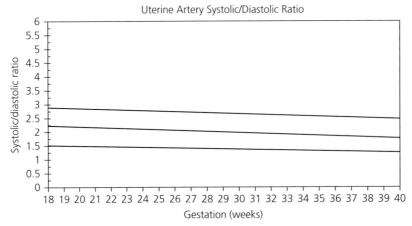

Figure A-4 Uterine artery systolic/diastolic ratio throughout gestation. Source: Ferrazzi E, Bulfamante G, Barbera A, Moneghini L, Pavesi A, Buscaglia M. Placental pathology and perinatal outcomes of fetuses with asymmetric growth alteration and abnomal uteroplacental Dopler waveforms. *It J Gynaec Obstet* 1992;3:89–92.

APPENDIX B

Laboratory Values in Normal Pregnancy

F. Gary Cunningham

University of Texas Southwestern Medical Center, Department of Obstetrics and Gynecology, Dallas, TX, USA

There are a number of profound physiological changes that result during normal pregnancy. Some of these can induce significant alterations in laboratory values that in a non-pregnant woman would be considered distinctly abnormal. Common examples are the lower hematocrit and hemoglobin concentrations that reach a nadir at the end of the second trimester. Another is that a seemingly normal serum creatinine value of 1.1 mg/dL signifies that almost half of the nephron mass is dysfunctional. And there are myriad other examples.

Even though these common pregnancy-induced laboratory aberrations are well recognized, very few laboratories routinely provide normal values for pregnant women. Indeed, many laboratories do not even report normal values for 'females', much less for pregnant women. Most reports of pregnancy-induced variations in laboratory values are studies of a limited number of analytes, while others are found within reference books that are not easily accessible. Presented in the following tables are normal reference ranges for some common laboratory test values that were determined across pregnancy. For comparison, normal values for non-regnant women are listed when available. These values have been summarized from the Appendix of normal laboratory values in the 23rd edition of *Williams Obstetrics* which was published in *Obstetrics & Gynecology*.

Protocols for High-Risk Pregnancies, 5th edition. Edited by J.T. Queenan, J.C. Hobbins and C.Y. Spong. © 2010 Blackwell Publishing Ltd.

Table B-1 Hematology

	Non-pregnant adult[a]	First trimester	Second trimester	Third trimester
Erythropoietin[b] (U/L)	4–27	12–25	8–67	14–222
Ferritin[b] (ng/mL)	10–150[d]	6–130	2–230	0–116
Folate, red blood cell (ng/mL)	150–450	137–589	94–828	109–663
Folate, serum (ng/mL)	5.4–18.0	2.6–15.0	0.8–24.0	1.4–20.7
Hemoglobin[b] (g/dL)	12–15.8[d]	11.6–13.9	9.7–14.8	9.5–15.0
Hematocrit[b] (%)	35.4–44.4	31.0–41.0	30.0–39.0	28.0–40.0
Iron, total binding capacity (TIBC)[b] (μg/dL)	251–406	278–403	Not reported	359–609
Iron, serum[b] (μg/dL)	41–141	72–143	44–178	30–193
Mean corpuscular hemoglobin (MCH) (pg/cell)	27–32	30–32	30–33	29–32
Mean corpuscular volume (MCV) (μm^3)	79–93	81–96	82–97	81–99
Platelet ($\times$ 10^9/L)	165–415	174–391	155–409	146–429
Mean platelet volume (MPV) (μm^3)	6.4–11.0	7.7–10.3	7.8–10.2	8.2–10.4
Red blood cell count (RBC) ($\times$ 10^6/mm^3)	4.00–5.20[d]	3.42–4.55	2.81–4.49	2.71–4.43
Red cell distribution width (RDW) **(%)**	<14.5	12.5–14.1	13.4–13.6	12.7–15.3
White blood cell count (WBC) ($\times$ 10^3/mm^3)	3.5–9.1	5.7–13.6	5.6–14.8	5.9–16.9
Neutrophils ($\times$ 10^3/mm^3)	1.4–4.6	3.6–10.1	3.8–12.3	3.9–13.1
Lymphocytes ($\times$ 10^3/mm^3)	0.7–4.6	1.1–3.6	0.9–3.9	1.0–3.6
Monocytes ($\times$ 10^3/mm^3)	0.1–0.7	0.1–1.1	0.1–1.1	0.1–1.4
Eosinophils ($\times$ 10^3/mm^3)	0–0.6	0–0.6	0–0.6	0–0.6
Basophils ($\times$ 10^3/mm^3)	0–0.2	0–0.1	0–0.1	0–0.1
Transferrin (mg/dL)	200–400	254–344	220–441	288–530
Transferrin, saturation without iron (%)	22–46[b]	Not reported	10–44	5–37
Transferrin, saturation with iron (%)	22–46[b]	Not reported	18–92	9–98

[a]Unless specified, normal reference values are from the 17th edition of *Harrison's Principles of Internal Medicine* (2008).

[b]Range includes references with and without iron supplementation.

[c]Reference value from *Laboratory Reference Handbook,* Pathology Department, Parkland Hospital, 2005.

[d]Normal reference range is specific range for females.

[e]Reference values are from the 15th edition of *Harrison's Principles of Internal Medicine* (2001).

Table B-2 Coagulation studies

	Non-pregnant adult[a]	First trimester	Second trimester	Third trimester
Antithrombin III, functional (%)	70–130	89–114	88–112	82–116
D-Dimer (µg/mL)	0.22–0.74	0.05–0.95	0.32–1.29	0.13–1.7
Factor V (%)	50–150	75–95	72–96	60–88
Factor VII (%)	50–150	100–146	95–153	149–2110
Factor VIII (%)	50–150	90–210	97–312	143–353
Factor IX (%)	50–150	103–172	154–217	164–235
Factor XI (%)	50–150	80–127	82–144	65–123
Factor XII (%)	50–150	78–124	90–151	129–194
Fibrinogen (mg/dL)	233–496	244–510	291–538	373–619
Homocysteine (µmol/L)	4.4–10.8	3.34–11	2.0–26.9	3.2–21.4
INR	0.9–1.04	0.89–1.05	0.85–0.97	0.80–0.94
Partial thromboplastin time, activated (aPTT) (sec)	26.3–39.4	24.3–38.9	24.2–38.1	24.7–35.0
Prothrombin time (PT) (sec)	12.7–15.4	9.7–13.5	9.5–13.4	9.6–12.9
Protein C, functional (%)	70–130	78–121	83–133	67–135
Protein S, total (%)	70–140	39–105	27–101	33–101
Protein S, free (%)	70–140	34–133	19–113	20–65
Protein S, functional activity (%)	65–140	57–95	42–68	16–42
von Willebrand factor (%)	75–125	Not reported	Not reported	121–260

[a]Unless specified, normal reference values are from the 17th edition of *Harrison's Principles of Internal Medicine* (2008).

[b]Range includes references with and without iron supplementation.

[c]Reference value from *Laboratory Reference Handbook,* Pathology Department, Parkland Hospital, 2005.

[d]Normal reference range is specific range for females.

[e]Reference values are from the 15th edition of *Harrison's Principles of Internal Medicine* (2001).

Table B-3 Blood chemistry

	Non-pregnant adult[a]	First trimester	Second trimester	Third trimester
Alanine transaminase (ALT) (U/L)	7–41	3–30	2–33	2–25
Albumin (g/dL)	4.1–5.3[d]	3.1–5.1	2.6–4.5	2.3–4.2
Alkaline phosphatase (U/L)	33–96	17–88	25–126	38–229
Alpha-1 antitrypsin (mg/dL)	100–200	225–323	273–391	327–487
Amylase (U/L)	20–96	24–83	16–73	15–81
Anion gap (mmol/L)	7–16	13–17	12–16	12–16
Aspartate transaminase (AST) (U/L)	12–38	3–23	3–33	4–32
Bicarbonate (mmol/L)	22–30	20–24	20–24	20–24
Bilirubin, total (mg/dL)	0.3–1.3	0.1–0.4	0.1–0.8	0.1–1.1
Bilirubin, unconjugated (mg/dL)	0.2–0.9	0.1–0.5	0.1–0.4	0.1–0.5
Bilirubin, conjugated (mg/dL)	0.1–0.4	0–0.1	0–0.1	0–0.1
Bile acids (μmol/L)	0.3–4.8	0–4.9	0–9.1	0–11.3
Calcium, ionized (mg/dL)	4.5–5.3	4.5–5.1	4.4–5.0	4.4–5.3
Calcium, total (mg/dL)	8.7–10.2	8.8–10.6	8.2–9.0	8.2–9.7
Ceruloplasmin (mg/dL)	25–63	30–49	40–53	43–78
Chloride (mEq/L)	102–109	101–105	97–109	97–109
Creatinine (mg/dL)	0.5–0.9[d]	0.4–0.7	0.4–0.8	0.4–0.9
Gamma-glutamyl transpeptidase (GGT) (U/L)	9–58	2–23	4–22	3–26
Lactate dehydrogenase (U/L)	115–221	78–433	80–447	82–524
Lipase (U/L)	3–43	21–76	26–100	41–112
Magnesium (mg/dL)	1.5–2.3	1.6–2.2	1.5–2.2	1.1–2.2
Osmolality (mOsm/kg H_2O)	275–295	275–280	276–289	278–280
Phosphate (mg/dL)	2.5–4.3	3.1–4.6	2.5–4.6	2.8–4.6
Potassium (mEq/L)	3.5–5.0	3.6–5.0	3.3–5.0	3.3–5.1
Prealbumin (mg/dL)	17–34	15–27	20–27	14–23
Protein, total (g/dL)	6.7–8.6	6.2–7.6	5.7–6.9	5.6–6.7
Sodium (mEq/L)	136–146	133–148	129–148	130–148
Urea nitrogen (mg/dL)	7–20	7–12	3–13	3–11
Uric acid (mg/dL)	2.5–5.6[d]	2.0–4.2	2.4–4.9	3.1–6.3

[a] Unless specified, normal reference values are from the 17th edition of *Harrison's Principles of Internal Medicine* (2008).

[b] Range includes references with and without iron supplementation.

[c] Reference value from *Laboratory Reference Handbook,* Pathology Department, Parkland Hospital, 2005.

[d] Normal reference range is specific range for females.

[e] Reference values are from the 15th edition of *Harrison's Principles of Internal Medicine* (2001).

Table B-4 Endocrine and metabolic values

	Non-pregnant adult[a]	First trimester	Second trimester	Third trimester
Aldosterone (ng/dL)	2–9	6–104	9–104	15–101
Angiotensin converting enzyme (ACE) (U/L)	9–67	1–38	1–36	1–39
Cortisol (μg/dL)	0–25	7–19	10–42	12–50
Hemoglobin A$_{1C}$ (%)	4–6	4–6	4–6	4–7
Parathyroid hormone (pg/mL)	8–51	10–15	18–25	9–26
Parathyroid hormone-related protein (pmol/L)	<1.3[e]	0.7–0.9	1.8–2.2	2.5–2.8
Renin, plasma activity (ng/mL/h)	0.3–9.0[e]	Not reported	7.5–54.0	5.9–58.8
Thyroid stimulating hormone (TSH) (μIU/mL)	0.34–4.25	0.60–3.40	0.37–3.60	0.38–4.04
Thyroxine-binding globulin (mg/dL)	1.3–3.0	1.8–3.2	2.8–4.0	2.6–4.2
Thyroxine, free (fT$_4$) (ng/dL)	0.8–1.7	0.8–1.2	0.6–1.0	0.5–0.8
Thyroxine, total (T$_4$) (μg/dL)	5.4–11.7	6.5–10.1	7.5–10.3	6.3–9.7
Triiodothyronine, free (fT$_3$) (pg/mL)	2.4–4.2	4.1–4.4	4.0–4.2	Not reported
Triiodothyronine, total (T$_3$) (ng/dL)	77–135	97–149	117–169	123–162

[a] Unless specified, normal reference values are from the 17th edition of *Harrison's Principles of Internal Medicine* (2008).

[b] Range includes references with and without iron supplementation.

[c] Reference value from *Laboratory Reference Handbook,* Pathology Department, Parkland Hospital, 2005.

[d] Normal reference range is specific range for females.

[e] Reference values are from the 15th edition of *Harrison's Principles of Internal Medicine* (2001).

Table B-5 Vitamins and minerals

	Non-pregnant adult[a]	First trimester	Second trimester	Third trimester
Copper (µg/dL)	70–140	112–199	165–221	130–240
Selenium (µg/L)	63–160	116–146	75–145	71–133
Vitamin A (retinol) (µg/dL)	20–100	32–47	35–44	29–42
Vitamin B12 (pg/mL)	279–966	118–438	130–656	99–526
Vitamin C (ascorbic acid) (mg/dL)	0.4–1.0	Not Reported	Not Reported	0.9–1.3
Vitamin D, 1,25-dihydroxy (pg/mL)	25–45	20–65	72–160	60–119
Vitamin D, 24,25-dihydroxy (ng/mL)	0.5–5.0	1.2–1.8	1.1–1.5	0.7–0.9
Vitamin D, 25-hydroxy (ng/mL)	14–80	18–27	10–22	10–18
Vitamin E (α-tocopherol) (µg/mL)	5–18	7–13	10–16	13–23
Zinc (µg/dL)	75–120	57–88	51–80	50–77

[a] Unless specified, normal reference values are from the 17th edition of *Harrison's Principles of Internal Medicine* (2008).
[b] Range includes references with and without iron supplementation.
[c] Reference value from *Laboratory Reference Handbook,* Pathology Department, Parkland Hospital, 2005.
[d] Normal reference range is specific range for females.
[e] Reference values are from the 15th edition of *Harrison's Principles of Internal Medicine* (2001).

Table B-6 Autoimmune and inflammatory mediators

	Non-pregnant adult[a]	First trimester	Second trimester	Third trimester
C3 complement (mg/dL)	83–177	62–98	73–103	77–111
C4 complement (mg/dL)	16–47	18–36	18–34	22–32
C-reactive protein (CRP) (mg/L)	0.2–3.0	Not reported	0.4–20.3	0.4–8.1
Erythrocyte sedimentation rate (ESR) (mm/h)	0–20[d]	4–57	7–47	13–70
IgA (mg/dL)	70–350	95–243	99–237	112–250
IgG (mg/dL)	700–1700	981–1267	813–1131	678–990
IgM (mg/dL)	50–300	78–232	74–218	85–269

[a] Unless specified, normal reference values are from the 17th edition of *Harrison's Principles of Internal Medicine* (2008).
[b] Range includes references with and without iron supplementation.
[c] Reference value from *Laboratory Reference Handbook,* Pathology Department, Parkland Hospital, 2005.
[d] Normal reference range is specific range for females.
[e] Reference values are from the 15th edition of *Harrison's Principles of Internal Medicine* (2001).

Table B-7 Sex hormones

	Non-pregnant adult[a]	First trimester	Second trimester	Third trimester
Dehydroepiandrosterone sulfate (DHEAS) (μmol/L)	1.3–6.8[e]	2.0–16.5	0.9–7.8	0.8–6.5
Estradiol (pg/mL)	<20–443[d]	188–2497	1278–7192	6137–3460
Progesterone (ng/mL)	<1–20[d]	8–48		99–342
Prolactin (ng/mL)	0–20	36–213	110–330	137–372
Sex hormone binding globulin (nmol/L)	18–114[d]	39–131	214–717	216–724
Testosterone (ng/dL)	6–86[d]	25.7–211.4	34.3–242.9	62.9–308.6
17-Hydroxyprogesterone (nmol/L)	0.6–10.6[d,e]	5.2–28.5	5.2–28.5	15.5–84

[a]Unless specified, normal reference values are from the 17th edition of *Harrison's Principles of Internal Medicine* (2008).
[b]Range includes references with and without iron supplementation.
[c]Reference value from *Laboratory Reference Handbook,* Pathology Department, Parkland Hospital, 2005.
[d]Normal reference range is specific range for females.
[e]Reference values are from the 15th edition of *Harrison's Principles of Internal Medicine* (2001).

Table B-8 Lipids

	Non-pregnant adult[a]	First trimester	Second trimester	Third trimester
Cholesterol, total (mg/dL)	<200	141–210	176–299	219–349
HDL-Cholesterol (mg/dL)	40–60	40–78	52–87	48–87
LDL-Cholesterol (mg/dL)	<100	60–153	77–184	101–224
VLDL-Cholesterol (mg/dL)	6–40[e]	10–18	13–23	21–36
Triglycerides (mg/dL)	<150	40–159	75–382	131–453
Apolipoprotein A-I (mg/dL)	119–240	111–150	142–253	145–262
Apolipoprotein B (mg/dL)	52–163	58–81	66–188	85–238

[a]Unless specified, normal reference values are from the 17th edition of *Harrison's Principles of Internal Medicine* (2008).
[b]Range includes references with and without iron supplementation.
[c]Reference value from *Laboratory Reference Handbook,* Pathology Department, Parkland Hospital, 2005.
[d]Normal reference range is specific range for females.
[e]Reference values are from the 15th edition of *Harrison's Principles of Internal Medicine* (2001).

Table B-9 Cardiac peptides and enzymes

	Non-pregnant adult[a]	First trimester	Second trimester	Third trimester
Atrial natrieuretic peptide (ANP) (pg/mL)	Not reported	Not reported	28.1–70.1	Not reported
B-type natrieuretic peptide (BNP) (pg/mL)	<167 (age and gender specific)	Not reported	13.5–29.5	Not reported
Creatine kinase (U/L)	39–238[d]	27–83	25–75	13–101
Creatine kinase-MB (U/L)	<6	Not reported	Not reported	1.8–2.4
Troponin I (ng/mL)	0–0.08	Not reported	Not reported	0–0.064 (intrapartum)

[a]Unless specified, normal reference values are from the 17th edition of *Harrison's Principles of Internal Medicine* (2008).
[b]Range includes references with and without iron supplementation.
[c]Reference value from *Laboratory Reference Handbook*, Pathology Department, Parkland Hospital, 2005.
[d]Normal reference range is specific range for females.
[e]Reference values are from the 15th edition of *Harrison's Principles of Internal Medicine* (2001).

Table B-10 Acid–base and blood gases

	Non-pregnant adult[a]	First trimester	Second trimester	Third trimester
Bicarbonate (HCO$_3$) (mEq/L)	22–26	Not reported	Not reported	16–22
PCO$_2$ (mmHg)	38–42	Not reported	Not reported	25–33
PO$_2$ (mmHg)	90–100	93–100	90–98	92–107
pH	7.38–7.42 (arterial)	7.36–7.52 (venous)	7.40–7.52 (venous)	7.41–7.53 (venous)
				7.39–7.45 (arterial)

[a]Unless specified, normal reference values are from the 17th edition of *Harrison's Principles of Internal Medicine* (2008).
[b]Range includes references with and without iron supplementation.
[c]Reference value from *Laboratory Reference Handbook*, Pathology Department, Parkland Hospital, 2005.
[d]Normal reference range is specific range for females.
[e]Reference values are from the 15th edition of *Harrison's Principles of Internal Medicine* (2001).

Table B-11 Renal function

	Non-pregnant adult[a]	First trimester	Second trimester	Third trimester
Effective renal plasma flow (mL/min)	492–696[d, e]	696–985	612–1170	595–945
Glomerular filtration rate (GFR) (mL/min)	106–132[d]	131–166	135–170	117–182
Filtration fraction (%)	16.9–24.7	14.7–21.6	14.3–21.9	17.1–25.1
Osmolarity, urine (mOsm/kg)	500–800	326–975	278–1066	238–1034
24-h albumin excretion (mg/24 h)	<30	5–15	4–18	3–22
24-h calcium excretion (mmol/24 h)	<7.5[e]	1.6–5.2	0.3–6.9	0.8–4.2
24-h creatinine clearance (mL/min)	91–130	69–140	55–136	50–166
24-h creatinine excretion (mmol/24 h)	8.8–14[e]	10.6–11.6	10.3–11.5	10.2–11.4
24-h potassium excretion (mmol/24 h)	25–100[e]	17–33	10–38	11–35
24-h protein excretion (mg/24 h)	<150	19–141	47–186	46–185
24-h sodium excretion (mmol/24 h)	100–260[e]	53–215	34–213	37–149

[a]Unless specified, normal reference values are from the 17th edition of *Harrison's Principles of Internal Medicine* (2008).

[b]Range includes references with and without iron supplementation.

[c]Reference value from *Laboratory Reference Handbook,* Pathology Department, Parkland Hospital, 2005.

[d]Normal reference range is specific range for females.

[e]Reference values are from the 15th edition of *Harrison's Principles of Internal Medicine* (2001).

Suggested reading

Hytten FE, Lind T. *Diagnostic Indices in Pregnancy.* Summit, NJ: Ciba-Geigy Corporation, 1975.

Larsson A, Palm M, Hansson L-O, *et al.* Reference values for clinical chemistry tests during normal pregnancy. *Br J Obstet Gynaecol* 2008;115:874.

Lockitch G. *Handbook of Diagnostic Biochemistry and Hematology in Normal Pregnancy.* Boca Raton, FL: CRC Press, 1993.

APPENDIX C

Evaluation of Fetal Defects and Maternal Disease

Lynn L. Simpson

Department of Obstetrics and Gynecology, Columbia University Medical Center, New York, NY, USA

Protocols for High-Risk Pregnancies, 5th edition. Edited by J.T. Queenan, J.C. Hobbins and C.Y. Spong. © 2010 Blackwell Publishing Ltd.

Table C-1 Risk of karyotypic abnormalities related to maternal age at delivery. (From Hook EB, Cross PK, Schreinemachers DM. Chromosomal abnormality rates at amniocentesis and in live-born infants. *JAMA* 1983;249:2034.)

Maternal age (years)	Incidence of trisomy 21 Live birth	Amniocentesis	Incidence of any chromosomal abnormality Live birth	Amniocentesis
20	1/1734	1/1231	1/526	–
25	1/1250	1/887	1/476	–
30	1/965	1/685	1/385	–
31	1/915	1/650	1/385	–
32	1/794	1/563	1/322	–
33	1/639	1/452	1/286	–
34	1/496	1/352	1/238	–
35	1/386	1/274	1/192	1/83
36	1/300	1/213	1/156	1/76
37	1/234	1/166	1/127	1/67
38	1/182	1/129	1/102	1/58
39	1/141	1/100	1/83	1/49
40	1/100	1/78	1/66	1/40
41	1/86	1/61	1/53	1/32
42	1/66	1/47	1/42	1/26
43	1/52	1/37	1/33	1/21
44	1/40	1/29	1/26	1/19
45	1/31	1/22	1/21	1115
46	1/24	1/17	1/16	1/12
47	1/19	1/13	1/13	1/20
48	1/15	1/10	1/10	1/18
49	1/11	1/8	1/8	1/16

Table C-2 Frequency of chromosome aberrations in newborns. (Modified from a summary of six surveys (Hook and Hamerton, 1977) including 56 952 newborns.)

Aberration	Incidence	
Numerical		
Sex chromosomes		
47,XYY	1/1000	MB
47,XXY	1/1000	MB
Other (males)	1/1350	MB
45,X	1/10,000	FB
47,XXX	1/1000	FB
Other (female)	1/2700	FB
Autosomes		
*Trisomies**		
No. 13 to 15 (group D)	1/20,000	LB
No. 16 to 18 (group E)	1/8000	LB
No. 21 to 22 (group G)	1/800	LB
Other	1/50,000	LB
Structural		
Balanced		
Robertsonian		
t(Dq; Dq)	1/1500	LB
t(Dq; Gq)	1/5000	LB
Reciprocal translocations	1/7000	LB
and insertional inversions		
Unbalanced		
Robertsonian	1/14,000	LB
Reciprocal and insertional	1/8000	LB
Inversions	1/50,000	LB
Deletions	1/10,000	LB
Supernumeraries	1/5000	LB
Other	1/8000	LB
Total	1/160	LB

FB, female births; LB, livebirths; MB, male births.

*Because most surveys did not use banding techniques, individual chromosomes within a group could not always be differentiated. However, group D trisomies are generally no. 13, group E no. 18, and group G no. 21.

Table C-3 Available prenatal diagnosis for common disorders. (Modified from Wapner RJ, Jenkins TM, Khalek N. Prenatal diagnosis of congenital disorders. In: Maternal-Fetal Medicine: Principles and Practice, 6th Edition, Creasy RK, Resnik R, Iams JD (editors). Saunders, Philadelphia, 2009: 248.)

Disorder	Mode of inheritance	Molecular diagnosis
α_1-Antitrypsin deficiency	AR	Determine PiZZ allele
α-Thalassemia	AR	α-Hemoglobin gene mutation
Adult polycystic kidney	AD	PKD1 and PKD2 gene mutations
β-Thalassemia	AR	β Hemoglobin gene mutation
Congenital adrenal hyperplasia	AR	CYP21A2 gene mutations and deletions
Cystic fibrosis	AR	CFTR gene mutation
Duchenne/Becker muscular dystrophy	XLR	Dystrophin gene mutation
Fragile X syndrome	XLR	CGG repeat number
Hemoglobinopathy (SS, SC)	AR	β-Chain gene mutation
Hemophilia A	XLR	Factor VIII gene inversion and mutations
Huntington disease	AD	CAG repeat number
Marfan syndrome	AD	Fibrillin (FBN-1) gene mutation
Myotonic dystrophy	AD	CTG expansion in the DMPK gene
Neurofibromatosis type 1	AD	NF1 gene mutation
Phenylketonuria	AR	Common mutations
Tay-Sachs disease	AR	Enzyme absence and gene mutation

AD, autosomal dominant; AR, autosomal recessive; XLR, X-linked recessive.

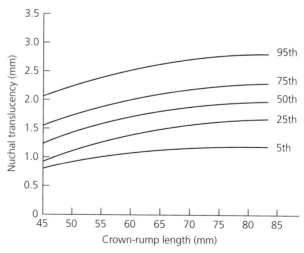

Figure C-1 Nuchal translucency measurements between 11 and 14 weeks' gestation. Nuchal translucency >95th percentile associated with risk of trisomy 21. (From Nicolaides KH, Sebire NJ, Snijders RJM. *The 11–14 Week Scan*. New York, Parthenon, 1999.)

Table C-4 Prevalence of major cardiac defects by nuchal translucency thickness in chromosomally normal fetuses. (From Hyatt J, Perdu M, Sharland G, *et al.* Using fetal nuchal translucency to screen for major congenital cardiac defects at 10–14 weeks of gestation: population based cohort study. *BMJ* 1999;318:81.)

Nuchal translucency	*n*	Major cardiac defects	Prevalence per 1000
<95th percentile	27,332	22	0.8
≥95th percentile–3.4 mm	1,507	8	5.3
3.5–4.4 mm	208	6	28.9
4.–5.4 mm	66	6	90.0
≥5.5 mm	41	8	195.1
Total	29,154	50	1.7

Table C-5 Increased risk for neural tube defect (NTD)

Sibling with NTD	2%
Parent with NTD	2%
Sibling with spinal dysraphism	4%
Sibling with multiple vertebral anomalies	2%
Cousin with NTD	0.5%
Sibling with communicating hydrocephalus	1%
Elevated maternal serum alpha-fetoprotein	10%

Table C-6 White's classification of diabetes during pregnancy

Class	Definition
A	Abnormal glucose tolerance test
B	Onset after age 20 and duration less than 10 years
C	Onset at age 10–20 years or duration of 10–20 years
D	Onset before age 10 or duration of 20 or more years; benign retinopathy
F	Renal disease
H	Coronary artery disease
R	Proliferative retinopathy
T	Renal transplant

Table C-7 Diagnostic criteria for 100-g 3-h oral glucose tolerance test. No data from clinical trials to determine which values are superior for diagnosis. (Modified from Report of the Expert Committee on the Diagnosis and Classification of Diabetes Mellitus. Diab Care 2000;23:S4.)

Time (h)	Carpenter/Coustan values* Glucose level (mg/dL)	O'Sullivan/Mahan values* Glucose level (mg/dL)
Fasting	95	105
1	180	190
2	155	165
3	140	145

*If two or more of the glucose levels are equal to or higher than the values listed, gestational diabetes is diagnosed.

Table C-8 Drugs associated with congenital malformations in humans. (Modified from Chambers C, Weiner CP. Teratogenesis and environmental Exposure. In: Creasy RK, Resnik R, Iams JD (eds) *Maternal-Fetal Medicine: Principles and Practice*, 6th edn. Philadelphia: Saunders, 2009: p. 351.)

Drug	Potential effects	Comments
ACE inhibitors	Calvarial hypoplasia, renal dysgenesis, oligohydramnios, IUGR, and neonatal renal failure	Risk increases with use in second and third trimester
Alcohol	Syndrome: prenatal and postnatal growth restriction, microcephaly, craniofacial dysmorphology (1–4/1000 live births); renal, cardiac, and other major malformations	Risk not limited to first trimester; late pregnancy use associated with IUGR and developmental delay; incidence of defects 4–44% among 'heavy drinkers'
Antidepressants (SSRIs)	Possible cardiac defects, NTD, omphalocele; neonatal pulmonary hypertension and withdrawal syndrome	—
Aminopterin and methotrexate	Syndrome: calvarial hypoplasia, craniofacial abnormalities, limb defects; possible developmental delay	Syndrome associated with methotrexate >10 mg/wk
Androgens and norprogesterones	Masculinization of external female genitalia	Labioscrotal fusion can occur with exposure; up to 50% of those exposed are affected
Carbamazepine	NTD (1%); possible facial hypoplasia and developmental delay	—
Corticosteroids	Cleft lip/palate increased threefold to sixfold; IUGR increased with high doses	—

(Continued)

Table C-8 (Continued)

Drug	Potential effects	Comments
Diethylstilbestrol	Clear cell adenocarcinoma of the vagina, vaginal adenosis, abnormalities of the cervix and uterus, testicular abnormalities, and male/female infertility	—
Isotretinoin	Syndrome: CNS malformations, microtia/anotia, micrognathia, thymus abnormalities, cleft palate, cardiac abnormalities, eye anomalies, limb reduction defects (28%); miscarriage (22%), developmental delay (47%)	—
Lithium	Small increase in Ebstein cardiac anomaly	—
Penicillamine	Cutis laxa with chronic use	—
Phenytoin	Syndrome: IUGR, microcephaly, facial hypoplasia, hypertelorism, prominent upper lip (10%); possible developmental delay	Full syndrome in 10%; up to 30% exhibit some features
Streptomycin	Hearing loss, eighth nerve damage	—
Tetracycline	Discoloration of deciduous teeth and enamel hypoplasia	Risk only in second and third trimester
Tobacco	Oral clefts: relative risk, 1.22–1.34; IUGR, IUFD, abruption	—
Trimethadione	Syndrome: oral clefts, craniofacial abnormalities, developmental delay (80%)	—
Valproic acid	NTD (1–2%); facial hypoplasia, possible developmental delay	—
Warfarin	Syndrome: nasal hypoplasia, stippled epiphyses, growth restriction (6%); also increased microcephaly, Dandy-Walker syndrome, IUGR, preterm birth, mental retardation	Greatest risk at 6–9 weeks

ACE, angiotensin-converting enzyme; CNS, central nervous system; IUFD, intrauterine fetal demise; IUGR, intrauterine growth restriction; NTD, neural tube defect; SAB, spontaneous abortion, SSRIs, selective serotonin reuptake inhibitors.

Table C-9 Food and Drug Administration categories for drug labeling. The Food and Drug Administration has established five categories of drugs based on their potential for causing birth defects in infants born to women who use the drugs during pregnancy. By law, the label must set forth all available information on teratogenicity.

Category A:	Well-controlled human studies have not disclosed any fetal risk. Possibility of fetal harm appears to be remote.
Category B:	Animal studies have not disclosed any fetal risk, or have suggested some risk not confirmed in controlled studies in women, or there are not adequate studies in women.
Category C:	Animal studies have revealed adverse fetal effects; there are no adequate controlled studies in women. Drugs should be given only if the potential benefit justifies the potential risk to the fetus.
Category D:	Evidence of human fetal risk, but benefits may outweigh risk (e.g., life-threatening illness, no safer effective drug). Patient should be warned of risk.
Category X:	Fetal abnormalities in animal and human studies; risk of the drug not outweighed by benefit. *Contraindicated in pregnancy.*

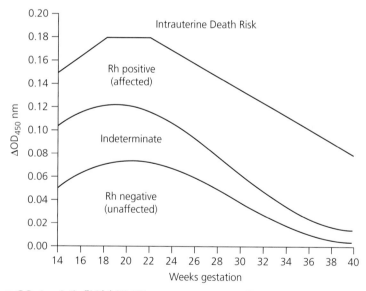

Figure C-2 Amniotic fluid ΔOD450 management zones. (From Queenan JT, Tomai TP, Ural SH, et al. Deviation in amniotic fluid optical density at a wavelength of 450 nm in Rh-immunized pregnancies from 14 to 40 weeks gestation: a proposal for clinical management. Am J Obstet Gynecol 1993;168:1370.)

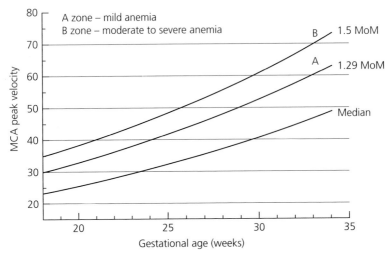

Figure C-3 Middle cerebral artery (MCA) Doppler peak velocities. Peak MCA Doppler velocity >1.5 MoM for gestational age predictive of fetal anemia. (From Moise KJ. Modern management of Rhesus alloimmunization in pregnancy. Obstet Gynecol 2002;100:600.).

Table C-10 Hemolytic disease resulting from irregular antibodies. (Modified from Weinstein L. Irregular antibodies causing hemolytic disease of the newborn: a continuing problem. *Clin Obstet Gynecol* 1982;25:321.)

Blood group system	Antigen	Severity of hemolytic disease	Blood group system	Antigen	Severity of hemolytic disease
Rh subtype	C	+ to +++	Lutheran	Lua	+
	Cw	+ to +++		Lub	+
	c	+ to +++	Diego	Dia	+ to +++
	E	+ to +++		Dib	+ to +++
	e	+ to +++	P	P	−
					+ to +++
Lewis	Lea	−		PPIPk (Tja)	+ to +++
	Leb	−			
I	I	−	Xg	Xga	+
Kell	K	+ to +++	Public antigens	Yta	+ to ++
	k	+		Ytb	+
	Ko	+		Lap	+
	Kpa	+		Ena	+ to +++
	Kpb	+		Ge	+
	Jsa	+		Jra	+
	Jsb	+		Coa	+ to +++
Duffy	Fya	+ to +++		Coab	+
	Fyb	−	Private antigens	Batty	+
	Fy3	+		Becker	+
Kidd	Jka	+ to +++		Berrens	+
	Jkb	+ to +++		Biles	+ to ++
	Jk3	+		Evans	+
MNSs	M	+ to +++		Gonzales	+
	N	−		Good	+ to +++
	S	+ to +++		Heibel	+ to ++
	s	+ to +++		Hunt	+
	U	+ to +++		Jobbins	+
	Mia	++		Radin	+ to ++
	Mta	++		Rm	+
	Vw	+		Ven	+
	Mur	+		Wrighta	+ to +++
	Hil	+		Wrightb	+
	Hut	+		Zd	+ to ++

−, not a proven cause of hemolytic disease of the newborn, no change in management.

+, mild, expectant management with no further diagnostic testing or intervention until delivery.

++, moderate, serial evaluations with middle cerebral Dopplers or amniotic fluid ΔOD_{450}.

+++, severe, serial evaluations with middle cerebral Dopplers or AF ΔOD_{450}.

Table C-11 Fetal blood sampling

Test	Tube type	Minimum amount (mL)
Complete blood count, differential, reticulocyte count	Purple	0.3
Type and cross	Dry Bullet (Salmon)	0.5
Direct/indirect Coombs'	Dry Bullet (Salmon)	0.5
Total immunoglobulin M (IgM)	Red	0.5
Toxoplasma and cytomegalovirus CMV IgM	Red	0.5
Rubella IgM	Red	0.5
Parvovirus IgG and IgM	Red	1.0
CMV blood culture	Red	1.0
Bilirubin (total and direct)	Red	0.5
Total protein and albumin	Red	0.5
Chem-7	Red	0.5
Chem-20	Red	1.0
Kleihauer-Betke stain	Purple	0.5
Prothrombin time/partial thromboplastin time	Blue	1.8
Clotting factor level	Blue (on ice)	1.8
Venous blood gas	Heparinized TB	0.3
Arterial blood gas	Heparinized TB	0.3
Chromosomes	Green	1.0
FISH	Green	1.0
Cystic fibrosis DNA testing	Green	3–4
Polymerase chain reaction	Purple/Green	0.5

CMV, cytomegalovirus; FISH, fluorescence in situ hybridization; Ig, immunoglobulin; TB, tuberculin syringe.

APPENDIX D

The Newborn: Reference charts and tables

Adam Rosenberg

Department of Pediatrics, University of Colorado Denver School of Medicine and The Children's Hospital, Aurora, CO, USA

Protocols for High-Risk Pregnancies, 5th edition. Edited by J.T. Queenan, J.C. Hobbins and C.Y. Spong. © 2010 Blackwell Publishing Ltd.

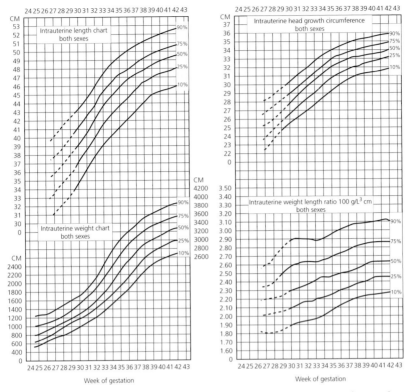

Figure D-1 Intrauterine growth curves for weight, length and head circumference for singleton births in Colorado. Reproduced with permission from Lubchenco LO, *et al.* Intrauterine growth in length and head circumference as estimated from live births at gestational ages from 26–42 weeks. *Pediatrics* 1966;37:403.

Table D-1 Relative timing and developmental pathology of certain malformations

System	Malformation	Embryology	Timing	Comment
Central nervous system	Anencephaly	Closure of anterior neural tube	26 days	Subsequent degeneration of forebrain
	Meningomyelocele	Closure in a part of posterior neural tube	28 days	80% lumbosacral
Face	Cleft lip	Closure of lip	36 days	42% with cleft palate
	Cleft maxillary palate	Fusion of maxillary palatal shelves	10 weeks	
	Branchial sinus and/or cyst	Resolution of branchial cleft	8 weeks	Preauricular; anterior to the sternocleidomastoid

(Continued)

Table D-1 (Continued)

System	Malformation	Embryology	Timing	Comment
Gastrointestinal	Esophageal atresia/ tracheoesophageal fistula	Lateral septation of foregut into trachea and foregut	30 days	
	Rectal atresia with fistula	Lateral septation of cloaca into rectum and urogenital sinus	6 weeks	
	Duodenal atresia	Recanalization of duodenum	7–8 weeks	Associated incomplete or aberrant mesenteric attachments
	Malrotation	Rotation of intestinal loop so cecum lies to the right	10 weeks	
	Omphalocele	Return of midgut from yolk sac to abdomen	10 weeks	
	Meckel diverticulum	Obliteration of vitelline duct	10 weeks	May contain gastric or pancreatic tissue
	Diaphragmatic hernia	Closure of pleuroperitoneal canal	6 weeks	Associated with lung hypoplasia
Genitourinary	Bladder exstrophy	Migration of infraumbilical mesenchyme	30 days	Associated mullerian and wolfian duct defects
	Bicornuate uterus	Fusion of lower part of mullerian ducts	10 weeks	
	Hypospadius	Fusion of urethral folds	12 weeks	
	Cryptorchidism	Descent of testes into scrotum	7–9 months	
Cardiac	Transposition of great vessels	Directional development of bulbus cordis septum	34 days	
	Ventricular septal defect	Closure of ventricular septum	6 weeks	
Limb	Aplasia of radius	Genesis of radial bone	38 days	Often accompanied by other defects of radial side of distal limb
	Syndactyly, severe	Separation of digital rays	6 weeks	

Adapted from Jones KL. *Smith's Recognizable Patterns of Human* Malformation, 6th edn. Elsevier Saunders, 2006.

Table D-2 Types of genetic abnormalities

Gene dosage effects	Chromosomal maldistribution	Aneuploidy Trisomies 21, 18, 13 etc
	Chromosomal rearrangements	Translocations, fragility, duplications, deletions, submicroscopic deletions
Major mutant genes	Autosomal dominant Autosomal recessive X-linked Mitochondrial	Over 6000 individually rare disorders
Multifactorial inheritance	Major and minor genes determining susceptibility interacting with the environment	Common isolated malformations, schizophrenia, coronary artery disease, hypertension, diabetes mellitus, other common disorders

Adapted from Jones KL. *Smith's Recognizable Patterns of Human* Malformation, 6th edn. Elsevier Saunders, 2006.

Table D-3 Assessment of gestational age using the Ballard examination

Neuromuscular Maturity

Neuromuscular Maturity Sign	Score							Record Score Here
	−1	0	1	2	3	4	5	
Posture								
Square window (wrist)	>90°	90°	60°	45°	30°	0°		
Arm recoil		180°	140° to 180°	110° to 140°	90° to 110°	<90°		
Popliteal angle	180°	160°	140°	120°	100°	90°	<90°	
Scarf sign								
Heel to ear								

Total Neuromuscular Maturity Score

Physical maturity

Physical Maturity Sign	Score							Record Score Here
	−1	0	1	2	3	4	5	
Skin	Sticky, friable, transparent	Gelatinous red, translucent	Smooth pink, visible veins	Superficial peeling &/or rash; few veins	Cracking pale areas rare veins	Parchment, deep cracking; no vessels	Leathery cracked, wrinkled	
Lanugo	None	Sparse	Abundant	Thinning	Bald areas	Mostly bald		
Plantar surface	Heel toe 40–50 mm: −1 <140 mm: −2	>50 mm: no crease	Faint red marks	Anterior transverse crease only	Creases anterior 2/3	Creases over entire sole		
Breast	Imperceptible	Barely perceptible	Flat areola; no bud	Stippled areola; 1- to 2-mm bud	Raised areola; 3- to 4-mm bud	Full areola; 5- to 10-mm bud		
Eye/Ear	Lids fused loosely: −1 tightly: −2	Lids open; pinna flat; stays folded	Slightly curved pinna; soft; slow recoil	Well-curved pinna; soft; but ready recoil	Formed & firm instant recoil	Thick cartilage; ear stiff		
Genitals (male)	Scrotum flat, smooth	Scrotum empty; faint rugae	Testes in upper canal; rare rugae	Testes descending; few rugae	Testes down; good rugae	Testes pendulous; deep rugae		
Genitals (female)	Clitoris prominent & labia flat	Prominent clitoris & small labia minora	Prominent clitoris & enlarging minora	Majora & minora equality prominent	Majora large; minora small	Majora cover clitoris & minora		

Total Physical Maturity Score

Maturity	Score	−10	−5	0	5	10	15	20	25	30	35	40	45	50
Rating	Weeks			20	22	24	26	28	30	32	34	36	38	40	42	44

The examination evaluates physical and neurological characteristics of the infant. Reproduced with permission from Ballard JL, et al. New Ballard score, expanded to include extremely premature infants. *J Pediatr* 1991;119:417.

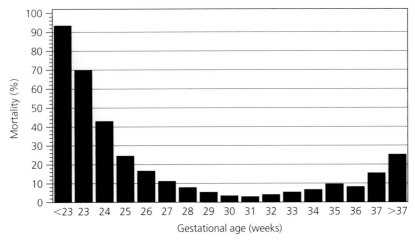

Figure D-2 Mortality rates before discharge by gestational age in 2007. Population consists of over 50,000 infants from nearly 700 centers worldwide reporting data on births <1500 grams to the Vermont Oxford Network. Reproduced with permission from the Vermont Oxford Network, 2008.

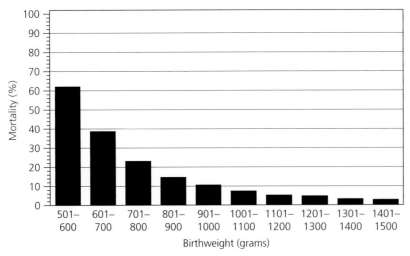

Figure D-3 Mortality rates reported by 100 g birthweight groups in 2007. Population consists of over 50,000 infants from nearly 700 centers worldwide reporting data on births <1500 grams to the Vermont Oxford Network. Reproduced with permission from the Vermont Oxford Network, 2008.

Table D-4 Incidence of common complications in preterm infants

Complication	501–700 g	701–900 g	901–1100 g	1101–1300 g	1301–1500 g
Respiratory distress syndrome	93%	90%	79%	67%	52%
Mechanical ventilation	90%	89%	79%	62%	47%
Late onset sepsis/meningitis	23%	18%	11%	7%	5%
Patent ductus arteriosus	52%	52%	39%	27%	17%
Necrotizing enterocolitis	9%	9%	7%	4%	2%
Severe IVH	24%	16%	9%	6%	3%
Periventricular leukomalacia	5%	5%	3%	2%	2%
Severe ROP	36%	20%	7%	1%	1%
Chronic lung disease	79%	53%	32%	19%	11%

Cumulative data reported to the Vermont Oxford Neonatal Network. This represents information on 32 339 infants reported from 408 centers with a birthweight <1500 g. Severe IVH is a grade 3 or 4 intraventricular hemorrhage and severe ROP is retinopathy of prematurity at prethreshold or threshold for treatment.

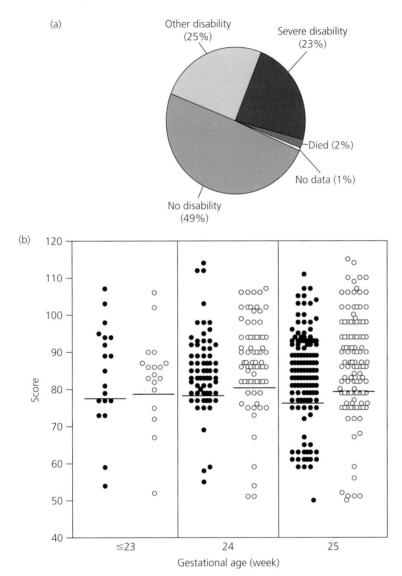

Figure D-4 Neurodevelopmental outcome in infants born at 23–25 weeks' gestation.
(a) Disability includes cerebral palsy, cognitive and behavioral disorders. The incidence
of neurodevelopmental handicap is less at higher gestational ages with infants of
28–32 weeks' gestational age at birth experiencing a <10% rate of severe disability. (b)
Represents scores on the Bayley scales of infant development at 30 months for 23–25
week gestational age survivors. The open circles are scores on the psychomotor portion
and the closed circles scores on the mental portion of the test. The mean score for a
normal term population is 100; the means here are 1 standard deviation below that
level.

(c)

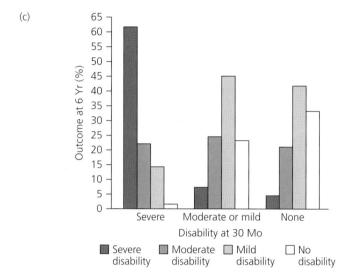

Figure D-4 (c) Thirty-month Bayley scores correlate well with school age outcome. Reproduced with permission from Wood NS, *et al.* Neurologic and developmental disability after extremely preterm birth. *N Engl J Med* 2000;343:378 and Marlow NM, *et al.* Neurologic and developmental disability at six years of age after extremely preterm birth. *N Engl J Med* 2005;352:9.

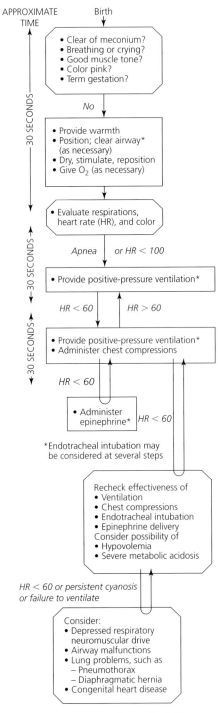

Figure D-5 Neonatal resuscitation program schema for delivery room management of the newborn. Reproduced with permission from the American Heart Association, American Academy of Pediatrics. *Neonatal Resuscitation Textbook*, 5th edition, 2005.

Table D-5 Traumatic birth injury in the newborn

Type of injury	Examples
Soft-tissue injuries	Abrasions, bruising, fat necrosis, lacerations
Extracranial bleeding	Cephalohematoma, subgaleal bleed
Intracranial bleeding	Subarachnoid, epidural, subdural, cerebral, cerebellar
Nerve injuries	Facial, cervical nerve roots (brachial plexus palsies, phrenic), Horner syndrome, recurrent laryngeal
Spinal cord injuries	Epidural hemorrhage of the cervical cord
Fractures	Clavicle, humerus, femur, skull
Dislocations	
Torticollis (sternocleidomastoid bleeding)	
Eye injuries	Subconjunctival and retinal hemorrhages
Solid organ injury	Liver, spleen

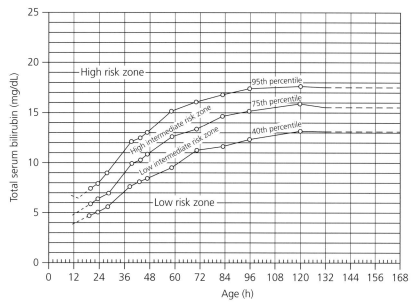

Figure D-6 Risk designation of term and near-term newborns based on their hour-specific bilirubin values. Infants with a total serum bilirubin greater than the 95th percentile for age in hours have a 40% risk of developing subsequent significant hyperbilirubinemia. Reproduced with permission from Bhutani VK, *et al.* Predictive ability of a predischarge hour-specific serum bilirubin test for subsequent significant hyperbilirubinemia in healthy term and near-term newborns. *Pediatrics* 1999;103:6.

Table D-6 Guidelines for successful breastfeeding

	First 8 Hours	8–24 Hours	Day 2	Day 3	Day 4	Day 5	Day 6 Onward
Milk supply	You may be able to express a few drops of milk.	Milk should come in between the second and fourth days.				Milk should be in. Breasts may be firm or leak milk.	Breasts should feel softer after feedings.
Baby's activity	Baby is usually wide-awake in the first hour of life. Put baby to breast within 30 minutes after birth.	Wake up your baby. Babies may not wake up on their own to feed.	Baby should be more cooperative and less sleepy.	Look for early feeding cues such as rooting, lip smacking, and hands to face.			Baby should appear satisfied after feedings.
Feeding routine	Baby may go into a deep sleep 2–4 hours after birth.		Use chart to write down time of each feeding. Feed your baby every 1½ – 3 hours or as often as wanted—at least 8–10 times a day.			May go one longer interval (up to 5 hours between feeds) in a 24-hour period.	
Breast feeding	Baby will wake up and be alert and responsive for several more hours after initial deep sleep.	As long as Mom is comfortable, nurse at both breasts as long as baby is actively sucking.	Try to nurse both sides each feeding, aiming at 10 minutes per side. Expect some nipple tenderness.	Consider hand expressing or pumping a few drops of milk to soften the nipple if the breast is too firm for the baby to latch on.	Nurse a minimum of 10–15 minutes per side every 2–3 hours for the first few months of life.		Mom's nipple tenderness is improving or is gone.
Baby's urine output		Baby must have a minimum of one wet diaper in first 24 hours.	Baby must have at least one wet diaper every 8–11 hours.	You should see an increase in wet diapers (up to four to six) in 24 hours.	Baby's urine should be light yellow.	Baby should have six to eight wet diapers per day of colorless or light yellow urine.	
Baby's stool		Baby should have a black-green (meconium) stool.	Baby may have a second very dark (meconium) stool.	Baby's stools should be in transition from black-green to yellow.		Baby should have three or four yellow, seedy stools a day.	The number of stools may decrease gradually after 4–6 weeks of life.

Reproduced with permission from Gabrielski, L. Lactation support services. The Childrens Hospital, Denver, 1994.

APPENDIX E

Medications

Catalin S. Buhimschi[1] and Carl P. Weiner[2]

[1] Department of Obstetrics, Gynecology and Reproductive Sciences, Yale University School of Medicine, New Haven, CT, USA
[2] University of Kansas School of Medicine, Departments of Obstetrics and Gynecology and Molecular & Integrative Physiology

Over 4.0 million live births are registered in the United States annually. The most common primary exposure categories are over-the-counter medication, psychiatric and gastrointestinal medication, herbals, vitamins, antibiotics and topical products. It is critical that clinicians become familiar with all the aspects of the drugs they recommend and consult with a maternal fetal medicine specialist so thus the best possible evidence-based counseling and treatments be provided. The purpose of this appendix is to provide a quick resource of drugs commonly used for pregnant and lactating women. The information provided in this appendix is concise, user friendly and will allow rapid access to the drug-related questions mentioned in this text. A short note was included for several FDA category B, C and all D and X medication drugs to emphasize the most common maternal and fetal risks associated with these agents.

Acetaminophen (Tylenol)
Type: Analgesic, antipyretic; *Class:* Pregnancy: B   Lactation: S
Note: Link with Acetaminophen, gastroschisis and small bowel atresia reported
Dose: Pain and/or fever: 650–1000 mg PO/PR q 4–6 h; max 4 g/d

---

Acyclovir (Zovirax)
Type: Antivirals; *Class:* Pregnancy: B   Lactation: S
Dose: Genital herpes, recurrent: 200 mg PO 5 × /d × 10 d; *Genital herpes, suppressive:*
400 mg PO bid for up to a year, or during pregnancy, from 36 w onward; with HIV, 400–800 mg PO 2– × × /d, or IV 5–10 mg/kg q 8 h × 5–10 d; *Varicella, acute:* 800 mg PO qid × 5 d; *Herpes zoster:* 800 mg PO 5 × /d × 7–10 d; *Ocular herpes:* 3% ointment 5 × /d × 7–10 d

---

Albuterol (Proventil)
Type: Adrenergic agonists; Bronchodilators; *Class:* Pregnancy: C   Lactation: S
Dose: Bronchospasm: 1–2 puffs metered dose inhaler q 4–6 h, max 12 puffs/d or 2–4 mg PO tid/qid; *Exercise-induced asthma:* 2 puffs metered dose inhaler × 1 given 15–30 min before exercise

---

(Continued)

Protocols for High-Risk Pregnancies, 5th edition. Edited by J.T. Queenan, J.C. Hobbins and C.Y. Spong. © 2010 Blackwell Publishing Ltd.

Amantadine (Contenton)
Type: Antiviral, extrapyramidal movement disorder; *Class:* Pregnancy: C   Lactation: U
Dose: Influenza A – treatment: 200 mg PO qd until 24–48 h after symptoms resolve;
Influenza A – prophylaxis: 200 mg PO qd beginning immediately after exposure and continuing
at least 10 d; *Extrapyramidal reactions:* 100 mg PO qd to tid (max 300 mg/d); *Parkinsonism:*
begin 100 mg PO qd, increase to bid after 1 w, max 400 mg/d; reduce to 100 mg/d if taking
other anti-parkinsonism drugs

Aminophylline (Aminophylline)
Type: Antiasthmatics, Bronchodilators; Xanthine derivatives; *Class:* Pregnancy: C   Lactation: U
Note: Serum levels should be periodically monitored and maintained between 10 and 20 μg/mL
Dose: Bronchospasm: 0. 3–0.8 mg/kg/h IV preceded by a variety of recommended loading doses
(0. 3–6 mg/kg over 12 h IV); alternatively 10–16 mg/kg/d PO

Amoxicillin/clavulanate (Augmentin)
Type: Antibiotics; Penicillins; *Class:* Pregnancy: B   Lactation: S
Note: Combined with either Clarithromycin and Lansoprazole/Omeprazole
Dose: Bacterial infection: 250–500 mg PO tid, or 500–750 mg PO bid (see note); *Gonorrhea
uncomplicated:* 3 g PO × 1; *Chlamydia trachomatis:* 500 mg PO tid × 7 d;*Endocarditis
prophylaxis:* 2 g PO × 1, 0.5–1 h prior to the procedure; *H. pylori infection:* 1 g PO bid ×
10–14 d

Ampicillin (Unasyn)
Type: Antibiotics; Penicillins; *Class:* Pregnancy: B   Lactation: S
Note: Coupling to the beta-lactamase inhibitor, sulbactam enhances the spectrum of coverage
Dose: Bacterial infection: 1.5–3 g IV/IM q 6 h; max 8 g/d

Anakinra (Kineret)
Type: Anti-interleukin 1; *Class:* Pregnancy: B   Lactation: U
Dose: Rheumatoid arthritis: SC 100 mg every other week

Atenolol (Alinor)
Type: Antiadrenergics; Beta blockers; *Class:* Pregnancy: B   Lactation: NS
Dose: Hypertension: 50 mg PO qd; increase to 100 mg qd after 7 d; *Myocardial infarction:* begin
5 mg IV over 5 min × 2 (10 min apart), then 50 mg PO q 12 h × 7 d, then 100 mg qd; *Angina:*
50 mg PO qd, max 200 mg qd

Atropine (Atropen)
Type: Anesthesia, adjunct; Antiarrhythmics; Antidotes; Cycloplegics; Mydriatics; Ophthalmics
Class: Pregnancy: C   Lactation: U
Note: May be combined with either Difenoxin, Diphenoxylate, or Hyoscyamine, Scopolamine and
Phenobarbital (Donnatal)
Dose: Symptomatic bradycardia: 0.5–1 mg IV q 3–5 min prn, max 2 mg (see note);
Organophosphate poisoning: 1–2 mg IM/IV q 20–30 min until muscarinic symptoms resolve;
Adjunct to anesthesia: 0.4 mg IM/SC 30–60 min preoperatively to dry oral secretions before
expected difficult airway management. Also given with anticholinesterase (atropine plus
neostigmine when reversing neuromuscular paralysis at the end of surgery)

(Continued)

Azathioprine (Imuran)

Type: Immunosuppressants; *Class:* Pregnancy: D   Lactation: U

Note: No clear pattern of malformations was detectable. Isolated skeletal defects, IUGR and fetal leukopenia have been reported

Dose: Transplant rejection: begin 3–5 mg/kg/d PO/IV qd; maintenance 1–3 mg/kg/d (transplant protocols vary); *Crohn's disease and ulcerative colitis:* begin 50 mg PO qd increasing to 150–250 mg PO qd; max 2.5 mg/kg/d; *Rheumatoid arthritis:* begin 1 mg/kg PO qd; increase 0.5 mg/kg/d after 6–8 w; max 2.5 mg/kg/d

Azithromycin (Aruzilina; Zithromax)

Type: Antibiotics; Macrolides; *Class:* Pregnancy: B   Lactation: S (likely)

Dose: Bacterial infection: 500 mg PO load × 1, then 250 mg PO qd × 6 d; *Chlamydia or chancroid:* 1 g PO × 1; *Uncomplicated gonorrhea:* 2 g PO × 1 (or 1 g PO × 1 plus fluoroquinolone or ceftriaxone or cefixime); *Pelvic inflammatory disease:* 500 mg IV qd × 2 d, then 250 mg PO qd × 6 d; *Community-acquired pneumonia:* 500 mg IV qd × 2–5 d, then 500 mg PO qd for a total 7–10 d

Beclomethasone (Beclovent)

Type: Corticosteroids; *Class:* Pregnancy: C   Lactation: U

Note: Each metered inhalation delivers 42 μg of aerosolized drug

Dose: Asthma: 4–16 inhalations/d (see note); *Rhinitis:* 1–2 inhalations in each nostril qd; max 336 μg/d; *Nasal polyp prophylaxis:* 1–2 inhalations in each nostril qd; max 336 μg/d

Betamethasone (Celestone)

Type: Corticosteroids; *Class:* Pregnancy: C   Lactation: U

Note: A single rescue course of ACS before 33 w improves neonatal outcome Repeat courses of corticosteroid was accompanied by a reduction in birthweight and an increase in the prevalence of small-for-gestational-age infants

Dose: Prevention of RDS in preterm neonates in women with preterm labor < 34 w: 12.5 mg IM × 2 doses 24 h apart; *Bursitis/ tendonitis:* 1 mL into the tendon sheath or joint combined with a local anesthetic agent; *Rheumatoid arthritis or osteoarthritis:* 0.5–2 mL into the joint

Bromocriptine (Parlodel)

Type: Antiparkinson agents; Dopaminergics; Ergot alkaloids and derivatives;

Class: Pregnancy: B   Lactation: NS

Dose: Parkinson disease: 10–40 mg PO qd; *Amenorrhea:* 5–7.5 mg PO qhs; *Acromegaly:* 20–30 mg PO qd

Budesonide (Budecort)

Type: Corticosteroids; inhalation; *Class:* Pregnancy: C   Lactation: S (likely)

Note: Preferred steroid for treatment of asthma during pregnancy

Dose: Asthma: 0.5–1 mg/d inhalation; *Rhinitis:* metered dose 50 μg/puff inhalation

Bupivacaine (Bupivacaine HCl; Marcaine)

Type: Anesthetics, local; *Class:* Pregnancy: C   Lactation: S

Dose: Local anesthesia: varies, max 2 mg/kg, 400 mg/d; onset 2–10 min, duration 3–6 h; *Conduction anesthesia:* varies, recommend consulting a specialty text

(Continued)

Bupropion (Zyban; Wellbutrin)
Type: Antidepressants; SSRI; *Class:* Pregnancy: B   Lactation S (likely)
Note: Patients quit smoking after 5–7 d of treatment.
Dose: Depression: 100 mg PO tid; max dose 150 mg PO tid; *Smoking cessation:* 150–300 mg PO bid; 2nd dose should not be later than 6 pm and at least 8 h after 1st dose

Butorfanol (Stadol)
Type: Analgesics, narcotic agonist-antagonist
Dose: Pain: 0.5–2 mg IV q 3–4 h prn pain; begin 1 mg IV or 2 mg IM; *Preoperative sedation:* 2 mg IV before induction; *Epidural anesthesia:* consult a specialty text

Carbamazepine (Tegretol)
Type: Anticonvulsants; *Class:* Pregnancy: C   Lactation: S (likely)
Note: The fetal "carbamazepine syndrome" includes: facial dysmorphism, developmental delay, spina bifida, distal phalange and fingernail hypoplasia
Dose: Seizure disorder: 400–600 mg PO bid (or 12–25 mg/kg/d); max 600 mg PO bid; *Trigeminal neuralgia:* 200–400 mg PO bid

Carboprost (Hemabate)
Type: Abortifacients; Oxytocics; Prostaglandins; Stimulants, uterine contractility
Class: Pregnancy: C   Lactation: U
Dose: Pregnancy termination: begin 100 μg IM test dose, then 250 μg IM q 90–120 min; max 12 mg total or use no longer than 2 d; *Uterine atony:* 250 μg IM × 1, may repeat q 15–90 min; max 2 mg

Cefazolin (Ancef)
Type: Antibiotics; Cephalosporins, 1st-generation; *Class:* Pregnancy: B   Lactation: S
Dose: Acute infection: 25–100 mg/kg/d IV/IM q 8 h; *Cesarean section prophylaxis:* 1 g IV at umbilical cord clamping; *Bacterial endocarditis:* 1 g IV/IM 30 min before procedure

Cefotaxime (Claforan; Zetaxim)
Type: Antibiotics; Cephalosporins, 3rd-generation; *Class:* Pregnancy: B   Lactation: S
Note: Renal dosing
Dose: Bacterial infection: 1–2 g IM or IV q 8 h (see note); *Gonorrhea:* 1 g IM × 1; *Surgical prophylaxis:* 1 g IV/IM 30–90 min preoperatively

Cefoxitin (Cefxitin; Mefoxin)
Type: Antibiotics; Cephalosporins, 2nd-generation; *Class:* Pregnancy: B   Lactation: S
Dose: Bacterial infection: 1–2 g IV q 6–8 h; alternatively for severe infection, 2 g q 4 h or 3 g q 6 h; *Perioperative prophylaxis:* 2 g IV, 30–60 min preoperatively

Ceftriaxone (Rocephin)
Type: Antibiotics; Cephalosporins, 3rd-generation; *Class:* Pregnancy: B   Lactation: S
Dose: Gonorrhea: 250 mg IM × 1 (see CDC STD guidelines); *Bacterial infection:* 1–2 g IV qd; *Preoperative prophylaxis:* 1 g IV

Cephalexin (Biocef; Carnosporin)
Type: Antibiotics; Cephalosporins, 1st-generation; *Class:* Pregnancy: B   Lactation: S
Dose: Bacterial infection: 250 mg–1 g PO q 6 h

(Continued)

Cetirizine (Alltec; Zyrtec)
Type: Allergy; Antihistamines; *Class:* Pregnancy: B   Lactation: U
Dose: Allergic rhinitis: 5–10 mg PO qd; max 10 mg qd; *Urticaria:* 5–10 mg PO qd; max 10 mg qd

Chlorpromazine (Thorazine)
Type: Antiemetics; Antivertigo; Antipsychotics; Phenothiazines; Tranquilizers
Class: Pregnancy: B   Lactation: S (likely)
Note: see Imipenem
Dose: Psychosis: 200–800 mg IM qd; divide dose tid or qid; *Nausea:* 10–25 mg PO q 4–6 h;
Hiccups: 25–50 mg PO tid or qid; if no response PO, may be given IM/IV; *Tetanus:* 25–50 mg
IM/IV q 6–8 h; *Porphyria (acute):* 25–50 mg IM tid or qid

Clarithromycin (Biaxin)
Type: Antibiotics; Macrolides; *Class:* Pregnancy: C   Lactation: U
Dose: Bacterial infection: 250–500 mg PO bid; *Mycoplasma avium cellulare infection:* 15 mg/kg
PO qd; dose divided q 12 h; *Coxiella burnetii (Q fever) during pregnancy:* 250–500 mg PO bid

Clavulanate
Type: Antiinfectives; *Class:* Pregnancy: B   Lactation: S
Note: see Penicillin, Amoxicillin and Ticarcillin
Dose: Clavulanate is combined with Penicillin, Amoxicillin, and Ticarcillin to broaden their
antibacterial spectrum to include certain gram-negative bacteria

Clindamycin (Cleocin)
Type: Antibiotics; Dermatologics; Lincosamides; *Class:* Pregnancy: B   Lactation: S
Dose: Bacterial infections: 150–450 mg PO qid × 7–14 d; max 4.8 g/d; alternatively, 300–900 mg
IV q 6–12 h; *Bacterial vaginosis:* 1 applicator PV qhs × 3–7 d; *Acne vulgaris:* apply 1% gel
topically bid

Clomiphene citrate (Clomid)
Type: Hormones; Stimulants, ovarian; *Class:* Pregnancy: X   Lactation: U
Note: No clear pattern of malformations is detectable. Rare ocular abnormalities (persistent
hyperplastic primary vitreous and retinal aplasia) have been reported in the offspring
Dose: Ovulation induction: 50 mg PO qd for 5 d (menstrual cycle day 5–10); max 100 mg PO qd

Cromolyn (Cromoglicic Acid; Cromogloz)
Type: Antiasthmatics; Ophthalmics; Mast cell stabilizers; *Class:* Pregnancy: B   Lactation: S
Dose: Mastocytosis: 200 mg PO qid; *Food allergy:* 200 mg PO qid; *Inflammatory bowel disease:*
200 mg PO qid; *Asthma and exercise:* induced asthma (chronic treatment) 20 mg NEB qid;
Allergic rhinitis: 1 puff per nostril bid or tid (5.2 mg/spray); *Allergic conjunctivitis, vernal keratitis:*
1 gtt OS/OD 4–6 × /d

Cyclophosphamide (Cytokan)
Type: Antineoplastics; Antirheumatics; Alkylating agents; *Class:* Pregnancy: D   Lactation: NS
Note: No clear pattern of malformations was detectable. Neonatal hematologic suppression and
secondary malignancies have been reported in the offspring; Hydration is essential
Dose: Chemotherapy: varies depending on tumor and protocol; *Mycosis fungoides:* 2–3 mg/kg
PO qd; *Rheumatoid arthritis:* 1.5–3 mg/kg PO qd

(Continued)

Cyclosporine (Ciclosporin)
Type: Immunosuppressants; *Class:* Pregnancy: D   Lactation: S (likely)
Note: No clear pattern of malformations was detectable. Some studies report a higher incidence of stillbirth and IUGR in transplant patients
Dose: Prevention of transplant rejection: 5–10 mg/kg/d PO in 2 divided doses; 5–6 mg/kg IV 4–12 h before surgery

Danazol (Danocrine)
Type: Hormones, other gynecologic; *Class:* Pregnancy: X   Lactation: NS
Note: An androgenic effect on female fetuses (vaginal atresia, clitoral hypertrophy, labial fusion, ambiguous genitalia) is possible. In pregnancies exposed to Danazol there is no reason a priori to terminate pregnancy
Dose: Endometriosis: begin 200–400 mg PO bid depending on severity; continue for 3–6 mo trial; *Fibrocystic breast disease:* 50–200 mg PO bid for 2–6 mo, then adjust dose; *Hereditary angioedema:* 200 mg PO tid until response, then half dose for 1–3 mo

Dapsone (Danocrine)
Type: Antimycobacterials; *Class:* Pregnancy: C   Lactation: S (likely)
Dose: Pneumocystis carinii pneumonia: 100 mg PO qd; usually given with trimethoprim (20 mg/kg qd × 3 w); *Dermatitis herpetiformis:* begin 50 mg PO qd, increase to 300 mg qd as needed; *Malaria suppression:* 100 mg PO qw, give with pyrimethamine 12.5 mg PO qw; *Leprosy prophylaxis:* 100 mg PO qd × 24 mo; *Leprosy treatment:* 50 mg PO qd

Dexamethasone (Corotason)
Type: Corotason; Curson; *Class:* Pregnancy: C   Lactation: U
Note: A single rescue course of steroids before 33 w improves neonatal outcome
Dose: Prevention of RDS in preterm neonates: 6 mg IM q 12 h × 4 doses; *Cerebral edema:* 10 mg IV, then 4 mg IM q 6 h; *Adrenal insufficiency:* 0.03–0.15 mg/kg PO, IV, IM qd; *Inflammatory states:* 0.75–9 mg PO, IV, IM qd; *Inflammatory ocular:* 1–2 gtt q 1–6 h; *Congenital adrenal hyperplasia:* 0.5 mg and 2 mg PO qd; *Allergic reactions:* 0.75–9 mg PO qd; *Shock:* 1–6 mg/kg IV q 2–6 h prn; *Diagnostic test for Cushing disease:* 2.0 mg of dexamethasone PO q 6 h for 48 h; 24-h urine collection required to calculate 17-hydroxycorticosteroid production; *Postoperative N/V:* 4–5 mg IV

Diazepam (Tranquil; Valitran; Valium)
Type: Anxiolytics; Benzodiazepine; Muscle relaxants; *Class:* Pregnancy: C   Lactation: U
Dose: Anxiety: 2–10 mg IV, IM tid/qid; *Alcohol withdrawal:* 5 mg PO tid/qid prn; *Seizure disorder:* 2–10 mg PO bid/qid; *Status epilepticus:* 5–10 mg IV q 10–15 min; *Muscle spasm:* 2–10 mg PO bid/qid

Dicloxacillin (Dycill; Dynapen)
Type: Antibiotics; Penicillins; *Class:* Pregnancy: B   Lactation: S
Dose: Skin infection: 125–500 mg PO q 6 h 1 h before or after a meal; *Osteomyelitis:* 250–500 mg PO q 6 h before or after a meal; *Mastitis:* 250–500 mg PO q 6 h before or after a meal

Dimenhydrinate (Amosyt; Biodramina)
Type: Anticholinergics; Antiemetics; Antivertigo; *Class:* Pregnancy: B   Lactation: S
Dose: Motion sickness: 50–100 mg PO, IM, IV q 4–6 h; begin at least 30 min before anticipated activity, max 400 mg/d *Migraine:* 50–100 mg PO

(Continued)

Dinoprostone (Cervidil; Prepidil; Prostin E2)

Type: Oxytocics; Prostaglandins; *Class:* Pregnancy: C   Lactation: S

Note: May augment the activity of other oxytocic agents and their concomitant use is not recommended. A 6- to 12-h interval is recommended

Dose: Cervical ripening: 0.5 mg gel PV endocervical, may repeat q 6 h $\times$ 2; alternatively, 10 mg insert PV into the posterior fornix (remain supine 2 h), remove with onset of labor or uterine hyperstimulation

---

Diphenhydramine (Amidryl)

Type: Antihistamines; *Class:* Pregnancy: B   Lactation: S

Dose: Antihistaminic: 25–50 mg PO/IV/IM q 6 h prn; *Anaphylaxis:* 1–1.25 mg/kg PO/IV/IM q 4–6 h; max 300 mg/d; *Dystonic reactions:* 25–50 mg PO tid/qid; max 300 mg/d; *Sedation:* 25–50 mg PO qid prn; *Insomnia:* 50 mg PO qhs; *Motion sickness:* 25–50 mg PO q 4–6 h prn; max 300 mg/d

---

Dopamine (Intropin)

Type: Adrenergic agonists; Inotropes; *Class:* Pregnancy: C   Lactation: NS

Dose: Adjunct for shock: 1–50 µg/kg/min IV; max 20–50 µg/kg/min; • 2–5 µg/kg/min primarily dopaminergic receptor effects, but may exhibit a pressor effect; • 5–10 µg/kg/min primarily beta-adrenergic effects with inotropy and chronotropy; • >10 µg/kg/min primarily alpha-adrenergic effects with peripheral vasoconstriction; *Refractory CHF:* 1–3 µg/kg/min IV

Doxycycline (Doxy; Doxy-100)

Type: Antibiotics; Tetracyclines; *Class:* Pregnancy: D   Lactation: NS

Note: Exposure of the fetus during the 3rd trimester, infancy, and in children less than 8 years can cause permanent discoloration of the teeth

Dose: Gonorrhea, uncomplicated: 100 mg PO bid $\times$ 7 d; *Chlamydia:* 100 mg PO bid $\times$ 7 d; *Pelvic inflammatory disease:* 100 mg PO bid $\times$ 10–14 d with another agent such as ceftriaxone 250 mg IM; *Malaria:* 100 mg PO qd beginning 1–2 d before departure and continuing through 4 w after exposure; *Lyme disease:* 100 mg PO bid $\times$ 14–21 d (28 d if associated with arthritis); *Anthrax:* 100 mg IV, PO q 12 h; post-exposure, 100 mg PO q 12 h for 60 d or until disease excluded

---

Doxylamine (Nyquil)

Type: Antihistamines; *Class:* Pregnancy: B   Lactation: S

Dose: Allergies: 12.5 to 25 mg PO q 4–6 h; prn; *Hyperemesis gravidarum:* 12.5 mg PO q 6–8 h; prn

---

Droperidol (Inapsine)

Type: Anesthetics, adjunct; Antivertigo; Anxiolytics; Sedatives; *Class:* Pregnancy: C   Lactation: S

Dose: Nausea and vomiting (perioperative): 0.625–1.25 mg IM/IV q 3–4 h prn

---

Efavirenz (Sustiva)

Type: Antivirals; Non-nucleoside reverse transcriptase inhibitors

Class: Pregnancy: D   Lactation: S

Note: Efavirenz was reported to be associated with CNS malformations in primates and humans; Astemizole, Midazolam, Triazolam, Cisapride, ergot derivatives should not be administered with Efavirenz

Dose: HIV infection: 600 mg PO qd

(Continued)

Enoxaparin (Lovenox)
Type: Anticoagulants; Low-molecular-weight heparins; *Class:* Pregnancy: B   Lactation: S (likely)
Note: Consult a specialty text such as *High Risk Pregnancy: Management Options*
Dose: Prophylaxis DVT: begin at 20–40 mg SC qd (see note); *Antiphospholipid syndrome:* begin at 20–40 mg SC qd; *Cesarean section:* at least 40 mg SC qd until patient is active; *Treatment of acute thrombosis:* 1–1.5 mg/kg SC q 12 h

Ephedrine (Ephedrine)
Type: Adrenergic agonists; Bronchodilators; Decongestants, nasal; *Class:* Pregnancy: C
Lactation: S
Dose: Decongestant: 25–50 mg PO q 6 h (max 150 mg/d)

Epinephrine (Adrenalin Chloride)
Type: Adrenergic agonists; Bronchodilators; Inotropes; Ophthalmics; Pressors;
Class: Pregnancy: C   Lactation: S
Dose: Severe asthma: 0.1–0.5 mg SC q 10–15 min; *Anaphylaxis:* 0.1–0.5 mg SC q 10–15 min (or 0.1–0.25 mg IV over 5–10 min); *Cardiac arrest:* 0.5–1 mg IV q 3–5 min prn (or 1 mg via ET tube, 0.1–1 mg intracardiac); may follow with 1–4 μg/min constant infusion

Erythromycin (Akne-Mycin; C-Solve-2)
Type: Antibiotics; Dermatologics; Macrolides; Ophthalmics; *Class:* Pregnancy: B   Lactation: S
Dose: Bacterial infection: 250–500 mg PO q 6–12 h; *Preterm PROM:* 250 mg PO qid × 10 d

Etanercept (Enbrel)
Type: Antitumor necrosis factor alpha; *Class:* Pregnancy: B   Lactation: U
Dose: Rheumatoid arthritis: SC 40 mg every other week

Famciclovir (Famvir)
Type: Antivirals; *Class:* Pregnancy: B   Lactation: U
Dose: Genital herpes (1st episode): 250 mg PO tid × 7 d; *Genital herpes (recurrent):* 125 mg PO bid × 5 d; *Genital herpes (prophylaxis):* 250 mg PO bid; *Herpes zoster:* 500 mg PO tid × 7 d

Fentanyl (Fentanyl Oralet)
Type: Analgesics; Narcotics; Anesthetics; general; *Class:* Pregnancy: C   Lactation: S
Dose: Preoperative analgesia: 50–100 μg IV 30–60 min prior to surgery; *Anesthesia, adjunct:* 2–50 μg/kg IV depending on needs; *Labor epidural anesthesia:* approximately 25 μg intrathecal; 40–50 μg epidural: usually followed by a dose of 20–30 μg/h mixed in solution of dilute local anesthetics (consult a specialty text); *Labor analgesia (IV):* begin 50 μg IV, thereafter 25 μg q 20–30 min prn; *Postoperative pain relief:* 50–100 μg IV q 1–2 h prn

Flunisolide (AeroBid; Nasalide; Nasarel)
Type: Corticosteroids, inhalation; *Class:* Pregnancy: C   Lactation: U
Dose: Asthma prophylaxis: 2 puffs INH bid (approx 50 μg per puff); *Allergic rhinitis:* 2 sprays/nostril bid/tid

Fluticasone (Cutivate; Flonase)
Type: Corticosteroids, inhalation; Corticosteroids, topical; Dermatologics;
Class: Pregnancy: C   Lactation: S
Dose: Asthma prophylaxis: begin 88 μg bid if on bronchodilator alone; max 880 μg bid, taper to lowest effective dose

(Continued)

Formoterol (Foradil Aerolizer)
Type: Adrenergic agonists; Bronchodilators; *Class:* Pregnancy: C   Lactation: S
Dose: Asthma prophylaxis: 12 µg INH (inhalation) q 12 h; *Treatment of exercise:* induced
asthma: 12 µg INH 15–30 min prior to exercise; may repeat q 12 h prn, max 24 µg/d; *COPD
maintenance:* 12 µg INH q 12 h; max 24 µg/d

Furosemide (Lasix)
Type: Diuretics, loop, thiazide diuretics; *Class:* Pregnancy: C   Lactation: S (likely)
Dose: Pulmonary edema: begin at 40 mg IV × 1 slowly, assess response; may increase to 80 mg
IV q 1 h prn; *Peripheral edema:* 20–80 mg PO qd to bid; max 600 mg qd; *Hypertension:* 40 mg
PO bid; max 600 mg qd; *Hypercalcemia:* 80–100 mg IV q 1–2 h, or 120 mg PO qd

Foscarnet (Foscavir)
Type: Antivirals; *Class:* Pregnancy: C   Lactation: U
Dose: Acyclovir-resistant HSV: 40 mg/kg IV given over 1h q 8 h for 2–3 w; *CMV retinitis,
AIDS:* begin at 60 mg/kg IV given over 1 h q 8 h; administer maintenance dose × 2–3 w

Gentamicin (Garamycin; Genoptic)
Type: Aminoglycoside; Antibiotics; Dermatologics; Ophthalmics; Otics;
Class: Pregnancy: C   Lactation: S
Dose: Bacterial infection: 1–3 mg/kg/d in 3 divided doses to achieve a peak 5–10 µg/mL and
trough <2 µg/mL; *Endocarditis prophylaxis:* 1.5 mg/kg IV 30–60 min prior to the procedure

Glyburide (DiaBeta; Micronase)
Type: Hypoglycemics; Sulfonylureas; *Class:* Pregnancy: B   Lactation: U
Dose: Diabetes mellitus, type 2: begin 2.5–5 mg PO with first main meal of the day; usual
maintenance dose 2.5–5.0 mg/d; max 20 mg qd (micronized 1.5–3.0 mg/d; usual maintenance
dose 0.75–1.25 mg/d)

Haloperidol (Haldol)
Type: Antipsychotics; *Class:* Pregnancy: B   Lactation: U
Dose: Psychosis: 0.5–5 mg PO bid/tid; max 100 mg/d; or 2.5 mg IV/IM q 4–8 h; *Tourette's
syndrome:* begin 0.5–1.5 mg PO tid, increase 2 mg/d prn; typically 9 mg/d; *Acute psychosis:*
0.5–50 mg IV (slow, at 5 mg/min)

Heparin (Heparin Flush; Heparin Lok-Pak)
Type: Anticoagulants; *Class:* Pregnancy: B   Lactation: S
Note: Keep aPTT 1.5–2.5 times control
Dose: Thromboembolic disease treatment: 80 U/kg IV × 1, then 18 U/kg/h IV to achieve an aPTT
1.5–2 × baseline (see note); *Thromboembolic disease prophylaxis:* 5000 U SC bid 1st trimester,
7500 U SC bid 2nd trimester, 10,000 U SC bid 3 rd trimester; *Antiphospholipid syndrome:* 81 mg
PO qd aspirin plus 5000 U SC bid 1st trimester, 7500 U SC bid 2nd trimester, 10,000 U bid 3 rd
trimester

Hydralazine (Apresoline; Apresrex)
Type: Antihypertensives; Vasodilators; *Class:* Pregnancy: C   Lactation: S
Dose: Hypertension (moderate to severe): begin 10–50 mg PO qid × 2–4 d, then 25 mg PO qid × 1 w;
max 100 mg PO qid; alternatively, 5–40 mg IV/IM q 4–6 h; for chronic use, switch to PO ASAP;
CHF: begin 50–75 mg PO × 1, then 50–150 mg PO qid; max 3000 mg/d

(Continued)

Hydroxychloroquine (Plaquenil)

Type: Antimalarials; Antiprotozoals; Antirheumatics; Immunomodulators;

Class: Pregnancy: C   Lactation: S

Dose: Systemic lupus erythematosus: 400 mg PO qd/bid; *Malaria treatment:* begin 800 mg PO bid × 1, followed 6–8 h later by 400 mg PO, then 400 mg PO qd × 2; *Malaria prophylaxis:* begin 400 mg PO qw × 2 w prior to exposure, continue 4–6 w after exposure; *Rheumatoid arthritis:* begin 400–600 mg PO qd × 4–12 w, then 200–400 mg PO qid

---

Hydroxyzine (Atarax; Atazina)

Type: Antiemetics; Antihistamines, H1; Antivertigo; Anxiolytics; Hypnotics; Sedatives;

Class: Pregnancy: C   Lactation: U

Dose: Anxiety: 50–100 mg PO or IM q 6 h prn; max 600 mg/d; *Pruritus:* 25–100 mg PO q 6–8 h prn; *Nausea, vomiting:* 25–100 mg IM q 4–6 h prn; max 600 mg/d; *Sedation adjunct:* 25–100 mg IM × 1; *Insomnia:* 50–100 mg PO qhs

---

Imipenem (Primaxin)

Type: Antibiotics; Carbapenems; *Class:* Pregnancy: C   Lactation: S

Dose: Serious bacterial infection: 250–1000 mg IM/IV q 12 h; max 50 mg/kg/d or 4000 mg/d

---

Indomethacin (Indocin)

Type: Analgesics, non-narcotic; Antiarthritics; NSAID; Antiinflammatory;

Class: Pregnancy: B   Lactation: S

Note: Indomethacin is closing the ductus arteriosus and may induce oligohydramnios and fetal renal failure

Dose: Dysmenorrhea: 25 mg PO tid/qid; *Mild to moderate pain:* 25–50 mg PO tid prn; *Osteoarthritis or rheumatoid arthritis:* begin 25 mg PO bid/tid, or 50 mg prn qid, increase by 25–50 mg q 7 d; max 200 mg/d; *Tocolysis:* 50 mg PR or PO load, then 25 mg PO/PR q 6 h × 2 d

---

Infliximab (Remicade)

Type: Antiinflammatory; Antirheumatics; Inflammatory bowel disease; Tumor necrosis factor modulators; *Class:* Pregnancy: C   Lactation: S (likely)

Note: Women on remission therapy can continue their Inflixumab given the disease may flare if the therapy is stopped

Dose: Crohn disease, moderate to severe: 5 mg/kg IV × 1 (see note); *Crohn disease, fistulizing:* 5 mg/kg IV × 1 for weeks 0, 2, 6; *Rheumatoid arthritis:* begin 3 mg/kg IV × 1 for weeks 0, 2, 6; may increase dose to 10 mg/kg or increase dose up to 10 mg/kg

---

Insulin, recombinant human (Humulin R, L, N and U)

Type: Antidiabetic agents; Hypoglycemics; *Class:* Pregnancy: B   Lactation: S

Dose: Diabetes mellitus:; *SC: R(egular):* 0.5–1 U/kg SC qd in 3–4 divided doses: give 30–60 min qac, onset 0.5 h, peak 2–4 h, duration 6–8 h; *L(ente):* give 30 min before meal or qhs, onset 1–3 h, peak 8–12 h, duration 18–24 h; *N(PH):* give 30–60 min before breakfast, onset 1–2 h, peak 6–12 h, duration 18–24 h; *U(ltralente):* 0.5–1 U/kg/d SC in 1–2 divided doses: give 30–60 min before meal; onset 4–8 h, peak 16–18 h, duration > 36 h; *Diabetic ketoacidosis:* begin 0.1 U/kg IV bolus of R, then 0.1 U/kg/h infusion; decrease infusion rate when glucose <275 mg/dL

(Continued)

Interferon alpha 2a (Roferon A)

Type: Antineoplastics, interferon; Antivirals, interferon; Immunomodulators;

Class: Pregnancy: B   Lactation: S

Dose: Chronic hepatitis C with compensated liver disease: 3 million U/d SC/IM 3 × /w for 52 w; *AIDS-associated Kaposi sarcoma:* begin 36 million U/d SC/IM × 10–12 w, then 3 × /w; *Hairy cell leukaemia:* begin 3 million U/d × 16–24 w, then 3 × /w

Ipratropium bromide (Atrovent; Disne-Asmol)

Type: Anticholinergics; Bronchodilators; *Class:* Pregnancy: B   Lactation: S

Note: Available in bronchial and nasal (0.03 and 0.06%) inhalers

Dose: Bronchospasm: 2–3 puffs INH tid-qid; alternatively 500 μg NEB q 6–8 h; *Rhinitis:* 2 sprays/nostril bid/tid (0.03%); *Rhinorrhea associated with cold:* 2 sprays/nostril tid/qid (0.06%)

Labetalol (Coreton; Normadate)

Type: Adrenergic antagonists; Alpha and beta blocker; Anti-hypertensives

Class: Pregnancy: C   Lactation: S

Dose: Hypertension: begin 100 mg PO bid, increase 100 mg bid q 2–3 w; max 2.4 g/d; *Acute hypertension:* if diastolic BP >105 mmHg, administer incremental dosing of 5–10 mg IV, with a cumulative dose of 40–80 mg IV over 20 min; max 300 mg IV

Lamotrigine (Lamictal)

Type: Anticonvulsants; *Class:* Pregnancy: C   Lactation: S (likely)

Note: Lamotrigene levels vary widely during pregnancy, and patients may experience a lose of seizure control without close monitoring

Dose: Seizures: begin 50 mg/d, then increase up to 50–250 mg PO bid; max 500 mg/d

Leflunomide (Arava)

Type: Antirheumatics; Immunomodulators; *Class:* Pregnancy: X   Lactation: U

Dose: Rheumatoid arthritis: begin 100 mg PO qd × 3 d, then 10–20 mg PO qd

Levofloxacin (Cravit; Lesacin)

Type: Antibiotics; Quinolones; *Class:* Pregnancy: C   Lactation: NS

Dose: Bacterial infections: 250–500 mg PO/IV qd

Lidocaine (Alphacaine; Leostesin)

Type: Anesthetics, local; Anesthetics, topical; *Class:* Pregnancy: B   Lactation: S

Note: Caution should be used in patients receiving class I antiarrhythmic drugs (e.g., Mexiletin, Tocaidine)

Dose: Ventricular arrhythmia: begin 1–1.5 mg/kg IV; may repeat bolus in 5 min, then begin infusion 1–4 mg/min IV; max 300 mg × 1 h; *Local anesthesia:* infiltrate IM/SC; max 300 mg; *Postherpetic neuralgia:* apply topically q 12 h

(Continued)

Magnesium sulfate (Tis U Sol)

Type: Anticonvulsants; Electrolyte replacements; Tocolytics;

Class: Pregnancy: A   Lactation: U

Note: Recent studies suggest that Magnesium sulphate holds a significant neuroprotective effect on premature neonates; Renal dosing; measure serum magnesium every 4–6 h if infusion >2g/h or oliguria or maternal symptoms of toxicity; maintain between 4 and 7 mEq/L (4.8–8.4 mg/dL)

Dose: Ventricular arrhythmia: 3–20 mg/min IV continuous IV × 6–48 h; *Eclampsia, prevention and treatment:* begin 4 g IV × 1 over 30 min; then 2 g/h IV maintenance rate for at least 24 h postpartum, or during diuresis >200 mL/h; alternatively, 10 g IM loading dose followed by 5 g IM q 4 h until at least 24 h postpartum; *Tocolysis:* begin 6 g IV × 1 over 30 min, then 2–4 g/h IV × 48 h; *Hypomagnesemia:* 1 g IM q 4–6 h; alternative 5 g mixed in 1 L NS IV over 3 h

Meclizine (Antivert; Ancolan)

Type: Antiemetics; Antihistamines, H1; Antivertigo; *Class:* Pregnancy: B   Lactation: S

Dose: Nausea, vomiting and dizziness due to motion sickness: 25–50 mg PO qd 1 h before travel; repeat q 24 h

Medroxyprogesterone (Amen; Aragest)

Type: Antineoplastics, hormone; Contraceptives; Hormones; *Class:* Pregnancy: X   Lactation: S

Note: Exposure of the male fetus in utero may double the risk of hypospadias

Dose: Amenorrhea: 5–10 mg PO qd × 5 on days 16–21 of the cycle or q mo; *Dysfunctional uterine bleeding:* 5–10 mg PO qd × 5 on days 16–21 of the cycle or q mo; *Hormone replacement:* 5–10 mg PO qd × 12–14 d; *Contraception:* 150 mg IM q 3 mo

Meperidine (Demerol; Doloneurin)

Type: Analgesics, narcotic; Anesthetics, adjunct; *Class:* Pregnancy: B   Lactation: S

Note: 75 mg parenteral Meperidine = 10 mg parenteral morphine

Dose: Pain: 50–150 mg PO/SC/IM q 3–4 h; IM preferred over SC/IV; *Preoperative sedation:* 50–100 mg SC/IM × 1, 30–60 min before surgery; *Obstetrical analgesia:* 50–100 mg SC/IM/IV q 3–4 h

Methacholine (Provocholine)

Type: Cholinergics; Diagnostics, nonradioactive; *Class:* Pregnancy: C   Lactation: S

Note: Diagnostic purpose only. Methacholine inhalation challenge should be performed only under the supervision of a physician trained in and thoroughly familiar with all aspects of the technique

Dose: Diagnosis of bronchial airway hyper-reactivity: 5 breaths (neb); measure FEV$_1$ at baseline and after 5 breaths

Methimazole (Antitroide-GW; Favistan)

Type: Antithyroid agents; Hormones; *Class:* Pregnancy: D   Lactation: S (likely)

Note: Methimazole and can induce fetal goiter and even cretinism in a dose-dependent fashion. Aplasia cutis is a rare complication of maternal therapy

Dose: Hyperthyroidism: begin 5–20 mg PO q 8h, then 5–15 mg PO qd

(Continued)

Methotrexate (Abitrexate; Emtexate)
Type: Antineoplastics, antimetabolite; Antirheumatics; *Class:* Pregnancy: X   Lactation: NS (likely)
Note: 1st trimester exposure to Methotrexate increases the risk of malformations (craniofacial, axial skeletal, cardiopulmonary, gastro-intestinal abnormalities and developmental delay) though most pregnancies exposed to low doses are unaffected
Dose: Ectopic pregnancy: 50 mg/m² IM × 1; may be repeated in 1 w if hCG rising; *Trophoblastic disease:* 15–30 mg PO/IM qd × 5 d; repeat × 3–5 at >1 w intervals; administer with folic acid 1 mg PO qd or leukovorin 5 mg qw; *Rheumatoid arthritis:* 7.5–25 mg PO/IM/SC qw; alternatively 2.5–7.5 mg PO q 12 h 3 × /w; max 30 mg/w; *Psoriasis:* 10–25 mg PO/IM/SC qw; alternatively 2.5–7.5 mg PO q 12 h 3 × /w; max 30 mg/w; *Mycosis fungoides:* 5–50 mg PO/IV qw; alternatively 15–37.5 mg PO 2 × /w; *Chemotherapy:* numerous dosing schedules depending on disease, response, and concomitant therapy

Methyldopa (Aldomet; Alfametildopa)
Type: Adrenergic antagonists, central; Antihypertensives; *Class:* Pregnancy: B   Lactation: S
Dose: Hypertension: 250–500 mg PO bid; begin 250 mg PO bid and adjust q 2d; max 3 g/d; alternative 250–500 mg IV q 6 h × 4, then PO

Methylergonovine (Methergine)
Type: Ergot alkaloids; Oxytocics; Uterine stimulants; *Class:* Pregnancy: C   Lactation: S
Dose: Postpartum bleeding – emergent: 0.2 mg IM q 2–4 h; max 5 doses; *Postpartum bleeding – on-emergent:* 0.2–0.4 mg PO q 6–12 h; max duration 7 d

Methylprednisolone (Medlone; Medrol)
Type: Corticosteroids; *Class:* Pregnancy: C   Lactation: S
Note: 4 mg Methylprednisolone = 5 mg Prednisolone
Dose: Inflammatory disorders: 2–60 mg PO qd; *Congenital adrenal hyperplasia:* 2–60 mg PO qd; *Rheumatic disorders, adjunctive treatment:* 2–60 mg PO qd; *Collagen vascular diseases:* 2–60 mg PO qd; *Allergy:* 2–60 mg PO qd; *Respiratory diseases:* 2–60 mg PO qd; *Hematologic disorders:* 2–60 mg PO qd; *Multiple sclerosis:* acute exacerbations 200 mg PO qd × 7 d, then 80 mg PO qod × 1 m

Metoclopramide (Reglan)
Type: Antiemetics; Antivertigo; Gastrointestinals; *Class:* Pregnancy: B   Lactation: S
Dose: Nausea, vomiting: 5–10 mg PO/IM/IV q 6–8 h; *Nausea, vomiting (chemo):* 1–2 mg/kg IV/PO q 2–4 h; *Gastroesophageal reflux disease:* 5–15 mg PO/IV/IM qac, qhs; *Gastroparesis (diabetes):* 10 mg IV/PO qac, qhs

Metronidazole (Flagyl)
Type: Antibiotics; Antiprotozoals; Dermatologics; *Class:* Pregnancy: B   Lactation: S
Dose: Bacterial infections: 500 mg PO q 6–8 h × 7–14 d; alternative 15 mg/kg/IV × 1 followed by 7.5 mg/kg IV q 5h; max 1 g/dose; *Amebic abscess:* 500–750 mg PO tid × 5–10 d; *Bacterial vaginosis:* 2 g PO × 1, alternative 500 mg PO bid × 7 d; *Giardiasis:* 250 mg PO tid × 5–7 d; alternative 2 g PO qd × 3 d; *C. difficile colitis:* 500 mg PO tid × 7–14 d; alternative 250 mg PO qid × 7–14 d; *Rosacea:* topical gel application bid × 9 w; *Vaginal trichomoniasis:* 2 g PO × 1; alternative 500 mg PO bid × 7 d, 1 g PO bid × 1 d (partner treatment is critical)

(Continued)

Misoprostol (Cytotec)

Type: Abortifacients; Gastrointestinals; Oxytocics; Prostaglandins; Stimulants, uterine;

Class: Pregnancy: X   Lactation: U

Note: Contraindicated in women with prior uterine scar

Dose: NSAID-induced gastric ulcers: 100–200 μg PO qid; *Constipation:* 600–2400 μg/d PO bid-qid; *Cervical ripening:* 25 μg vaginally q 3–6 h; wait at least 4 h before initiating oxytocin; max 50 μg/dose; *Abortion:* 400 μg PO × 1; may repeat q 4–6 h

---

Montelukast (Singulair)

Type: Antileukotriene; *Class:* Pregnancy: B   Lactation: NS

Dose: Asthma: 10.4 mg PO qd

Morphine (Avinza; Kadian)

Type: Analgesics, narcotic; *Class:* Pregnancy: C   Lactation: S

Dose: Pain: 2.5–10 mg IV slowly over 5–15 min; alternative 5–20 mg IM/SC or 10–30 mg PO q 4 h; *Post-cesarean section analgesia:* intrathecal 100–250 μg, epidural 2–5 mg

---

Nalbuphine (Nubain)

Type: Analeptics; Narcotic agonist-antagonists; *Class:* Pregnancy: B   Lactation: S

Dose: Pain: 10 mg IV/IM/SC q 3–6 h prn; max 20 mg/dose or 160 mg/d; *Anesthesia (adjunct):* 0.25–0.5 mg/kg prn; begin 0.3–3 mg/kg IV

Naloxone (Narcan)

Type: Antidotes; Narcotic agonist-antagonists; *Class:* Pregnancy: B   Lactation: S

Dose: Opiate overdose: 0.4–2 mg SC/IV/IM q 2–3 min; if no response by 10 min, the diagnosis should be questioned; *Postoperative opiate reversal:* 0.1–0.2 mg IV q 2–3 min prn

---

Nevirapine (Viramune)

Type: Antivirals; Non-nucleoside reverse transcriptase inhibitors;

Class: Pregnancy: C   Lactation: NS

Note: Should be initiated in pregnant women with CD4 counts >250 cells/mm ^{3} only if benefits outweighs risk due to potential for hepatotoxicity

Dose: HIV infection: 200 mg PO qd × 14 d; continue treatment with 200 mg PO bid in combination with nucleoside antiretrovirals

---

Nicardipine (Cardene)

Type: Antiarrhythmics; Antihypertensives; Calcium-channel blockers;

Class: Pregnancy: C   Lactation: U

Dose: Hypertension: 20–40 mg PO tid; max 40 mg PO tid; *Angina:* begin 20 mg PO tid; max 40 mg PO tid; *Acute hypertension:* 5 mg/h, increase 2.5 mg/h q 5–15 min prn, titrate down to effect

---

Nifedipine (Adalat; Procardia XL)

Type: Antiarrhythmics; Antihypertensives; Calcium-channel blockers;

Class: Pregnancy: C   Lactation: S (likely)

Dose: Hypertension: begin 10 mg PO tid, titer to effect; max 180 mg/d; *Angina, Prinzmetal's:* begin 10 mg PO tid, titer to effect; max 180 mg/d; *Angina variant:* begin 10 mg PO tid, titer to effect; max 180 mg/d

---

(Continued)

Nitrofurantoin (Macrodantin; Macrobid)
Type: Antibiotics; Nitrofurans; *Class:* Pregnancy: B   Lactation: S (likely)
Dose: Urinary tract infection: 100 mg PO bid; alternative 50–100 mg PO qid; *Urinary tract infection suppression:* 50–100 mg PO qhs

Nitroglycerin (Nitro-Dur; Nitrolingual)
Type: Vasodilators; *Class:* Pregnancy: C   Lactation: U
Dose: Angina, acute: 0.3–0.6 mg SL q 5 min; max 3 doses within 15 min; *Angina, prophylaxis:* 0.3–0.6 mg SL × 1; take 5–10 min before strenuous activity

Ondansetron (Zofran)
Type: Antiemetics; Serotonin receptor antagonists; *Class:* Pregnancy: B   Lactation: U
Dose: Severe nausea and vomiting – postoperative: 4 mg IM/IV × 1; pre-chemotherapy: 24 mg PO or 32 mg IV 30 min before initiating chemotherapy; *Severe nausea and vomiting – radiation therapy:* begin 8 mg PO 1–2 h before radiation, continue q 8 h × 2 d

Oseltamivir (Tamiflu)
Type: Antivirals; *Class:* Pregnancy: C   Lactation: U
Note: Pregnancy should not be considered a contraindication to Oseltamivir (http://www.cdc.gov/h1n1flu/recommendations.htm)
Dose: Influenza A/B; H1N1 (swine flu) – prophylaxis: 75 mg PO qd; initiate at outbreak; *Influenza A/B; H1N1 (swine flu) – treatment:* 75 mg PO bid × 5 d beginning within 48 h of symptoms

Oxcarbazepine (Trileptal)
Type: Anticonvulsants; *Class:* Pregnancy: C   Lactation: S (likely)
Dose: Seizure disorder: begin at 300 mg PO bid, increasing by 300 mg/d q 3 d; max 2400 mg/d

Oxytocin (Pitocin; Syntocinon; Xitocin)
Type: Hormones/hormone modifiers; Oxytocics; Stimulants, uterine;
Class: Pregnancy: X   Lactation: S (likely)
Note: Oxytocin is used only to end pregnancy and poses only labor-associated risk to the fetus; Oxytocin is the drug of choice for labor augmentation. Should not be used less than 4 h after Misoprostol
Dose: Labor induction: 1–2 mIU/min IV; double q 20–30 min until 8 mIU/min, then increase by 1–2 mIU/min; max 200 mIU/min; *Postpartum bleeding:* 10–40 IU/L at a rate titrated to control bleeding; *Lactation aid:* 1–2 sprays per nostril 2–3 min before feeding or pumping during the 1st week after delivery

Pancuronium (Pavulon)
Type: Neuromuscular blockers, nondepolarizing; *Class:* Pregnancy: C   Lactation: U
Dose: Paralysis: 0.04–0.1 mg/kg IV; *Paralysis, fetal:* 0.03 mg/kg fetal IM or IV into the umbilical vein

Penciclovir (Denavir)
Type: Antivirals; Dermatologics; *Class:* Pregnancy: B   Lactation: S (likely)
Dose: Herpes labialis: apply q 2 h × 4 d

(Continued)

Penicillamine (Cuprimine; Depen; Mercaptyl)

Type: Antirheumatics; Cystine-depleting agents; *Class:* Pregnancy: D   Lactation: U

Note: Congenital cutis laxa and associated defects (micrognathia, contractures, CNS abnormalities) have been reported

Dose: Wilson disease: 250–500 mg PO tid/qid 30 min before meals; *Cystinuria:* 250–1000 mg PO qid 30 min before meals; *Rheumatoid arthritis (unresponsive to conventional agents):* 250 mg PO bid/tid 30 min before meals; requires 3–6 mo for max effect; *Heavy metal poisoning:* 125–600 mg PO tid 30 min before meals

Penicillin G (Bicillin LA; Pen-Di-Ben; Permapen)

Type: Antibiotics; Penicillins; *Class:* Pregnancy: B   Lactation: S

Dose: Systemic infection (moderate to severe): 4 million units IM/IV q 4 h; *Anthrax:* 4 million units IV q 4 h as part of a multidrug regimen × 60 d for oral, GI or inhalational; 4 million units IV q 4 h × 7–10 d for cutaneous, then switch to PO for 60 d; *Neurosyphilis:* 18–24 million units qd IV × 10–14 d

Perphenazine (Trilifan; Trilafon)

Type: Antiemetics; Antipsychotics; Antivertigo; Phenothiazines; *Class:* Pregnancy: C   Lactation: U

Dose: Psychosis: 8–16 mg PO bid/qid; max 64 mg/d; *Severe nausea and vomiting:* begin 5 mg IM or PO (avoid IV); max 24 mg/d

Phenobarbital (Barbita; Dormiral; Luminal Sodium)

Type: Anticonvulsants; Barbiturates; Preanesthetics; Sedatives/ hypnotics;

Class: Pregnancy: D   Lactation: S (likely)

Dose: Seizure disorder: load with 15–20 mg/kg IV, then 60 mg PO bid/tid; *Status epilepticus:* 10–20 mg/kg IV × 1; may repeat if necessary; *Sedation:* 10–40 mg PO/IM/IV tid

Phenytoin (Dilantin; Hydantol)

Type: Anticonvulsants; Hydantoins; *Class:* Pregnancy: D   Lactation: S

Dose: Seizure disorder: load with 400 mg, 300 mg, and 300 mg PO 2–4 h apart, then 300–400 mg PO qd (or divided bid), alternatively, 10–20 mg/kg; IV × 1, then 4–6 mg/kg IV qd; *Status epilepticus:* 15–20 mg/kg IV q 30 min prn; max 1500 mg/d

Piperacillin (Pipracil)

Type: Antibiotics; Penicillins; *Class:* Pregnancy: B   Lactation: S

Note: Renal dosing; may be combined with the beta-lactamase inhibitor tazobactam (Tazosyn; Zosyn)

Dose: Bacterial infections (pseudomonas, intraabdominal or sepsis): 3–4 g IV/IM q 4–6 h × 3–10 d; *Post-gynecologic or cesarean prophylaxis:* 2 g IV 30 min preoperatively or at umbilical cord clamping, then q 4–6 h × 2; *Gonorrhea, uncomplicated:* 1 g probenecid PO 30 min before 2 g IM × 1

Piperacillin-tazobactam (Tazosyn; Zosyn)

Type: Antibiotics; Penicillins; *Class:* Pregnancy: B   Lactation: S (likely)

Dose: Bacterial infections (pseudomonas, intra-abdominal, or sepsis): 3.375 g IV q 6 h × 3–10 d; *Postpartum endomyometritis or pelvic inflammatory disease:* 3.375 g IV q 6 h × 3–10 d; *Community-acquired pneumonia:* 3.375 g IV q 6 h × 3–10 d

(Continued)

Prednisone (Adasone, Deltasone)

Type: Corticosteroids; *Class:* Pregnancy: B   Lactation: S

Dose: Inflammatory disorders: 5–60 mg PO qd; *Relapsing multiple sclerosis:* begin 200 mg PO qd × 1 w, then 80 mg PO qod × 1 m; *Pneumocystic pneumonia:* begin 40 mg PO bid × 5 d, then 40 mg qd × 5 d, then 20 mg qd; *Adrenal insufficiency:* 4–5 mg/m^2 PO qd

---

Primidone (Midone; Mylepsin)

Type: Anticonvulsants; *Class:* Pregnancy: B   Lactation: NS

Dose: Seizure disorder: begin 100–125 mg PO qhs × 3 d, 100–125 mg PO bid × 3 d, then 250 mg PO tid-qid; max 2 g/d; *Essential tremor:* begin 12.5–25 mg PO qhs, increase 12.5–25 mg/d qw; max 750 mg/d

---

Probenecid (Benemid; Panuric)

Type: Antigouts; Uricosurics; *Class:* Pregnancy: B   Lactation: S

Dose: Adjunct to penicillin therapy: 500 mg PO qid; *Gout:* begin 250 mg PO bid × 7 d; max 2–3 g/d

---

Procaine (Novocain)

Type: Anesthetics, local; *Class:* Pregnancy: C   Lactation: S (likely)

Dose: Local and regional anesthesia: dose varies; max 10 mg/kg

---

Prochlorperazine (Compazine; Cotranzine)

Type: Antiemetics; Antipsychotics; Antivertigo; Phenothiazines;

Class: Pregnancy: C   Lactation: U

Dose: Nausea, vomiting: 5–10 mg PO/IM tid-qid, or 25 mg PR bid, or 5–10 mg IV over 2 min; max 40 mg/d; *Psychosis:* 5–10 mg PO tid/qid; max 150 mg/d

---

Progesterone (Crinone)

Type: Contraceptives; Hormones; Progestins; *Class:* Pregnancy: D Lactation: S

Note: Recent studies suggest that administration of progesterone (vaginal gel or cream) or 17-α-hydroxyprogesterone caproate administered weekly IM decrease the incidence of preterm birth

Dose: Infertility, progesterone deficiency: 1 applicator 8% PV qd; continue through 10-12 w of pregnancy; *Prevention of idiopathic preterm birth:* 1 applicator 8% PV qod or bid; 17-α-hydroxyprogesterone caproate, 250 mg/wk from 16 to 20 wks up to 36 wks of gestation

---

Promethazine (Phenergan; Phenerzine)

Type: Antiemetics; Antihistamines; Phenothiazines; *Class:* Pregnancy: C   Lactation: S

Note: May be combined with Codeine

Dose: Nausea, vomiting: 12.5–25 mg PO/PR/IM q 4–6 h prn; *Motion sickness:* 25 mg PO bid; *Sedation:* 25–50 mg PO/PR/IM q 4–6 h prn; *Allergic rhinitis:* 12.5–25 mg PO q 6 h, or 25 mg PO qhs

---

Propranolol (Inderal)

Type: Adrenergic antagonists; Antiarrhythmics class II; Beta blockers;

Class: Pregnancy: C   Lactation: S

Dose: Hypertension: begin 40 mg PO bid, increasing q 3–7 d; max 640 mg/d; *Migraine headache prophylaxis:* begin 20 mg PO qd; increase gradually to 40–60 mg PO qid; *Supraventricular tachycardia:* begin 1–3 mg IV at 1 mg/min; may repeat 2 min later; if control, then 10–30 mg PO tid/qid beginning 4 h later; *Angina:* 80–120 mg PO bid; may increase q 7–10 d

---

(Continued)

Propylthiouracil (PTU)
Type: Antithyroid agents; Hormone modifiers; Hormones; *Class:* Pregnancy: D   Lactation: S
Note: An FDA warning was issued in 2009 given that there is an increased risk of hepatotoxicity with Propylthiouracil when compared to Methimazole (MMI) (http://www.fda.gov/Safety/MedWatch/SafetyInformation/SafetyAlertsforHumanMedicalProducts/ucm164162.htm)
Dose: Hyperthyroidism (Graves disease): begin 100–125 mg PO tid; 200–300 mg PO qid if thyroid storm

---

Protamine (Protamine)
Type: Antidotes; Bleeding disorders; *Class:* Pregnancy: C   Lactation: S (likely)
Dose: Heparin reversal: 1–1.5 mg IV per 100 U heparin estimated to remain in the body; if 0–30 min from last dose, give 1–1.5 mg/100 U, if 30–60 min give 0.5–0.75 mg/100 U, if >2 h, give 0.25–0.375 mg/100 U

Pyrimethamine (Daraprim; Eraprelina)
Type: Antiprotozoals; *Class:* Pregnancy: C   Lactation: S (likely)
Dose: Malaria treatment: 50 mg PO qd × 2 w in combination with sulfadiazine and quinine; use in chloroquine-resistant areas; *Malaria prophylaxis:* 25 mg PO qw for 10 w after exposure; use in chloroquine-resistant areas; *Toxoplasmosis:* begin 50–75 mg PO qd × 1–3 w, then 25–50 mg PO qd × 4–5 w in combination with sulfadoxine and folinic acid; *Toxoplasmosis with HIV:* begin 200 mg PO × 1, then 50–100 mg PO qd × 4–8 w, then maintenance; *Isosporiasis:* 50–75 mg PO qd

---

Ranitidine (Ranitiget; Zantac)
Type: Antihistamines, H2; Antiulcer; Gastrointestinals; *Class:* Pregnancy: B   Lactation: S (likely)
Dose: Duodenal or gastric ulcer: 150 mg PO bid; *Erosive esophagitis:* 150 mg PO qid; *Gastroesophageal reflux disease:* 150 mg PO bid; *Dyspepsia:* 75 mg PO qd/bid

---

Ribavirin (Rebetol; Viramid)
Type: Antivirals; *Class:* Pregnancy: X   Lactation: U
Note: Rodent studies reveal an increase prevalence of limb, eye and brain defects
Dose: Chronic hepatitis C: 400 mg PO q a.m. and 600 mg q p.m. if <75 kg; 600 mg PO bid if >74.9 kg

---

Ritodrine (Yutopar)
Type: Adrenergic agonists; Beta agonists; Tocolytics; *Class:* Pregnancy: B   Lactation: S
Dose: Preterm labor: begin 0.05 mg/min, increase by 0.05 mg/min q 10 min (unless maternal heart rate >130 bpm) until contractions stop; continue that dose for 12 h after contractions end; max 0.35 mg/min

---

Ropivicaine (Naropin)
Type: Anaesthetic, local; *Class:* Pregnancy: B   Lactation: S (likely)
Dose: Epidural analgesia: 2 mg/mL continuous infusion

Salmeterol (Serevent; Serevent Diskus)
Type: Adrenergic agonists; Beta agonists; Bronchodilators; *Class:* Pregnancy: C   Lactation: S
Dose: Asthma prophylaxis: 2 puffs INH q 12 h; *Exercise-induced asthma:* 2 puffs INH × 1; *COPD:* 2 puffs INH q 12 h

---

(Continued)

Scopolamine (Scopoderm; Isopto Hyoscine)

Type: Anesthetics, adjunct; Anticholinergics; Antiemetics; Cycloplegics; Gastrointestinals; Motion sickness; Mydriatics; Ophthalmics; Vertigo; *Class:* Pregnancy: C   Lactation: S

Dose: Motion sickness: 1 patch behind the ear 4 h prior to need; may replace in 3 d; *Obstetric amnesia or preoperative sedation:* 0.32–0.65 mg SC/IM; *Intraoperative amnesia:* 0.4 mg IV

Spiramycin (Rovamycine)

Type: Antibacterial, Antiprotozoal; *Class:* Pregnancy: B   Lactation: S (likely)

Note: Not available in the US

Dose: Toxoplasmosis: 1–2 g (3–6 million International Units [IU]) PO bid or 500 mg IV q 8 h; *Toxoplasmosis – alternative regimen:* 500 mg to 1 gram (1.5–3 million IU) three times a day.; *Toxoplasmosis – severe infections:* 2–2.5 g (6–7.5 million IU) bid

Sufentanil (Sufenta)

Type: Analgesics, narcotic; Anesthesia, general; *Class:* Pregnancy: C   Lactation: S

Dose: General anesthesia: begin 2–8 μg/kg IV when used with inhalational anesthetics; up to 30 μg/kg when used with amnestic and oxygen alone: titrate additional smaller doses to desired effect; *Epidural during labor:* several regimens including 10–15 μg sufentanil plus 10 mL 0.125% bupivacaine; *Intrathecal during labor:* several regimens including 5–7.5 μg with or without Bupivacaine

Sulfadiazine (Microsulfon)

Type: Antibiotics; Sulfonamides; *Class:* Pregnancy: C   Lactation: S (likely)

Dose: Toxoplasmosis: 2–8 g PO qd in 3–4 divided doses × 4 w plus pyrimethamine 25 mg/d

Sulfamethoxazole (Gamazole; Gantanol)

Type: Bacteriostatic; inhibits dihydropteroate synthesis; *Class:* Pregnancy: C   Lactation: U

Dose: Bacterial infection: begin 2 g PO × 1, then 1 g PO bid

Sulindac (Antribid)

Type: Analgesics, non-narcotic; NSAID; *Class:* Pregnancy: C   Lactation: S

Dose: Osteoarthritis or rheumatoid arthritis: 150–200 mg PO bid; max 400 mg/d; *Anti-inflammatory:* 200 mg PO bid × 7–14 d; max 400 mg/d; *Ankylosing spondylitis:* 150–200 mg PO bid; max 400 mg/d; *Acute gout:* 150–200 mg PO bid; max 400 mg/d

Terbutaline (Brethaire; Brethancer)

Type: Adrenergic agonists; Beta agonists; Bronchodilators; *Class:* Pregnancy: B   Lactation: S

Dose: Asthma: 5 mg PO q 6 h prn; max 15 mg/d; or, 2 puffs INH q 4–6 h; or 0.25 mg SC q 15–30 min × 2; *Tocolysis:* 0.25 mg SC q 30 min; max 1 mg/4 h; or, 2.5–10 μg/min IV, max 30 μg/min

Tetracycline (Telmycin; Tetocyn)

Type: Antibiotics; Dermatologics; Ophthalmics; Tetracyclines; *Class:* Pregnancy: D   Lactation: S

Note: Exposure of the fetus during the 3rd trimester, infancy, and in children less than 8 years can cause permanent discoloration of the teeth

Dose: Bacterial infection: 1–2 g qd divided bid or qid at least 1 h before or 2 h after meals; *Chlamydia infection:* 500 mg PO qid at least 1 h before or 2 h after meals × 7 d; *Acne vulgaris:* 250–500 mg PO qid at least 1 h before or 2 h after meals

(Continued)

Thalidomide (Thalomid)

Type: Dermatologics; Immunomodulators; *Class:* Pregnancy: X   Lactation: U

Note: A common effect of Thalidomide is either duplication (preaxial polydactyly of hands and feet) or deficiency (absence of thumb)

Dose: Restricted access in United States: call 1-888-423-5436 for information; *Erythema nodosum leprosum:* begin 100–00 mg PO × 2 w or until symptoms improve, then decrease by 50 mg/d q 2–4 w; *HIV wasting:* 100–300 mg PO qhs; *Aphthous ulcer:* 200 mg PO qd

---

Theophylline (Theo-Dur)

Type: Bronchodilators; Xanthine derivatives; *Class:* Pregnancy: C   Lactation: S (likely)

Note: therapeutic level 10–20 µg/mL; exists in multiple formats with varying release rates. Dosing quoted for theophylline only

Dose: Chronic asthma: begin 300 mg PO qd in divided doses bid/tid × 3 d, then 400 mg/d × 3 d, then 600 mg/d if tolerated; *COPD (maintenance):* begin 300 mg PO qd in divided doses bid/tid × 3 d, then 400 mg/d × 3 d, then 600 mg/d if tolerated

---

Ticarcillin (Ticar; Timentin)

Type: Antibiotics; Penicillins; *Class:* Pregnancy: B   Lactation: S

Dose: Bacterial infection: 3–4 g IV/IM q 4–6 h, or 200–300 mg/kg IV div q 4–6 h; max 24 g/d

---

Topiramate (Topamax)

Type: Anticonvulsants; *Class:* Pregnancy: C   Lactation: S

Dose: Seizures, adjunct therapy: 25–50 mg PO qd, increase 25–50 mg/w; usual dose 400 mg/d in divided doses

---

Triamcinolone (Aristcort)

Type: Corticosteroids; *Class:* Pregnancy: C   Lactation: S

Dose: Adrenal insufficiency: 4–12 mg PO qd; *Inflammatory disorders:* 4–48 mg PO in divided doses qd; *Chronic asthma:* 2 puffs INH tid/qid, rinse mouth after use; max 16 puffs qd; *Allergic rhinitis:* 1–2 sprays/nostril qd; max 2 sprays/nostril qd; discontinue after 3 w if no improvement; *Steroid-responsive dermatitis:* apply sparingly to affected area bid/qid

---

Trimethadione (Tridione)

Type: Anticonvulsants; *Class:* Pregnancy: D   Lactation: U

Note: The fetal "trimethadione syndrome" includes: septal defect, patent ductus, mental retardation, simian crease, malformations of the hand, club foot, microcephaly, hypospadias, ambiguous genitalia

Dose: Seizure disorder (petit mal): 300 mg tid

Trimethobenzamide (Arrestin; Benzacot)

Type: Anticholinergics; Antiemetics; Antivertigo; *Class:* Pregnancy: C   Lactation: U

Dose: Nausea/ vomiting: 300 mg PO tid/qid, or 200 mg PR/IM tid/qid

---

Trimethoprim (Bactin)

Type: Antibiotics; Folate antagonists; *Class:* Pregnancy: C   Lactation: S

Dose: UTI: 100 mg PO q 12 h × 10 d; *UTI prophylaxis:* 100 mg PO qhs × 6–24 w; *Traveler's diarrhea:* 200 mg PO bid × 5 d; *Pneumocystis carinii pneumonia treatment:* 20 mg/kg/d PO in divided doses

---

(Continued)

Valacyclovir (Valtrex)
Type: Antivirals; *Class:* Pregnancy: B   Lactation: S
Dose: Genital herpes – primary: 1000 mg PO bid × 10d; *Genital herpes – recurrent:* 500 mg PO bid × 3 d; prophylaxis, 1000 mg PO qd; *Herpes zoster:* 1000 mg PO tid × 7 d

---

Valproate (Depacon; Epival)
Type: Anticonvulsants; *Class:* Pregnancy: D   Lactation: S
Note: The fetal "valproate syndrome" includes a distinct craniofacial appearance, limb abnormalities, heart defects, coupled with a cluster of minor and major anomalies and central nervous system dysfunction
Dose: Seizures: 10–15 mg/kg/d IV in divided doses qd/tid, increase by 5–10 mg/kg/d q 7 d to achieve therapeutic trough of 50–100 μg/mL; max 60 mg/kg/d

---

Vancomycin (Balcorin; Edicin)
Type: Antibiotics; Glycopeptides; *Class:* Pregnancy: B   Lactation: S
Dose: Bacterial infections: 500 mg IV q 6 h; peak 25–40 μg/mL, trough 5–10 μg/mL; *Endocarditis prophylaxis:* 1 g slow IV over 1 h

---

Warfarin (Coumadin)
Type: Anticoagulants; Thrombolytics; *Class:* Pregnancy: X   Lactation: U
Note: The fetal "warfarin syndrome" includes a various spectrum of manifestations that include: nasal hypoplasia, micropthalmia, hypoplasia of the extremities, IUGR, heart disease, scoliosis, deafness, and mental retardation
Dose: Acute therapy of thromboembolic disease: begin 2.5 mg, increase gradual over 2–4 d to achieve desired INR; *Prosthetic cardiac valves or atrial fibrillation:* 2.5–10 mg PO qd, INR should be maintained between 2.5–3.0 depending on the valve type

---

Zafirlukast (Accolate)
Type: Antiasthmatics; Leukotriene antagonists; *Class:* Pregnancy: B   Lactation: S (likely)
Dose: Asthma prophylaxis: 20 mg PO 1 h before or 2 h after meals bid

---

Zanamivir (Relenza)
Type: Antivirals; *Class:* Pregnancy: C   Lactation: U
Dose: Uncomplicated influenza: begin within 48 h of symptoms, 10 mg INH q 2–4 h × 2, then 12 h × 5 d

---

Zidovudine (Aviral; AZT; Retrovir; Retrovis)
Type: Antivirals; Nucleoside reverse transcriptase inhibitors; *Class:* Pregnancy: C   Lactation: U
Dose: HIV during pregnancy: begin 100 mg PO 5 × /d after 14 w until onset of labor; in intrapartum period: 2 mg/kg IV over 1 h, then 1 mg/kg/h until cord clamping; *HIV in non-pregnant women:* 300 mg PO q 12 h, or 1 mg/kg IV q 4 h

---

Zileuton (Zyflo)
Type: Antiasthmatics; Leukotriene antagonists; *Class:* Pregnancy: C   Lactation: U
Dose: Asthma: 600 mg PO qid; max 2400 mg/d

(Continued)

Zonisamide (Zonegran)
Type: Anticonvulsants; *Class:* Pregnancy: C   Lactation: U
Dose: Partial seizures: begin 100 mg PO qd, increasing q 2 w or greater for control; max dose 600 mg/d in divided doses if necessary

Suggested reading

Weiner CP, Buhimschi CS. *Drugs for Pregnant and Lactating Women*, 2nd edn. Philadelphia: Elsevier Saunders, 2009.

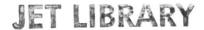

Index

Page numbers in **bold** refer to tables and those in *italics* refer in figures.